MUSIC THERAPY HANDBOOK

CREATIVE ARTS AND PLAY THERAPY

Cathy A. Malchiodi and David A. Crenshaw,
Series Editors

This series highlights action-oriented therapeutic approaches that utilize art, music, dance/movement, drama, play, and related modalities. Emphasizing current best practices and research, experienced practitioners show how creative arts and play therapies can be integrated into overall treatment for individuals of all ages. Books in the series provide richly illustrated guidelines and techniques for addressing trauma, attachment problems, and other psychological difficulties, as well as for supporting resilience and self-regulation.

Creative Arts and Play Therapy for Attachment Problems
Cathy A. Malchiodi and David A. Crenshaw, Editors

Play Therapy: A Comprehensive Guide to Theory and Practice
David A. Crenshaw and Anne L. Stewart, Editors

Creative Interventions with Traumatized Children, Second Edition
Cathy A. Malchiodi, Editor

Music Therapy Handbook
Barbara L. Wheeler, Editor

Play Therapy Interventions to Enhance Resilience
David A. Crenshaw, Robert Brooks,
and Sam Goldstein, Editors

MUSIC THERAPY
Handbook

edited by

Barbara L. Wheeler

THE GUILFORD PRESS
New York   London

© 2015 The Guilford Press
A Division of Guilford Publications, Inc.
370 Seventh Avenue, Suite 1200, New York, NY 10001
www.guilford.com

Paperback edition 2017

Printed in the United States of America

This book is printed on acid-free paper.

Last digit is print number: 9   8   7   6

The authors have checked with sources believed to be reliable in their efforts to
provide information that is complete and generally in accord with the standards
of practice that are accepted at the time of publication. However, in view of the
possibility of human error or changes in behavioral, mental health, or medical
sciences, neither the authors, nor the editors and publisher, nor any other party who
has been involved in the preparation or publication of this work warrants that the
information contained herein is in every respect accurate or complete, and they are
not responsible for any errors or omissions or the results obtained from the use of
such information. Readers are encouraged to confirm the information contained in
this book with other sources.

Library of Congress Cataloging-in-Publication Data

Music therapy handbook / edited by Barbara L. Wheeler.
     pages cm—(Creative arts and play therapy)
   Includes bibliographical references and index.
   ISBN 978-1-4625-1803-6 (hardcover : alk. paper)
   ISBN 978-1-4625-2972-8 (paperback : alk. paper)
   1. Music therapy.   I. Wheeler, Barbara L.
   ML3920.M89776 2015
   615.8′5154—dc23

                                                                        2014040684

About the Editor

Barbara L. Wheeler, PhD, MT-BC, is Professor Emerita at Montclair State University in New Jersey, where she taught from 1975 to 2000. Dr. Wheeler initiated the music therapy program at the University of Louisville in 2000, retiring in 2011. She presents and teaches in the United States and internationally, with current faculty appointments at the Department of Social Studies, University of Applied Sciences Würzburg Schweinfurt, Würzburg, Germany; and the Karol Szymanowski Academy of Music, Katowice, Poland. She has been an active clinician throughout her career, working with a diverse clientele. Dr. Wheeler has edited and authored several chapters, articles, and books, including *Music Therapy Research* (now in its third edition) and *Clinical Training Guide for the Student Music Therapist*. She is a past president of the American Music Therapy Association and former Interview Coeditor for *Voices: A World Forum for Music Therapy*.

Contributors

Brian Abrams, PhD, MT-BC, LCAT, LPC, is an analytical music therapist, a Fellow of the Association for Music and Imagery, and Associate Professor and Coordinator of Music Therapy at the John J. Cali School of Music at Montclair State University in New Jersey. A music therapist since 1995, he has worked in various clinical contexts. His international scholarship includes the development of theoretical perspectives on humanistic music therapy.

Ruthlee Figlure Adler, BS, MT-BC, is a music therapist and consultant in Bethesda, Maryland, and has over 50 years of experience working with children and adults with varying abilities and disabilities at the Ivymount School, the National Institutes of Health, and in private practice. She is the author of numerous music therapy publications, including *Target on Music: Activities to Enhance Learning through Music.*

Felicity A. Baker, PhD, RMT, is Associate Professor and Australia Research Council Fellow at the Centre for Music, Mind, and Wellbeing at the University of Melbourne, Australia, and National President of the Australian Music Therapy Association. She has research interests in songwriting, neurorehabilitation, and therapeutic choirs, and has published widely on these topics.

Debbie Bates, MMT, MT-BC, is a Music Therapist II in the Arts and Medicine Institute at the Cleveland Clinic, where she has clinical, research, and supervisory responsibilities. She is a PhD student in Music Therapy at Temple University and presents regularly on the topic of professional ethics in music therapy at national and regional conferences in the United States.

Ronald M. Borczon, MT-BC, is Professor of Music Therapy at California State University, Northridge. He has authored three books and has garnered many of the highest professional awards in the field. He is known for his innovative treatment approaches in working with survivors of mass trauma and is often asked to present these interventions at professional conferences.

Cynthia A. Briggs, PsyD, MT-BC, is Associate Professor and Director of the Music Therapy Program at Maryville University in St. Louis. Dr. Briggs is a past president of the American Association for Music Therapy (now the American Music Therapy Association [AMTA]) and a past chairperson of the National Coalition of Arts Therapies Associations. She is one of the creators of Kids Rock Cancer.

Debra S. Burns, PhD, MT-BC, is Associate Professor, Coordinator of the Music Therapy Program, and Chair of the Department of Music and Arts Technology in the Purdue School of Engineering and Technology at Indiana University–Purdue University. Her research program focuses on the evaluation of music-based interventions delivered to adult cancer survivors throughout the disease trajectory and at the end of life.

John A. Carpente, PhD, MT-BC, LCAT, is a Nordoff–Robbins music therapist, Associate Professor of Music Therapy at Molloy College in Rockville Centre, New York, and Executive Director of The Rebecca Center for Music Therapy and Center for Autism and Child Development at Molloy. Dr. Carpente has authored several music therapy publications, including the *Individual Music-Centered Assessment Profile for Neurodevelopmental Disorders (IMCAP-ND): A Clinical Manual.*

Sandra L. Curtis, PhD, MTA, MT-BC, is Professor and Graduate Music Therapy Program Director at Concordia University in Montreal. She has more than 30 years' experience in clinical practice, education, and research, and specializes in work with survivors of violence, people with differing abilities, and palliative care. Her current research interests include feminist music therapy and community music therapy.

William Davis, PhD, MT-BC, Emeritus Professor at Colorado State University, has been active in the AMTA for many years, serving as Historian and now Archivist. He has published numerous articles on the history of music therapy and coedited *An Introduction to Music Therapy: Theory and Practice.* In 2013, Dr. Davis received AMTA's Lifetime Achievement Award.

Paige A. Robbins Elwafi, MMT, MT-BC, is a music therapist in Cincinnati who works with babies, children, and adults who have blindness and visual impairment. She also enjoys contributing to the research on music therapy and cultural competence, and is the author of recent book chapters on music therapy and visual impairment, as well as Muslim cultures.

Lucy Forrest, MMus (Ethno), BMus (Therapy), RMT, is Senior Music Therapist at Mercy Palliative Care and a PhD student at the University of Melbourne. She has worked in palliative care music therapy for 20 years, and her clinical and research interests include pediatric palliative care, neuropalliative care, cultural issues in practice, and supervision.

Lisa Gallagher, MA, MT-BC, is Music Therapy Program Manager for the Arts and Medicine Institute at the Cleveland Clinic in Ohio. She is a presenter and researcher, has published articles and book chapters, and has served on the boards of the Great Lakes Region of the AMTA and the Certification Board for Music Therapists. She has also received awards for her service and research at state, regional, and international levels.

Susan Gardstrom, PhD, MT-BC, is Professor and Coordinator of Music Therapy at the University of Dayton in Ohio. She is a frequent presenter and has published in multiple journals. Dr. Gardstrom has served as an editor of *Qualitative Inquiries in Music Therapy* and is the author of the textbook *Music Therapy Improvisation for Groups: Essential Leadership Competencies.*

Greta E. Gillmeister, MT-BC, is a contractual music therapist in Louisville, Kentucky. She provides individual and group music therapy services to children in the public and private schools of the central Kentucky area and is an active presenter and clinician who specializes in working with children who are deaf or hard of hearing.

Nina Guerrero, MA, MT-BC, LCAT, is a Nordoff–Robbins music therapist who served as Research Coordinator at New York University's Nordoff–Robbins Center from 2008 to 2013, overseeing diverse projects including a collaborative study with the Rusk Institute for Rehabilitation at NYU Medical Center. She currently works as part of a newly formed multidisciplinary clinical liaison team at the Queen's Medical Center in Honolulu.

Susan Hadley, PhD, MT-BC, is Professor and Director of Music Therapy at Slippery Rock University in Slippery Rock, Pennsylvania. Dr. Hadley is the author of numerous music therapy publications, including *Experiencing Race as a Music Therapist: Personal Narratives.* She is also Coeditor-in-Chief of *Voices: A World Forum for Music Therapy.*

Suzanne Hanser, EdD, MT-BC, chairs the Music Therapy Department at Berklee College of Music in Boston. She is past president of the World Federation of Music Therapy and the National Association for Music Therapy and established the music therapy service at the Dana–Farber Cancer Institute. Dr. Hanser is the author of *The New Music Therapist's Handbook* and *Manage Your Stress and Pain.*

Deanna Hanson-Abromeit, PhD, MT-BC, is Assistant Professor at the University of Kansas. Her clinical and research focus is on preventive music-based interventions with infants who are neurodevelopmentally at risk. She coedited two monographs on hospital-based music therapy, has authored book chapters and peer-reviewed articles, and serves on the editorial boards for the *Journal of Music Therapy* and *Music Therapy Perspectives.*

James Hiller, PhD, MT-BC, is Lecturer in Music Therapy at the University of Dayton in Ohio, where he also provides clinical supervision. Dr. Hiller's scholarly interests include exploration of the theoretical foundations of music therapy practice, music as a therapeutic medium, emotion in music, and clinical improvisation methods.

Kathleen M. Howland, PhD, MT-BC, CCC-SLP, is a Neurologic Music Therapist–Fellow and Professor of Music Therapy at the Berklee College of Music in Boston. She also maintains a private practice in music therapy with neurogenic populations and lectures frequently in medical settings.

Marcia Humpal, MEd, MT-BC, is semiretired after a long career with the Cuyahoga County Board of Developmental Disabilities in Cleveland. An adjunct faculty member at Cleveland State University, she also works part-time for the Rock and Roll Hall of Fame's Toddler Rock program. Among her many publications is the book *Early Childhood Music Therapy and Autism Spectrum Disorders.*

Corene P. Hurt-Thaut, PhD, MT-BC, is Research Associate at the Center for Biomedical Research in Music at Colorado State University and Continuing Education Coordinator and head clinical faculty for the Unkefer Academy for Neurologic Music Therapy (NMT). She is internationally recognized for her teaching in NMT and has written numerous book chapters and research articles on this topic.

Connie Isenberg, PhD, MTA, MT-BC, a Fellow of the Association for Music and Imagery, is Founding Professor of Music Therapy at the University of Québec in Montreal. A Charter Member of the Canadian Association for Music Therapy, she was awarded a Lifetime Membership in recognition of her contributions to the field. Music therapist, psychologist, psychoanalyst, and marriage and family therapist, she has published extensively and presents her work nationally and internationally.

Sarah B. Johnson, MM, MT-BC, recently retired as a neurologic music therapist for University Colorado Health Systems, the program she founded in 1987. She has been co-coordinator of NMT community outreach classes and continues to teach for the online Master's program at Colorado State University. She presents internationally on her clinical work, and has been awarded the Professional Practice Award from the AMTA.

Seung-A Kim, PhD, LCAT, MT-BC, an analytical music therapist, is Associate Professor of Music Therapy at Molloy College in Rockville Centre, New York. She is also an Article Editor on *Voices: A World Forum for Music Therapy* and serves on the AMTA Diversity Committee and Assembly of Delegates. She developed a music therapy program for Korean immigrant families in New York.

Robert E. Krout, EdD, MT-BC, is Professor and Chair of the Music Therapy Department at Southern Methodist University in Dallas. He taught previously at Massey University in New Zealand, The State University of New York, New Paltz, and Georgia College. Dr. Krout was Music Therapy Manager and Internship Director at Hospice of Palm Beach County, Florida, where he also worked with grieving children, teens, and adults.

A. Blythe LaGasse, PhD, MT-BC, is Associate Professor of Music Therapy at Colorado State University in Fort Collins, Colorado. She also maintains a private practice where she provides music therapy for persons on the autism spectrum. Dr. LaGasse has published numerous articles on topics including NMT and music therapy for persons on the autism spectrum.

Gillian Stephens Langdon, MA, MT-BC, LCAT, retired from the Bronx Psychiatric Center after 41 years. She teaches in New York University's Steinhardt Music Therapy Graduate Program and at Molloy College in Rockville Centre, New York. She is the author of numerous music therapy publications including a coauthored chapter in *Music Therapy and Trauma: Bridging Theory and Clinical Practice* and a chapter in *Music Therapy Supervision*.

Anne W. Lipe, PhD, MT-BC, is Adjunct Associate Professor of Music Therapy at Shenandoah University in Winchester, Virginia. She has taught in four academic music therapy programs and has worked clinically with older adults and individuals in hospice and medical settings. Her assessment tool, the Music-Based Evaluation of Cognitive Functioning (MBECF), is the subject of several research publications and numerous presentations.

Joanne Loewy, DA, LCAT, MT-BC, is Director of the Louis Armstrong Center for Music and Medicine, Associate Professor at Albert Einstein College of Medicine, a Founding Member of the International Association for Music and Medicine, and Coeditor in Chief of *Music and Medicine*. She is a graduate music therapy professor at New York University, Drexel University, Molloy College, and the University of Barcelona, and has authored and edited numerous books and articles.

David Marcus, MMus, MA, CMT, a Nordoff–Robbins music therapist, is the founder and clinical director of Creative Music Therapy Studio, a private Nordoff–Robbins music therapy practice in New York City. He is the author or coauthor of numerous music therapy publications, including scholarly articles, book chapters, and the revision and expansion of the seminal textbook *Creative Music Therapy*.

Katrina Skewes McFerran, PhD, RMT, is Associate Professor and Head of Music Therapy at the University of Melbourne in Australia. Dr. McFerran has published extensively about working with young people in schools, hospitals, palliative care, and community settings, including her book, *Adolescents, Music and Music Therapy*.

Cathy H. McKinney, PhD, LCAT, MT-BC, is Professor and Coordinator of Music Therapy at Appalachian State University in Boone, North Carolina, where she has a small Bonny Method of Guided Imagery and Music (GIM) practice. A Fellow of the Association for Music and Imagery, her research has focused on the effects of GIM on mood and physiology and of music on imagery.

Beth McLaughlin, MSE, LCAT, MT-BC, is Coordinator of Music Therapy Services at the Wildwood School in Schenectady, New York. She is a contributing author to numerous music therapy publications and a frequent presenter at local and national conferences. She is an advocate for music therapy in special education and provides services to students from more than 50 school districts throughout upstate New York.

Anthony Meadows, PhD, MT-BC, LPC, is a Fellow of the Association for Music and Imagery and Associate Professor and Chair for the Graduate Music Therapy Program at Shenandoah University in Winchester, Virginia. He is Editor of *Music Therapy Perspectives* and has published on a range of topics. He has twice received the Arthur Flagler Fultz Research Award from the AMTA.

Kathleen M. Murphy, PhD, MT-BC, is Assistant Professor of Music Therapy at the University of Evansville in Evansville, Indiana. She is an active clinician, supervisor, and researcher, with research interests in the area of substance abuse prevention and treatment across the lifespan. Dr. Murphy has authored several book chapters and articles on substance abuse and other topics.

Clare O'Callaghan, PhD, RMT, is a music therapist at Caritas Christi Hospice, St. Vincent's Hospital in Melbourne, and a Senior Research Associate in Palliative Care, Cabrini Education and Research Project, Cabrini Health in Victoria, Australia. Her honorary positions include Associate Professor in the Department of Medicine and Principal Fellow at the Melbourne Conservatorium of Music at the University of Melbourne, and Research Fellow at the Peter MacCallum Cancer Centre in Melbourne. Dr. O'Callaghan's research, theoretical findings, and perspectives are widely published in music therapy, palliative medicine, psycho-oncology, and social work refereed journals and texts.

Hanne Mette Ridder, PhD, Professor of Music Therapy at Aalborg University, Denmark, is Head of the Doctoral Programme in Music Therapy and head of the Research Team at the 5-year training course in music therapy at Aalborg University. Dr. Ridder is President of the European Music Therapy Confederation. Her research mainly focuses on music therapy in dementia care.

Benedikte B. Scheiby, MA, is a Certified Licensed Creative Arts Music Psychotherapist, Body Psychotherapist, and Mindfulness-Based Stress Reduction Trainer in New York City. She is also Adjunct Professor in the New York University Music Therapy Graduate Program, Director of Intern Training and Supervision and Senior Clinician at the Institute for Music and Neurologic Function in the Bronx, and Director of the Postgraduate Training Institute in Analytical Music Therapy in New York City.

Helen Shoemark, PhD, RMT, is a researcher at the Murdoch Children's Research Institute and Senior Music Therapist (Neonatology) at The Royal Children's Hospital in Melbourne. She is also Adjunct Professor at the University of Queensland and a Senior Fellow with the Department of Paediatrics and Melbourne Conservatorium of Music at the University of Melbourne.

Carol Shultis, PhD, LPC, MT-BC, is a Fellow of the Association for Music and Imagery and Assistant Professor of Music Therapy at Converse College in Spartanburg, South Carolina. She also provides medical music therapy to patients of the Spartanburg Regional Health System (adult medical/surgical, pediatrics, and hospice care), is a frequent continuing education course instructor, and is coauthor of *Clinical Training Guide for the Student Music Therapist.*

Suzanne Sorel, DA, LCAT, MT-BC, a Nordoff–Robbins music therapist, is Associate Dean and Director of Graduate Music Therapy at Molloy College in Rockville Centre, New York. She is also Director of Nordoff–Robbins Training at The Rebecca Center for Music Therapy in Rockville Centre. Dr. Sorel's interests relate to clinical improvisation, supervision, and training of music therapists, educators, and students.

Brynjulf Stige, PhD, Professor and Head of Research at GAMUT–The Grieg Academy Music Therapy Research Centre at the University of Bergen and Uni Research Health, Bergen, Norway. His research interests include culture, community, practice, and philosophy. Dr. Stige founded the *Nordic Journal of Music Therapy* and is founding coeditor of *Voices: A World Forum for Music Therapy.*

Jeanette Tamplin, PhD, RMT, holds a Postdoctoral Research Fellowship in Music Therapy at the University of Melbourne and works as music therapist at Austin Health in Melbourne, Australia. Dr. Tamplin specializes in therapeutic singing and songwriting interventions in neurorehabilitation and is the author of numerous music therapy publications in this area, including the coauthored text *Music Therapy Methods in Neurorehabilitation.*

Concetta M. Tomaino, DA, MT-BC, LCAT, is Executive Director and Cofounder of the Institute for Music and Neurologic Function and Senior Vice President for Music Therapy at the CenterLight Health System in the Bronx, New York. Internationally known for her research in the clinical applications of music and neurologic rehabilitation, Dr. Tomaino is Professor at the Albert Einstein College of Medicine and Lehman College of the City University of New York.

Alan Turry, DA, MT-BC, LCAT, is a Nordoff–Robbins music therapist and Managing Director of the Nordoff–Robbins Center for Music Therapy at the Steinhardt School of Culture, Education, and Human Development at New York University. On several editorial boards and the author of numerous publications, he received the AMTA Arthur Flagler Fultz Research Award in 2012 to support the collaboration between the Nordoff–Robbins Center and Rusk Rehabilitation Institute to develop and research an integrated music therapy/occupational therapy stroke rehabilitation program.

Madelaine Ventre, MS, LCAT, MT-BC, is a Fellow of the Association for Music and Imagery and a Primary Trainer and graduate faculty member at several universities. She has taught Guided Imagery and Music nationally and internationally at the undergraduate, graduate, and postgraduate levels; has published in professional journals and books; has presented at national and international conferences; and maintains a private practice in Forestburgh, New York.

Margareta Wärja, MA, is a licensed psychotherapist and group psychotherapist, a Fellow of the Association for Music and Imagery, a Primary Trainer, and Director of Expressive Arts in Stockholm, Sweden. She is a faculty member of the Graduate Music Therapy Program at the Royal College of Music in Stockholm, and of the graduate Expressive Arts Therapy Program at University College of Buskerud and Vestfold in Norway. Her research focuses on the use of receptive music therapy and expressive arts in oncology rehabilitation.

Yun Wen, MA, is a Registered Music Therapist and Project Officer with the Chinese Community Social Services Centre in Victoria, Australia. She is currently conducting a government-funded project called *Home-Based Preferred Music Listening Program* for elderly Chinese immigrants in Australia. She is interested in exploring the adaptation of music therapy in a multicultural context.

Barbara L. Wheeler. See "About the Editor."

Annette Whitehead-Pleaux, MA, MT-BC, is a clinical music therapist and researcher at Shriners Hospitals for Children—Boston, working with children who are burn survivors. She is also Adjunct Professor of Music Therapy at Saint Mary-of-the-Woods College in Saint Mary of the Woods, Indiana, and the author of several music therapy articles and chapters that focus on pain and anxiety, trauma, technology, and multicultural music therapy.

Elizabeth York, PhD, MT-BC, is Professor of Music Therapy and Chair of the Department of Music Education and Music Therapy at Converse College in Spartanburg, South Carolina. Dr. York has contributed many scholarly works to the field of music therapy and served in leadership capacities, including as President of the Southeastern Region of the American Music Therapy Association and Co-Chair of the AMTA Ethics Board.

Series Editors' Note

The epigram "Where words leave off, music begins" is most frequently attributed to the 19th-century German poet Heinrich Heine. How prescient Heine was more than 200 years before neuroscience, trauma research, and the study of the brain demonstrated how music, a core domain of the creative arts, can reach deeply into the human soul and provide healing when words cannot. David Dubal, when discussing the nine symphonies of Beethoven in *The Essential Canon of Classical Music*, quoted the biographer André Maurois: "Everything that I had thought and been unable to express was sung in the wordless phrases of these symphonies—when that mighty river of sound began to flow, I let myself be carried on its waters. My soul was bathed and purified . . . Beethoven called me back to kindness, charity, and love" (Dubal, 2001, p. 126). Partly because of the transformative power of the medium, music therapy has an integral role to play in contemporary healing arts guided by new understandings, including modern attachment theory, neurobiological research, and relational therapy.

As coeditors of the Guilford series *Creative Arts and Play Therapy*, we are pleased to see music therapy take its rightful place at the table of meaningful right-hemisphere-dominant therapies in the midst of the persistent focus in recent decades on cognitive, language-based, left-hemisphere therapies. Cognitive therapy and language-dependent therapies of many forms and shapes also have a role in modern healing arts. What neurobiological research reveals, however, is that the sequence and timing of therapeutic approaches is critically important if they are to be effective, as illustrated in Bruce Perry's Neurosequential Model of Therapeutics.

The profession of music therapy is a development of the past 65 years, but music has been used for thousands of years in many cultures as a pathway to healing. The ability of music to activate forces of healing and resilience was well illustrated by Dubal when discussing Beethoven's work. Dubal stated, "Beethoven struggled for over four years with the Fifth Symphony in C Minor (Op. 67), the most loved and widely performed symphony of all time. The work seems to exemplify the defiant spirit of the human race to continue to strive against adversity" (p. 127). Listening to or making music can "soothe the brain stem" (which Perry says is essential to treating an early-life trauma before more traditional approaches to therapy can work), or rouse in an individual the innate fighting spirit and resilience that Ann Masten refers to as "ordinary magic"; in either case, music therapy is potentially a powerful modality. Music is a mode of expression that creates a kind of receptive consciousness that can also speak to the unconscious in human beings. Music therapy has its own special footprint, bears its own signature, and has unique benefits.

Barbara Wheeler and her outstanding chapter contributors have made the history, theory, and practical applications of music therapy available in readable form to all of us, whether music therapists or allied mental health practitioners or students in play therapy or the creative arts. This book indeed is a true gift. This volume is a long overdue and breakthrough contribution on one of the important creative forms of the healing arts.

CATHY A. MALCHIODI, PhD
Trauma-Informed Practices
and Expressive Arts Therapy Institute

DAVID A. CRENSHAW, PhD, ABPP
Children's Home of Poughkeepsie

REFERENCE

Dubal, D. (2001). *The essential canon of classical music.* New York: North Point Press.

Acknowledgments

I would like to thank a number of people who have made this book possible. First and foremost, I acknowledge the chapter authors, all outstanding music therapy clinicians and educators, who have brought their experiences and perspectives to their chapters. All authors have been respectful, patient, and considerate in writing and revising the chapters. The results of their efforts make the book both interesting and educational.

Thank you to Cathy Malchiodi, art therapist colleague and friend, who, when I was exploring ways of continuing my professional activity after I retired from full-time teaching, suggested this book and facilitated the collaboration with The Guilford Press. Her encouragement and advice have been essential in bringing the book to fruition.

I am grateful also to the staff members of The Guilford Press, who were willing to take a risk on Guilford's first music therapy book. My editor, Rochelle Serwator, in particular, has guided me, helped to work out issues that have come up, and encouraged me during the process.

Finally, I would like to acknowledge and thank the clients with whom music therapists work. Music therapy does amazing things, and this is most evident through its impact on those we serve. It is only through the work with clients that music therapy comes to life. They are, of course, the reason that music therapy exists.

Contents

PART II. ORIENTATIONS AND APPROACHES

PART III. CLINICAL APPLICATIONS

Section A. *Music Therapy for Children and Adolescents*

Section B. Music Therapy for Adults

Section C. Medical Music Therapy

Purchasers of this book can download audio
files illustrative of the Nordoff–Robbins model
from *www.guilford.com/wheeler-materials*.
For information about the audio files,
see Chapter 15.

PART I

OVERVIEW AND ISSUES

INTRODUCTION

The *Music Therapy Handbook* introduces the reader to the fascinating field of music therapy. Because each chapter has a different author, various perspectives are presented, giving a broad and diverse overview of music therapy. Although music has been used in healing for many centuries and has been a formal discipline for more than 70 years, many people do not really understand what music therapy entails—indeed, some people even think that it is a brand new approach to treatment. This book introduces the reader to a number of important concepts and issues in music therapy, and this section provides background information on this exciting field.

Chapter 1, "Overview of Music Therapy as a Profession," includes a definition of music therapy and distinctions among music therapy and other uses of music, an overview of the history of music therapy, information on clientele with whom music therapists work and the settings in which music therapy may occur, an overview of the treatment process and how music therapy fits into it, the education and clinical training that is required to become a music therapist, the importance of research and evidence-based practice in music therapy, publications, an international perspective, interdisciplinary collaboration, some of the recent publicity about music therapy, and some issues confronting music therapy and music therapists.

This foundation is followed by "A History of Music Therapy" (Chapter 2), which provides an account of the emergence of music therapy from a global perspective, beginning with the use of music for healing purposes in ancient times, in various cultures, and extends to the present. The chapter includes information on the development of more formal music therapy approaches throughout the 20th century, including the establishment of the National Association for Music Therapy in 1950 in the United

States and the establishment of professional music therapy training programs and organizations around the world after that time.

"Aesthetic Foundations of Music Therapy: Music and Emotion" (Chapter 3) examines the ubiquitous and often essential therapeutic component of music therapy—
emotion—by focusing on a client's active music-making processes, wherein emotions
are consciously and unconsciously expressed in or through music rather than those elicited by music. It considers and explores sources of emotion, where emotions might be
located within music-making processes, and theories that explain how musical expressions of emotions might occur.

In "Music Therapy and the Brain" (Chapter 4), the way that music is processed
in the brain and its connections to the rest of the neurological system are examined
and discussed. The fields of music perception and cognitive neuroscience are bringing
new understanding as to how music is perceived and processed in the human brain,
and this information can help music therapists better understand the implications of
using music to impact human function as well as to know how changes in the brain may
impact an individual's ability to respond to it. The last decades have seen tremendous
growth in our understanding of these relationships, and this chapter presents them as
well as implications for music therapy.

Chapter 5, "Music Therapy and Cultural Diversity," examines cultural issues in
relation to the practice of music therapy. Music is a universal phenomenon that can
be found across cultures. Since our choice of music represents our identities and the
culture to which we belong, culture has significant implications for music therapy. The
chapter discusses the development of cultural diversity in music therapy and the importance of cultural awareness, examines music therapists' own stereotyping and ethnocentrism, and highlights cultural empathy and the role of music in facilitating a culturally informed music therapy.

Chapter 6, "Ethics in Music Therapy," examines and explores many aspects of ethics. It presents ethical foundations, including types of ethics, core ethical principles,
and differences in codes of ethics internationally. Ethical issues related to confidentiality, multiple relationships, and social media are emphasized, and a number of ethical
issues and dilemmas are explored.

Assessment is part of the music therapy process. Assessment is aimed at understanding the client and planning treatment. Various types assessments are reviewed in
Chapter 7, "Music Therapy Assessment," including an examination of their psychometric properties, and general issues concerning assessment are discussed.

"Music Therapy Research" (Chapter 8) provides a rationale for connecting research
and clinical practice in music therapy. It includes an overview of music therapy research
methods, including quantitative, qualitative, and mixed methods. Examples of music
therapy research using each method are included. The importance of the research
question, and how it evolves to a design for a research study, are included.

"Evidence-Based Practice in Music Therapy" (Chapter 9) includes a definition and
discussion of what is accepted as evidence in music therapy and the process of utilizing
evidence-based practice. It includes the need to include qualitative as well as quantita-

tive evidence. Information on music therapy as an evidence-based practice is presented, including discussion of the evidence that is available for music therapy and an overview of Cochrane reviews that include music therapy and music medicine.

"Music Therapy Methods" (Chapter 10) defines four methods: receptive (or listening), composition, improvisation, and re-creative (or performance). Each method refers to a different way in which clients encounter music as a feature of the therapeutic process. The chapter includes descriptions of variations, or applications, of these four methods, illustrated with case examples of a wide range of clientele.

Although each of these chapters covers an important topic related to music therapy, more information is available on every topic. Articles, chapter, and entire books have been written about most of them and will continue to be written to develop and update the information. Readers who find that they want more information on any of the areas can find ample additional information.

CHAPTER 1

Music Therapy as a Profession

Barbara L. Wheeler

Music therapy helps people to develop skills, adapt behavior, and overcome obstacles in their lives. Music therapists use different kinds of musical experiences, including improvising, performing, composing, and listening, along with talking about people's experiences, to meet clients' needs by utilizing the unique relationship between the client, the music, and the therapist. The profession of music therapy began in the 1950s in the United States and has grown into a dynamic, ever-expanding form of health care in educational, hospital, mental health, and private practice settings. This chapter provides an overview of the profession and discusses central elements in defining the broad array of practices in the field.

Music therapy can be defined in numerous ways. The American Music Therapy Association (AMTA) defines it as "the clinical and evidence-based use of music interventions to accomplish individualized goals within a therapeutic relationship by a credentialed professional who has completed an approved music therapy program" (*www.musictherapy.org*). Bruscia (1998) says, "Music therapy is a systematic process of interven-tion wherein the therapist helps the client to promote health, using music experiences and the relationships that develop through them as dynamic forces of change" (p. 20). The music therapy associations of many countries publish their own definitions, as does the World Federation of Music Therapy (WFMT; *www.musictherapyworld.net*).

Music therapists use the unique qualities of music and a relationship with a therapist to access emotions and memories, structure behavior, and provide social experiences in order to address clinical goals. Music therapy methods can be both active and receptive. Active methods involve the client *doing* something with the music; receptive methods mean that the client is *receiving* the music, generally through some form of listening. All methods may include verbal processing of feelings and experiences, particularly with adults.

Bruscia (1998) divides the uses of music in therapy into four methods: (1) improvising, (2) performing or re-creating, (3) composing, and (4) listening experiences. Improvising occurs when the client makes up music using any medium. Performing or re-creating takes place when the client learns or performs precomposed music. Composing experiences involve the client writing songs, lyrics, or instrumental pieces. In listening experiences, or receptive music therapy, the client listens to music and responds. The therapist facilitates all of these experiences.

Music in Healing Throughout History

Music has been used in healing throughout history. Many are familiar with the story of David playing the harp to rid King Saul of an evil spirit, using rituals incorporating music and dance with trance dancing, or with shamans driving demons from people's bodies in primitive societies. As views on health have evolved, the place of music in promoting health has also changed, with music being used to improve health in many cultures and in many ways. The evolution of music and music therapy throughout history is described from a multicultural perspective in a chapter in this book.

In the 1900s early forms of music therapy emerged in the United States and various associations formed to encourage its growth, although they were short-lived. More formal music therapy emerged in the United States in response to the need to help hospitalized soldiers from World War II and the discovery that music, played by professional musicians in Veterans Administration (VA) hospitals, was helpful to them. Michigan State was the first university to offer a music therapy curriculum in 1944, with other universities, including the University of Kansas, Chicago Musical College, College of the Pacific in Stockton, California, and Alverno College in Milwaukee, following suit (see *www.musictherapy. org*). The first U.S. music therapy association, the National Association for Music Therapy (NAMT), was formed in 1950. The profession of music therapy has seen steady growth in the United States throughout the last 60 years or so. Music therapy emerged in Great Britain in similar ways, and the

Society for Music Therapy and Remedial Music was founded in 1958, with the object of promoting the use and development of music therapy. Formal music therapy associations developed in other countries in the next decades, and music therapy continues to develop around the world.

Music Therapy Today

Clientele and Settings

Music therapy can be used with children or adults with physical or emotional problems, or with healthy people to achieve higher levels of awareness. Music therapists work with clients who have a range of diagnoses. The client groups listed in Tables 1.1 and 1.2, representing only some of the many client groups that music therapists see, are arranged according to those with whom music therapists work more frequently to those with whom they work less frequently and indicate the number of people who responded in each category. Both tables reflect this information for the United States (AMTA, 2013).

The Treatment Process

The treatment process for music therapy involves a number of phases. According to Gfeller and Davis (2008), these include (1) referral, (2) assessment, (3) treatment planning, (4) documentation of progress, and (5) evaluation and termination of treatment.

The first step, a referral to music therapy, often comes from another professional—perhaps a psychologist who suggests music therapy to a client who is having difficulty expressing herself verbally or a teacher who feels that a child's fine motor coordination or breathing could be helped by learning an instrument. These referrals can occur in the community or in an institution. Examples of referrals that might take place in an institution are a nurse suggesting music therapy for a patient who is very anxious

TABLE 1.1. Populations Served by Music Therapists

Developmentally disabled: 215	Substance abuse: 91
Autism spectrum disorders: 204	Learning disabled: 89
Mental health: 182	Posttraumatic stress disorder: 79
Alzheimer's/dementia: 165	Head injured: 78
Behavioral disorders: 159	Music therapist college students: 78
Elderly persons: 152	Medical/surgical: 69
School-age populations: 132	Parkinson's disease: 69
Terminally ill: 127	Visually impaired: 75
Emotionally disturbed: 119	Hearing impaired: 59
Neurologically impaired: 118	Chronic pain: 49
Multiply disabled: 105	Forensic: 34
Physically disabled: 103	Rett syndrome: 28
Early childhood: 103	Abused/sexually abused: 24
Speech impaired: 100	Nondisabled: 22
Cancer: 98	Eating disorders: 17
Dual diagnosed: 95	Comatose: 17
Stroke: 94	

Note. Respondents could list as many categories as appropriate, so the total number of responses could exceed the number of survey respondents.

about an upcoming surgical procedure, and a social worker suggesting involvement in music therapy for a client in a psychiatric institution who is isolated and could benefit from music therapy sessions that provide opportunities for contact with others within the context of a structured, music-based group experience. These are just two examples of many ways in which a referral can occur. Clients may also self-refer to music therapy, contacting the music therapist directly with particular needs in mind.

The next step in the music therapy process, assessment, is aimed at understanding the client's unique strengths and challenges and determining whether the client may benefit from music therapy treatment. Assessment can also provide guidelines for treatment planning. Occurring in many forms, assessment is sometimes systematic,

TABLE 1.2. Work Settings for Music Therapists

School, K–12: 105	Children's day care/preschool: 29
Nursing home/assisted living: 102	Forensic facility: 28
Hospice/bereavement services: 88	Group home: 23
University/college: 71	Early intervention program: 23
Inpatient psychiatric unit: 65	Day care/treatment center: 22
Self-employed/private practice: 62	Geriatric psychiatric unit: 19
Community-based service: 50	Intermediate care facility/dual diagnosis: 19
Children's hospital or unit: 42	Outpatient clinic: 19
General hospital: 39	Geriatric facility, not nursing: 18
Private music therapy agency: 36	Drug/alcohol program: 16
State agency: 36	Veterans Affairs facility: 16
Adult day care: 34	Wellness program/center: 16
Physical rehabilitation: 31	Oncology: 15
Child/adolescent treatment center: 29	

Note. Respondents could list as many categories as appropriate, so the total number of responses could exceed the number of survey respondents.

wherein the client engages with music so that the therapist can observe and evaluate his or her responses. Assessment may also include less formal forms of inquiry such as observation, a verbal interview, speaking with others who know the client, or reading the medical or educational records, including the referral to music therapy.

Treatment planning occurs next. Goals and objectives are determined at this stage, generally based on what was listed in the referral and what has been determined by the assessment. This phase is often implemented as part of an interdisciplinary team effort and preferably with input from the client. The music therapist, though, is also able to plan treatment based on the client's needs and interests, and sometimes does this with minimal input from others.

The treatment then occurs, based on the goals and objectives that were outlined during the treatment planning stage. Treatment may involve a number of different methods, often involving, as outlined above, improvisation, composition, re-creation, and listening or receptive experiences. Much of the music therapy literature describes these treatments.

During treatment, some type of evaluation is conducted regarding the goals and objectives that were established earlier. Evaluation is aimed at determining client progress or the effectiveness of the therapy method after a given period of treatment. Evaluation is ongoing and may occur prior to, during, and at the end of therapy. Termination is the final step and may occur because the therapy goals have been met, because of a lack of satisfactory progress, or because the client or therapist is leaving the facility or area.

Music Therapy, Music Medicine, Music Education, and Other Practices

Music therapists are not the only people who use music as a part of a process of helping people or healing. Based upon an analysis of articles published in the journal *Music and Medicine,* Dileo (2013) found that the practices that emerge from the interface of the fields of music and medicine fall into four categories: (1) treatment of musicians (by medical personnel and by music therapists); (2) music in medical and health education (in medical humanities, in medical education, and in health education); (3) music practices for patients and staff (by musicians, by medical personnel, and by music therapists); and (4) foundational research. An important distinction is noted for the third category of music practices for patients and staff, wherein the "use of music by medical personnel to reduce anxiety, pain, and autonomic reactivity and improve the status and well-being of medical patients" (p. 113) is referred to as *music medicine.* Prerecorded music, selected by either the patient or the medical professional, is most often used in this situation. Dileo goes on to explain that, "Although it is possible that a relationship exists between these two persons, this relationship does not evolve through the music experience but has its basis in the medical care provided" (p. 113). Addressing foundational research, Dileo describes a range of topics investigated, including "the neuroscience of music (neuroanatomy of music processing and production, effects of music on the brain, music perception, memory for music, brain plasticity, relationships between music and attention, learning, memory, speech, language, motor functioning, and spirituality), physiological responses to music, and psychological responses to music" (pp. 114–115). She also suggests that this category includes "musical characteristics, attributes, preferences, and abilities of special populations" (p. 115). The International Association for Music and Medicine was founded in 2009 to promote an integrative perspective to the application of music in health care, including directing attention toward the integration of a wide range of research initiatives and contemporary practices in the uses of music in the health care arena.

Another use of music by those concerned with improving health is through the arts in health care, a relatively new area that aims to transform "health and healing by connecting people with the arts at key moments in their lives" (Society for the Arts in Healthcare, 2011). Musicians who use their art in health care settings bring their music to those who are in need or seek better health.

Music education and music therapy share common aspects. Although music education is not typically concerned with improving health, those who are involved in music education often use music in some of the same ways that music therapists use it. The primary goals, though, are different. Whereas improving health could be seen as the primary goal for music therapy, improving music skills (e.g., performing, listening, appreciating) is the most basic goal of music education. Those participating in music therapy very often also improve their music skills, and those participating in music education often improve aspects of their health—but the primary goals are different.

In addition to these disciplines involved with health care, many others use music and study topics related to music therapy. Music educators, music psychologists, music sociologists, and neuromusicologists (who perhaps should be labeled as neurologists who study music responses) deal with some of the same areas that are of interest and concern to music therapists. Music educators, for instance, are interested in aspects of music therapy when they work with children with special needs or when they seek evidence that music can assist with learning or promote language skills. Music psychologists provide much of the foundational research for music therapy—research that provides the basis for what music therapists do. An example of this would be research indicating that rhythm can help to organize movement, which is then applied to music therapy techniques designed to help the movement of people with neurological problems. Music sociologists are interested in sociological aspects of music and may help music therapists understand how music can be used to influence groups of people. And neuromusicologists help us understand how the brain processes music, which is beneficial in articulating what occurs in the brain while a person is involved with music and the implications for music therapy. Phenomenal progress has been made in recent years in understanding the role of the brain and central nervous system in processing music, and the research and newfound understanding has broad implications for music therapy assessment, treatment, and practice. Those who study physiological responses and aspects of human anatomy may be concerned with the effects of music, since music can affect blood pressure, respiration rate, muscle tension, and many other bodily responses. Increased understanding of these responses applies to a number of medical areas, where the impact of music on such responses can contribute to improved health.

Education and Clinical Training

Educational requirements for music therapists differ from country to country. Clinical training is always an essential part of the education.

In the United States, AMTA establishes standards and oversees music therapy education and training. Music therapy training is offered at the bachelor's level or higher at over 70 approved educational institutions. Bachelor's-level training leads to entry-level competencies in musical, clinical, and music therapy foundations and principles, acquired through academic coursework and 1,200 hours of clinical training that includes a supervised internship. Many universities offer master's and doctoral degrees in music therapy. Music therapists may also obtain graduate degrees in related fields, such as special education, social work, or gerontology.

Many countries have developed formal education and clinical training requirements governing the process of becoming a music therapist. The WFMT (1999; Wheeler & Grocke, 2001) developed guidelines for education and training, intended to direct countries in their development of music therapy educational programs.

Specialized trainings are offered in some areas of music therapy. These are typically provided as postgraduate training and generally include a certification of some sort that recognizes the additional training and skills of the practitioner. Such trainings and designations are offered in Nordoff–Robbins Music Therapy, Analytical Music Therapy, Guided Imagery and Music, and Neurologic Music Therapy. The approaches underlying all of these trainings are included in chapters of this book. Music therapists may also receive advanced training in a variety of related areas.

Board Certification and Licensure

Because music therapy has developed in various ways in different countries and because countries have their own requirements for practicing, what is required in order to practice music therapy varies from country to country. This variation encompasses training protocols, qualification requirements, and governmental or other statutory regulators of music therapy. In many countries, for instance, music therapy must have formal recognition by the government in order for therapists to practice or to be paid for their services. Sometimes the music therapy association handles the regulation of music therapy. In some countries where government recognition has not yet been achieved and there are thus no accepted requirements for practicing music therapy, people may call themselves music therapists regardless of their training or qualifications. There are frequently concerns about people who call themselves music therapists without training or formal qualifications, but the way of dealing with such concerns varies depending upon the specifics of the country.

The Certification Board for Music Therapists (CBMT; *www.cbmt.org*) establishes competencies for music therapists to become board certified music therapists (MT-BC), the credential necessary to practice music therapy, and requires continuing education to ensure that music therapists' skills are up to date.

Some requirements for practice are regulated by the state. Licensure, for example, is a state-by-state process. A few states have established licenses for music therapists. In some states, music therapists can qualify to be licensed as counselors or in other related areas.

Music therapists may work as creative arts therapists, implying a broader approach than just using music. In New York State, many music therapists are also licensed creative arts therapists (LCATs), signifying that they are qualified to use the creative arts in psychotherapy. Some music therapists work as part of a creative arts or expressive arts team, allying themselves closely with art, dance/movement, and drama therapists.

Research and Evidence-Based Practice

Research is an important aspect of the discipline of music therapy. Research has been linked with practice and theory since Gaston (1968) suggested that theory, clinical practice, and research form a tripod, each "leg" necessary for the other to stand. Research has been defined as "a systematic, self-monitored inquiry which leads to a discovery or new insight which, when documented and disseminated, contributes to or modifies existing knowledge or practice" (Bruscia, 1995, p. 21). Through research, music therapists can gather information on their work and its effectiveness, learn more about the process that is involved, or explore other aspects that they find interesting. Research is very important for the growth of music therapy.

Numerous research methods are used in music therapy. Quantitative research has been employed since the beginning of the development of music therapy as a profession. Qualitative research began assuming increasing importance in the 1980s and now contributes greatly to the understanding of music therapy from various perspectives. Mixed methods research is used increasingly, as researchers attempt to gather information that can best be sought through both quantitative and qualitative means. Additional methods of research include philosophical and historical approaches as well as methods for investigating music.

Evidence-based practice (EBP) is defined as the "conscientious, explicit, and judicious use of current best evidence in making decisions about care of individual patients. The practice of evidence based medicine means integrating individual clinical expertise with the best available external clinical evidence from systematic research" (Sackett, Rosenberg, Gray, Haynes, & Richardson, 1996, p. 71). EBP represents the combined use of (1) systematic reviews of the scientific literature, (2) practitioner experience and opinion, and (3) patient/client preferences and values for making clinical decisions and treatment/intervention planning.

All health care professions are called to follow principles of EBP, and music therapy is no exception. Indeed, the definition of music therapy that is provided by AMTA and that was given earlier includes "evidence-based use of music interventions."

The importance of research to music therapy was recognized in the United States when the first of the original six objectives of NAMT, founded in 1950, was stated: "to encourage and report research projects" (Gilliland, 1952, p. v). Research continues to hold a very important role in the development of music therapy.

Publications

Music therapy publications include journals as well as books. Journals published in related disciplines also contain information related to music therapy.

Music therapy journals published regularly in English include the *Journal of Music Therapy* and *Music Therapy Perspectives* from the United States, the *Canadian Journal of Music Therapy*, the *British Journal of Music Therapy*, the *Australian Journal of Music Therapy*, the *New Zealand Journal of Music Therapy*, the *Nordic Journal of Music Therapy*, and *Voices: A World Forum for Music Therapy*. All of these, except for the *Nordic Journal of Music Therapy* and *Voices*, are published by the music therapy associations of their respective countries. Some articles in *Voices* are translated into languages other than, but including, English. In addition to journals published in English, the German journal, *Musiktherapeutische Umshcau*, plays an important role in the development of music therapy in Germany.

The Arts in Psychotherapy, an international journal that includes all of the arts therapies, includes a substantial number of articles on music therapy. *Music and Medicine: An Interdisciplinary Journal* includes articles on music therapy, music medicine, and other aspects of music and medicine. It is sponsored by the International Association of Music and Medicine and includes abstracts in several languages. In addition, the *Journal of the Association of Music and Imagery* (AMI) focuses on the Bonny Method of Guided Imagery and Music (BMGIM or GIM), which is closely related to music therapy.

Levels of Practice

Music therapists sometimes find it useful to delineate the level or depth at which they are working or from which their clients will benefit. Previously, I (Wheeler, 1983; Houghton et al., 2005) proposed that, based on levels of psychotherapy presented by Wolberg (1977), music therapy as psychotherapy may occur at three levels. In *supportive, activities-oriented music therapy*, goals are achieved through the use of therapeutic activities (including verbalization when appropriate). Music therapists who work at this level support clients in establishing and maintaining adaptive behaviors. Insight into why a behavior occurs is not considered important.

In *reeducative, insight-, and process-oriented music therapy*, the focus is on the exposition and discussion of feelings, which leads to insight that improves functioning. Music can be used to elicit emotional and/or cognitive reactions necessary for the therapy. This type of music therapy relies on what Zwerling (1979) considers one of the unique features of the creative arts therapies: their ability to tap into deeper emotional levels than are normally accessible. The feelings that are discussed in insight-oriented music therapy with reeducative goals are relatively close to consciousness and can therefore be elicited through attention to the here and now, including personal feelings and interpersonal reactions.

In *reconstructive, analytically, and catharsis-oriented music therapy*, music therapy techniques are employed to elicit unconscious material, which is then utilized in an effort to promote reorganization of the personality. The ability of music to tap deeper levels of emotion is utilized to reach this unconscious material. The goal is to work through situations that were inadequately lived/resolved as the person grew up. Working at this level of music therapy requires training beyond that typically offered in a music therapy degree program, although advanced training in certain music therapy methods (e.g., Analytical Music Therapy or Guided Imagery with Music) helps in developing the skills.

International Scope

As noted, music therapy has developed differently in different countries. It is well established in many parts of the world, and many countries (in addition to the United States) have standards for educating and training music therapists, governmental regulations for music therapy, and active music therapy associations. The Country of the Month section of *Voices* (*www.voices.no*) is a good place to gain an overview of the status of music therapy in various countries.

The Internet has facilitated communication among music therapists everywhere so that, today, music therapists communicate regularly with their colleagues around the world. It is easy to find information on music therapy anywhere in the world. The websites mentioned here, as well as other sites, provide international networking opportunities for music therapists and others interested in music therapy and assist in increasing awareness and communication.

The WFMT is dedicated to the promotion and development of music therapy worldwide (*www.musictherapyworld.net*). The website includes a great deal of information on music therapy around the world, including an international library of music, a global calendar, and a section in which students share their experiences from around the world.

In addition to the WFMT, several confederations of music therapy associations exist. One is the European Music Therapy Confederation (EMTC; *emtc-eu.com*), which was founded in 1990 as a forum for exchange between music therapists in Europe. The EMTC works to promote the development of professional practice in Europe and to foster exchange and collaboration among member countries. The EMTC sponsors a European music therapy conference every 3 years, offering an opportunity for European music therapists and others to exchange ideas and share their work.

The Latin American Committee of Music Therapy (CLAM) was formed in 1993 to promote collaborative work in the region as well as equal participation in the world music therapy context. CLAM sponsors a conference every 3 years in one of the member countries.

Internet Communication

The Internet has revolutionized communication in all aspects of music therapy, not only international communication. Music therapists communicate among themselves and with the general public through many Internet sources. Online communication is in a constant state of flux and change, with new methods of exchanging information emerging on a regular basis. These change so rapidly that there is little point in listing them for any type of permanent retrieval. At the present time, music therapists and others share information through blogs, podcasts, Facebook groups, LinkedIn, Pinterest, Skype, YouTube, e-books, online journals, and other methods. Individual music therapists, music therapy clinics, university programs, and national and regional organizations interact in various ways via websites, Internet programs, and social media. Music therapy professionals and organizations provide regular online updates about topics such as clinical protocols and experiences; resources; research results; breaking news; and reviews about music, music instruments, and other materials related to music therapy. Online journals, e-books, online workshops, webinars, professional mentoring services, and self-study e-courses for continuing education credit are available on the Internet for music therapy professionals, interns, and students (C. Knoll, personal communication, March 23, 2013).

Interdisciplinary Collaboration

Music therapists collaborate with people from other disciplines in many settings. Working in schools, music therapists often work with children for whom music therapy has been determined to be important to their education and written into their individualized education programs (IEPs). Music therapy is considered a related service as part of the Individuals with Disabilities Education Act (IDEA) and, after proper referral and assessment, may be included as part of a child's education. In this situation music therapists work with other members of an interdisciplinary or multidisciplinary team to determine the goals for music therapy and to implement these goals. A similar model may be followed in other settings, although the IEP may not be the document that is used for planning. For example, in early childhood education (from birth to age 3), the individualized family service plan (IFSP) is used. In work with adults with developmental disabilities, an individual program plan (IPP) is often used. In all of these, though, the intent is to provide a coordinated treatment plan for the client.

Music therapists working in hospitals are usually part of an interdisciplinary team that consists of physicians; nurses; occupational, speech, and physical therapists; and other professionals. Working with other professionals, with each contributing his or her own expertise, benefits the patients, and these other professionals usually provide the referrals to music therapy.

Music therapists working in psychiatric settings, both institutions and community-based programs, are also part of an interdisciplinary team. Along with other team members, the music therapist will help to determine the needs of the clients and how and when music therapy may be helpful in meeting these needs.

Public Awareness of Music Therapy

Music therapy has received unprecedented publicity in the last few years. Gabrielle Giffords, the congresswoman from Arizona who received a traumatic brain injury (TBI) when she was shot in the head in 2011, benefited greatly from music therapy and credits it with helping her regain her speech. A number of news agencies reported on this, sharing video clips of her music therapy sessions and describing the positive effects of music therapy.

Several novels with music therapists as main characters have also been published. The most prominent of these was *Sing You Home* by Jodi Picoult (2011). Another novel, *I Think I Love You*, by Allison Pearson (2011), also featured a music therapist, and *A White Wind Blew*, by James Markert (2013), is a fictional account of a physician who treats patients with tuberculosis using music. A movie, *The Music Never Stopped* (Moritz & Kohlberg, 2011), based on a case study and essay titled "The Last Hippie," by Dr. Oliver Sacks (1995), depicts the work of music therapist Concetta Tomaino. Nathanial Ayers, an outstanding musician who has a severe psychiatric illness, is featured in the movie *The Soloist* (Foster, Krasnoff, & Wright, 2009), bringing attention to the role of music in helping people with mental illness, and *Young at Heart* (George & Walker, 2008) is a documentary about a chorus of senior citizens from Massachusetts. Oliver Sacks, prominent neurologist and author, has put the power of music in the public eye by spotlighting the role of music with neurological and related problems in books such as *The Man Who Mistook His Wife for a Hat* (1985) and *Musicophilia* (2007).

The past few years have included the publication of a number of Cochrane reviews of music and music therapy (*www.cochrane. org/cochrane-reviews*), with ensuing publicity. Music therapy was featured in a series of lectures in the Music and the Brain II Series at the Library of Congress. There have been regular articles on music therapy in the *Huffington Post* and frequent coverage of music therapy in various newspapers, magazines, and television and radio programs (e.g., see *www.musictherapy.org/ events/media*). These and numerous television and radio features on music therapy are just some of the ways that music therapy has become more visible.

Issues in Music Therapy

Many issues pertinent to the field of music therapy are of concern to music therapists. These issues are dealt with around the world, although certainly there are variations in different countries, due to both the culture of the countries and to the level of development of music therapy in different places. These issues are discussed individually.

Recognition of Music Therapy

One issue of concern to music therapists is a lack of recognition and understanding of what music therapy is and its benefits. Although the increased publicity that was just mentioned *has* made a difference in people's awareness of music therapy, many people still have not heard of the profession. This lack of awareness includes the general public but also other professionals, including those who would be in a position to support music therapy in various ways. Related to this awareness is a lack of understanding of how music therapy works. Because it is often enjoyable, and people participating in a music therapy session may look as though they are having fun (which very well may be the case), sometimes the observer misses the clinical goals that are being worked toward or the therapy that is occurring. Even when music therapists try to educate others about what is actually occurring in music therapy, people do not always understand.

Various issues arise concerning formal recognition of music therapy by government agencies or, as sometimes conceived, accreditation. These issues also affect how funding is provided for music therapy. In the United States, AMTA and CBMT have organized task forces in many states to promote state recognition of music therapy. These task forces have led to a number of positive changes for music therapists, including job descriptions for music therapists and licenses in several states.

As was also discussed earlier, there is a call in many areas of health care for EBP. Although the effectiveness of music therapy is increasingly evidence-based, there is a need for more documented evidence. There are many issues involved in producing evidence in a discipline such as music therapy, including the difficulty (and perhaps inadvisability) of developing protocols for what occurs in music therapy. A protocol for a music therapy session would specify the sequence of what is to occur in a session. Such a protocol is necessary for many research studies to ensure that what occurs in the session is consistent and can be reported. However, few actual music therapy sessions follow such a set structure, leading many to point out that using a protocol in research makes the music therapy session in a research study very different from an actual session and to question the validity of research based on such a protocol. In addition, there are not many music therapists and even fewer who are in a position to do research, and the clients or research subjects for such research are usually not plentiful. All of these are potential obstacles in developing an evidence base for music therapy. An additional concern is that not all ways of doing music therapy are in line with the demands of evidence-based practice, as was discussed earlier.

Looking forward, it seems that music therapy is experiencing growth worldwide. Recognition by many states in the United States and national regulating agencies in some countries adds to its credibility. Research is increasing, also adding to its credibility.

ACKNOWLEDGMENT

I wish to thank the following colleagues for feedback on this chapter: Anthony Meadows, Virginia Driscoll, Claire Ghetti, Cathy Malchiodi, and Suzanne Sorel.

REFERENCES

American Music Therapy Association. (2013). *A descriptive statistical profile of the AMTA membership*. Retrieved from *www.musictherapy.org/assets/1/7/13WorkforceAnalysis.pdf*.

Bruscia, K. E. (1995). The boundaries of music therapy research. In B. L. Wheeler (Ed.), *Music therapy research: Quantitative and qualitative perspectives* (pp. 17–27). Gilsum, NH: Barcelona.

Bruscia, K. E. (1998). *Defining music therapy* (2nd ed.). Gilsum, NH: Barcelona.

Dileo, C. (2013). A proposed model for identifying practices: A content analysis of the first 4 years of *Music and Medicine*. *Music and Medicine, 5*(2), 110–118.

Foster, G., & Krasnoff, R. (Producers), & Wright, J. (Director). (2009). *The soloist*. United States: DreamWorks.

Gaston, E. T. (1968). *Music in therapy*. New York: Macmillan.

George, S. (Producer), & Walker, S. (Director). (2008). *Young at heart*. United Kingdom: Fox Searchlight Pictures.

Gfeller, K. E., & Davis, W. B. (2008). The music therapy treatment process. In W. B. Davis, K. E. Gfeller, & M. H. Thaut (Eds.), *An introduction to music therapy: Theory and process* (3rd ed., pp. 429–486). Silver Spring, MD: American Music Therapy Association.

Gilliland, E. (1952). The development of music therapy as a profession. In E. Gilliland (Ed.), *Music therapy 1951* (pp. v–xvi). Waukegan, IL: North Shore Printers.

Houghton, B. A., Scovel, M. A., Smeltekop, R. A., Thaut, M. H., Unkefer, R. F., & Wilson, B. L. (2005). Taxonomy of clinical music therapy programs and techniques. In R. F. Unkefer & M. H. Thaut (Eds.), *Music therapy in the treatment of adults with mental disorders* (pp. 181–206). Gilsum, NH: Barcelona.

Markert, J. (2013). *A white wind blew*. Naperville, IL: Sourcebooks Landmark.

Moritz, N. (Producer), & Kohlberg, J. (Director). (2011). *The music never stopped*. United States: Essential Pictures.

Pearson, A. (2011). *I think I love you*. New York: Knopf.

Picoult, J. (2011). *Sing you home*. New York: Atria Books.

Sackett, D. L., Rosenberg, W. M. C., Gray, J. A. M., Haynes, R. B., & Richardson, W. D. (1996). Evidence based medicine: What it is and what it isn't. *British Medical Journal, 312*, 71–72.

Sacks, O. (1985). *The man who mistook his wife for a hat*. New York: Touchstone Books.

Sacks, O. (1995). The last hippie. In O. Sacks (Ed.), *An anthropologist on Mars: Seven paradoxical tales* (pp. 42–76). New York: Knopf.

Sacks, O. (2007). *Musicophilia*. New York: Vintage Books.

Society for the Arts in Healthcare. (2011). *What is*

arts and health? Retrieved from *http://thesah.org/doc/Definition_FINALNovember2011.pdf*.

Wheeler, B. L. (1983). A psychotherapeutic classification of music therapy practices: A continuum of procedures. *Music Therapy Perspectives, 1*(2), 8–12.

Wheeler, B. L., & Grocke, D. E. (2001). Report of the World Federation of Music Therapy Commission on Education, Training, and Accreditation Symposium. *Music Therapy Perspectives, 19*, 63–67.

Wolberg, L. R. (1977). *The technique of psychotherapy* (3rd ed., Pt.1). New York: Grune & Stratton.

World Federation of Music Therapy. (1999). Guidelines for music therapy education and training. Retrieved from *www.musictherapyworld.net/WFMT/Education_and_Training_files/WFMT%20Education%20Guidelines%201999.pdf*.

Zwerling, I. (1979, December). The creative arts therapist as "real therapies." *Hospital and Community Psychiatry, 30*, 841–844.

CHAPTER 2

A History of Music Therapy

William Davis
Susan Hadley

Seated at the roaring loom of time, for six thousand years man[kind]
has woven a seamless garment. But that garment is invisible and
intangible save where the dyes of written history fall upon it, and
forever preserve it as a possession of generations to come.
                                              —ALLAN NEVINS

I have always held that the history of music therapy is a forgotten
history, one of the "small narratives" threading its way along other
grand narratives about philosophy, music and medicine.
                                              —EVEN RUUD

No one has created or invented music therapy; however
many individuals have discovered its theories, ideologies and
methodologies.
                                              —ROLANDO BENENZON

The task of writing a history of music therapy within a short chapter is certainly a daunting one. In the three epigraphs above, it is apparent that what we find in history is but a thread in the garment of human experience. What we get is information that fits a particular historian's interests and needs. And much of the history of music therapy is submersed by larger narratives, such as those of philosophy, musicology, and medicine, of which music therapy is a part. Adding to the difficulty of writing this chapter is that we were tasked with taking a global approach to the history of music

therapy. Gouk (2000) notes that delineating a historical perspective presupposes a set of categories and assumptions that we need to make explicit if we want to create a truly cross-cultural approach (p. 5). She suggests that the nature and purpose of history "has traditionally been to hold up individuals, groups or nations as examples to propagate moral and religious values" (p. 5). As such, many of the historical accounts of music therapy have been influenced by a Western Christian cultural grounding. What we need to be careful of in our accounts is what Horden (2000) describes as "the danger [of] 'first-world' music therapy [being] privileged over 'traditional' forms of musical healing" (p. 316).

Several books provide insight into a global approach to the history of musical healing or the therapeutics of music. These include Horden's (2000) *Music as Medicine: The History of Music Therapy Since Antiquity*, Gouk's (2000) *Musical Healing in Cultural Contexts*, and Dileo Maranto's (1993) *Music Therapy: International Perspectives*. Each brings different insights: The first two comprise contributions largely from anthropologists, musicologists, and historians—that is, primarily those outside of the profession of music therapy. These texts are viewed by the editors, Gouk and Horden, as companion texts, both having grown out of symposiums in London in 1997, organized by the respective editors: "Music, Healing and Culture: Towards a Comparative Perspective," and "Music and Medicine: The History of Music Therapy since Antiquity." The beauty of these texts is that the authors bring their expertise in historical, cultural, and musicological research to bear on traditions of musical healing and music as medicine. While they are cognizant that what they are writing about extends outside of what has been considered the professionalization of music therapy, the historical perspectives are certainly pertinent to the emergence of music therapy as a fully accredited profession. Dileo Maranto's (1993) text, in contrast, is a compilation of narratives by music therapists about music therapy as practiced in 38 countries (although notably missing is Germany), each including historical perspectives. In addition to Dileo Maranto's text, many historical accounts of music therapy, as practiced in a large number of countries, are found in the Country of the Month section of *Voices: A World Forum for Music Therapy* (*www.voices.no*).

In this chapter we provide a fine thread in the fabric of history as it relates to the emergence of music therapy from a global perspective. For more in-depth treatises, we encourage readers to turn to the literature we cite throughout the chapter.

Early Concepts of Music Therapy: A Multicultural Perspective

Across cultural contexts, music has been associated with practices that seek greater health and wholeness. How music is conceptualized is dependent on the cultural context, as is the conceptualization of health and wholeness. As Gouk (2000) states, "There is a correlation between the way healers and their patients identify themselves and interact with each other, and the way they understand the human body and its relationship to the world more generally" (p. 10).

An analysis of the practices of medicine and psychiatry over many hundreds of years reveals that many forms of treatment, including the use of music, have been used to ameliorate physical and mental illnesses. Some forms of treatment are based on superstition (e.g., tarantism) or spiritual beliefs and practices (e.g., shamanism and holistic approaches), and some are based on scientific theories (e.g., modern music therapy). In each case, the concepts of how best to address treatment correspond to the cultural and theoretical contexts from which they emerge. Some premodern societies based their views of disease on the mysterious, not delineating between health care, the supernatural, and religion. For example, tarantism, which developed in the Middle Ages and was practiced in Italy and Spain, utilized music and dance to induce trance states for healing purposes (Horden, 2000, pp. 249–253). In other cultural contexts, disease was attributed to supernatural causes and treated by shamans (men or women with access to the spiritual realm), who in many instances included music in their ceremonies. Shamans are "an integral part of communal religious traditions, professionals who make use of personal supernatural experiences, especially trance, as a resource for the wider community's physical and spiritual wellbeing" (DuBois, 2009, p. i). Shamanic traditions "regard altered states of consciousness . . . as pivotal elements in human interactions with the supernatural" (p. 153). Music, along with dance, is one of the main tools employed in shamanism to achieve a trance state or an altered state of consciousness (p. 153). Shamanism was, and in many cases still is, practiced in many countries throughout the world. Today, there are music therapists who practice shamanism, including Barbara Crowe, who is a trained shamanic practitioner and has been practicing shamanic traditions since the mid-1980s (B. Crowe, personal communication, May 27, 2013).

More broadly, healing practices associated with altered states of consciousness can be found in parts of Africa, Asia, the Middle East, Europe, and the Americas. In music therapy today, an altered state of consciousness is induced in the practice of the Bonny Method of Guided Imagery and Music (BMGIM or GIM; Bruscia & Grocke, 2002) and in practices that use monochromatic sounds, such as the monochord, gong, didgeridoo, or Tibetan prayer bowl, "in order to open the healing potential of trance states for the therapy process" (Bossinger & Hess, 1993, p. 239).

Holistic forms of music and healing, based on spiritual values, can be seen in many indigenous cultures around the world. For example, the First Nations people in the Americas frequently employed, and in some contexts still employ, music as therapy for the treatment and prevention of disease, as well as a way of maintaining good health. What music therapists now consider basic tenets of music therapy, developed from European and American perspectives, have actually been in use by many Native American cultures for centuries. For example, healing ceremonies might focus on rehabilitation of physical disorders using stimulative music, whereas sedative music might be included in a ceremony devoted to the palliation of psychiatric disorders (Densmore, 1948).

Music healing practices, while varying from tribe to tribe, were an integral fabric of Native American life. Densmore (1948) described how music, employing rhythm as a primary mode of treatment, was used to treat physical and emotional disorders. Some of the shamans used music in conjunction with herbs and other medications, whereas others used music alone. A combination of songs and rhythm instruments was sometimes used, and at other times only singing was employed.

In early Western culture, as concepts of disease shifted from supernatural causes (e.g., due to the wrath of unhappy gods), the manner in which music was employed as a healing tool also changed. Then, with the rise of Greek culture about 600 years B.C.E., rational medicine superseded the supernatural and religious beliefs in the quest to explain the origins of physical and mental disorders. In fact, during the time of Hippocrates and Galen, the concept of the four cardinal humors became important to help explain disease from an empirical point of view; a healthy person was thought to be in perfect harmony or equilibrium, whereas illness indicated a disturbance of this balance (Boxberger, 1962). Music therapy as an academic discipline emerged within this Western biomedical model. In our Western history of music therapy, Ruud (1998) notes two concepts that run through from Ancient Greece to the 19th century: (1) how music relates to different concepts of illness (e.g., the theory of the four humors), and (2) how music can restore peace and harmony (e.g., within a hygienics framework) (p. 50). Thus, therapy has most often been associated with disease or illness and hence with our biology (p. 51).

A new pattern of health care emerged during the Middle Ages in Western civilization as Christianity became the dominant religion in Europe and, later, during the 17th century, with the arrival of the first settlers in the Americas. The physically ill were treated with compassion, whereas those suffering behavioral or emotional disturbances were frequently put into restraints, ostracized, and abused in other ways, due to a profound lack of understanding of the causes of mental disorders (Boxberger, 1962).

By 1800, the scientific method for diagnosing and treating disease began to take a more important role with the use of drugs and surgery. The employment of music therapy became more specific, leading to the development of techniques in use today. For example, the *iso principle* (mood vectoring) and the selection of patient-preferred music began to appear. During the late 19th century, more reports of music therapy practice began to emerge, including the use of music therapy with groups in institutional settings and in private practice (Davis, 1987).

The 20th century marks the beginning of the modern development of music therapy. Music therapy developed as a profession at different rates in various countries, but the second half of the century saw tremendous growth of music therapy in many parts of the world, with music therapy associations being founded to address the needs of an emerging profession, including the need to vigorously promote research, develop standards for university educational and clinical training programs, and publish journals and newsletters to keep the music therapy community abreast of developments affecting education and clinical practice. Today music therapy is recognized as a legitimate profession around much of the modern world.

Music Therapy during the European Romantic Era and in the Early American Republic

Music has long been important in the Western medical tradition. Two texts that trace this history are Schullian and Schoen's *Music and Medicine* (1948), which examines the use of music within the context of West-

ern medical science from Antiquity to the mid-20th century (Gouk, 2000, p. 3), and Kümmel's *Musik und Medizin* (1977), which examines theory and practice in music and medicine in Europe from 800 to 1800, covering themes such as "music and the pulse; music and medical education; the foundations of the dietetic–therapeutic functions of music; music as an aid to health, and its role in therapy" (Gouk, p. 4). This second text illustrates that "theorists and practitioners of all kinds, from all major European countries, and in almost every century, recommended listening or performing [music] as a means of preventing or alleviating ill health" (Horden, 2000, p. 23).

Although there was a long history of using music in medicine throughout the ages in Europe, music therapy was largely criticized in Europe in the 18th century on scientific grounds (Lecourt, 1993, pp. 222–223). However, in 1744 in Spain, Antonio Jose Rodriguez devoted a chapter in a medical text to establishing a scientific theory of music therapy, proposing that music could address the psychological and emotional aspects of a patient's illness (Blasco, 1993, p. 534).

During the same time period, with the end of the war against Great Britain, North Americans enjoyed the newly acquired political independence as an opportunity to compete with other countries for world leadership in medicine and psychiatry. One of the influential figures during this time was Benjamin Rush, who was given the moniker of *American Father of Psychiatry*. Rush was deeply involved with moral and humanitarian causes and championed changes in the way that behavioral and emotional disorders were viewed. Though he employed then-contemporary practices such as bleeding and the use of emetics and restraints, Rush also advocated for gentler forms of treatment for his clients, including gardening, sewing, self-reflection, and music (Davis, 1987).

Though there is no evidence that Rush practiced music therapy or was even a musician, he understood the power of music as a complementary therapy. Two medical students under his guidance, Edwin Atlee (1776–1852) and Samuel Mathews (birth and death dates unknown), produced short dissertations 2 years apart on the influence of music on disease. Atlee, writing in 1804, noted that music could be used to treat a variety of psychiatric disorders. Observing that there was a strong connection between mind and body, he advocated the use of music from the patient's culture to elicit pleasant memories (extramusical associations).

Samuel Mathews followed closely with his dissertation, written in 1806. He focused specifically on a psychiatric disorder referred to as *phantasm* (likely schizophrenia) and a physical disease, chorea, which would probably be described today as Huntington's disease. Mathews championed the use of live music and, like Atlee, noted the important mind–body connection when treating illness. Additional concepts that appeared in the two dissertations that are sometimes used in contemporary music therapy practice include (1) the use of the *iso principle*, (2) acknowledging differences in responding to musical stimuli between musicians and nonmusicians, (3) involving the patient as a participant in the music therapy process, and (4) the use of client-preferred music (Davis, 1987).

During the same period of time, music therapy was being used in educational institutions for persons with disabilities. The Perkins Institute for the Blind in Massachusetts reported the use of music therapy as early as 1832. Samuel Gridley Howe implemented a strong music curriculum, employing professional musicians from the Boston area to teach piano and voice. Other examples include music instruction at the New York School for the Blind and at the American Asylum for the Deaf in Connecticut. Music therapy programs also appeared in a few schools for persons with physical disabilities (Darrow & Heller, 1985).

Late-19th-Century Music Therapy: The Influence of the Medical and Psychiatric Communities

During the final three decades of the 19th century, three important reports documenting music therapy practice appeared in medical journals. The first was a brief article titled "Music as Mind Medicine," which was published in the *Virginia Medical Monthly* of 1878. The essay chronicled a series of experiments describing reactions of persons with psychiatric illness to live vocal and instrumental music. Prominent soloists and ensembles from New York City took part in the sessions, which were carried out at Blackwell's Island (now Roosevelt Island), an infamous, overcrowded facility designed to care for impoverished women with emotional and/or behavioral disturbances. Nine documented visits to the island provided women with either a concert or, for a few fortunate individuals, a one-on-one session. The goal of the individual sessions was to test changes in heart and respiration rates of individuals to Western classical music. This attempt at using live music to relieve suffering of women with psychiatric illnesses is important because it is likely the first example in U.S. history of music therapy used in a large institution (Davis, 1987).

A second late-19th-century account of music therapy was authored by prominent psychiatrist and mental health advocate George Alder Blumer. His paper, "Music in Its Relation to the Mind," appeared in the *American Journal of Insanity* in 1892. The principal emphasis of Blumer's program was to support music therapy at Utica State Hospital, a large institution for persons with psychiatric disorders. Blumer believed so much in music as therapy that he hired immigrant musicians to perform for patients at this hospital, where he was chief administrator (Davis, 1987).

The third example of substantial music therapy practice to appear during the 19th century focused on an interesting private practice. James Leonard Corning, a prominent New York City neurologist, conducted a notable series of experiments using music in combination with visual imagery, and occasionally medication, to treat clients suffering from mild psychological and emotional disorders. Corning believed that by listening to music both before and during sleep, cognitive processes would be suspended, thereby permitting the saturation of *musical vibrations* into the subconscious. He believed that his use of classical music facilitated the transfer of positive images and emotions into a patient's waking hours and that they, in turn, would replace negative thoughts and feelings and improve the quality of sleep and a client's outlook on life (Davis, 2012).

Still during the 19th century, new developments in music therapy emerged in Europe with the introduction of modern psychiatry. In France, medical doctors such as Esquirol, Leuret, Dupre, Nathan, and Bourneville conducted clinical research in hospitals using music listening, music performance, and music instruction of hospital patients, with the aim of reducing anxiety and regulating mood and behavior (Lecourt, 1993, p. 223). At this time, a precursor to community music therapy was seen in the creation of musical societies aimed at social and political organizations, the effects of harmony being thought to both *civilize the masses* and to *influence the psyches* of those with mental illnesses. It was also around this time that the German writer, Novalis, is reputed to have said that every illness is a musical problem and that its cure is a musical solution (Horden, 2000, p. 3). And in 1891 in England, Canon Harford founded The Guild of St. Cecilia, the aim of which was for accomplished musicians to play sedative music to patients in hospitals in London (Davis, 1988). Although this program gained great support and media attention, it also received harsh criticism. Due to lack of funds and the declining health of Harford, the guild soon folded. Therapeutic uses of music were also recorded in the late 1800s in Hungary, particularly with emotionally disturbed children (Konta & Varga, 1993, p. 265), and in Finland, especially in psychiatric hospitals (Lehtonen, 1993, p. 212).

Music Therapy in the Early 20th Century: Musicians as Advocates

The practice of music therapy in the 19th century, though sporadic and experimental, is important because it clearly shows an interest in using music as an alternative treatment to the harsh, sometimes cruel methods used to incarcerate persons with disabilities. The dissemination of these ideas was primarily the provenance of physicians and psychiatrists, which unfortunately limited the scope of influence, due to the restricted audience of exclusively medical professionals. The trend of physicians advocating for music therapy changed dramatically with the turn of the 20th century.

During the first years of the 20th century, music therapy clinical practice in North America was promoted more vigorously than ever before due to the efforts of musicians and, to a lesser degree, physicians. Eva Augusta Vescelius, Isa Maud Ilsen, Harriet Ayer Seymour, and Willem van de Wall were all determined, well-trained musicians who developed interesting personal philosophies concerning the use of music in therapy. They all enthusiastically advocated for music therapy, with Vescelius, Ilsen, and Seymour establishing short-lived organizations founded to promote music therapy to musicians and health care professionals (Davis, 1993).

Eva Augusta Vescelius, a classically trained vocalist, was the first of the three to practice music therapy. Borrowing ideas from the New Thought movement (a controversial nonliturgical religion) and her considerable talents as a musician, she blended music and mental imagery to treat clients with varying mental and physical illnesses.

Her methods were unique in that she did not believe in interacting with her clients during music therapy sessions; instead she would perform classical music, selecting each piece personally and employing a small group of instrumentalists and vocalists, while using mental imagery to convey positive thoughts.

In 1903 Vescelius founded the first organization devoted to promoting music therapy, the National Society of Music Therapeutics. Her goal was to "encourage the study of music in its relation to life, and the promotion of its use as a curative agent in homes, hospitals, asylums, and prisons" (Vescelius, 1913, p. 8). In addition to an organization promoting music therapy, she also must be credited with publishing the first journal devoted to music therapy, *Music and Health* (Davis, 1993). In the 1920s, a branch of the International Society for Musical Therapeutics was also established in Sydney, Australia (O'Callaghan, 2002).

Slightly overlapping Vescelius in time, Isa Maud Ilsen, a trained nurse, advocated for a style of music therapy that is much more accepted today. Unlike Vescelius, Ilsen believed in establishing a therapeutic relationship with her clients. She was interested in employing music to treat a variety of clinical populations, including persons with physical, psychological, and intellectual disabilities. Her music therapy activities carried over to providing services to injured World War I veterans and to teaching a short course in music therapy at Columbia University in 1919.

In 1926, Ilsen founded the second American organization for music therapy, the National Association for Music in Hospitals. Though she had some unusual ideas, such as avoiding the use of the cello, trumpet, or portable organ in sessions (she approved of the violin, voice, and harp), other ideas were better thought out. For example, she advocated for training musicians in proper hospital protocol, cooperating with doctors and nurses, and, as noted, establishing a therapeutic relationship with her clients (Davis, 1993).

Harriet Ayer Seymour, an educator and music therapist, began her career much like Vescelius and Ilsen: by developing music therapy techniques through experience. Seymour was also an accomplished author, publishing a number of books about music education and, later, music therapy. Her spiritual preferences were similar to Vescelius's; she relied on her musicianship and positive thoughts to shape her music therapy practice. Though she initially felt that little interaction was necessary with clients, she changed her philosophy later in her career working with World War II veterans and encouraged an active role between therapist and client. Seymour also founded an organization, the National Foundation of Musical Therapy, to promote music therapy to the public. Her major achievement, though, was an attempt at authoring the first text about music therapy. Written about 1944, shortly before her death, *An Instructional Course in the Use and Practice of Musical Therapy* was never published (Davis, 1993).

A number of physicians were also using music therapeutically in the operating room in the United States during the early years of the 20th century. As early as 1915, reports surfaced in medical journals promoting the use of the recently available phonograph to aid relaxation in patients undergoing surgery.

In 1918, Columbia University initiated a course called Musicotherapy, taught by Margaret Anderton, a British musician who had experience working with Canadian soldiers in World War I (Columbia University to Heal Wounded by Music, 1919). And as early as 1926 Willem Van de Wall was teaching classes that included Institutional Music, Music in Mental and Social Therapy, and Problems in Institutional Music at Teachers College, Columbia University. These classes included demonstrations and clinical practice in New York institutions. By 1929 classes in the Psychology of Music and Dalcroze Eurythmics (a system of music education developed during the early 20th century by Emile Jaques-Dalcroze that uses movement to teach musical concepts to children) were also offered through Teachers College (Columbia University, Teachers College Announcement, 1926–1927; S. Hanser, personal communication, June 18, 2013). In 1929 Duke University reported the effectiveness of music not only in operating and recovery arenas, but also in children's and adults' wards. In 1930 J. A. McGlinn enthusiastically endorsed the use of music during anesthesia to relax patients and doctors alike. Erdman later experimented successfully with the use of headphones to block unwanted operating room sounds from patients undergoing surgery (Taylor, 1981).

Similarly, in Germany in the first half of the 20th century, medical doctor Karl-Heinz Polter wrote about ways that he used music in treating neurological, psychiatric, and psychosomatic diseases. He published these in his 1934 text, *Music as a Medium of Healing* (Wosch, 2003).

Despite an increase in the use of music therapy during the first 40 years of the 20th century, there was still uncertainty (in the United States) that music therapy would be widely accepted as a treatment modality. It would not be until the decade of the 1940s that a number of individuals, government agencies, and music organizations began working in concert to found an organization that would represent music therapy on a national level (Boxberger, 1963).

Emerging Professionalism: Rapid Growth of Music Therapy during the Mid-20th Century

By the end of World War II, momentum was gathering toward creating a professional association in the United States that would assist in the development of the rigorous standards needed to assure that musicians were adequately trained to work in

hospitals and schools as music therapists. A number of professional music associations, charitable organizations, and the Veterans Administration (VA) provided the important groundwork for this to occur. The National Federation of Music Clubs, the Music Teachers National Association, and the American Red Cross represented just a few of the organizations involved with organizing volunteer musicians to work with returning World War II veterans, raising funds for the purchase of musical instruments and music, or encouraging much-needed research. Many of the volunteers worked in VA hospitals, helping returning soldiers with mental and physical disabilities (Boxberger, 1963). The Red Cross in Australia also introduced music therapy in various hospitals at the end of World War II (O'Callaghan, 2002).

In addition to groups coming together to support music therapy during the war years, educational programs were also being developed at Michigan State College (now University) and at the University of Kansas. Other U.S. schools quickly followed, with undergraduate programs started at the University of the Pacific (Stockton, CA), Boston School of Occupational Therapy, Chicago Musical College, and Alverno College (Milwaukee, WI). Clinical training was also becoming a requirement for a degree in music therapy. In conjunction with the program at Michigan State College, the first U.S. internship site was developed at Wayne County General Hospital. Other internships quickly followed, and soon other universities were adding a required 6-month clinical training component (Boxberger, 1963).

As the profession of music therapy continued to grow in stature in the United States, it became clear that the guidance of a professional organization was needed to develop standards of education and clinical training and to assure professional competence through a registration process.

At this time, music therapy was also being established outside of the United States. In

Argentina, music therapy clinical practice was begun in 1948, and in 1949 the first training course for special music educators was developed (Wagner & Benenzon, 1993).

Music Therapy Matures into a Profession for the 21st Century

At a 1947 meeting of the Music Teachers National Association, a U.S. organization, Roy Underwood summarized the status of music therapy by stating that, in addition to having no formal organization, there was a lack of understanding of the true function of music therapy, no publications, a paucity of good research, and the need to standardize curriculum and clinical training standards. Underwood's sentiments were backed by an important survey conducted by the National Music Council. The 1944 survey found that hospital administrators, for the most part, found music beneficial to improve the physical and mental health of children and adults (Van de Wall, 1944).

The stage was thus set for the founding of a permanent organization to represent the professional interests of music therapy in the United States. The initial meeting to found the National Association for Music Therapy (NAMT) took place in June of 1950 at the annual Music Teachers National Association conference in New York City. Over the next decade, work was completed to standardize undergraduate and graduate educational curriculum, set guidelines for clinical training, encourage research, and produce research and clinical publications (Boxberger, 1963).

During the 1950s and 1960s, outside of the United States, more music therapy associations were established and more training programs were developed. In Britain, following the work of the Entertainments National Services Association that took music to British servicemen during World War II, the Council for Music in Hospitals was set up after the war. One of the earliest musi-

cians to work in the hospitals in Britain was Juliette Alvin, a professional cellist from France who married an Englishman and, after moving to England, performed in hospitals, institutions, and special schools (Tyler, 2000, p. 381). In 1958 Alvin formed the British Society for Music Therapy. The *British Journal of Music Therapy* was also established in 1958 (Ansdell, Bunt, & Hartley, 2002). Ten years later, Alvin began the first training program in the United Kingdom at the Guildhall School of Music and Drama in London (Bunt & Hoskyns, 2002, p. 12). Later, in 1980, another training program was developed at Southlands College, Roehampton Institute for Higher Education (Bunt & Hoskyns, 2002, p. 12), directed by Elaine Streeter.

Also in the United Kingdom in 1958, Paul Nordoff and Clive Robbins met and forged a team, based on anthroposophical concepts, using improvisational music with children with multiple disabilities (Hadley, 1998). In 1960, they began to spread their creative music therapy approach, traveling through many parts of the United Kingdom and Europe, and then in the United States. By 1966, they had begun training sessions in their approach to music therapy, teaching courses in Scandinavia, United Kingdom, Germany, Holland, Italy, and Greece (Hadley, p. 242). In 1974, they began teaching at Goldie Leigh Hospital in South London. Around this time, they also toured Australia and New Zealand for the first time (Hadley).

Also in the United Kingdom in the late 1960s and early 1970s, Mary Priestley was developing analytical music therapy (AMT) with Marjorie Wardell and Peter Wright (Hadley, 2001, 2003). After publishing a book describing this way of working, Europeans from Germany and the Netherlands sought her out for training in AMT. In the 1980s Priestley provided training in AMT at the University of Herdecke, Germany, alongside training by Clive Robbins in the approach that he and Paul Nordoff had developed (Hadley, 1998, p. 84). These pioneers were also influential in the development of music therapy in West Germany (Wosch, 2003).

Other developments were also occurring in music therapy in Europe in the mid-20th century. In the late 1950s, Christoph Schwabe developed what he called *regulative music therapy*, a receptive music therapy approach that he used in psychotherapy and in a psychiatry clinic at Leipzig University (Wosch, 2003). He also developed an active group music therapy approach based on the theory of psychodrama (Wosch). Later, in the 1970s, Gertrude Orff founded Orff music therapy, also a well-known specialization in Germany. In the 1940s and 1950s Franz Adalbert Fengler published the first German articles and a book about music therapy. He also began the first academic training program in music therapy in Berlin at the University of the Arts (Wosch). In 1958 the Austrian Society for Music Therapy was established, and Hildebrandt R. Teirich wrote *Music and Medicine*, one of the first books on European music therapy (Wosch). By 1959, the first music therapy course at the University of Vienna was developed. The first German music therapy congress was held in Leipzig in 1969 (Wosch).

The 1960s saw the spread of music therapy in Puerto Rico, Brazil (which developed a training program in 1969), Denmark, France, the Netherlands, Norway, Israel, and Uruguay (Dileo Maranto, 1993). Music therapy was also being established as a specific health profession in several Asian countries at this time. In the 1950s and 1960s, music therapy was being practiced by psychologists, psychiatrists, and musicians in Japan. Significant early pioneers traveled to Japan and shared their concepts of music therapy: Juliette Alvin visited in 1967, and Carol and Clive Robbins visited in 1984 (Okazaki-Sakaue, 2003). Early influential publications in music therapy were translated into Japanese in the late 1960s and early 1970s. At this time, doctors in Korea were also discussing music therapy theory (Ihm, 1993). Later, in the 1980s,

music therapy was established in China and Hong Kong.

In 1971 a second professional organization was established in the United States, the American Association for Music Therapy (AAMT). Initially called the Urban Federation for Music Therapists, AAMT developed policies and procedures on education, clinical training, and certification that differed from those of NAMT. In 1998 the two U.S. music therapy organizations, NAMT and AAMT, unified as a single association, the American Music Therapy Association (AMTA), to advocate for music therapy. With the unification of the two organizations, professional recognition of Music Therapy in the United States was finally at hand. The creation of standardized education and clinical training standards, clinical and research publications, and effective administration led to recognition of music therapy as the viable, respected profession of today (Davis & Gfeller, 2008).

In the 1970s music therapy spread widely around the world, with associations founded in Brazil, Columbia, Finland, South Africa, Canada, Australia, New Zealand, Israel, and Puerto Rico (Dileo Maranto, 1993). In 1974, the first World Congress of Music Therapy was held in Paris. In 1985, at the 5th World Congress of Music Therapy, held in Genoa, Italy, the World Federation for Music Therapy (WFMT) was founded in order to support a global music therapy network and to promote music therapy globally. The 10 founding members were Rolando Benenzon (Argentina), Giovannia Mutti (Italy), Jacques Jost (France), Barbara Hesser (United States), Amelia Oldfield (United Kingdom), Ruth Bright (Australia), Heinrich Otto Moll (Germany), Rafael Colon (Puerto Rico), Clementina Nastari (Brazil), and Tadeusz Natanson (Poland). Since 1990, a World Congress of Music Therapy has been held every 3 years in countries around the world (see series of interviews on World Congresses of Music Therapy in *Voices* [*www.voices.no*], beginning in 2008 [Vol. 8, No. 3]).

Since the 1950s music therapy has continued to spread internationally as an academic discipline and is now practiced in over 50 countries. Although many music therapists around the world have been trained in Western concepts of music therapy, some have included their own cultural concepts of music and health and the relationships between these in the way they understand and practice music therapy. The diversity of cultural contexts and practices makes for a richer understanding of the power of music to transform the lives of people throughout the world.

Conclusions

Throughout recorded history, music therapy has been recognized as a powerful tool with which to treat physical and mental illness. Beginning with premodern societies and up to present times, music was and is used in accordance with the prevailing attitudes toward health and the treatment of disease. Regardless of whether illness was believed to be the result of evil spirits, imbalance in the four humors, or understood from a "rational" medical perspective, music oftentimes played a significant role in a person's treatment.

Several pioneering medical doctors introduced the idea of music therapy in the United States and Europe at the turn of the 19th century, and during the next 100 years the concepts of group and private practice were advocated by physicians and psychiatrists. By the beginning of the 20th century, musicians began taking a central role in the development of music therapy as a recognized profession, creating organizations to promote music therapy and refining music therapy techniques.

In 1950 the first long-standing music therapy organization was founded in the United States to develop education and clinical training standards, promote research, and assure that practitioners met minimum standards before working with clients.

From the mid-20th century onward, music therapy associations and training programs have been established around the world. The pioneering efforts of women and men from many cultures to bring music therapy to those with debilitating illnesses must be credited with laying the groundwork for the professional development of music therapy throughout much of the world today. The advent of strong national organizations, continued emphasis on research, and the refining of techniques used by music therapists have led to wide acceptance of this unique profession among health care professionals around the world.

REFERENCES

Ansdell, G., Bunt, L., & Hartley, N. (2002). Music therapy in the United Kingdom. *Voices: A World Forum for Music Therapy*. Retrieved from *http://testvoices.uib.no/?q=country-of-the-month/2002-music-therapy-united-kingdom*.

Blasco, S. P. (1993). Music therapy in Spain (Part one). In C. Dileo Maranto (Ed.), *Music therapy: International perspectives* (pp. 534–546). Pipersville, PA: Jeffrey Books.

Bossinger, W., & Hess, P. (1993). Musik und außergewöhnliche Bewußtseinszustände [Music and extraordinary states of consciousness]. *Musiktherapeutische Umshau, 14*(3), 239–254.

Boxberger, R. (1962). Historical basis for the use of music in therapy. In E. H. Schneider (Ed.), *Music therapy 1961* (pp. 125–166). Lawrence, KS: National Association for Music Therapy.

Boxberger, R. (1963). A historical study of the National Association for Music Therapy, Inc. In E. H. Schneider (Ed.), *Music therapy 1962* (pp. 133–197). Lawrence, KS: National Association for Music Therapy.

Bruscia, K. E., & Grocke, D. E. (Eds.). (2002). *Guided Imagery and Music: The Bonny method and beyond*. Gilsum, NH: Barcelona.

Bunt, L., & Hoskyns, S. (2002). *The handbook of music therapy*. New York: Routledge.

Columbia University to heal wounded by music. (1919, March 1). *Literary Digest, 60*, 59–62.

Columbia University, Teachers College. (1926–1927). *Columbia University, Teachers College Announcement, 1926–1927*. New York: Author.

Darrow, A.-A., & Heller, G. N. (1985). Early advocates for music education for the hearing impaired: William Wolcott Turner and David Ely

Bartlett. *Journal of Research in Music Education, 33*, 269–279.

Davis, W. B. (1987). Music therapy in nineteenth-century America. *Journal of Music Therapy, 24*, 76–87.

Davis, W. B. (1988). Music therapy in Victorian England. *Journal of British Music Therapy, 2*(1), 10–17.

Davis, W. B. (1993). Keeping the dream alive: Profiles of three early twentieth-century music therapists. *Journal of Music Therapy, 30*, 34–45.

Davis, W. B. (2012). The first systematic experimentation in music therapy: The genius of James Leonard Corning. *Journal of Music Therapy, 49*, 102–117.

Davis, W. B., & Gfeller, K. E. (2008). Music therapy: Historical perspective. In W. B. Davis, K. E. Gfeller, & M. H. Thaut (Eds.), *An introduction to music therapy: Theory and practice* (3rd ed., pp. 17–39). Silver Spring, MD: American Music Therapy Association.

Densmore, F. (1948). The use of music in the treatment of the sick by American Indians. In D. M. Schullian & M. Schoen (Eds.), *Music in medicine* (pp. 25–46). New York: Henry Schuman.

Dileo Maranto, C. (Ed.). (1993). *Music therapy: International perspectives*. Pipersville, PA: Jeffrey Books.

DuBois, T. A. (2009). *An introduction to shamanism*. Cambridge, UK: Cambridge University Press.

Gouk, P. (2000). *Musical healing in cultural contexts*. Aldershot, UK: Ashgate.

Hadley, S. (1998). *Exploring relationships between life and work in music therapy: The stories of Mary Priestley and Clive Robbins* (doctoral dissertation). Available from ProQuest (UMI No. 9911013).

Hadley, S. (2001). Exploring relationships between Mary Priestley's life and work. *Nordic Journal of Music Therapy, 10*(2), 116–131.

Hadley, S. (2003). Meaning making through narrative inquiry: Exploring the life of Clive Robbins. *Nordic Journal of Music Therapy, 12*(1), 34–54.

Horden, P. (2000). *Music as medicine: The history of music therapy since antiquity*. Aldershot, UK: Ashgate.

Ihm, E. H. (1993). Music therapy in Korea. In C.

Dileo Maranto (Ed.), *Music therapy: International perspectives* (pp. 355–364). Pipersville, PA: Jeffrey Books.

Konta, I., & Varga, K. U. (1993). Music therapy in Hungary. In C. Dileo Maranto (Ed.), *Music therapy: International perspectives* (pp. 263–278). Pipersville, PA: Jeffrey Books.

Kümmel, W. F. (1977). *Musik und Medizin* [Music and medicine]. München, Germany: Alber.

Lecourt, E. (1993). Music therapy in France. In C. Dileo Maranto (Ed.), *Music therapy: International perspectives* (pp. 221–238). Pipersville, PA: Jeffrey Books.

Lehtonen, K. (1993). Music therapy in Finland. In C. Dileo Maranto (Ed.), *Music therapy: International perspectives* (pp. 211–220). Pipersville, PA: Jeffrey Books.

O'Callaghan, C. (2002). Australian music therapy. *Voices: A World Forum for Music Therapy*. Retrieved from *http://testvoices.uib.no/?q=country-of-the-month/2002-australian-music-therapy*.

Okazaki-Sakaue, K. (2003). Music therapy in Japan. *Voices: A World Forum for Music Therapy*. Retrieved from *http://testvoices.uib.no/?q=country/monthjapan_may2003*.

Ruud, E. (1998). *Music therapy: Improvisation, communication, and culture*. Gilsum, NH: Barcelona.

Schullian, D. M., & Schoen, M. (1948). *Music and medicine*. New York: Henry Schuman.

Taylor, D. B. (1981). Music in general hospital treatment from 1900–1950. *Journal of Music Therapy, 18*, 62–73.

Tyler, H. (2000). The music therapy profession in modern Britain. In P. Horden (Ed.), *Music as medicine: The history of music therapy since antiquity* (pp. 375–393). Aldershot, UK: Ashgate.

Van de Wall, W. (1944). Report on the survey. *National Music Council Bulletin, 5*, 9–13.

Vescelius, E. A. (1913). Music in its relation to life. *Music and Health, 1*, 8.

Wagner, G., & Benenzon, R. (1993). Music therapy in Argentina. In C. Dileo Maranto (Ed.), *Music therapy: International perspectives* (pp. 5–34). Pipersville, PA: Jeffrey Books.

Wosch, T. (2003). Music therapy in Germany. *Voices: A World Forum for Music Therapy*. Retrieved from *http://testvoices.uib.no/?q=country/monthgermany_march2003*.

CHAPTER 3

Aesthetic Foundations of Music Therapy: Music and Emotion

James Hiller

The subject of aesthetic experience as it relates to music embodies a vast and fascinating territory of philosophical thought. Ancient philosophers to modern musicologists have engaged in scholarly debate over the topic from many perspectives (Davies, 2010; Kivy, 1989). Not surprisingly, a similar intrigue surrounds questions regarding the *clinical* value of aesthetic aspects of music and of music making for health, healing, and human development (Aigen, 1995, 2007).

Numerous links between aesthetic experience and therapeutic processes are found in the music therapy literature. In fact, volumes could be filled with theories and philosophical arguments for and against the meaning and/or meaningfulness of aesthetic experiences in healing, such as those found in music therapy treatment processes. However, in this chapter, I delimit our exploration to an assortment of perspectives that address, arguably, one of the most clinically relevant aspects of the aesthetic music experience: that of emotion and its expression in or through music (Ee-

rola & Vuoskoski, 2013). More specifically, I focus on a client's active music-making processes wherein emotions might be expressed *in* or *through* music rather than being elicited *by* music. I consider sources of emotion and where emotions might be located within music-making processes. And finally I explore theories that variously explain how musical expressions of emotions might occur. These theories provide guidance for the music therapist who wishes to understand and respond to the potential emotional meanings of a client's music making. In fact, to gain insights about a client's emotional world via music making is a unique and clinically powerful facet of music therapy.

Expression of Emotion

Emotional Expression and Music Therapy

Aigen (2005) notes that, regardless of the nature of specific clinical goals in music therapy, emotion is always a relevant consideration in treatment. Before examining how a client might express emotions through music, we must consider how such emotional expressions might be clinically beneficial within a therapy process. What does it mean to the client, the therapist, and/or the therapeutic process when we say that a client expresses emotion while making music?

The notion of catharsis, or "release of difficult, repressed, or unconscious feelings," is found frequently in the music therapy literature when clinical focus is on emotion, particularly with regard to the symbolic nature of a client's expressive music making (Aigen, 2007, p. 115). But whereas cathartic release of emotional energies may be powerful experiences for a client, such experiences have been considered to be only temporarily beneficial toward healing if not linked to cognitions about the emotion expressed (Yalom, 2005). Nonetheless, such experiences undeniably take place, and it behooves a therapist to recognize their occurrence and understand the clinical implications and potentials for the treatment process.

In Priestley's (1994) analytical music therapy (AMT), an improvisational approach to music psychotherapy, a client's musical expressions are often recorded. The recordings are then reviewed by client and therapist and the material verbally processed. In assessment, this process aids in understanding the client's emotional well-being, whereas in treatment it helps a client to gain insight about, and work through, conscious and unconscious issues and related emotions. In AMT, the client's *process* while musically engaged is primary. In music psychotherapy there are times when a client may be unaware of, or uncertain about, emotions attached to specific events or relationships, and music making provides an avenue for identifying these. In considering a client's process of improvisational music making, I note that a client "may hear evidence in the music . . . that an emotion is somehow being expressed"

(Hiller, 2011, p. 122) and thereby gain clarity about it.

Bruscia (1987) highlights the usefulness of analyzing a client's improvised emotional expressions for assessment and treatment via the Improvisation Assessment Profiles (IAPs). Here, the *product* of the client's music making may take precedence in analysis and interpretation of meanings. Accordingly, the various musical elements, as played and combined by a client, are considered projections of aspects of personality and emotion.

In short, a client's music making may serve as a temporary release of emotional energy (catharsis), as a representation of the client's inner emotional world, or as a reflection of the way he or she expresses aspects of personality and emotional experiences. Each of these perspectives may benefit client and therapist toward gaining clarity about, and addressing, the client's emotional expressions in the musically based clinical situation.

Emotional Expression and Music Making

Throughout history, musicologists have declared that emotions may be found in, or expressed through, music (Juslin & Sloboda, 2010). Music therapists know that there is a relationship between emotions and music making, for we sometimes hear emotion manifested in a client's music or see emotion being expressed through a client's music-related actions. We may even feel a client's emotions as they are manifested in his or her music through experiences of transference, projective identification, and countertransference (Bruscia, 1998b). But how do internal human experiences such as emotions find their way into music? Where does the emotion come from, and how does it become apparent in music or a music-making process?

Musicologists most often have focused on the relationship between emotions and music from a listener's perspective; that is, they have tried to determine how it is that a music listener may be moved to experience emotion or recognize it in the music heard (Eerola & Vuoskoski, 2013). In music therapy, however, a client's experience is not just as a listener who may be moved by a therapist's music or a recording; the client is often an agent in the creation of meaningful musical sounds and interactions with a therapist and others through playing, singing, and composing. This means that emotions ascribed to music in the clinical situation may sometimes belong to the client him- or herself. It also means that the expression of emotion in the music is, in some way, of the client's doing; that is to say, an emotion is expressed, revealed, or manifested through the client's actions while making music. This seems an astounding actuality, given the severity of challenges faced by many clients in music therapy. Reviewing how musicologists have sought to explain these phenomena is our present endeavor.

A few researchers have examined how skilled performers imbue composed music with a given emotion for a musically trained audience to hear and recognize (Behrens & Green, 1993; Juslin, 2001; Juslin & Timmers, 2010). Yet music therapy clients, who are generally a musically untrained group, repeatedly exhibit a similar ability to express emotion within musical processes of re-creating, improvising, and composing. Before reviewing some select theories, let us examine how the concepts of emotion and expression might be defined and consider the notions of locations and sources of emotion in music.

Emotions and Emotion-Related Terms

What are emotions, and what do we mean when we say that one *expresses* them in music? Providing a definitive description of just what emotions are is an ongoing human enterprise. In fact, although emotion has been of philosophical and psychological interest throughout recorded time, it remains heavily researched across many fields of investigation, including aesthetics and the area of study known as the *affective sciences* (Lewis, Haviland-Jones, & Barnett, 2008). Let us begin our inquiry with definitions of a few emotion-related terms from Juslin and Sloboda's (2010) *Handbook of Music and Emotion: Theory, Research, and Applications* and Robinson's (2005) *Deeper Than Reason*.

Affect is an overarching term for all observable, emotion-related experiences. The term is meant generally to refer to experiences of emotion, but not as a reference to any specific emotion or emotional state. *Emotion*, on the other hand, refers to "a quite brief but intense affective reaction" (Juslin & Sloboda, 2010, p. 10) that is directed toward a specific object and that includes both physiological and cognitive components. An emotion may endure for a brief period of minutes or for hours and typically elicits an action response of some sort that might be expressed via facial appearance, bodily movements, and/or vocalizations. Action responses elicited by an emotion may be expressed intentionally and therefore consciously, or be manifested unintentionally and therefore unconsciously. Robinson (2005) stresses that emotions or emotional responses are processes that occur over time and stem from human interactions with the environment, with *environment* often meaning an interpersonal interaction. In that emotions are internal processes that occur over time, it seems that they possess an experiential or phenomenal flow that one may subsequently comprehend and recall.

A *feeling* is defined as "the subjective experience of an emotion or mood" (Juslin & Sloboda, 2010, p. 10), or the way our bodies and minds undergo an emotion. Feelings entail experiences of energy related to an emotion and movement related to that energy. The *feelingful* aspect of an emotional experience is of particular interest for investigating expressions through music, for it is a process that occurs over time with variations in flow and form, similar to the way that music unfolds. The feelingful aspects of emotions have been the basis from which many theorists have symbolically allied emotions and music.

Expression

Juslin and Timmers (2010) begin their chapter, "Expression and Communication of Emotion in Music Performance," by stating, "There is still no universally accepted definition of the concept of *expression*" (p. 454, emphasis original). We nonetheless require at least a working definition. *The New Oxford American Dictionary* (Jewell & Abate, 2001) defines expression as "the process of making known one's thoughts or feelings" (p. 600). Robinson (2005) believes that the "core notion of expression in the arts is derived from Romantic artists—primarily poets, composers, and painters—who thought of themselves as expressing their feelings and emotions in the artworks that they produced" (p. 232). Robinson further holds to the Romantic view that expression in the arts is *about* emotions, or more specifically, about experiences of emotional processes. She invokes Kant's and Hegel's support for the idea that artists, through their art, demonstrate a specialized sort of knowledge and insight about emotions and, more importantly, the ability to uniquely convey emotions through their particular media (Robinson, 2005, pp. 232–233). Although arguably not *artists* per se, clients in music therapy are nonetheless human agents working in and through an artistic medium and are therefore capable, on some level, of gaining access to, recognizing, comprehending, and expressing emotional material through interactions with the medium—that is, the musical elements.

Locations and Sources of Emotion in Music

The importance of location of emotion in music making should become evident as the reader reflects on each of the following questions: Can emotion be found in a client's musical products (songs or pieces), or is it found in the music-making processes that the client undergoes while playing, singing, or improvising? Can we recognize emotion in a client's physical actions while he or she makes music, or do we, rather, recognize emotion in the musical sounds thus produced? Does a client consciously express emotions in/through music, or is it the case that the way the client's music sounds reveals properties of emotions that are not necessarily in the client's conscious awareness? Can emotion be heard when listening to a recording of client-generated music rather than in a live rendering? Does a client need to feel an emotion while playing/singing in order for expression of that emotion to occur in the music? Interestingly, given the range of theorizing we encounter below, the answer to any of these questions can be *yes*. To summarize: Emotions may be found in a variety of locations during music engagement, including, but not limited to, musical products and processes, in bodily actions or in sounds produced through them, in or outside of a client's consciousness, in recordings, and/or in the moment of feeling an emotion or after a client's emotional experience has passed (i.e., from a memory of the experience).

From which source(s) of knowledge and/or experience might a client draw when expressing emotion through music? It seems that a client must first have some sense of the nature of emotions—for example, the different ways that emotions feel internally as they occur, or typical responses that people enact vocally, verbally, motorically, or via facial affect while feeling particular emotions. A client must also have experiences with musical examples that are related to emotions in some way. These subjective experiences, it seems, may accumulate simply through living in a world where music and emotions both exist (Robinson, 2005). Hence, it is apparent that a key source for emotional expression in clinical music making is the confluence of a client's subjective understanding of how emotions feel, physical responses to emotions of oneself or others, and musical sounds that are related in some way to emotional experiences (Hiller, 2011).

The concepts presented below are limited to a class of theories that rely on symbolism or representational thought and include somatic, expressive code, contour, expression, and gesture theories. An important caveat is that none of the theories is more right or wrong than any other, but each provides potentially useful concepts that a music therapist may draw upon toward understanding a client's emotional–musical processes and products.

Symbolic Theories of Emotion and Music

Symbolism is "the use of symbols to represent ideas or qualities" (Jewell & Abate, 2001, p. 1720). A symbol is the *thing* that represents something else. To *represent* is to "depict (a particular subject) in a picture or other work of art" (Jewell & Abate, p. 1445, parentheses in original). Many musicologists believe that music can indeed symbolize something about human emotions (Cumming, 2001; Robinson, 2005). Yet the processes of representation, as explained in the following theories, may occur in a variety of ways.

Somatic Theory: Music and Feelings

Music philosophers refer frequently to the writings of Hanslick (1885/1974) and Langer (1942) as foundational in addressing the symbolic relationship between music and emotions (Robinson, 2005). These authors focus on *felt* experiences of emotion, that is, the experience of changes internal to the human body. These may be termed *somatic* theories of emotion in music, referencing the Greek word *soma* (body). This frame of reference is akin to William James's (cited in Robinson, 2005, pp. 28–29) theoretical view of emotion as an inner, physiological moving or stirring. Music, it is theorized, resembles "the rhythm and pattern of [emotions'] rise and decline and intertwining" (Langer, 1942, p. 238). Moreover, Langer's belief, like Hanslick's, is that there exists a structural likeness between the way music unfolds over time and the way emotions are experienced internally. An oft-quoted statement by Langer helps to clarify this stance:

> There are certain aspects of the so-called "inner life"—physical or mental—which have formal properties similar to those of music— patterns of motion and rest, of tension and release, of agreement and disagreement, preparation, fulfillment, excitation, sudden change, etc. (1942, p. 228)

Hence, Langer believes that music sounds to us the way that emotions feel to us. In other words, our experience of a particular configuration of musical sounds may be so similar to our inner experience of feelings that the music may seem to us to possess an emotional character. In this regard, we may infer that emotion is located in the musical configurations that a client creates while making music.

Based on somatic theory, then, a client may construct musical representations of his or her emotions by using the musical elements in ways that imitate the feelings that are experienced internally; that is, inside the body. The client may intentionally use tempo, dynamics, and phrasing, for instance, to symbolize the flow of emotional energy experienced. As noted earlier, such configurations may also be manifested in music unintentionally and later be recognized by a therapist or the client as representative of particular emotions (Priestley, 1994). Further, a therapist may hear in the client's configurations certain sound structures that are reminiscent of the therapist's own experiences of emotional energy, and he or she may thereby interpret that the music represents the client's emotions.

With such awareness, the therapist may respond in a way that serves to validate and/or further explore the client's emotional materials, musically and otherwise.

Expressive Code Theory: Music, Emotions, and Expressive Vocal Inflections

Music psychologist Juslin (2001) and his collaborators aim to identify particular manipulation techniques (i.e., articulations and inflections) that performers use in communicating emotion to an audience via composed pieces. These researchers seek to explain a performer's *emotional communication* with an audience by comparing instrumental performance to the expressive nuances of human emotional vocal expression (Juslin & Timmers, 2010, pp. 470–471). A performer manipulates the musical elements in various ways by inflecting the music similarly to the way an emotion-laden verbal statement might be uttered. For example, a performer's use of *diminuendo* at the end of a particular phrase may mirror the way a person might vocally inflect a verbal statement of deep disappointment, as if concluding a statement with a sigh. Similarly, a performer may *clip* certain notes of a melodic phrase via staccato articulations, just as a person might vocally articulate an utterance in an almost stuttering manner while experiencing profound shock or dismay. The performer's manipulations are then to be comprehended by an audience, but not necessarily felt by those listeners. Accordingly, we may identify emotion as being located in the nuances of musical inflection rather than in the composed structures, in the composer or performer him- or herself, or in the listener. In other words, neither the composer nor the performer is actually feeling the emotion articulated in the musical inflections. Rather, the emotion is located in the inflection, which is drawn from knowledge of vocal emotional expressions.

Juslin and his colleagues refer to a performer's manipulations as the *expressive code* or acoustic cues (Gabrielsson & Juslin, 2003; Juslin, 2001). This particular research has focused on the following five *basic emotions* noted as those most often studied: tenderness, happiness, sadness, fear, and anger (Juslin, 2001). The researchers hypothesize that the effectiveness of the performer's expressive code is based on listeners' sharing of that same communicative code. The researchers further argue that the genesis of the code is in *innate brain programs* common in human vocal expression across cultures (p. 321). The acoustic cues (expressive code) include timbre, tone attacks, tone decays, intonation, articulation, vibrato, timing, tempo, sound levels, and pauses (Juslin & Timmers, 2010, p. 462). Coutinho and Dibben (2013) also include characteristics of sharpness/roughness as factors related to timbre. By way of example, Juslin and Timmers note that

> *sadness* expressions are associated with slow tempo, low sound level, legato articulation, small articulation variability, slow tone attacks, and soft timbre, whereas *happiness* expressions are associated with fast tempo, high sound level, staccato articulation, large articulation variability, fast tone attacks, and bright timbre. (pp. 462–463, emphasis in original)

According to *expressive code theory*, a client and therapist share a communicative code based on knowledge of the ways that emotionally charged verbal/vocal inflections sound. Thus, a client may emotionally inflect aspects of performed or improvised music in ways related to his or her experiences of vocal expressions. This seems the case because, as human beings, clients experience nearly constant, lifelong exposure to expressive inflections in the verbalizations/vocalizations of others and, in many cases, may themselves have learned to use such inflections. Presumably, these experiences of enculturation occur to a point where an individual's application of verbal/vocal inflections becomes a natural part of general sound-based communication.

Contour Theory:
Music and Emotion Resemblances

Davies (2010) and Kivy (1989) espouse variations of a theory that the emotional expressiveness of music involves the relationship between a work's "dynamic structures and behaviors or movements that, in humans, present emotion characteristics" (Davies, p. 31). The idea here is that the dynamic properties (e.g., movement in rhythm, melody, harmony, dynamic changes) found in renderings of composed music represent human behaviors and *comportments* (i.e., how one carries oneself) that are equated with expressions of human emotions. Or, said yet another way, dynamic (i.e., varying, changing) structures in music *sound like* what various emotion-based comportments of human beings *look like*. According to contour theory, therefore, emotion resides in the resemblances between characteristics of a piece of music and an observable behavioral appearance that generally reveals human emotion. Hence, the way a person's physical body posture and movement characteristics appear when grumpy or anxious are represented through the way music sounds. Importantly, contour theory stresses that music does not express emotion (because music is not a live, sentient being who can express emotion), but that music is *expressive of* emotion (Kivy, 1989).

Robinson (2005) wittily refers to contour theory as the *doggy theory* (p. 300), due to the fact that both Kivy and Davies use as examples the sad-appearing faces of St. Bernard and bassett hound dogs. For although people may find these dogs' faces sad looking, it is not necessarily the case that the animals actually feel the way that their faces appear; the dogs are not sad, they just look that way. Yet, Kivy (1989) tells us, we humans have a tendency to *animate*

things that we perceive (p. 59). With regard to music, then, contour theory holds that music may sound sad to a listener because of the way the elements work together, but the perceived sadness is simply a *trait* of the given music; the music itself is not expressing emotion, but rather it is *expressive of* emotion. The music is not sad—it is not in a state of sadness—it simply sounds that way, and therefore we may hear sadness in music.

Given the tenets of contour theory, it seems that a music therapy client may access memories of observing postures and/or comportments of others that reflect certain emotions to inform how to depict those emotions via singing and/or playing. For example, a client, drawing from the image of a highly anxious person—pacing, leaning forward with tense muscles, and wringing hands—may drum in a highly contained and intense manner to express the experience of anxiety, playing a constant and quick barrage of subdivisions. Or, referring to observations of others' depressed countenances—slumped shoulders, bowed head, and slow movements—a client may express such feelings on a xylophone via downward melodic motion, soft volume, and a series of slow *thuds* on the bars, rather than using the rebounded energy of the mallet head as used in a light, energetic stroke. Through such representations a therapist may recognize and respond to the emotional characteristics of a client's music making.

Expression Theory:
Music and Immediately
Occurring Emotions

Expression theory holds that emotions expressed in music belong to the composer or performer of a musical work, and that these emotions are drawn from the composer or performer's own immediate experiences of emotion during creation or re-creation of music (Davies, 1994, pp. 170–173). Robinson (2005), a strong advocate of expression theory, notes that expression of emotions via the arts shares the same processes as emotional expression in typical daily life. She believes that an individual's particular behaviors, enacted in response to an emotional experience, are indicative or evidence of that emotion. An observer may thus infer from an individual's actions the emotion from which those actions have their genesis (p. 258). For example, an individual's throaty, growling vocalizations may be considered reliable evidence of the immediate presence of anger or frustration. That is, when a person hears another person growling, he or she may infer that the person is angry or frustrated for some reason. Regarding music, therefore, a composer or performer's emotions should be recognizable from listening to their musical expressions.

Significant to the usefulness of expression theory is Robinson's (2005) acceptance of the idea of a *persona*, or imaginary person, to whom a music listener may attribute emotions heard in music, rather than attributing them to the performer of the work (p. 259). For example, we may not believe that a performer who is playing a piece on stage is, in that moment, *feeling* a particular emotion and that the emotion is revealed in the music. We may more likely accept the notion that an emotion heard in the music belongs to an imagined persona— someone who *could be* feeling that emotion right then. So, a performer may imagine the emotion that another person could be feeling and transmit that emotion through the music for the audience to hear. Or, a listener may infer emotional meanings from the music heard to an imagined persona rather than to the performer on stage or to the composer.

While making music, according to expression theory, a client may consciously transmit his or her own emotion or that of an imagined persona onto instruments, resulting in sounds that are artifacts of emotion-driven actions. The client does

this by choosing and articulating musical elements believed to most closely correspond to nonmusical emotional behaviors (Robinson, 2005, pp. 266–267). In clinical improvisation, for instance, clients are sometimes asked to improvise while in the role of a person with whom they are in conflict or from whom they need to gain understanding of that person's particular perspective—either instance necessarily includes emotional material. The client thus sounds the emotions of the imagined other through interactions with the instruments.

A music therapist's source for comprehending the client's expression is past experiences of witnessing others expressing emotion in various ways. The music therapist thus may hear *evidence* in the client's music that an emotion is being expressed and may attribute the emotion to the client or to a persona of the client's imagining.

Gesture Theory: Music and Communicative Gestures

Communicative gestures have been described as "any energetic shaping through time that may be interpreted as significant" (Hatten, 2006, p. 1), and they function when an interpreter recognizes the communicative intent of a given gesture. Imagine what may be communicated through a rapidly shaken fist or the slow reaching out of an open hand. These are simple examples of communicative gestures, each with a particular "envelope" or flow of energy from the beginning to the end of the gesture. In other words, each gesture has a rhythmic shape that, if repeated, reveals a recognizable pattern. Emotions, too, possess a flow of energy from the beginning of the emotional experience to the end. Hatten holds that the information conveyed through a gesture is often "affectively loaded" (p. 1); that is to say, it has to do with the expression of emotion. A communicative gesture, then, is a brief (but repeatable) movement scheme, irreducible to its constitutive parts without losing its meaning, and born of a single human impulse (Lidov, 1987, p. 77). Lidov hypothesizes the existence of a limited quantity of distinct gestures that humans consistently correlate with particular emotional messages, thereby making it possible for others to interpret our gestures.

In linking perception of music with gesture, Lidov (1987) hypothesizes that a listener's perception of the shape or pattern of grouped musical sounds is compatible with perception of the total rhythmic profile of particular gestures. He therefore argues for the existence of a link between (1) the *energy envelope* of an emotion, (2) the *rhythmic shape* of a bodily gesture that reveals the emotion, and (3) the *sound shape* of a musical/rhythmic expression (pp. 28–29). In other words, when a client seeks to express emotion musically, he or she may draw from a repertoire of communicative gestures and apply a gesture in the process of interacting with an instrument. The resulting sounds, then, reveal the manifestation of the emotion. The presence of the emotion thus becomes available for a therapist to hear and interpret or for the client to perceive and comprehend. For example, imagine a crowd of people rhythmically punching at the air as a collective expression of rage against an oppressor. A client may draw from the same sort of motion to beat on a drum toward expressing anger in/through music making. The resulting drum sounds are considered congruous with the emotion attached to the gesture used.

Cumming (2001) points out the rhythmically embodied nature of musical gestures, in contrast to the actuality of written musical notes, melodies, and/or phrases. Although an emotion may be inferred from a specific composed musical passage, it is the performer/client, drawing from a repertoire of emotions and bodily movement experiences (i.e., affectively loaded gestures), who uniquely inflects the music through particular uses of communicative gestures. This may explain why the inflection of, for instance, Yo Yo Ma's musical phrasing of a particularly wrenching pas-sage sounds different from that of other players; his emotional experience is different, as is the energy envelope of how he might apply gesture in communicating his emotion. Thus, a client's sounding of a musical pattern has to do, in large measure, with how the rhythmic aspects are enacted, meaning the unique energetic shaping of a musical action (pp. 136–137). This connection is the case due to the inextricable link between rhythm and bodily movement and gestures, which contain emotional information (Hatten, 2006; Seivers, Polansky, Casey, & Wheatley, 2013).

Emotion, according to gesture theory, is located in the particular energetic flow of the physical actions used when making music, either with instruments or vocally. While interacting musically or listening to a client's music making, a music therapist may conceptualize the client's musical sounds as related to expressive movement schemes (i.e., gestures). The therapist may thus witness and interpret the potential affective meanings contained in the client's sounds toward understanding the emotional nature of the musical expressions.

Conclusions

It is not an exaggeration to say that belief in the emotionally expressive potential of music is thousands of years old. Modern theorizing on the subject has brought us numerous ways of understanding how human emotions may be rendered and communicated through musical sounds. It seems noteworthy that many musicological theories relating emotion with musical expression rely on the potential of music to function as a symbolic form of human expression. Somatic theories allow us to relate the inner unfolding of emotional energies with the flow of musical and rhythmic expressions. In expressive code theory, we might relate musical expressions to the way verbal or vocal inflections of emotions commonly occur, thus providing a point of inference regarding an individual's emotions. Contour theory, on the other hand, stresses that music can be expressive of emotion through its resemblance to the way humans carry themselves physically while feeling particular emotions. The belief that emotion is expressed during the moments of the creative process—for instance, of instrumental improvising—is the foundation of expression theory. The sounds created are thus considered specialized representations of the expresser's immediate emotional state. And lastly, gesture theory links the energetic envelope of particular physical gestures that humans use to express emotion with their application in producing musical sounds. For instance, using certain movement schemes that mimic emotional communicative gestures in order to sound instruments leads to potential communication of emotion through the music produced.

Whereas musicologists seek answers to questions of how human emotions are expressed through music largely as a scholarly pursuit, music therapists apply such theorizing to enhance a client's healing, growth, and development. Music therapists are indeed uniquely positioned to apply concepts from theories of music and emotion to more deeply understand and bring benefit to humans in their change processes. This benefit is due to the intimate roles that both music and music therapists play within the therapeutic relationship. Yet, it is important to understand that none of the theories presented herein is more or less true than any other, but that each has potential utility for comprehending how and when a client expresses—makes known—aspects of his or her emotional world through music making. By thinking in an integral fashion and thereby drawing from the most clinically useful theoretical stance in a given therapy situation, music therapists gain access to a great depth and breadth of knowledge about clients' emotions toward understanding and assisting in the change process (Bruscia, 2014).

REFERENCES

Aigen, K. (1995). An aesthetic foundation of clinical theory: An underlying basis of creative music therapy. In C. B. Kenny (Ed.), *Listening, playing, creating: Essays on the power of sound* (pp. 233–257). Albany: State University of New York Press.

Aigen, K. (2005). *Music-Centered Music Therapy.* Gilsum, NH: Barcelona.

Aigen, K. (2007). In defense of beauty: A role for the aesthetic in music therapy theory: Part I. The development of aesthetic theory in music therapy. *Nordic Journal of Music Therapy, 16*(2), 112–128.

Behrens, G. A., & Green, S. B. (1993). The ability to identify emotional content of solo improvisations performed vocally and on three different instruments. *Psychology of Music, 21,* 20–33.

Bruscia, K. E. (1987). *Improvisational models of music therapy.* Springfield, IL: Charles C Thomas.

Bruscia, K. E. (1998a). *Defining music therapy* (2nd ed.). Gilsum, NH: Barcelona.

Bruscia, K. E. (Ed.). (1998b). *The dynamics of music psychotherapy.* Gilsum, NH: Barcelona.

Bruscia, K. E. (2014). *Defining music therapy* (3rd ed.). University Park, IL: Barcelona.

Coutinho, E., & Dibben, N. (2013). Psychoacoustic cues to emotion in speech prosody and music. *Cognition and Emotion, 27*(4), 658–684.

Cumming, N. (2001). *The sonic self: Musical subjectivity and signification.* Bloomington, IN: Indiana University Press.

Davies, S. (1994). *Musical meaning and expression.* Ithaca, NY: Cornell University Press.

Davies, S. (2010). Emotions expressed and aroused by music: Philosophical perspectives. In P. Juslin & J. Sloboda (Eds.), *Handbook of music and emotion* (pp. 15–43). New York: Oxford University Press.

Eerola, T., & Vuoskoski, J. K. (2013). A review of music and emotion studies: Approaches, emotion models, and stimuli. *Music Perception, 30*(3), 307–340.

Gabrielsson, A., & Juslin, P. (2003). Emotional expression in music. In R. Davidson, K. Scherer, & H. Goldsmith (Eds.), *Handbook of affective sciences* (pp. 503–534). New York: Oxford University Press.

Hanslick, E. (1974). *The beautiful in music* (G. Cohen, Trans.). New York: Da Capo Press. (Original work published 1885)

Hatten, R. (2006). A theory of musical gesture and its application to Beethoven and Schubert. In A. Gritten & E. King (Eds.), *Music and gesture* (pp. 1–23). Burlington, VT: Ashgate.

Hiller, J. (2011). *Theoretical foundations for understanding the meaning potential of rhythm in improvisation* (Doctoral dissertation). Available from ProQuest Dissertations and Theses database (UMI No. 3457829).

Jewell, E. J., & Abate, F. R. (Eds.). (2001). *The new Oxford American dictionary*. New York: Oxford University Press.

Juslin, P. N. (2001). Communicating emotion in music performance: A review and theoretical framework. In P. Juslin & J. Sloboda (Eds.), *Music and emotion: Theory and research* (pp. 309–337). New York: Oxford University Press.

Juslin, P. N., & Sloboda, J. A. (Eds.). (2010). *Handbook of music and emotion: Theory, research, and applications*. New York: Oxford University Press.

Juslin, P. N., & Timmers, R. (2010). Expression and communication of emotion in music performance. In P. N. Juslin & J. A. Sloboda (Eds.), *Handbook of music and emotion: Theory, research, and applications* (pp. 453–489). New York: Oxford University Press.

Kivy, P. (1989). *Sound sentiment*. Philadelphia: Temple University Press.

Langer, S. (1942). *Philosophy in a new key: A study in the symbolism of reason, rite, and art*. Cambridge, MA: Harvard University Press.

Lewis, M., Haviland-Jones, J. M., & Barnett, L. F. (2008). *Handbook of emotions* (3rd ed.). New York: Guilford Press.

Lidov, D. (1987). Mind and body in music. *Semiotica, 66*(1), 70–97.

Priestley, M. (1994). *Essays on analytical music therapy*. Gilsum, NH: Barcelona.

Robinson, J. (2005). *Deeper than reason*. New York: Oxford University Press.

Seivers, B., Polansky, L., Casey, M., & Wheatley, T. (2013). Music and movement share a dynamic structure that supports universal expressions of emotion. *Proceedings of the National Academy of Sciences of the United States of America, 110*(1), 70–75.

Yalom, I. D. (2005). *The theory and practice of group psychotherapy* (5th ed.). New York: Basic Books.

CHAPTER 4

Music Therapy and the Brain

Concetta M. Tomaino

Music is a powerful and complex stimulus that affects us on many levels. A working knowledge of how music listening as well as active music making influence brain activity is important, since all human function is mediated by the brain. The fields of music perception and cognitive neuroscience are bringing new understanding to how music is perceived and processed in the human brain. This emerging information can help music therapists better understand the implications of using music to impact human function as well as to know how changes in the brain may impact an individual's ability to respond to music. To appreciate the scope of how music stimulates, organizes, and affects human function, it is important to understand some of the basics of how music is processed.

Making Sense of Sound

From the Outside In

The diagram in Figure 4.1 illustrates how sound moves from the outside in and through the multiple levels of brain analysis. As you can see, music is much more than the sum of its parts. Every music experience brings with it layers of information, from vibrational frequencies to the emotional and historical context in which we experience it. *Sound waves* enter the ear as pressure and then move through a series of processes that transform the wave signals into electrical impulses that reach the brain via the auditory nerve. Figure 4.2 shows how the *outer ear*, the folds of cartilage or pinna we recognize as the *ear*, captures sound waves from the environment as directional information, as well as high and low air pressure.

These vibrational waves then move through the auditory canal to the *middle ear*. The middle ear is an air-filled canal that begins at the eardrum or tympanic membrane. The wave information travels across the middle ear cavity via a series of delicate bones, or ossicles (hammer, stirrup, and anvil), that convert the lower pressure vibrations to higher pressure vibrations. Higher pressure is needed to enable these vibrations to pass through the next area, the *inner ear*, which is liquid rather than air (Kandel, Schwartz, & Jessell, 2000, pp. 591–624). The sound information is converted in the inner ear within

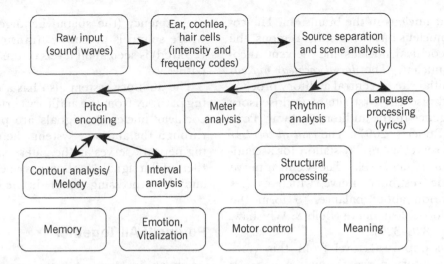

FIGURE 4.1. The path of sound moving through the levels of brain analysis. Reprinted with permission of Felipe Gerhard.

the *cochlea*, where fluid waves travel across a membrane (organ of Corti) that converts wave frequencies into nerve impulses. The organ of Corti has little hair cells (inner hair cells) across its membrane that then convert the vibrational waves into electrical signals that travel within nerve fibers of the cochlear nerve (or auditory/acoustic nerve) and then connect to various networks in the brain.

Making Connections

The *cochlear nerve* from each ear has connections on the same side of the brain as well as similar or homologous areas on the contralateral side. This bilateral representation and processing of sound is important because it allows for the engagement of multiple neural networks and brain areas. The cochlear nerve connects first with the

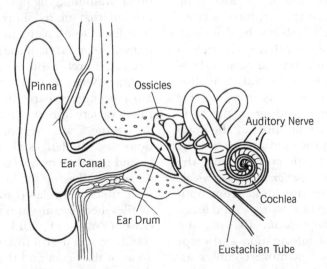

FIGURE 4.2. The human ear. Illustration by Denis Barbulat.

cochlear nucleus in the brainstem. The cochlear nucleus has two distinct regions, the
dorsal cochlear nucleus and the ventral cochlear nucleus. The *dorsal cochlear nucleus*
is an initial site of central auditory processing and also the first site of multisensory
convergence in the auditory pathway (Portfors & Roberts, 2007). The *ventral cochlear
nucleus* serves as a relay station for ascending auditory nerve cells. The cochlear nerve
joins the vestibular nerve, which carries
information about balance, to form the
vestibulocochlear nerve (Kolb & Whishaw,
2011, pp. 328–329).

Nerve impulses travel from this combined auditory nerve through a network
of brain areas, each further processing the
sound information. The auditory nerve has
connections to the most primitive parts of
the brain (superior olivary complex of the
brainstem) and the inferior colliculus of the
midbrain, before eventually reaching the
thalamus and then the primary auditory
cortex in the temporal lobe. The auditory
brainstem is able to maintain most of the
temporal and low frequencies of the original sound, as evident from electroencephalogram (EEG) measures of the auditory
brainstem response (Skoe & Kraus, 2010).

Although complex networks interact
throughout, the picture of the ascending
pathway of the central auditory nervous
system (see Figure 4.3) shows the main connections. It can be seen that each cochlea
connects to networks on the same side as
well as the opposite or contralateral side,
though the bulk of neurons from one ear
crosses over when ascending to the auditory cortex. As a result, most of the auditory information processed on one side of
the brain is sent by the cochlea from the
opposite side. The *superior olivary complex*,
the first area to receive input from both
ears, contributes to processing sound localization. The *inferior colliculus* (IC) is a site
for convergence of information and helps
with the processing of more complex aspects of sound. A *tonotopic* representation

of frequency (the spatial arrangement of
where sound is perceived, transmitted, or
received) is seen at all levels of the auditory
pathway.

The auditory system also has a descending pathway from the auditory cortex to the
cochlear nuclei. As signals are processed
through the auditory system, the descending network serves as the gatekeeper to either inhibit signals or allow passage to other
auditory processing centers in the brain.

Putting It All Together

As shown in Figure 4.4, the *cortex* is comprised of several distinct regions that contribute to our ability to make sense of a
work of music, be it a popular song or a
symphony. For example, the temporal lobes
process the actual tones we hear, but it is
the frontal lobe that provides the short-
term attention to stream those tones into
a melody, and it is the parietal lobe that
helps us associate the melody with personal
experiences. Our understanding of how
these areas share responsibility for music
perception is still being explored through
neuroscience research and use of *functional
magnetic resonance imaging* (fMRI) as well as
other brain-imaging devices. It is becoming
evident that many shared networks work
in consort to allow us to process sound as
music. No one area of the brain works alone
but rather relies on inputs from complementary networks to integrate information.
Most recently, research in this area indicates
that a variety of network *hubs* helps to coordinate the brain's response to novel situations and challenges. These processes are
bound together by a web of a dozen major
networks, allowing the brain to execute distinct functions related to auditory, visual,
tactile, memory, attention, and motor processes (Cole et al., 2013). With this understanding, it is useful to know about various
areas of the brain and their role in perception and action.

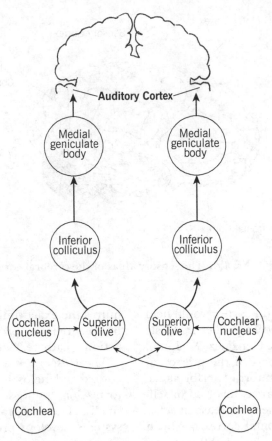

FIGURE 4.3. Schematic diagram of the bilateral central auditory pathway.

The *prefrontal cortex* is located in the front of the brain and plays a role in executive function and decision making. It is often referred to as the brain's CEO (chief executive officer) because it helps us to interact effectively with our environment. It is involved in focusing attention, organizing thoughts, solving problems, foreseeing and weighing possible consequences of behavior, considering the future and making predictions, forming strategies and planning, balancing short-term rewards with long-term goals, shifting and adjusting behavior when situations change, controlling impulses and delaying gratification, modulating intense emotions, inhibiting inappropriate behavior and initiating appropriate behavior, and considering multiple streams of information when faced with complex and challenging information.

The *prefrontal cortex* is one of the last areas of the brain to develop, with much of the development occurring during adolescence. Latent development of this region is why many teenagers are unable to see the implications of their actions and why they have difficulty interpreting what others say to them (Bunge & Wright, 2007). Because it is involved in short-term and working memory, the prefrontal cortex is one of the first areas to be affected by dementia and Alzheimer's disease. It provides relays to other areas of the brain to help us make quick responses or plan ahead. The prefrontal cortex plays a role in creation and expectation. For example, if a note is wrong in

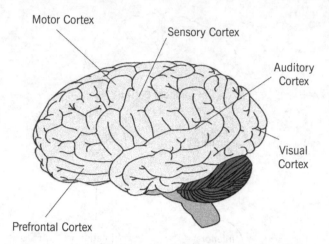

FIGURE 4.4. The sensory areas of the cerebral cortex.

a melody, the prefrontal cortex would help us *hear* that error. Recent studies in music improvisation (López-González & Limb, 2012) show that the part of the prefrontal cortex involved in monitoring performance shuts down, whereas areas involved in self-initiation and spontaneity increase in activity. The medial prefrontal cortex has been identified in studies by Janata (2009) as active in converging information about songs that have autobiographical importance and may explain why people with dementia still recognize and respond to songs of personal significance.

The *motor cortex* lies just behind the frontal cortex and is responsible for coordinating voluntary motor function. The motor cortex receives information from other areas of the brain to help in creating strategies for the best motor response. Networks in the motor cortex contribute to the control of fine motor activity as well as motor aspects of speech. Rich connections to other areas of the brain—the basal ganglia and the cerebellum as well as the auditory cortex—are also involved in motor function. In music, the motor cortex helps in planning fine finger and arm movements during performance. Unlike other sensory motor activities, music performance re-

quires the exact timing of multiple levels of brain activity to produce highly organized actions (Zatorre, Chen, & Penhune, 2007).

The *sensory cortex* lies behind the motor cortex and helps integrate all sensory information (sight, sound, touch, taste, and smell). The integration of these sensory systems develops progressively from birth. This process of multisensory integration is highly adaptive. It brings together information from different sensory networks to allow the brain to amplify minimal signals and reduce ambiguity when detecting, identifying, and reacting to environmental events. Having multiple sensory systems has obvious benefits because one sensory input, such as sound, can inform another sensory input, such as vision, by providing information on direction or distance. Also, the integration of these systems consolidates information to help the brain respond quickly or allow the information to be properly identified. Stein and his team at Wake Forest University (Liping, Rowland, & Stein, 2010) investigate models of sensory integration, particularly two neural models: one in the *midbrain superior colliculus* (SC) and one in the *association cortex*. They have found the midbrain SC to be the most effective model for sensory integration. The sensory cortex also plays a large role in integrating the multiple tactile sensations that comprise active music making, from finger positions to immediate adjustments of tuning to the force applied to produce the sound. These processes become almost automatic with the advanced training of the musician.

The *primary auditory cortex* is the first cortical region of the ascending auditory pathway and processes the sound we hear. It is located in the temporal lobes and helps in the processing of pitch and volume. The frequencies of sound are processed in a tonotopic map, where specific points along the temporal lobe are responsible for perceiving specific pitches. The temporal lobes are involved in aspects of speech perception and execution, depending on whether it is the left or right side of the brain. Areas in the frontal and parietal lobes (involved in associative memory function) also contribute to auditory processing. The primary auditory cortex relays impulses to subcortical areas in the midbrain as well as the brainstem. These connections to lower brain areas explain why there are automatic responses

to sound, such as changes in respiratory function, even when a person may not be consciously aware of this. The automatic and quick processing of melodic properties occurs in the *secondary auditory cortex*. The detection of incongruities in pitch may actually be processed automatically in the secondary auditory cortex, suggesting that incoming information is quickly compared against previously learned musical properties, including culturally influenced musical properties such as scales and harmonies (Brattico, Tervaniemi, Naatanen, & Peretz, 2006). The location of the auditory cortex on the surface of the brain is shown in Figure 4.5.

The *cerebellum* is the central processor for motor control and is often called the *little brain*. It receives input from sensory systems of the spinal cord as well as other parts of the brain. By processing these inputs, it fine-tunes motor activity to help with coordination and accuracy of movements. If the cerebellum is damaged, problems with posture, balance, and fine motor activity will result. Because the auditory system has rich

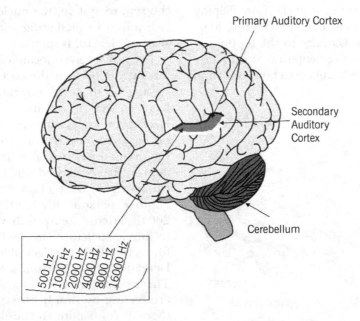

FIGURE 4.5. The primary auditory cortex in humans.

connections to the cerebellum, it is involved in automatic motor responses such as foot tapping.

The *limbic system* (see Figure 4.6) is the set of brain structures that form the inner border of the cortex on both sides of the thalamus. It includes the cerebrum, hippocampus, and amygdala, among other structures, and is involved in processes related to our emotions as well as forming and retrieving memories. When the music we listen to is perceived as emotional, rapid responses occur in these limbic structures. Connections to and processes by the temporal lobes and parietofrontal areas of the cortex add semantics and syntax to what is heard (Sel & Calvo-Merino, 2013). Depending on the type of emotion being processed (whether it is attached to past experiences or is a spontaneous response to new music), various networks will be involved in processing it and its connections to associations and memories (Tomaino, 1993).

The *hippocampus* is located in both the right and left medial temporal lobes just below the cortical surface. It is part of the limbic system and plays a major role in memory processing, especially in helping consolidate short-term memories into long-term memories. Damage to the hippocampus will lead to disorientation and eventually memory loss. Damage to both right and left hippocampi will cause anterograde amnesia, leaving a person unable to make or retain new memories. The damage to people with Alzheimer's disease usually starts in this area of the brain. The hippocampus, because of its role in memory processing, helps connect music memories with life experiences.

The *amygdala* is the brain's fight-or-flight system that regulates fear responses and autonomic responses such as the freezing. In this regard, the amygdala signals the hypothalamus to activate the sympathetic nervous system to allow for the body's quick response to potential danger. For this reason, it plays a role in pairing memories with emotionally charged events. Consequently, it is involved in how we process emotion related to music listening. Research studies have shown that damage to the amygdala impairs emotion recognition in music (Gosselin, Peretz, Johnsen, & Adolphs, 2007).

The *nucleus accumbens* is a brain structure that is key to our internal reward system. This structure releases the neurochemical *dopamine* when we have pleasant responses to music. In addition to its function with the reward system, the nucleus accumbens is involved in mediating addictive, aggressive, and fearful responses.

The *visual cortex*, located in the occipital lobe at the back of the cortex, allows processing of all visual information and also has connections to motor timing areas. Recent research has revealed the existence of *mirror neurons* in the visual cortex and the premotor cortex. A mirror neuron is a neuron that is excited when we do a physical activity and we observe that activity in another person (Rizzolatti & Craighero, 2004). Mirror neurons have connections to limbic structures in the brain, allowing for us to mimic and feel what we see (Wan, Demaine, Zipse, Norton, & Schlaug, 2010). These neurons enable us to *feel* what others are feeling by simply observing them and thereby contribute to the development of empathy as well as our ability to learn by observation.

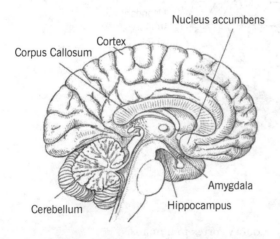

FIGURE 4.6. The limbic system.

Implications for Music Therapy

The fields of cognitive neuroscience and music perception are contributing increasingly to a new understanding of how we process and are influenced by music. This knowledge is important for music therapists because it can inform our engagement with clients who have developmental, psychological, and/or neurological problems. For example, a person who has incurred damage to the frontal cortex may not be able to plan out his or her actions. Including verbal processing and/or verbal cues may add a level of complexity that forces the patient into an impaired cognitive mode.

How can the music therapist use specific elements of music (e.g., rhythm, tone, dynamics) to engage this person in such a way as to allow for spontaneous responses with little or no need for the patient's mental planning? Spontaneous response draws from the person's innate or preserved musical skills rather than the cognitive task of following a verbal instruction. For the music therapist working with children, can an understanding of sensory integration processes help to better assess the child who withdraws or becomes hyperaroused during the music therapy session? Such knowledge can help the therapist realize that the child isn't showing a dislike for the music but may perceive it as distorted noise. How would this child respond to simple sounds or individual tones, rather than chords or to rhythm without melody? Are multiple sensory cues, such as tactile sensation along with sound, too much? What is the lowest common denominator that will allow for the child's engagement without adverse response or withdrawal? Will the child's tolerance of the sound increase if he or she performs it rather than passively listens to it? The sounds one creates are sometimes perceived differently than those created by others. You may observe a child who pulls away when you play a drum but then plays the drum alone without any signs of withdrawal or unease. Music can provide meaning for a child with autism who is not able to understand emotional meaning in facial expressions. Exploring the range of music expression available to the child and matching it to facial expressions may help the child form a connection between sound expressions, facial expressions, and meaning. The music therapist needs to have knowledge of music perception and brain function to truly understand how to make the most of the therapeutic interaction.

In human development a fetus at 5 months gestation already has auditory memory (Winkler et al., 2003). Immediately after birth, the newborn is able to distinguish the temporal aspects of sound (i.e., can feel the beat; Honing, Ladinig, Winkler, & Háden, 2009). Infants do not passively take in sound but actively engage with it as a prelinguistic form of communication with the people and world around them (Trevarthen, 2002). As these interactions occur, the brain develops further to make sense of the auditory signals, forming emotional, spatial, linguistic, and other associations with the sounds. Trehub's (2001) research has shown how this ability to process temporal and tonal aspects of sound enables infants to learn the rules of their native language.

The more emotionally charged the musical experience, the more likely a strong memory is connected to it. As associations, including feelings, memories, and images, become paired with music, the information becomes encoded in such a way that the next time there is a similar experience, such as hearing the song again, an instantaneous response, both conscious and subconscious, is drawn from the previous experience. The limbic system, comprised of several brain areas, including the hippocampus and amygdala, has long been considered to be primarily responsible for processing emotions and long-term memory, as noted previously. However, current neuroscientists, such as LeDoux (2000, 2012), theorize that there are different levels of emotional processes that recruit brain areas differently depending on the type of emotion. This encoding process, which continues throughout life, eventually gives us a repertoire of emotional responses, musical preferences, perceptual skills, long-term memories, and so forth.

Because music provides cues for memories and associations, it can prime or stimulate neural networks to react at a faster and more efficient pace. Think about how quickly we recall past experiences with music or how we can prompt lyrics to a song with just a few introductory notes. Music-based cues such as these can inform many areas of physical and cognitive function, making it an excellent tool in rehabilitative medicine. For example, superimposing a strong rhythmic pulse on intoned spoken phrases can provide the temporal structure and oral–motor coordination needed to help a person with dysarthria (a motor speech problem) to speak more intelligibly. Many shared networks serve both singing and speaking (Patel, 2008), making music a strong habilitative and rehabilitative tool for persons with speech deficits. For a person with Broca's (nonfluent or expressive aphasia), who can sing words but not speak them, being prompted to fill in the blanks to a verse of a familiar song may help with priming word retrieval for nonmusical words (Tomaino, 2012). A child who does not understand the structural rules of language may learn linguistic prosody through the use of words in melody. For the music therapist, understanding the similarities between language and music will guide the musical elements included in the treatment plan.

Some individuals are born with, or acquire through brain injury or disease, the inability to perceive the correct frequencies of music or the ability to remember melodies. This problem with the perception of music is termed *amusia*. Peretz has studied this phenomenon extensively and has created an amusia test, the Montreal Battery of Evaluation of Amusia (MBEA; Peretz, Champod, & Hyde, 2003). It is estimated that 4% of the population has this disorder. It is important for the music therapist to assess when a patient is not able to process certain musical elements, be it tone and or rhythm (beat deafness), and determine whether or not this was a preexisting condition or the result of the clinical problem being treated (e.g., traumatic brain injury [TBI], stroke, developmental delay).

Another important implication of music and the brain is the effect of music improvisation on exciting and inhibiting responses in the brain. Music improvisation is often a fundamental part of music therapy interventions. This dynamic, interactive, and personalized engagement often reveals abilities in individuals who seem quite unable to exhibit those same abilities outside of the music. This specific responsiveness may result from the arousal of subcortical areas and neural networks that stimulate action and inhibit self-monitoring (Tomaino, 2013). People who have had a brain injury or neurological disease often have to think hard about how to move a paretic arm or leg; similarly, a person who has had a stroke may have trouble with word retrieval but may find the word easier to retrieve after singing a song. Those with some type of brain injury, whether by trauma, disease, or stroke, often have trouble with multistep planning, attention, and mental flexibility—all aspects of *executive function*. Understanding what the improvising brain looks like can offer some insights as to why a patient with impaired executive function shows ability when engaged in spontaneous activity. From their research in music and creativity, Limb and Braun (2008) describe that, during improvisation, the prefrontal cortex of the brain undergoes an interesting shift in activity in which a broad area, the *lateral prefrontal* region, shuts down, with a significant inhibition of the prefrontal cortex. These areas are involved in conscious self-monitoring, self-inhibition, and evaluation of what is correct or incorrect for the action that will be implemented. Simultaneously, another part of the prefrontal cortex, the *medial prefrontal cortex*, turns on. This region has been implicated in autobiographical narrative abilities and sense of self. This research corroborates findings by Janata (2009) that demonstrate the activation of this area when music of autobiographical significance is heard.

Our skills, musical and nonmusical, are developed over time, and our brain learns to apply our *repertoire* in an infinite array of possible outcomes. Basic motor skills can be applied to everyday tasks such as walking and dressing but can also be used for more advanced skills such as playing the violin or competing in gymnastics. The more advanced our skills, the more enriched the number of networks and brain areas that are used to produce the given outcome. Mental processes such as fear and uncertainty inhibit the freedom with which we apply these skills. Similarly, head trauma and disease can interfere with ability as well. Using spontaneous music making and improvisation within the music therapy session can help to disinhibit the self-monitoring or bypass this system to enable increased function in those with neurological deficits.

Introduced in 1995, the *polyvagal theory* (Porges, 1995, 2010), which relates autonomic function to behavior, should also be considered when considering how music affects the brain. This polyvagal perspective includes (1) an appreciation of the autonomic nervous system as a *system*, (2) the identification of neural circuits involved in the regulation of autonomic state, and (3) an interpretation of autonomic reactivity as adaptive within the context of the phylogeny of the vertebrate autonomic nervous system. The polyvagal theory emphasizes the neurophysiological and neuroanatomical distinction between the two branches of the vagus and autonomic nervous system (i.e., the tenth cranial nerve). Porges proposed that humans react to sounds in various frequency ranges based on autonomic nervous system response; for example, low frequencies convey a sense of danger whereas middle frequencies (the human voice is in this range) convey a sense of safety. Another aspect of his theory supports the importance of interactions, including facial expression and changes in facial muscles, in activating the neural network and the visceral and autonomic systems. Such engagement can lead to restoration of prosocial and more positive affective states of mind. This theory points to the fact that there are many neurological levels, both conscious and autonomic, that come into play as we develop behaviors and skills over a lifetime. Because music therapists incorporate music within a clinical, interpersonal context, it is important to understand not only the direct effect of music on brain function but also the impact of the interpersonal exchange that accompanies the musical interaction.

Conclusions

Understanding the various aspects of how music and the components of music affect brain function, both in developing infants and those with neurological problems, will enable music therapists to enrich their sessions and optimize clinical outcomes for their clients. Information about music and the brain is constantly unfolding. It is important for music therapists to keep current with scientific research on music and the brain, as this research can help validate standard practices in music therapy and provide needed evidence for how and why music therapy works.

REFERENCES

Brattico, E., Tervaniemi, M., Naatanen, R., & Peretz, I. (2006). Musical scale properties are automatically processed in the human auditory cortex. *Brain Research, 1117*(1), 162–174.

Bunge, S. A., & Wright, S. B. (2007). Neurodevelopmental changes in working memory and cognitive control. *Current Opinion in Neurobiology, 17*, 243–250.

Cole, M. W., Reynolds, J. R., Power, J. D., Repovs,

G., Anticevic, A., & Braver, T. S. (2013). Multitask connectivity reveals flexible hubs for adaptive task control. *Nature Neuroscience, 16*, 1348–1355.

Gosselin, N., Peretz, I., Johnsen, E., & Adolphs, R. (2007). Amygdala damage impairs emotion recognition from music. *Neuropsychologia, 45*(2), 236–244.

Honing, H., Ladinig, O., Winkler, I., & Háden, G. (2009). Is beat induction innate or learned?: Probing emergent meter perception in adults and newborns using event-related brain potentials (ERP). *Annals of the New York Academy of Sciences, 1169*, 93–96.

Janata, P. (2009). The neural architecture of music-evoked autobiographical memories. *Cerebral Cortex, 19*(11), 2579–2594.

Kandel, E., Schwartz, J., & Jessell, T. (2000). *Principles of neural science* (4th ed.). New York: McGraw-Hill.

Kolb, B., & Whishaw, I. Q. (2011). *An introduction to brain and behavior* (3rd ed.). New York: Worth.

LeDoux, J. E. (2000). Emotion circuits in the brain. *Annual Review of Neuroscience, 23*, 155–184.

LeDoux, J. E. (2012). Rethinking the emotional brain. *Neuron, 73*(4), 653–676. Erratum in *Neuron* (2012), *73*(5), 1052.

Limb, C. J., & Braun, A. R. (2008). Neural substrates of spontaneous musical performance: An fMRI study of jazz improvisation. *PLoS ONE, 3*(2), e1679.

Liping, Y., Rowland, B. A., & Stein, B. E. (2010). Initiating the development of multisensory integration by manipulating sensory experience. *Journal of Neuroscience, 30*(14), 4904–4913.

López-González, M., & Limb, C. J. (2012). Musical creativity and the brain. *Cerebrum, 2*, 1–30.

Patel, A. D. (2008). *Music language and the brain.* New York: Oxford University Press.

Peretz, I., Champod, S., & Hyde, K. (2003). Varieties of musical disorders: The Montreal Battery of Evaluation of Amusia. *Annals of the New York Academy of Sciences, 999*, 58–75.

Porges, S. W. (1995). Orienting in a defensive world: Mammalian modifications of our evolutionary heritage: A Polyvagal Theory. *Psychophysiology, 32*(4), 301–318.

Porges, S. W. (2010). Music therapy and trauma: Insights from the Polyvagal Theory. In K. Stewart (Ed.), *Symposium on music therapy and trauma:*

Bridging theory and clinical practice (pp. 3–15). New York: Satchnote Press.

Portfors, C. V., & Roberts, P. D. (2007). Temporal and frequency characteristics of cartwheel cells in the dorsal cochlear nucleus of the awake mouse. *Journal of Neurophysiology, 98*(2), 744–756.

Rizzolatti, G., & Craighero, L. (2004). The mirror-neuron system. *Annual Review of Neuroscience, 27*, 169–192.

Sel, A., & Calvo-Merino, B. (2013). Neuroarchitecture of musical emotions. *Revista de Neurologia, 56*(5), 289–297.

Skoe, E., & Kraus, N. (2010). Auditory brainstem response to complex sounds: A tutorial. *Ear and Hearing, 31*(3), 302–324.

Tomaino, C. M. (1993). Music and the limbic system. In F. J. Bejjani (Ed.), *Current research in arts medicine* (pp. 393–398). Chicago: A Cappella Books.

Tomaino, C. M. (2012). Effective music therapy techniques in the treatment of nonfluent aphasia. *Annals of the New York Academy of Sciences, 1252*, 312–317.

Tomaino, C. M. (2013). Creativity and improvisation as therapeutic tools within music therapy. *Annals of the New York Academy of Sciences, 1303*, 84–86.

Trehub, S. E. (2001). Musical predispositions in infancy. *Annals of the New York Academy of Sciences, 930*, 1–16.

Trevarthen, C. (2002). Origins of musical identity: Evidence from infancy for musical social awareness. In R. A. R. Macdonald, D. Miell, & D. J. Hargreaves (Eds.), *Musical identities* (pp. 21–38). Oxford, UK: Oxford University Press.

Wan, C. Y., Demaine, K., Zipse, L., Norton, A., & Schlaug, G. (2010). From music making to speaking: Engaging the mirror neuron system in autism. *Brain Research Bulletin, 82*(3–4), 161–168.

Winkler, I., Kushnerenko, E., Horváth, J., Čeponiené, R., Fellman, V., Huotilainen, M., et al. (2003). Newborn infants can organize the auditory world. *Proceedings of the National Academy of Sciences, 100*(20), 11812–11815.

Zatorre, R. J., Chen, J. L., & Penhune, V. B. (2007). When the brain plays music: Auditory–motor interactions in music perception and production. *Nature Reviews Neuroscience, 8*(7), 547–558.

CHAPTER 5

Music Therapy and Cultural Diversity

Seung-A Kim
Annette Whitehead-Pleaux

In the preface to Stige's (2002) *Culture-Centered Music Therapy*, Bruscia states that the *culture-centeredness* perspective is regarded as the fifth force in music therapy. For music therapists, culture has a particularly significant meaning because the work entails understanding the self and the client. The main modality in music therapy is *music*—the representation of a specific culture, or more aptly, the self and the society to which the individual belongs. In addition, cultural misunderstanding can take place any time during the course of music therapy—during assessment, treatment, or termination (Estrella, 2001). Misunderstanding can adversely affect the development of a therapeutic relationship and the establishment of an effective treatment plan.

Culture refers to "those beliefs, actions and behaviors associated with sex, age, location of residence, educational status, social economic status, history, formal and informal affiliations, nationality, ethnic group, language, race, religion, disability, illness, developmental handicap, lifestyle, and sexual orientation" (Dileo, 2000, p. 149). To date, statistics on the number of clients of different cultures that receive music therapy services have been unavailable to us. However, as the demographics of the U.S. population become increasingly diverse, it is likely that music therapists will work with more diverse populations. For example, population projections show a significant change in the racial and ethnic profile of Americans. In 2050, European Americans will no longer maintain their majority status, with the number of Hispanics rising from 42 million to 128 million, and of Asians from 14 million to 41 million (Population Reference Bureau, 2008). On the other hand, the American Music Therapy Association (AMTA, 2013a) reports that music therapists and students in the United States are predominantly European American and female. This discrepancy further heightens the need for discussion of cultural diversity in music therapy.

Historical Perspectives

As the world became increasingly globalized, music therapy was making a timely entrance on the global stage as a profession seeking a more articulate and unified effort. In the 1970s, there was an increasing interest in dialoguing about music therapy among professionals from around the world; they began to exchange ideas about music therapy and trainings, and a few international gatherings were organized for this purpose. The First International Music Therapy Congress took place in Paris in 1974 (Wheeler, 2008), followed by other international conferences. Later, two noteworthy symposia were held: the International Symposium of Music Therapy Training, held in Herdecke, Germany, in 1978 (Wheeler, 2003), and an international symposium, Music in the Life of Man, held at New York University in 1982. At the time, international communication rarely occurred among music therapists, so, following the New York symposium, Kenneth Bruscia (1983) initiated the *International Newsletter of Music Therapy*, writing, "I sincerely hope that as the newsletter develops and improves, it will serve an important communication function in the world community of music therapists" (p. 3). These events and others began the communication that eventually led to a broader international perspective and consideration of cultural issues (Barbara L. Wheeler, personal communication, February 12, 2013).

Although progress was slow initially, a collective effort paved the way for a discussion of cultural issues that has become an integral component of music therapy. There has been steadfast effort by music therapists and scholars to bring this topic to light (Chase, 2003a). Some of the relevant topics that appear in music therapy literature include the importance of multicultural competencies and ethics (Dileo, 2000); music therapists' worldviews (Wheeler & Baker, 2010); work with diverse clients (Whitehead-Pleaux & Clark, 2009); the impact of music therapists' religious beliefs (Elwafi, 2011); ethnic music in music therapy (Moreno, 1988) and training (Shapiro, 2005); community music therapy (Pavlicevic & Ansdell, 2004; Stige & Leif, 2012); international music therapy students and acculturative stress (Kim, 2011); ethnicity and race (Hadley, 2013; Kenny, 2006); feminist perspectives (Curtis, 2013b; Hadley, 2006); sexual orientation and gender identity (Whitehead-Pleaux et al., 2012, 2013); and cross-cultural supervision (Kim, 2008; Young, 2009). As the work of music therapists gained momentum and a more concerted effort, further information and discourse were disseminated through institutes for multicultural music therapy at the AMTA conferences (Kim, 2012; Whitehead-Pleaux, 2012); the first international conference on gender, health, and the creative arts therapies in Montreal, Canada, in 2012 (Curtis, 2013a); the World Congress of Music Therapy conferences, held triennially around the world; and through *Voices: A World Forum for Music Therapy*, an electronic journal. Furthermore, in 2011, AMTA formed a diversity committee to address cultural issues in the music therapy profession in a more systemic and organized way. As a result of the cumulative efforts of music therapy professionals from around the world, the World Congress of Music Therapy has been held every 3 years, and carries the overarching theme of "cultural diversity in music therapy, practice, research, and education."

Music: Universal and/or Relative?

Music therapy and culture are intrinsically connected and are topics of significant interest to music therapists (Stige, 2002). The interconnection of these two leaves us with many questions. For example, what type of music and music therapy interventions would be more effective in treating clients from diverse cultures? Western classical music is usually used in guided imagery and music (GIM) and has proven to be an effective medium (Burns, 2000). Would this be the case when working with a client coming from Latin America, Asia, or Africa as well?

We can also examine improvisation, one of the main music experiences that the music therapist employs in sessions. Would the meaning of improvisation be the same to a client who is not accustomed to Western European and American music and improvisation? Westerners are accustomed to diatonic scales and harmonic structures, and to them, music from a variety of cultures may seem out of tune. As a matter of fact, the banding sound often used in music from a variety of cultures does not even exist in Western scales. While practicing music therapy in Africa, Pavlicevic (2004) noted that she experienced the Africans' *musicking* as going "on, and on and on—often with not too much variation in tempo, phrasing, melody or harmony and with slow build-ups of intensity over time" (p. 46), because she was accustomed to the "Western-trained musical mind." She proposed that this response may have been influenced by her expectations about improvisation: "Is this a compromise of our western heritage of improvisation in music therapy—where the client's music may well lead us to the edge of our being?" (p. 182). More specifically, would Western European and American music provide the same results to a client from India who has just arrived in America? Can you imagine a client who has never heard the piano in his or her own country being asked to improvise on the piano for the first time in a music therapy session? Moreover, how uncomfortable would it be for a client, raised within a structured society, to be asked to make something up freely in music? Such a client would expect the therapist to display full command and supply comprehensive instruction. He or she may interpret this approach as a sign of weakness or a lack of preparation.

On the other hand, an Indian immigrant who has lived in the United States for more than 20 years may enjoy jazz more than ragas (Indian traditional improvised music). Still another consideration: Music and dance are inseparable for some cultures. Some people may feel more natural making improvised movements through their body with music rather than just improvising solely on musical instruments. For them, it is natural to use their body as the main instrument.

Stereotyping and Ethnocentrism in the Use of Music

Although music is culture-specific, some musical elements found in other countries can also be found in America, and vice versa. For example, some Western classical composers, such as Debussy and Schönberg, integrated Asian and Spanish musical elements into their compositions. In addition, modern technology and globalization have influenced music. Many children around the world grew up with Disney films, which are riddled with stereotypes. Most Disney movies are based on white characters and tend to display strong stereotypical patriarchal/gender roles (e.g., the bad lion in *The Lion King* had many stereotypical gay male traits). Non-Westerners may perceive Western cultures in a certain way because their only exposure to Western cultures has occurred through movies. It is noteworthy that individual differences among members of the same cultural groups also need to be considered.

As Moreno (1988) pointed out, "American music therapists tend to be more ethnocentric and to use music in therapy that primarily derives from western-oriented classical, popular, and folk traditions" (p. 18). He emphasized that music from a variety of cultures is not only a tool for contacting clients from these other cultures but also a vehicle from which Western-based music therapy clients could benefit. The purpose of using music from a variety of cultures is to build clients' identities and increase their feelings of self-worth (Shapiro, 2005). Music therapists should consider music from other cultures based on the traditions and cultural practices of their cultures.

Culturally Informed Therapeutic Relationship

Music therapists have explored effective ways of establishing therapeutic relationships with clients from diverse cultures (Dileo & Magill, 2005; Kim, 2013b). An effective therapeutic relationship is essential to bringing about positive outcomes. Without a cultural understanding of their clients, therapists would have a hard time empathizing with many situations. For this crucial reason, Dileo and Magill (2005) emphasize the following:

> Music therapists must: commit themselves to learning about the [client's] various cultural needs and musical preferences; examine their own personal cultural values and how they may be in conflict with those of the [client]; and develop authentic skills in multicultural empathy. (p. 228)

Current music therapy theories and methods of therapy are also oriented primarily toward European American middle- to upper-class populations. Westerners value separation–individuation, autonomy, self-assertiveness, and verbal articulateness. These values are culturally encapsulated in our therapy orientations. How, then, can we possibly apply these values to the clients who come from collectivist societies? In Eastern collectivist-oriented countries, key figures in the community assume the role of the therapist—family members, relatives, close friends, and religious leaders. Such figures do not easily discuss personal issues outside of the family. Delving into the personal lives of others is regarded as shameful for the entire family, especially if an individual has had a troubled past.

If the client's values and belief systems differ from our own, then therapy treatment plans—including goals, assessments, and evaluations—should all be revised according to the individual's cultural values. Given that all therapists (ideally) strive for the betterment of the client within the value system of that individual, the reality of diversity has profound implications for therapy. It means that the definition of a better life is a *culturally subjective* determination. How well do our current methods of therapy work for non-Westerners? What type of therapeutic approaches would be effective? Would individual therapy help clients from different cultures open up to personal issues? Another complication: Music therapists are finding that more and more clients do not speak English as a first language. When verbal communication does not work well, how can we build a therapeutic relationship effectively?

To answer these questions, alternative approaches to music therapy have been proposed (Chase, 2003b; Stige, 2002). Stige (2002) developed a culture-centered theory, and Stige and others have developed community music therapy (CoMT; Pavlicevic & Ansdell, 2004; Stige, Ansdell, Elefant, & Pavlicevic, 2010; Stige & Leif, 2012). CoMT emphasizes that music therapy always takes place *in context*. Thus, individuals can be understood fully only within a context and culture as an "individual–communal continuum" (Pavlicevic & Ansdell, 2004, p. 23). Stige (2002) explained:

> It is quite possible that other music therapists may see it differently. . . . I can only tell you what Community Music Therapy is for me, and perhaps for some other people in the hope that this will help you work it out for yourself. In an effort to bridge the gap between client and community, community music therapists made the profession rethink and resituate the traditional definitions of music therapy and ethical considerations. Community music therapists are "musicking community workers" in order to bring out "social and cultural change." (pp. 92–93)

As reviewed above, a cultural understanding of all clients, an assessment of musical and nonmusical characteristics incorporating their acculturation history, and a shift in our methods to accommodate their worldviews must be taken into consideration for effective treatment. It is important that music therapists approach their work in a way that integrates the clients into the music therapy process, rather than dictating what is best for clients based on the dominant culture. In essence, we are describing a Culturally Informed Music Therapy (CIMT) (Kim, 2010). Through humility (Whitehead-Pleaux, 2012), seeking information, and learning about the culture of each client, music therapists can create music therapy treatment that is relevant to each client's worldview and life. The goals and interventions of music therapy should incorporate clients' cultural music so that each individual's therapy is tailored to his or her background and needs. In the next section, music therapy methods of addressing cultural diversity issues are described.

Culturally Informed Music Therapy

CIMT is a music therapy approach designed for clients who have experience with two or more cultures and addresses clients' cultural well-being through music (Kim, 2010). Flexibility when applying therapy principles and techniques is a cornerstone of CIMT. To better understand the CIMT approach, AMTA (2013c) delineated several steps in the *Standards of Clinical Practice*: assessment, treatment planning, implementation, documentation and evaluation, and termination. In addition, recommendations for best practices in culturally informed clinical music therapy are explored. The *AMTA Standards of Clinical Practice* state: "The music therapy assessment will explore the client's culture. This can include but is not limited to race, ethnicity, language, religion/spirituality, social class, family experiences, sexual orientation, gender identity,

and social organizations" (2.2). Similarly, *AMTA Professional Competencies* (AMTA, 2013b) state that the music therapist is to

select and implement effective culturally based methods for assessing the client's assets and problems through music. (16.4)

Select and implement effective culturally based methods for assessing the client's musical preferences and level of musical functioning or development. (16.5)

When assessing a client, it is essential for the music therapist to engage in culturally informed practices. The assessment is not only a time to learn more about the client's clinical needs, but also to learn about his or her culture. The following case example illustrates a culturally informed assessment.

Assessment

As I (Annette Whitehead-Pleaux) was cleaning my instruments one afternoon a few years ago, my coworker, a nurse, came into the office and told me about a new admission. She was a 4-year-old girl from Senegal who was injured a year prior. She spoke Wolof and knew very little English. My coworker felt that music therapy would be a good match for her, as she was exhibiting signs of trauma and was very anxious with all medical personnel.

I grabbed my guitar and cautiously stepped into her room. I saw a tiny child curled up in a bed, crying with the covers pulled up to her chin. Her father sat next to her looking very haggard, while the interpreter looked anxious and uncomfortable. I was immediately struck with the realization that my assistance would be limited, as I knew nothing about Senegalese music, Senegalese culture, the social norms and mores of the culture, and the role music plays in the Senegalese culture. I had no idea what a Senegalese children's song might sound like. How could I introduce music therapy to this father and his daughter in a way that would be both pertinent to her needs and effective for her treatment? How could I fully explain the basis for music therapy with no knowledge of their background

pecially when the music therapist focuses on the music culture with which the client identifies. Learning the client's cultural identity is crucial in the assessment because he or she may not identify with the music culture of his or her heritage and actually find that music offensive.

Juan, a teenage boy, was admitted to the hospital at 8 P.M. Friday, after my shift had ended. I (Annette Whitehead-Pleaux) was not returning until the following Monday, so I wanted to leave some CDs in his room to aid in his transition to the hospital. From his chart, I learned that he was from Honduras. I left a variety of CDs that reflected many of the popular Latin genres of music, such as salsa, reggaeton, romantica, and ranchera. Monday morning I went to Juan's room and introduced myself. Immediately he told me how someone had left a bunch of music in his room that he did not like at all, and that I was to take it away this instant. He preferred Michael Jackson and Justin Bieber. As I gathered up the CDs, I apologized for guessing incorrectly what music he likes, saying it was not included in his medical chart from the Honduran hospital. He began to laugh, and we joked about other information that may not be included in the chart, including his sister's name and how many chickens his family owns.

Expanding the assessment to include culture not only increases the music therapist's understanding of the client, but also affects the rest of the music therapy process from treatment planning to intervention design to evaluation of progress. The extra time spent learning more about the client creates an environment (1) wherein the client feels valued for who he or she is, (2) that builds the therapeutic relationship faster, and (3) that creates a greater rapport between the music therapist and the client. In addition to the music therapy goals that address the universal domains, the CIMT goals include therapists' development of increased cultural awareness; acknowledgment of own cultural identity; resolution of cultural conflicts within the context of the client's culture; formulation of needed coping skills for the client; management of client's acculturative stress; and development of preventive methods (Kim, 2010).

Treatment Plan

Once the assessment is completed, the treatment plan must be created. Through a thorough synthesis of the information collected during the assessment, the music therapist identifies the client's needs, strengths, interests, and music preferences. This information helps the music therapist to craft the goals, objectives, and interventions for future sessions. Although not articulated specifically, *AMTA Professional Competencies* (AMTA, 2013b) states that music therapists must select and adapt musical instruments and equipment consistent with the strengths and needs of the client:

Select and adapt musical instruments and equipment consistent with strengths and needs of the client. (17.7)

Select and implement effective culturally based methods for assessing the client's musical preferences and level of musical functioning or development. (16.5)

When these competencies are interpreted through a CIMT lens, the idea of music preferences and musical instruments can become the music and instruments of the client's culture(s), which then can be interwoven through the interventions. The music therapist can learn the melodies, songs, or musical idioms of the client's preferred musical genres. Recorded music from that culture can be incorporated into the sessions. Instruments from the culture or similar sounding instruments can be utilized as well. Handheld electronic music devices such as tablets or MP3 players that use apps are an easy way to bring the sounds of instruments from other cultures to the session at a minimal cost (Whitehead-Pleaux, 2012).

In addition to music and instrument selection, the music therapist must also work closely with clients from less dominant cultures to ensure that practices are conducted in a culturally sensitive manner. In the lesbian, gay, bisexual, transgender, and questioning (LGBTQ) best practices, for example, Whitehead-Pleaux et al. (2012) describe culturally sensitive behaviors that include creating a safe space where hate speech is not allowed, avoiding assumptions about the client, treating "all diverse clients, family members, and support people equally and with respect" (p. 160), being "open and affirming to LGBTQ clients" (p. 160), and practicing culturally appropriate language in speech and writing. When working with individuals from cultures that have experienced oppression and discrimination, the clinician must understand that different terms have different meanings to these individuals based on historical events, generational factors, and cultural associations. Thus, the therapist should always ask the client what terms he or she should use when discussing issues related to the client's cultural identity (Whitehead-Pleaux et. al., 2012). This final point is especially relevant if the music therapist is either a member of, or perceived to be a member of, the dominant culture. The history of domination and oppression runs deep through many cultures and, as therapists, we must be aware of these histories through not just the view of our own cultural lens but also through that of individuals from these oppressed cultures.

Openness and Humility: The Qualities of the Culturally Informed Music Therapist

It is vital that the music therapist get to know the client fully, for it is human connection and trust that allow for the greatest growth and well-being. A culturally informed music therapist is "a kind of culture bearer, a person who learned their songs and some of their languages, archived, and elicited this material, when appropriate" (Shapiro, 2005, p. 31).

Approaching the client with openness, humility, and a genuine interest in knowing who he or she is helps to strip away the power inequity, allowing for the strengths, knowledge, and worldview of the client to enter into the sessions. Through this deeper understanding of the client, the music therapist can better serve and meet the client's clinical needs. With these principles in mind, it is important for music therapists to design intake forms and assessments that give voice to the diversity of all cultures other than the dominant culture.

The best practices for LGBTQ recommend that all music therapists "develop intakes, assessments, consents, releases, and other documents that provide for optional self-identification regarding gender identity; sexual orientation; and marital, partnership, and family status" (Whitehead-Pleaux et al., 2012, p. 160). This best-practice principle can be applied to a larger cultural view that also includes race, ethnicity, religion/spirituality, socio-economic class, family experiences, ability, and social organizations. Changing these important forms will help to set the tone with the client that this therapeutic process is one that seeks to validate who he or she is, rather than limit his or her expression to that which is acceptable to the dominant culture. The music therapy space must be a space that is safe for *all* clients.

Self-Awareness

One aspect of CIMT practice that is not always discussed is that of self-exploration and the learning of cultural competencies. Moreno (1988) emphasized that ethnic music was not only a tool for contacting clients from other cultures but also a vehicle through which mainstream music therapy clients could also benefit.

As we are profoundly influenced by the culture surrounding us, much of what we see, hear, and feel is imprinted in our minds. It is through this cultural lens that we view our world. Unfortunately, some of these messages with which we interpret the world contain biases, and we carry them into our sessions with our clients. To practice CIMT, we must embark on a journey of self-exploration to uncover these biases and work through them (Chase, 2003b). This journey is one that is best taken on with a supervisor who is well trained in this area. Supervision is a must for music therapists who work with clients from cultures other than their own (Estrella, 2001). The threefold approach of open communication with the client, information seeking, and supervision will aid the music therapist in providing the highest quality of care for clients from different cultures.

Ethical Considerations

Since 1982, the American Counseling Association and the American Psychological Association have mandated multicultural education in their training. These mandates include awareness of personal beliefs and/or attitudes about culturally diverse clients, knowledge of diverse cultures, and the ability to use intervention skills or techniques that are culturally appropriate. (The American Psychological Association [2003] also documented "Guidelines on Multicultural Education, Training, Research, Practice, and Organizational Change for Psychologists" in 2003).

There has been an effort to increase sensitivity to ethical issues in music therapy (Dileo, 2000). However, *AMTA Professional Competencies* (AMTA, 2013b) should include more on the subject of diverse cultural populations, specifically articulated for both entry and advanced levels of music therapists. Dileo (2000) made several suggestions, including the need for a certification program to train and evaluate supervisors in supervisory competence, sensitivity to gender, and multicultural issues of supervisees and clients. It is crucial to delve

deeper into, and facilitate discussions of, these competencies in dealing with a diverse clientele. Therefore, both the supervisor and supervisee should openly discuss their expectations about the training and supervision process. As cultural empathy is an important element in building a trusting supervisory relationship, it is important to acknowledge and learn more about the cultural differences between the two people in question.

Cultural Diversity Education and Training

Cultural issues have significant implications for music therapy education and training (Dileo, 2000; Kim, 2008). Researchers have identified a variety of cross-cultural difficulties and found that multicultural issues are not adequately addressed in music therapy education and supervision, including internships. Although there have been more presentations on this topic at conferences, the curricula of current music therapy training programs are not sufficient to meet the requirements of preparing culturally sensitive music therapists (Dileo, 2000). This deficit is partially due to the lack of multicultural theories and resources available to the profession.

Kim (2011) surveyed international music therapy students in the United States and found the strongest predictors of acculturative stress to be degree of English proficiency, neuroticism, and music therapy education stress. Eight percent of the respondents were identified as a high-risk group. Asian international students were more likely to have high levels of acculturative stress compared with their European counterparts. Educators and supervisors need to closely monitor these students and advise them at an earlier stage.

Music therapists believe that it is important to be informed about multicultural considerations in their work and to be able to utilize cross-cultural skills. Seventy-five percent of respondents to a survey by Darrow and Malloy (1998) reported that they learned about multiculturalism through their work experience. Similar results were found a decade later by Young (2009), who surveyed 104 internship supervisors in the United States and Canada to examine the extent to which multicultural issues were being addressed in music therapy internships. She found that many internship supervisors had little formal training in multicultural music therapy and that multicultural issues were not being consistently addressed in music therapy internships.

In a phenomenological study, Kim (2008) studied supervisees' experiences in cross-cultural music therapy supervision. Seven music therapy supervisees with diverse cultural backgrounds were interviewed and asked to describe significant misunderstood and understood experiences in cross-cultural music therapy supervision. The results of the study showed that the most important indicators of effective cross-cultural music therapy supervision were cultural empathy, openness, and a nonjudgmental attitude on the part of the supervisor. Specific cultural factors, including language and cultural barriers, racial and gender issues, and the experience of prejudice, were noted. Supervisors should openly discuss cultural issues to help supervisees integrate their sense of cultural identity. Because there is an inherent power imbalance between the supervisor and supervisee, the supervisor should take the responsibility of bringing up these cultural issues relating to the clinical work.

In reviewing music therapy literature, it is also apparent that the topic of cultural diversity is still lacking (Estrella, 2001; Kim, 2008), although it is discussed in the following articles. A variety of age groups with different diagnoses (Rilinger, 2011) have been studied; however, very few articles have investigated the use of music therapy with immigrants (Kim, 2013b) or the cultural implications for music therapy in palliative care (Dileo & Magill, 2005; Forrest,

2000, 2011). In addition, literature on religions (Elwafi, 2011), ethnicity (Kim, 2013b), race (Hadley, 2013), gender issues (Hadley, 2006; Curtis, 2013b), sexual orientation and gender identity issues (Whitehead-Pleaux et al., 2012), disability (Humpal, 2012), and cross-cultural supervision and training (Kim, 2008; Young, 2009) has scarcely been touched. Research studies also do not always include the information about cultural diversity that the National Institutes of Health (2013) requires.

What methods would be effective in multicultural training for music therapists? Kim (2013a) suggested that music may be useful in increasing cultural awareness, enhancing cognitive–emotional flexibility, and learning about diverse cultures. Since music is a reflection of culture, by learning ethnic songs we can experience not only the music but also the cultural background relating to the song. For example, when an immigrant learns "God Bless America," he or she learns more about American culture through the lyrics and background of the song. The meaning of this song can vary every time he or she sings it, depending on his or her own experiences. Also, he or she may realize that there are some similarities between this song and the songs from his or her own culture through lyrics, harmonies, and other patriotic songs. Music can be a vehicle for increasing one's self-awareness and for learning about the cultural aspects of a particular music.

However, as an effective method in multicultural training, music needs to be studied further. The differences between professional and student needs regarding multicultural training should also be examined. Interesting results were found in Kim's (2013a) multicultural training study: Although cultural knowledge increased over time and participants retained the knowledge, cultural awareness did not change. This lacuna may be due to participants' belief that they are already adequately aware of cultural issues, or to their denial of the core issues or their blind spot.

Conclusions

Although music therapists value diversity in their practices and have worked to serve their culturally diverse clients more effectively, the development of solutions to address diversity issues has been slow. More guidelines for multicultural and ethical considerations in practice and supervision are required. In addition, multicultural education should become a requirement for the core curriculum in music therapy, and more resources for cultivating cross-cultural knowledge and skills need to be made available to students, educators, and supervisors. There is a need to further develop multicultural music therapy theories and multicultural competencies. Many questions regarding cultural diversity in music therapy need to be further researched.

As society becomes more diverse, the cultural implications for music therapy are more significant than ever, given that music and culture are closely interrelated. The continued and collaborative effort among music therapists, educators, and researchers will help the music therapy profession prepare well for the future.

REFERENCES

American Music Therapy Association (AMTA). (2013a). *A descriptive statistical profile of the AMTA membership.* Retrieved from *www.musictherapy.org/assets/1/7/13WorkforceAnalysis.pdf.*

American Music Therapy Association (AMTA). (2013b). *AMTA professional competencies.* Retrieved from *www.musictherapy.org/about/competencies.*

American Music Therapy Association (AMTA). (2013c). *AMTA standards of clinical practice.* Retrieved from *www.musictherapy.org/about/standards.*

American Psychological Association. (2003). Guidelines for multicultural education, training, research, practice, and organizational change for psychologists. *American Psychologist, 58,* 377–402.

Bruscia, K. E. (1983). *International newsletter of music therapy, 1.* New York: American Association for Music Therapy.

Burns, D. (2000). The effect of classical music on the absorption and control of mental imagery. *Journal of the Association for Music and Imagery, 7,* 34–43.

Chase, K. M. (2003a). Multicultural music therapy: A review of literature. *Music Therapy Perspectives, 21,* 84–88.

Chase, K. M. (2003b). *The multicultural music therapy handbook.* Columbus, MS: Southern Pen.

Curtis, S. L. (2013a). Sorry it has taken so long: Continuing feminist dialogues in music therapy. *Voices: A World Forum for Music Therapy, 13*(1). Retrieved from *https://normt.uib.no/index.php/voices/article/view/688.*

Curtis, S. L. (2013b). On gender and the creative arts therapies. *Arts in Psychotherapy, 40,* 371–372.

Darrow, A., & Malloy, D. (1998). Multicultural perspectives in music therapy: An examination of the literature, educational curricula, and clinical practices in culturally diverse cities of the United States. *Music Therapy Perspectives, 16,* 27–32.

Dileo, C. (2000). *Ethical thinking in music therapy.* Cherry Hills, NJ: Jeffrey Books.

Dileo, C., & Magill, L. (2005). Song writing with oncology and hospice adult patients from a multicultural perspective. In F. Baker & T. Wigram (Eds.), *Songwriting: Methods, techniques, and clinical applications for music therapy clinicians, educators and students* (pp. 226–245). London: Jessica Kingsley.

Elwafi, P. R. (2011). The impact of music therapists' religious beliefs on clinical identity and professional practice. *Qualitative Inquiries in Music Therapy, 6,* 155–191.

Estrella, K. (2001). Multicultural approaches to music therapy supervision. In M. Forinash (Ed.), *Music therapy supervision* (pp. 39–66). Gilsum, NH: Barcelona.

Forrest, L. C. (2000). Addressing issues of ethnicity and identity in palliative care through music therapy practice. *Australian Journal of Music Therapy, 11,* 23–37.

Forrest, L. C. (2011). Supportive cancer care at the end of life: Mapping the cultural landscape in palliative care and music therapy. *Music and Medicine, 3,* 9–14.

Hadley, S. (2006). *Feminist perspectives in music therapy.* Gilsum, NH: Barcelona.

Hadley, S. (2013). *Experiencing race as a music therapist: Personal narratives.* Gilsum, NH: Barcelona.

Humpal, M. (2012, October). Culture of disability. In A. Whitehead-Pleaux & X. Tan (Eds.), *Multicultural Music Therapy Institute: The intersections of music, health, and the individual manual.*

American Music Therapy Association National Conference, St. Charles, IL.

Kenny, C. B. (2006). The earth is our mother: Reflections on the ecology of music therapy from a native perspective. In S. Hadley (Ed.), *Feminist perspectives in music therapy* (pp. 81–96). Gilsum, NH: Barcelona.

Kim, S. A. (2008). The supervisee's experience in cross-cultural music therapy supervision. *Qualitative Inquiries in Music Therapy, 4,* 1–44.

Kim, S. A. (2010). *Culturally informed music therapy.* Unpublished manuscript, Temple University, Philadelphia.

Kim, S. A. (2011). Predictors of acculturative stress among international music therapy students in the U.S. *Music Therapy Perspectives, 29,* 126–132.

Kim, S. A. (2012, March). *When a paradigm shifts: Therapeutic applications of music therapy across cultures.* Paper presented at the conference of the Mid-Atlantic Region of AMTA, Baltimore, MD.

Kim, S. A. (2013a, April). *Multicultural training for the healthcare professionals and students.* Poster presented at the conference of the Mid-Atlantic Region of AMTA, Scranton, PA.

Kim, S. A. (2013b). Re-discovering voice: Korean immigrant women in group music therapy. *Arts in Psychotherapy, 40,* 428–435.

Moreno, J. (1988). Multicultural music therapy: The world music connection. *Journal of Music Therapy, 25*(1), 17–27.

National Institutes of Health. (2013). *Clear communication: A NIH national literacy initiative.* Retrieved from *www.nih.gov/clearcommunication/culturalcompetency.htm.*

Pavlicevic, M. (2004). Music therapy in South Africa: Compromise or synthesis? In M. Pavlicevic & G. Ansdell (Eds.), *Community Music Therapy* (pp. 179–182). London: Jessica Kingsley.

Pavlicevic, M., & Ansdell, G. (Eds.). (2004). *Community Music Therapy.* London: Jessica Kingsley.

Population Reference Bureau. (2008). *Data sheet.* Retrieved from *www.prb.org/Publications/Datasheets.aspx.*

Rilinger, R. L. (2011). Music therapy for Mexican American children: Cultural implications and practical considerations. *Music Therapy Perspectives, 29,* 78–85.

Shapiro, N. (2005). Sounds in the world: Multi-cultural influences in music therapy in clinical practice and training. *Music Therapy Perspectives, 23,* 29–35.

Stige, B. (2002). *Culture-Centered Music Therapy.* Gilsum, NH: Barcelona.

Stige, B., Ansdell, G., Elefant, C., & Pavlicevic, M. (2010). *Where music helps: Community Music Therapy in action and reflection.* Farnham, UK: Ashgate.

Stige, B., & Leif, E. A. (2012). *Invitation to community music therapy.* New York: Routledge.

Wheeler, B. L. (2003). First International Symposium on Music Therapy Training: A retrospective examination. *Nordic Journal of Music Therapy, 12,* 54–66.

Wheeler, B. L. (2008). Edith Lecourt interviewed by Barbara Wheeler. *Voices: A World Forum for Music Therapy, 8*(3). Retrieved from *https://normt.uib.no/index.php/voices/article/view/425/349.*

Wheeler, B. L., & Baker, F. A. (2010). Influences of music therapists' worldviews on work in different countries. *Arts in Psychotherapy, 37,* 215–227.

Whitehead-Pleaux, A. (2012, October). The role of technology in multicultural music therapy practice. In A. Whitehead-Pleaux & X. Tan (Eds.), *Multicultural Music Therapy Institute: The intersections of music, health, and the individual manual.* Presented at the American Music Therapy Association National Conference, St. Charles, IL.

Whitehead-Pleaux, A., & Clark, S. (2009, November). *Changing keys: Moving from ethnocentrism to multiculturalism.* Paper presented at the American Music Therapy Association Conference, San Diego, CA.

Whitehead-Pleaux, A., Donnenwerth, A., Robinson, B., Hardy, S., Forinash, M., Oswanski, L., et al. (2012). Best practices in music therapy: LGBTQ. *Music Therapy Perspectives, 30,* 158–166.

Whitehead-Pleaux, A., Donnenwerth, A., Robinson, B., Hardy, S., Oswanski, L., Forinash, M., et al. (2013). Music therapists' attitudes and actions regarding the LGBTQ community: A preliminary report. *Arts in Psychotherapy, 40,* 409–414.

Young, L. (2009). Multicultural issues encountered in the supervision of music therapy internships in the USA and Canada. *Arts in Psychotherapy, 36,* 191–201.

CHAPTER 6

Ethics in Music Therapy

Debbie Bates

Ethics is _____. Take a moment to consider how you would fill in that blank—and be honest. Boring? Intimidating? Essential? Fun? Say the word ethics and people respond in many ways: groans, sighs—and sometimes a sense of excitement. Regardless of your response, it is important to recognize that ethics is at the heart of every facet of a music therapist's work, from advertising to assessment, treatment to termination, and documentation to data collection. Ethics affects every interaction in which a music therapist engages on a daily basis.

Ethics is broad topic that changes as clinical practice evolves. Just as it is nearly impossible for a code of ethics to address every possible ethical issue and dilemma, it is also nearly impossible to comprehensively cover every aspect of music therapy ethics in one chapter. Instead, consider this a brief introduction to ethics in music therapy. Following this introduction, foundational aspects of ethics are presented. Brief ethical dilemmas related to confidentiality, multiple relationships, and technology are described. The ethical issues

within the dilemmas are explored within the context of music therapy ethics in the United States.

Despite its importance, there is a dearth of literature about music therapy ethics, especially in music therapy journals. Only one book, Ethical Thinking in Music Therapy (Dileo, 2000), is entirely devoted to the topic. Given the vastness of the topic, highlighting ethical issues related to specific topics within music therapy is also valuable. Ethics chapters appear in several books, including Music Therapy Supervision (Forinash, 2001), Guided Imagery and Music: The Bonny Method and Beyond (Bruscia & Grocke, 2002), Music Therapy Research (Wheeler, 2005), and Feminist Perspectives in Music Therapy (Hadley, 2007). In 2011, the U.S. Certification Board for Music Therapists implemented a three-credit ethics requirement for every recertification cycle. It is anticipated that this requirement will increase the awareness of and interest in music therapy ethics and lead to more published articles and books on the topic.

Ethical thinking is a skill that develops over time and requires ongoing awareness, constant questioning, and personal responsibility (Pope & Keith-Spiegel, 2008). The multiple obligations and responsibilities, as one deals with an ethical dilemma or in day-to-day work, can make ethical awareness seem overwhelming. Time and experience enhance ethical thinking skills, so it is critical to begin developing these skills as early as possible. Developing ethical thinking skills and awareness helps music therapists to recognize the potential for an ethical dilemma and to seek resolution before the issue becomes truly problematic.

An ethical dilemma presents when equally relevant principles are in conflict with no clear solution (Greenfield & Jenson, 2010). Ethical dilemmas often have more than one viable option for resolution. The manner in which a person resolves a dilemma today might differ from how the same person would resolve the matter 5 years later. Most music therapists strive to uphold the highest ethical standards and to act in the best interest of their clients. However, Pope and Keith-Spiegel (2008) recognize that even the most experienced professional can make mistakes, overlook something, work from a limited perspective, reach an incorrect conclusion, or hold onto a misguided but cherished belief. Similarly, it is important to recognize that a perfect music therapist does not exist; nonetheless, music therapists should always strive to provide services and make decisions that are in the client's best interest.

Ethical Foundations

Merriam-Webster (n.d.) defines ethics as

> the discipline dealing with what is good and bad and with moral duty and obligation; a set of moral principles: a theory or system of moral values; the principles of conduct governing an individual or a group, such as professional ethics; a guiding principle; a consciousness of moral importance; a set of moral issues or aspects (as rightness).

Using this definition, it is not surprising that ethics may seem intimidating, as the responsibilities of ethical practice can feel daunting. However, music therapists, as helping professionals, have a responsibility to behave in an ethical manner (Dileo, 2000). Since right or wrong is rarely as clear as black or white, the challenge of ethical dilemmas frequently lies in the gray areas where the best resolution may be more right or less wrong. Whose right and whose wrong are under consideration? One music therapist might choose one resolution to an ethical dilemma, whereas another might take a completely different approach; both may be valid and feasible. The resolution that is in the client's best interest might conflict with a state law or institutional policy. Such areas that may be in conflict increase the complexity of the ethical decision-making process.

As implied by the definition, there are different types of ethics, and all are relevant to music therapy. Professional ethics are those behaviors and conduct that regulate professional practice (Calley, 2009) and encompass principle ethics, which focus on standards of clinical practice, such as those found within codes of ethics (Barnett, Behnke, Rosenthal, & Koocher, 2007). Virtue ethics are those that address underlying ethical principles and provide general guidance in decision making (Barnett et al.).

Similarly, there are many ethical principles to help guide professional behavior. These include beneficence ("do good"), nonmaleficence ("do no harm"), autonomy (patients' right to make decisions), and justice (the need for fairness and equality), which are consistently identified across literature (Barnett et al., 2007; Dileo, 2000; Greenfield & Jenson, 2010). Additionally, Dileo identified fidelity (honoring commitments), veracity (honesty), acknowledging dignity, acting with caring and compassion, striving for excellence, and acknowledging accountability (pp. 7–8) as core ethical principles for music therapists.

Let us consider these core ethical principles within a clinical context:

Jennifer is an 8-year-old oncology patient in a pediatric hospital. You have worked with her in music therapy during numerous admissions throughout her treatment. Her prognosis is very poor. Her parents adamantly refuse to tell her of the gravity of her condition so that she does not "lose hope." They tell the multidisciplinary team not to tell her, either. One afternoon during an individual session, Jennifer asks, "Am I going to die?"

The ethical principle of veracity suggests that music therapists must be honest and tell the truth. The principle of autonomy respects Jennifer's right to make choices about her own welfare and to be aware of her medical condition. However, fidelity requires that music therapists fulfill responsibilities and honor the commitments made to others; therefore, there is also an obligation to honor and respect the wishes of Jennifer's parents, who are the decision makers since Jennifer is a minor. Unfortunately, American Music Therapy Association's (AMTA; 2013a) Code of Ethics does not provide direct guidance for this particular dilemma, and the ethical principles previously identified conflict with each other. This is truly an ethical dilemma. If the code of ethics cannot provide guidance for every situation, why does it exist?

Ethical standards exist to protect clients, guide professional behavior, ensure professional autonomy, elevate the status of the profession, instill client and community trust in the profession, and outline collegial conduct among professionals (Calley, 2009). Like other helping professions, music therapists have a code of ethics that can help to guide ethical their decision making. It is important to understand that codes of ethics are created and adopted by professional associations. As a result, music therapy codes of ethics differ from country to country, and sometimes even within a country, if the country has more than one professional association. In countries where music therapy is still developing, codes of ethics may not yet exist.

To illustrate just one difference between codes, let's look at the applicability of codes of ethics. In the United States, AMTA Code of Ethics (AMTA, 2013a) applies only to its members and students/interns under the auspices of music therapy educators and internship directors. The Code of Ethics of the Australian Music Therapy Association is applicable only to its members; however, all registered music therapists must be members of the association (G. Thompson, personal communication, March 28, 2013). The Canadian Association for Music Therapy's (1999) Code of Ethics applies to members, although nonmembers are advised that courts or other public bodies could apply expectations for conduct contained within the Code of Ethics. The European Music Therapy Confederation (EMTC; 2005) requires compatibility of member organizations' codes of ethics with its Ethical Code, and the EMTC's Code applies only to individual professional members. Finally, the World Federation of Music Therapy (WFMT) provides an introduction to ethical practice, offers guidelines for professional associations to create music therapy codes of ethics, and contains statements describing ethical practice in music therapy, specifically related to ethics and informed-consent requirements for music therapy research publications and music therapy-related Internet and privacy issues (WFMT, 2013). These examples only highlight the differences in applicability for codes of ethics, and one can imagine the subtle differences contained within the various documents. Although similarities exist across codes of ethics of music therapy associations, variations are necessary due to the differences in clinical practice and other aspects of the associations and the countries that they represent.

Ethical codes provide a framework with which to interpret specific forms of conduct to regulate ethical behaviors of members of professional organizations, thereby providing guidance to professionals in the field (Calley, 2009). Additionally, codes of ethics function to

provide a moral template for professional conduct, provide a common ethical language to discuss cases with ethical content, indicate to society and other healthcare professionals a willingness to elevate the standard of practice, articulate the fiduciary responsibilities to clients, and to accept social responsibility and our role in contemporary healthcare. (Greenfield & Jenson, 2010, p. 89)

A code of ethics is often the first resource to use when faced with an ethical dilemma, although, as we have already seen, a code cannot address every possible ethical issue. Ethical dilemmas must be considered within the full context of a particular situation. When dealing with an ethical dilemma, state or local laws, facility-specific policies, and other relevant practice guidelines—such as AMTA Standards of Clinical Practice (AMTA, 2013b) or the U.S. Certification Board for Music Therapists (2010) Scope of Practice or Code of Professional Practice—may provide additional guidance in resolving an ethical dilemma. These tools may help to inform, but will not always determine, a music therapist's final decision when faced with an ethical dilemma.

Ethics are also influenced by an individual's values, morals, beliefs, and culture. Ethical thinking therefore requires a process of critical self-reflection about our personal and professional core values (Greenfield & Jenson, 2010). We must be aware of what our values are and of how our personal and professional values may influence our feelings or decision making within the therapy setting, or if our personal and professional values are in conflict.

Amber is a music therapist who works on an inpatient oncology unit. She does not support marriage equality and is uncomfortable with these relationships. She receives a new referral for Jerry, who is gay. Jerry's partner, Sam, is at the bedside when Amber arrives for the assessment session.

As a professional, Amber has a responsibility to uphold core ethical principles to acknowledge dignity and act with caring and compassion. However, she is also charged with nonmaleficence, which means she will "do no harm" (Dileo, 2000, p. 7). Will Amber be able to act authentically with caring and compassion when her personal values are in conflict? Is she at risk to unintentionally cause harm to Jerry?

Ethical dilemmas inevitably stir emotions, sometimes very strong, within us. These feelings can color or influence our perspective of a situation. So despite all of the available tools, working through ethical dilemmas requires honest self-reflection, thinking, and feeling. There are many models for resolving ethical dilemmas within counseling and psychology literature. Integrating concepts from numerous ethical decision-making models, Dileo (2000) outlines a 12-step model for resolving ethical dilemmas. Decision making steps in the model include (1) identifying problems and issues; (2) identifying to whom obligations are owed; (3) assessing emotional responses; (4) considering ethical principles, codes, laws, etc.; (5) considering the context and setting; (6) considering personal beliefs as well as those of the client; (7) consulting with trusted colleagues; (8) considering how the virtuous music therapist might respond; (9) generating solutions; (10) evaluating solutions and making a decision; (11) implementation; and (12) evaluation (p. 17). Be cognizant of these steps as ethical dilemmas are presented within the remainder of the chapter.

An Overview of Ethical Issues in Music Therapy

As you read the dilemmas that follow, be aware of your reactions and responses to the situations presented. Consider Dileo's

12-step model. Is an ethical dilemma present? If so, what are the problems? Consider the issues within the context of your culture or country's professional association. Does your code of ethics differ from what is presented in the discussion? Keeping in mind that an ethical dilemma may be resolved in multiple ways, how might you respond if you were the music therapist in the situation?

Confidentiality

Danielle is a music therapist who lives in the small, rural community where she also works. She often sees clients while she is running errands, out for dinner, or at the local coffee shop. She is uncertain about how to acknowledge clients when she is in the community.

Megan is a music therapist in private practice and has a website for her business. She frequently takes photos of her clients "in action" during music therapy sessions to post on her website and business Facebook page. She occasionally identifies clients by first name. She has not obtained consent from the clients to be photographed or to use the pictures on her websites.

Confidentiality is a cornerstone of professionalism (Fisher, 2008); foundational for the client to build trust, empathy, and a working alliance with the therapist; and protects the privacy of client information obtained through the fiduciary nature of a therapeutic relationship (Younggren & Harris, 2008). Confidentiality differs from privacy, which describes how much information can be shared with another person (Dileo, 2000). Privileged communication specifies that without the client's permission, information shared by the client in sessions is protected from disclosure in courts of law (Dileo). Every U.S. state has provisions regarding privileged communication that differ in scope and exceptions (Younggren & Harris). A LexisNexis database search found no U.S. laws or other information suggesting that privileged communication exists for clients in music therapy relationships, so it is presumed that privileged communication does not apply in music therapy relationships.

Confidentiality is more complex an issue than not sharing information revealed by clients within the music therapy session. For example, what if a client reveals the intent to harm him- or herself within a music therapy session? Are the expectations for confidentiality the same if the client is a minor? There are times in therapy when—legally or ethically—confidentiality may need to be breached. Most music therapy codes of ethics outline specific circumstances under which confidential information may be shared. The AMTA Code of Ethics (AMTA, 2013a) includes circumstances of imminent danger, collaboration with other professionals who are working with the client, a client's consent to release information, and by court or administrative order or subpoena. Confidentiality may also be compromised when billing for music therapy services is completed, if done by someone other than the music therapist (Dileo, 2000). Clients have the right to know about the limits to confidentiality, and this right is also identified as an expectation within AMTA Code of Ethics. Because confidentiality and informed consent are closely related, guidelines for informed consent are now explored.

Informed Consent

When confidentiality is conditional, fully explaining these conditions promotes clients' rights to be informed about the risk that confidentiality might be breached and to give (or refuse) consent to accept the risk to receive services (Fisher, 2008). Informed consent (1) respects clients' autonomous decision making regarding entering the therapeutic relationship and accepting the risks, (2) reflects the collaborative nature of therapy, (3) emphasizes clients' agency in making treatment decisions, and (4) may reduce anxiety about the therapeutic process (Fisher & Oransky, 2008).

Completed in writing and reviewed in person, a thorough informed-consent process includes, but is not limited to:

- The nature of treatment: a description of treatment, session duration and frequency, length of treatment, general goals, and interventions.
- Fees and financial arrangements: cost of sessions, payment options and plans, accepted insurance or other reimbursement, sliding scale fees, payment schedule, cancellation and missed appointment policies, and late or delinquent payment policies.
- Limits of confidentiality: legal requirements for disclosure of confidential information, duty to warn and protect, and information sharing with third-party payers (Dileo, 2000; Fisher & Oransky, 2008).
- Information about the music therapist: certifications, licensures, specialized training, participation in supervision and consultation, and how confidentiality will be maintained in this circumstance (Dileo, 2000).

Special considerations for confidentiality and consent are also required for minor clients or adult clients with diminished capacity to provide consent (Fisher & Oransky, 2008). Music therapists should be familiar with state and local laws when working with minors, as these vary by location (Dileo, 2000). For clients who are unable to provide consent, assent to participate in treatment is encouraged. Initially introduced in pediatric medical settings to give children a role in decision making, assent helps the client achieve a developmentally appropriate understanding of the nature of his or her condition, tells the client what to expect from tests or treatment, assesses the client's understanding of the situation, and asks about the client's willingness to accept the proposed treatment (Lee, Havens, Sato, Hoffman, & Leuthner, 2006). Similar to the informed-consent process, assent reinforces the ethical principles of autonomy and acknowledging dignity, and also collaborates with the client for treatment.

Reconsider the ethical dilemmas involving Danielle and Megan, described at the beginning of this section. Is confidentiality at risk? How so? What steps could each music therapist take to maintain confidentiality? In Danielle's scenario, her clients' confidentiality could be at risk when she sees them in the community, outside of the music therapy setting. Clients may not always recognize that public interactions could breach the confidentiality of the therapy relationship. For example, if either party is with another person, introductions can become challenging. However, if Danielle ignores a client in public, his or her feelings may be hurt. After Danielle considers the different options for managing public encounters, one aspect of her informed-consent process might include an explanation of how confidentiality will be maintained and how inevitable public meetings will be handled.

Although many ethical dilemmas have gray areas, Megan's situation is rather straightforward. Photographing clients without consent is not acceptable, as a photograph is considered identifiable client information. Using the photos on a website or Facebook page breaches confidentiality. The inclusion of client first names breaches confidentiality. The AMTA Code of Ethics (AMTA, 2013a) is helpful in this scenario; obtaining consent prior to acquiring any type of identifiable client information is outlined in 3.12.5. Even with photographic consent, the use of identifiable information, such as client names, is discouraged. If Megan wishes to use client photos on her website and Facebook page, in addition to obtaining consent, it would be proactive of her to include a statement wherever the photographs appear indicating that consent was obtained to use the photos. What steps could Megan take to remedy this situation?

Multiple Relationships

Joseph is a music therapist who works with children who have diagnoses on the autism spectrum. In his community, there are several music therapists who provide services for these children. His wife's best friend asks Joseph to provide music therapy services for her son, who was recently diagnosed with autism. She thinks it will be easier for her son to relate to Joseph, since they already know each other.

Multiple relationships, also referred to as dual relationships, are created when a helping professional undertakes more than one role or relationship, either simultaneously or sequentially, with a client (Ringstad, 2008). Boundaries refer to limits that distinguish professional behaviors intended to serve the good of the patient within the context of the therapeutic relationship (Jain & Roberts, 2009). It is important to recognize that there are different types of boundary offenses that differ in severity. Boundary crossings are behaviors, practices, or decisions that are clearly different from usual therapeutic practices and create an uncertain impact on treatment, whereas boundary violations are behaviors, practices, or decisions that depart from usual practices and are clearly harmful or exploitative to the client (Jain & Roberts). Just as there are different types of boundary offenses, there are two primary types of multiple relationships, sexual and nonsexual, the latter of which can be created in a variety of ways.

There is agreement across helping professions that sexual relationships between therapists and patients or former patients are always unethical and unacceptable. However, some assert that nonsexual multiple relationships may not be harmful and could actually be beneficial (Pope & Keith-Spiegel, 2008). Nonsexual multiple relationships can be created in a variety of ways, but include the categories of role, time, place or space, money, gifts, services, clothing, language, self-disclosure, or physical contact (Gutheil & Gabbard, 1993). Meeting a client socially, consistently going beyond session time, sharing therapeutically irrelevant personal information, bartering, and accepting or giving gifts can all be ways of creating multiple relationships.

Multiple relationships are problematic for several reasons: There is an inherent power differential between the therapist and the client (Dileo, 2000), so conflicts of interest can be created, placing the client at risk for exploitation and compromising the therapist's objectivity, thus endangering the therapeutic process (Ringstad, 2008). Engaging in multiple relationships may compromise many ethical principles, including autonomy, justice, fidelity, and acknowledging accountability. Autonomy may be comprised if a client feels as though he or she cannot decline engagement in a multiple relationship because of the power differential. Justice is in question, since the therapist is not likely to engage in multiple relationships with all clients. If the therapist's objectivity is comprised, fidelity may be at risk, as the therapist may be unable to adequately fulfill professional responsibilities to the client. Of course, the relevant ethical principles will depend on the type of relationship in question and the context of the situation. In Joseph's scenario, his objectivity in making clinical decisions could be compromised due to the preexisting relationship with the child and the child's mother.

The AMTA Code of Ethics (2013a) advises this: "The music therapist will not enter into dual relationships with clients, students, or research subjects and will avoid situations that interfere with professional judgment or objectivity" (3.5). However, changes in clinical practice make multiple relationships more challenging to navigate. Like Danielle in the earlier scenario, many music therapists live and work in small or rural communities, and multiple relationships may be impossible to avoid. It is not uncommon for music therapists to be invited to social events that mark milestones in a client's life. In deciding whether to accept an invitation, one consideration may be the role and context in which the offer is extended. Upon self-reflection, if the music therapist perceives that the invitation is purely social, it may be best to decline. If the music therapist is being invited in a professional context, fewer ethical dilemmas may be present. For example, hospice music therapists frequently attend or provide music for clients' memorial services. Although the ritual has a social quality, the context is still within the professional realm of the music therapist. Multiple relationships are complex and do not have simple answers. Depending on the music therapist's decision to create a multiple relationship, additional ethical dilemmas or questions can arise. For this reason, it is important to brainstorm as thoroughly as possible through all of the possible outcomes when trying to make any ethical decision. Let's consider more closely how multiple relationships can be created in ways other than specific dual roles by examining another scenario.

Gifts

Bernadette operates a private practice in music therapy. For Christmas, one of her client's families gives her an electric guitar that can be used by all of the clients she serves. Two weeks later, the family requests a schedule change that would impact two other clients and considerably lengthen Bernadette's workday.

When a gift is low in monetary value—a token of appreciation—the decision to accept may not be as difficult; however, when a gift is high in monetary value, the decision to accept can become more difficult. Music therapists will sometimes accept larger gifts that may benefit other clients,

as in Bernadette's scenario. However, it is still necessary to consider the implications and potential risks of accepting larger gifts. For example, because of the gift Bernadette was given, will she feel obligated to comply with the family's request to change the session time, even though it impacts other clients and her own schedule?

Music therapists should consider in advance how they would respond to gifts, as this situation is almost inevitable. Herlihy and Corey (2006) recommend considering the client's motivation for offering a gift, the client's diagnosis, the monetary value of the gift, stage and length of therapy, as well as the therapist's motivation for accepting or declining the gift. They also suggest that gifts that may provide financial benefit for the therapist, such as financial planning or stock tips, are rarely appropriate. Additional considerations are warranted when the gift is from a child or an adult who lacks the cognitive ability to work through or process the refusal of a gift (Herlihy & Corey). It is also important to consider the cultural background of the client offering the gift, as gifts have different meanings in some non-Western cultures (Dileo, 2000).

The AMTA Code of Ethics (2013a) provides guidance in this area and advises that gifts that could interfere with the music therapist's decisions or judgments should not be accepted. Facilities may have existing policies about what gifts are permissible for employees to accept, and these policies will provide additional guidelines for the music therapist. In addition, music therapists are encouraged to create their own policies regarding gifts and to share these policies with clients. Bernadette is in an especially difficult situation, as she has already accepted the gift and must determine if she will honor the family's request to change the session time or not. Could Bernadette's judgment be impaired in this situation? What would you do? As with most ethical dilemmas, accepting a gift must be evaluated within the context of the particular situation.

Technology

Now let's consider an ethical issue within an emerging area of practice:

Teresa is a music therapist who works in a hospital. She also supervises practicum students. She has "friended" several of her patients and students on Facebook and frequently "tweets" about her day.

Herlihy and Dufrene (2011) observe that codes of ethics may not be helpful when guidance is needed around new or emerging areas of practice. Many helping professions' codes of ethics, such as those of the American Psychological Association and American Counseling Association, are updated every 7–10 years, so being current is nearly impossible (Herlihy & Dufrene). One advantage is that time is allowed for emerging practices to develop more fully, so that appropriate guidelines can be created. The AMTA Code of Ethics (AMTA, 2013a) is a living document and, through a designated process, can be revised yearly to reflect changes in practice. Even so, it is not always feasible to update the code of ethics when an emerging practice is still uncertain or incomplete, as the revisions may not adequately address all of the issues. For example, in 2003, AMTA Code of Ethics was revised to include the Internet in item 10.6, announcing services. At that time, using the term Internet was sufficient because websites were much simpler in content, design, and layout, and social media did not exist. As technology has advanced, identifying specific and appropriate Internet content and venues on which to announce services may be warranted for a future revision. Technology is one emerging area that is underaddressed in AMTA Code of Ethics, represented only in items 3.12.5 and 10.6 (both previously referenced in this chapter). In 2010, the WFMT approved a document titled "Reporting on Music Therapy Clients on the Internet and Privacy Issues," but it primarily focuses on the use of sharing client information in public presentations.

The topic of technology is broad and can include devices used within music therapy sessions, such as switches or iPads or social media, cloud computing, and Skype. The focus of technology in this chapter is limited to digital means by which music therapists may connect with each other, the public, and clients. Social media, Internet calls and video chat, cloud computing, and the increased use of websites for advertising have emerged as technological tools used by music therapists. Technological advances have benefits, but many ethical dilemmas exist as well.

Music therapists connect with each other via Facebook, but what if a client sends a friend request? Many private practice owners have Facebook pages for their businesses and use Twitter to advocate for music therapy. Is confidentiality at risk if, immediately following a session, the music therapist tweets "My client just had an awesome breakthrough!"? Skype is often used to provide clinical supervision services, but what about providing music therapy services via Skype? Dropbox, Google Docs, and iPad apps can store clinical documentation or be used for client scheduling. Although these programs and applications provide easy access for the music therapist and can reduce costs, what about the security of the documents?

Music therapy websites have grown in number, design complexity, and information provided. Does the information provided on many websites, including testimonials, conflict with the guidelines set forth for announcing services within AMTA Code of Ethics (AMTA, 2013a)? Entrepreneurial music therapists make original songs and intervention ideas available under members only sections of their websites or sell products online. Is this consistent with not engaging in commercial activities that conflict with responsibilities to clients or colleagues (AMTA, 2013a)? The ethical issues are numerous and complex; the benefits as well as the risks must be considered in emerging areas of practice. Ethical issues related to social media and computer-mediated music therapy are briefly explored next (although it is important to acknowledge that the information in this section of the chapter may also become quickly outdated!).

Social Media

With the broad use of social networking sites, both professionally and personally, a new type of professionalism has emerged: E-professionalism is the "impact of online behavior on one's professionalism" (Bradt, 2010, para. 1). Many possible relationship interactions exist for music therapists on social networking sites: clients, students, interns, employers, other professionals, and the general public. Although ethical implications may vary slightly depending upon the relationship, the broad ethical issues relate to privacy, confidentiality, boundaries, and multiple relationships that can be created through social media.

Although some clinicians in other helping professions believe that informal communication via social media humanizes the therapeutic relationship and increases practitioner accessibility (Reamer, 2013), multiple challenges are associated with online relationships. Because social networking is so prevalent, clients, students, or interns may not consider that interacting with a therapist, educator, or supervisor through this medium is inappropriate. Expectations associated with a relationship via social media may be different because social is in inherent in the name. Social networking interactions are often less formal or professional than interactions that occur in person. Known as the online disinhibition effect (Barros-Bailey & Saunders, 2010), there is a sense of anonymity when interacting online, which, for the client, student, or music therapist, could lead to problematic or unintended self-disclosures that may not have occurred during in-person interactions (Reamer, 2013; Taylor, McMinn, Bufford,

& Chang, 2010). Social media relationships may create interactions that are not part of the therapeutic relationship, do not prioritize the therapeutic interests of the client (or student), and may put confidentiality at risk, as clients may not recognize that they could be surrendering their anonymity by submitting a friend request to the therapist (Guseh, Brendel, & Brendel, 2009).

It is not uncommon for facilities or institutions to use social networking via Facebook, Twitter, or blogs. However, as employees, music therapists should be aware of organizational policies regarding personal social media use. Posting about workplace issues or making negative statements about an employer should be avoided. In addition to being unprofessional, incidences of employees being fired for inappropriate social media posts are growing in prevalence (Greysen, Kind, & Chretien, 2010). Music therapists are also cautioned that employers may use Internet search engines or read personal websites or blogs to learn about applicants or employees (Bradt, 2010). Music therapists are urged to be aware that their digital footprint—that is, the pieces of digital information that are left behind with some online interactions—is searchable and therefore may be visible to others (Greysen et al., 2010).

Music therapists are encouraged to consider in advance how they will manage interactions, such as accepting friend requests, with clients, students, or interns via social media, including consideration of what might be said in a conversation about engaging in social media or declining a friend request. Although privacy settings are not foolproof and change frequently, it is still wise to utilize them. Discretion is encouraged when adding personal information or posting on social networking sites (Guseh et al., 2009). Additionally, creating specific friend lists with limited accessibility may also help to prevent inadvertent information sharing (Taylor et al., 2010). Pseudonyms (Guseh et al., 2009), as well as altering the spelling of one's name (e.g., Ddebbie Bbates) or using an alternate e-mail address, may provide a degree of therapist anonymity from online or social networking search engines.

Conclusions

As mentioned previously, it is impossible for a code of ethics to address every possible ethical dilemma, so it is important to briefly consider how one might proceed if the code of ethics does not provide adequate guidance for an ethical dilemma. In the absence of clear guidelines from the code of ethics, it is important to be able to isolate the ethical issues at the center of the dilemma. Review the code of ethics for your professional association thoroughly and look for related items that may be relevant. Although the code may not specifically address an issue, related items may provide some guidance in decision making. If similar issues exist in other helping professions, search the literature for insight into your situation. Consult with trusted and knowledgeable colleagues. Seek clinical supervision and proceed with caution.

This chapter highlights some of the myriad ethical issues encountered in music therapy. Ethics in music therapy is a broad but fascinating topic that is foundational to the practice of music therapy. Ethical decision making is complex because it is guided by ethical principles, codes of ethics, laws, and institutional policies and is influenced by personal values and beliefs. Ethical reflection begins with critical self-reflection on personal and professional values (Greenfield & Jenson, 2010). Calley (2009) notes that "adopting a contextual understanding of the role of ethics within specific counseling settings requires that the counselor takes a proactive approach to ethics, spending time engaging in much 'process thinking,' exploring the various ways in which specific ethical issues may be translated into practice" (p. 478). Hopefully, this chapter has raised awareness of

music therapy ethics and encouraged you to begin honing your ethical thinking skills now. Like our musical skills, ethical thinking becomes more refined with practice.

REFERENCES

American Music Therapy Association (AMTA). (2013a). *Code of ethics*. Retrieved from *www.musictherapy.org/about/ethics*.

American Music Therapy Association (AMTA). (2013b). *AMTA standards of clinical practice*. Retrieved from *www.musictherapy.org/about/standards*.

Barnett, J., Behnke, S., Rosenthal, S., & Koocher, G. (2007). In case of ethical dilemma, break glass: Commentary on ethical decision making in practice. *Professional Psychology: Research and Practice, 38*(1), 7–12.

Barros-Bailey, M., & Saunders, J. (2010). Ethics and the use of technology in rehabilitation counseling. *Rehabilitation Counseling Bulletin, 53*(4), 255–259.

Bradt, J. (2010). E-professionalism. *Voices: A World Forum for Music Therapy*. Retrieved from http://testvoices.uib.no/?q=colbradt250110.

Bruscia, K. E., & Grocke, D. E. (Eds.). (2002). *Guided Imagery and Music: The Bonny method and beyond*. Gilsum, NH: Barcelona.

Calley, N. (2009). Promoting a contextual perspective in the application of the ACA Code of Ethics: The ethics into action map. *Journal of Counseling and Development, 87*(4), 476–482.

Canadian Association of Music Therapy. (1999). *Code of ethics*. Retrieved from *www.musictherapy.ca/documents/official/codeofethics99.pdf*.

Certification Board for Music Therapists. (2010). *Scope of practice*. Retrieved from *www.cbmt.org*.

Dileo, C. (2000). *Ethical thinking in music therapy*. Cherry Hill, NJ: Jeffrey Books.

Ethics. (n.d.). In *Merriam-Webster.com*. Retrieved from *www.merriam-webster.com/dictionary/ethics*.

European Music Therapy Confederation. (2005). *Ethical code*. Retrieved from *http://emtc-eu.com/ethical-code*.

Fisher, C., & Oransky, M. (2008). Informed consent to psychotherapy: Protecting the dignity and respecting the autonomy of patients. *Journal of Clinical Psychology: In Session, 64*(5), 576–588.

Fisher, M. (2008). Protecting confidentiality rights: The need for an ethical practice model. *American Psychologist, 63*(1), 1–13.

Forinash, M. (Ed.). (2011). *Music therapy supervision*. Gilsum, NH: Barcelona.

Greenfield, B., & Jenson, G. (2010). Beyond a code of ethics: Phenomenological ethics for everyday practice. *Physiotherapy Research International, 15,* 88–95.

Greysen, S., Kind, T., & Chretien, K. (2010). Online professionalism and the mirror of social media. *Journal of General Internal Medicine, 25*(11), 1227–1229.

Guseh, J., Brendel, R., & Brendel, D. (2009). Medical professionalism in the age of online social networking. *Journal of Medical Ethics, 35,* 584–586.

Gutheil, T., & Gabbard, G. (1993). The concept of boundaries in clinical practice: Theoretical and risk-management dimensions. *American Journal of Psychiatry, 150*(2), 188–196.

Hadley, S. (Ed.). (2007). *Feminist perspectives in music therapy.* Gilsum, NH: Barcelona.

Herlihy, B., & Corey, G. (2006). *Boundary issues in counseling: Multiple roles and responsibilities.* Alexandria, VA: ACA Press.

Herlihy, B., & Dufrene, R. (2011). Current and emerging ethical issues in counseling: A Delphi study of expert opinions. *Counseling and Values, 56,* 10–24.

Jain, S., & Roberts, L. (2009). Ethics in psychotherapy: A focus on professional boundaries and confidentiality practices. *Psychiatric Clinics of North America, 32*(2), 299–314.

Lee, K., Havens, P., Sato, T., Hoffman, G., & Leuthner, S. (2006). Assent for treatment: Clinician knowledge, attitudes, and practice. *Pediatrics, 118*(2), 723–730.

Pope, K., & Keith-Spiegel, P. (2008). A practical approach to boundaries in psychotherapy: Making decisions, bypassing blunders, and mending fences. *Journal of Clinical Psychology: In Session, 64*(5), 638–652.

Reamer, F. (2013). Social work in a digital age: ethical and risk management challenges. *Social Work, 58*(2), 163–172.

Ringstad, R. (2008). The ethics of dual relationships: Beliefs and behaviors of clinical practitioners. *Families in Society: The Journal of Contemporary Social Services, 89*(1), 69–77.

Taylor, L., McMinn, M., Bufford, R., & Chang, K. (2010). Psychologists' attitudes and ethical concerns regarding the use of social networking web sites. *Professional Psychology: Research and Practice, 41*(2), 153–159.

Wheeler, B. L. (Ed.). (2005). *Music therapy research* (2nd ed.). Gilsum, NH: Barcelona.

World Federation of Music Therapy. (2010). *Reporting on music therapy clients on the Internet and privacy issues.* Retrieved from *www.musictherapyworld.net/WFMT/Research_and_Ethics_files/Internet%20and%20Privacy%20Issues%20related%20to%20Music%20Therapy.pdf.*

World Federation of Music Therapy. (2013). *Commission: Research and Ethics.* Retrieved from *www.musictherapyworld.net/WFMT/Research_and_Ethics.html.*

Younggren, J., & Harris, E. (2008). Can you keep a secret?: Confidentiality in psychotherapy. *Journal of Clinical Psychology: In Session, 64*(5), 589–600.

CHAPTER 7

Music Therapy Assessment

Anne W. Lipe

Music therapists frequently find themselves in a creative tension between the art of *music* and the science of *therapy*. How do they balance these two elements in such a way that the strengths of both bear fruit in the lives of clients and in the growth of the profession? Feder and Feder (1988) note that both are necessary in the arts therapy arena: "Without science, therapy can degenerate to the practice of superstitious ritual, in which each practitioner owes allegiance only to his or her personal myth of existence. Without art, it can lose the very humanity it seeks to examine" (p. ix). To reframe this idea, without science, music therapy becomes indistinguishable from what might be offered by a well-meaning hospital staff member who plays the flute to assist in a support group on an oncology unit. Without art (in a generic sense), music therapy morphs into a form of occupational, speech, or physical therapy, albeit with music. It is my belief that well-constructed, well-validated music-based assessment tools and protocols allow music therapists to successfully practice within this creative tension.

We begin by examining the directives regarding assessment that are contained in professional documents and then setting these directives within a historical framework. Important terms are defined, and the central importance of *musicality* is discussed. Extended definitions of key terms associated with *psychometrics* are offered, and the role of this type of research in music therapy assessment is explored. Selected examples of assessment approaches in current music therapy practice are presented and evaluated, guidelines for developing an assessment tool or protocol are offered, and reflections on the importance of *evidence-based* assessment conclude the chapter.

Why *music-based* assessment procedures? Some music therapy professionals have argued that since music experiences are generally pleasurable for most people, such experiences may reduce the anxiety associated with testing situations (Hanser, 1987). Music-based approaches also may offer opportunities for increased self-disclosure, for nonverbal and symbolic communication, and may allow clients to be observed "in process" (Bruscia, 1988, p. 7). Although these are important assumptions, other questions also need to be asked. What information do musical behaviors provide about a client's functional status? How do we understand what musical behaviors mean to the client and within the context of therapy? How do we accurately interpret this information to develop a successful treatment plan? Is there something unique about the music experience that has the potential to enable change? It is the job of the assessment process to answer these questions in ways that are ethical, that rely on scientific evidence, and that demonstrate professional accountability.

Music Therapy Assessment in Professional Documents

It is difficult to determine an exact point in the history of modern music therapy practice when a unique music therapy assessment became a part of a potential client's experience. A detailed discussion of early developments in assessment can be found in Wheeler (2013), where it is made clear that assessment has been an important part of music therapy practice since the early 1960s.

An examination of the contents of professional documents serves as a starting point for understanding the music therapist's obligations during the assessment process. According to Solomon (1985), there was an awareness of the need for professional standards of practice during the formative years (1950s–1960s) of the modern profession of music therapy in the United States, and efforts to develop such a document arose out of a desire of the young profession to establish itself in the medical community. According to Bryan Hunter (personal communication, December 6, 2012), the standards of practice used by occupational therapists were particularly well informed and helpful in guiding music therapists' efforts. The first Standards of Practice for the National Association for Music Therapy (NAMT) were adopted in November 1982 and have been revised several times, with the latest revision approved in 2013. The standards contain seven items relating to assessment, directing the music therapist to (1) identify general categories that the assessment should include, (2) be sensitive to client cultural and demographic characteristics, (3) select methods of assessment that reflect client preferences and functional ability, (4) appropriately and accurately interpret results of standardized tests and other aspects of the assessment situation, (5) include the results of music therapy assessment in the client's file, (6) make a final decision about the appropriateness of music therapy services, (7) if indicated, make appropriate referrals to other professionals, and (8) and (9) include current diagnosis and evaluate skill levels in several functional domains (American Music Therapy Association [AMTA], 2013).

Additional information on assessment can be found in the *Scope of Practice* of the Certification Board for Music Therapists (CBMT; 2010), which defines 30 specific skills that may be needed to properly conduct an assessment and interpret its results. These documents provide the practicing music therapist with sufficient guidance to develop assessment procedures that have professional integrity and that meet the needs of the client and the clinical environment.

Definitions, Purposes, and Types of Assessments

Definitions of assessment vary considerably depending upon the context in which the term is used. The *AMTA Standards of Practice* (AMTA, 2013) define it as "the process of determining the client's present level of functioning," and in the standard clinical process, it follows referral and precedes development of a treatment plan. Definitions of assessment in music therapy also emphasize musical engagement as a way to understand the client and to determine what needs and resources the individual brings to the therapeutic process (Bruscia, 1998). Meadows, Wheeler, Shultis, and Polen (2005) note that music therapy assessment can be formal or informal, should have a defined goal or purpose, should utilize appropriately chosen music tasks to provide information about a client's skills and abilities, and should be documented and communicated to the appropriate treatment team (p. 28).

Purposes of assessment and approaches to assessment vary from one setting to another. Traditionally, music therapy assessments have not performed a diagnostic function, although recent developments are moving the profession in this direction (Magee, Siegert, Daveson, Lenton-Smith, & Taylor, 2013). Bruscia (1998) indicates that music therapy assessments might be *interpretive*, in which there is an attempt to explain observations in terms of theory or other frames of reference; *descriptive*, in which observations provide an overall picture of a client's functional status in selected domains; *prescriptive*, in which observations suggest a direction for treatment goals and objectives; or *evaluative*, in which observations serve as a baseline to measure the effectiveness of the treatment interventions. Wheeler (2013) provides specific examples of music therapy assessments that reflect each of these purposes.

In most assessment situations, it is common to gather information using both informal methods, such as interviews and questionnaires, and formal methods such as standardized tests, tools, or inventories. Formal methods might include the use of Likert scales to evaluate musical preferences or to evaluate responses to music listening or performance tasks, or these methods may involve the use of standardized or norm-referenced tests. Information may be gathered directly from the client or from a family member or close friend. Systematic observation of musical behavior is another common method used in music therapy assessment, and may or may not include a scoring protocol.

Terms and Concepts Associated with Psychometrics

It is stating the obvious to note that *music experience* and its meaning are front and center in music therapy. Radocy and Boyle (1997) indicate that *music ability* involves the ability to "do something" with music (p. 334). They further define *musicality* as "a state of being 'musical,' of being sensitive to changes in a musical stimulus" (p. 335). In an earlier text, Radocy and Boyle (1988) differentiated musicality from other terms closely associated with it, such as talent, capacity, and aptitude. *Talent* implies exceptional music ability as determined by two factors: musical *capacity*, which includes genetic and maturational components, and *aptitude*, which involves a predisposition to musical talent shaped both by genetic and environmental determinants (Radocy & Boyle, 1988, pp. 295–296). All of these concepts are important for assessment because, as music therapists, we deal primarily with constructs, of which musicality is central. A *construct* is defined as a hypothetical psychological attribute that cannot be measured directly, so its presence must be inferred through observed behaviors (Crocker & Algina, 1986). We cannot directly observe musicality, so we infer its existence by designated behaviors such as singing, playing an instrument in rhythm, or moving rhythmically to music. In the assessment process, it is important that the construct of interest be clearly represented through the behaviors that are chosen to define it. When we are clear about defining a construct in the context of a specific clinical situation, then we are in a better position to measure that construct and to make reasonable inferences about the meaning of the behaviors that we observe.

Inventories, tools, tests, and *instruments* are terms that are frequently used interchangeably in the literature and refer to procedures that may have undergone psychometric research. This type of research uses statistical methods to examine an instrument's *reliability* and *validity.* When a researcher does a reliability study, the focus is on the degree to which the tool provides consistent, stable results over time. Detailed descriptions of reliability and validity and accompanying statistical methodology are found in Wheeler (2013) and in Boyle and Radocy (1987). The literature also contains reports of *interrater reliability* or *agreement.* These reports typically are used for tools that gather information based on systematic observation. The statistics reflect the degree of similarity with which different observers rate or score study participants on the tool's items (see Layman, Hussey, & Laing, 2002; Mahoney, 2010). Reliability of instruments used in music therapy assessment is important because when instruments are used to establish a baseline against which the effectiveness of treatment intervention can be measured, the therapist needs assurance that therapeutic change is indeed change and not simply an artifact of a mediocre tool.

When a psychometric researcher performs a validity study, he or she is interested in the degree to which the tool being tested actually measures what it is intended to measure. *Content validity* typically is done during the instrument's development stage and involves the degree to which the items on the instrument represent the *domain* of interest. Good descriptions of the content validity process are found in Douglass (2006) and York (1994). Next, the researcher considers *criterion-related validity,* which involves evaluating how well the new tool might predict behavior, or how well it reflects similar behaviors measured by existing, psychometrically stable tools. In va-

lidity testing of the newly developed Music-Based Evaluation of Cognitive Functioning (MBECF) for individuals with dementia, I (Lipe, 1995) selected three standard mental status tests: the Mini-Mental State Examination (MMSE; Folstein, Folstein, & McHugh, 1975), the Brief Cognitive Rating Scale (BCRS; Reisberg, Schneck, Ferris, Schwartz, & DeLeon, 1983), and the Severe Impairment Battery (Saxton & Swihart, 1989). Strong correlations between scores on the MBECF and these three measures demonstrated that the MBECF performs similar functions as do more established measures.

Construct validity involves evaluating the degree to which a tool accurately reflects an underlying psychological attribute and/or theoretical foundation. It requires precise definition and fleshing out of the construct of interest. Theory was implicitly present in the study described above (Lipe, 1995), as the MMSE, the oldest of these tools, was originally validated using the Wechsler Adult Intelligence Scale (Verbal and Performance scores). This test emerged out of Wechsler's view of intelligence as "a many-faceted entity, a complex of diverse and numerous components" (Wechsler, 1975, p. 135). In a later study, my colleagues and I (Lipe, York, & Jensen, 2007) found strong relationships between two music-based tools designed for use among older adults with dementia, and when compared with the MMSE (Folstein et al., 1975), concluded that these tools strongly represented *music cognition* in this population. We concluded that "'music cognition' is a multidimensional construct comprised of rhythm, singing and melodic skills which can be uniquely identified, but which are not independent of each other" (p. 381).

Why is it important for music therapy clinicians to understand validity? First, developing tools to use in assessment situations makes our lives easier. For example, we do not have to replicate what the speech or occupational therapist is doing, but can develop uniquely music-based tools that tap into similar skills. Validity testing is what demonstrates the strength of these connections. Second, without validity testing we do not have a strong foundation from which to draw extramusical inferences based on the responses we observe in our clients.

Psychometric testing is the process used to standardize our tools and procedures. Standardized tools can be an important part of the assessment process because they may provide baseline information against which progress toward goals and objectives can be measured. It is the use of these tools that connects assessment to the evaluative purpose identified by Bruscia (1998), since the same tool can be used at different points during therapy to determine progress toward treatment goals. Likewise, the use of standardized tools might make a stronger case in an interpretive context, since a theoretical framework is frequently part of the validation process.

Although not typically used in music therapy practice, *norm-referenced* tests of music ability or aptitude have appeared in the music therapy literature. Norm-referenced tools compare an individual's score to that of a large sample representative of a designated population (Boyle & Radocy, 1987; Crocker & Algina, 1986). Because these tools are frequently used in both psychological and educational settings, music therapists practicing in these areas need a working knowledge of how they are developed and how scores are interpreted. Researchers have used norm-referenced tests to describe music aptitude among children with hearing impairments (Darrow, 1987) and older adults (Gibbons, 1983a, 1983b), music perception among adult cochlear implant users (Gfeller & Lansing, 1992), and sound conceptualization among visually impaired students (Madsen & Darrow, 1989). The use of these tests in the music therapy literature is infrequent, and study samples are small. In all cases where they

are used, researchers draw upon the results of studies to make specific recommendations for clinical practice options.

Assessment in Music Therapy Practice

This section includes selected examples of music therapy assessments drawn from the literature (see Table 7.1). These examples are from scholarly journals or texts that have appeared in the last 20 years or so (1992–2012). Although this time range is somewhat arbitrary, the assessment literature prior to 1992 is limited, and it is difficult to determine whether these early tools are currently in use. Two exceptions are the Improvisation Assessment Profiles (IAPs) (Bruscia, 1987) and the three scales developed to evaluate children's musical responses using the Nordoff–Robbins approach (Nordoff & Robbins, 1977, 2007), discussed below.

In addition to hand searches of the *Journal of Music Therapy, Music Therapy Perspectives*, and several music therapy texts, computer searches were done on the *Nordic Journal of Music Therapy* (2000–2012), the *Canadian Journal of Music Therapy* (2009–2012), and the *Australian Journal of Music Therapy* (2003–2012). Included are references in which actual tools or processes are published. References that were excluded were those in which assessment procedures were described in general ways, or those that have appeared in conference presentations, dissertations, or theses. Several studies that appear in the literature present results of surveys on the assessment practices of clinicians working with various population groups (Cassity & Cassity, 1994; Chase, 2004; Codding, 2002; Silverman, 2007; Wilson & Smith, 2000); these also were excluded from the review.

Several conclusions can be drawn from an examination of this list. First, 50% of the assessments in this list are behavior checklists. In most cases, a rationale for the choice of behaviors that appears in the checklist is provided. In most instruments, the choice of a specific music protocol is left up to the individual therapist, although some authors offer suggestions for conducting the assessments, which usually follow a music therapy session format.

Second, several tools are extensive assessments that have been published separately. The Special Education Music Therapy Assessment Process (SEMTAP; Brunk & Coleman, 1999) is often referred to in the literature and appears to be widely used. A supplement to this tool, the recently published Music Therapy Special Education Assessment Scale (MT-SEAS) provides a scoring system for the SEMTAP and organizes its domains using developmental milestones (Bradfield, Carlenius, Gold, & White, 2014). Several references were found to the Individualized Music Therapy Assessment Profile (IMTAP; Baxter et al., 2007) and to the Musical Assessment of Gerontologic Needs and Treatment (MAGNET; Adler, 2001). These are extensive tools, and portions of them might be useful for specific purposes or in certain clinical situations. Practitioners need to be aware, though, that these assessments are not standardized in the way that the term was defined above.

Third, psychometric data are reported for six instruments (Bruscia, 2000; Daveson, Magee, Crewe, Beaumont, & Kenealy, 2007; Jeong & Lesiuk, 2011; Layman et al., 2002; Lipe, 1995; Lipe et al., 2007; Magee et al., 2013; Meadows, 2000; O'Kelly & Magee, 2013; York, 1994). All of these instruments contain a designated scoring system and, with the exception of the Beech Brook Music Therapy Assessment (Layman et al.), a specific music protocol. In order to successfully use these instruments, practitioners need to understand how to interpret the psychometric information provided and how to use that information to draw meaningful conclusions about client responses and subsequent music therapy treatment options. Practitioners who use these tools should also be cautioned not to add, delete, or change items, since doing so compromises the tool's psychometric integrity and jeopardizes any conclusions that may be drawn from results.

Nordoff–Robbins Music Therapy (NRMT) has been in use for several decades and is widely practiced in the United States and abroad. Mahoney (2010) found a "healthy degree" (p. 27) of interrater agreement on the Client–Therapist Relationship in Musical Activity Scale. NRMT also provides the foundation for the Individual Music-Centered Assessment Profile for Neurodevelopmental Disorders (IMCAP-ND; Carpente, 2013), which contains three separate scales, a 5-point scoring system for frequency of response, level of support needed, and medium of client response. To date, no psychometric testing has been done on this tool.

It also is important for music therapists to be knowledgeable about assessment instruments used by other professionals. Darrow (1989) presents detailed procedures for the assessment of auditory training, speech production, and language development among hearing-impaired children and suggests nine additional tests that might be used by music therapists in this type of assessment. Hobson (2006) describes testing procedures used by speech–language pathologists (SLPs) and recommends ways in which music therapists and SLPs can collaborate in the assessment process. She notes that SLP assessments require specialized training, but that music therapists should understand how to interpret and apply the results of these tests in formulating music therapy treatment goals (Hobson, 2006, p. 60). Weller and Baker (2011) reviewed the literature in music therapy and physical rehabilitation and identified areas of functioning that music therapists may or may not be trained to assess. Groen (2007) provides information on several standardized pain assessments used by both music therapists and registered nurses in palliative care settings.

TABLE 7.1. Selected Assessment Instruments: 1992–2013

Author(s)	Title	Purpose	Type of tool	No. of domains	Music protocol	Scoring	Psychometric information
Ko & Moon (2014)	Korean Music-Based Evaluation of Cognitive Functioning (K-MBECF)	Evaluate cognitive functioning in older adults with dementia	Systematic observation	1	19 specific singing, verbal, melodic, and rhythm tasks	0–3 for each task	Strong concurrent and known groups validity; strong internal consistency and inter-rater reliability
Betz & Held (2013a)	Betz Held Strengths Inventory for Children with Disabilities	Identify behavioral strengths in children with multiple severe disabilities	Video observation and behavior analysis	4	Suggestions provided for music therapy cues to elicit potential strengths	Detailed procedures provided for scoring in both cue and response categories	None
Betz & Held (2013b)	Betz Held Strengths Inventory for Infants and Toddlers	Identify emerging behavioral strengths in the development of infants and toddlers	Video observation and behavior analysis	5	Suggestions provided for 67 music and art cues to elicit 35 potential strengths	Detailed procedures provided for scoring in both cue and response categories	None
Norman (2012)	Music Therapy Assessment	Descriptive and prescriptive for nursing home residents	Behavior checklist	6	Recommendations provided	None	None
Jeong & Lesiuk (2011)	Music-Based Attention Assessment (MAA)	Evaluate attention in patients with TBI	Systematic observation	1	48 items; 3 subtests; various melodic contours	0–1	Acceptable item discrimination and difficulty; high internal consistency; confirmatory factor analysis on a 45-item revised test (MAA-R) identified five factors;

Author (Year)	Name of tool	Purpose	Type	Number	Items/tasks	Rating scale	Reliability/validity
							high internal consistency (Jeong, 2013)
Langan (2009)	Music Therapy Special Education Assessment Tool	Evaluate therapeutic process as related to curriculum goals	Behavior checklist	8	None—assessment attempts to reflect content of music therapy sessions	None	None
Snow (2009)	Music Therapy Assessment Tool for Adults with DD	Evaluative	Systematic observation	8 scales	6 specific tasks	1–5	Reliability and construct validity are mentioned, but no data are reported
Magee (2007)	Music Therapy Assessment Tool for Awareness in Disorders of Consciousness (MATADOC)	Diagnose and prescribe correct music therapy treatment for patients in minimally conscious states	Systematic observation	5	14 items in 3 subscales using designated musical stimuli. One assessment = 4 sessions within 10-day period	0–7; ratings differ from item to item	Strong concurrent validity (Daveson et al., 2007); strong diagnostic agreement with reference standard (O'Kelly & Magee, 2013); for Subscale I: good internal consistency, inter- and intrarater reliability, and strong first principal component (Magee et al., 2013)
Rohrbacher (2007)	Assessment of Functions of Music Therapy (AFMT)	Program design for older adults in community settings	Behavior checklist	6	None provided	1–5 throughout all domains	None
Baxter et al. (2007)	Individualized Music Therapy Assessment Profile (IMTAP)	Multilevel assessment for children and adolescents	Behavior checklist	10	None provided; case examples of sessions given	Rating scale based on % of time response is observed	None

(continued)

TABLE 7.1. *(continued)*

Author(s)	Title	Purpose	Type of tool	No. of domains	Music protocol	Scoring	Psychometric information
Maue-Johnson & Tanguay (2006)	Hospice Music Therapy Assessment	Descriptive and prescriptive	Behavior checklist	6	None provided	None	None
Douglass (2006)	Pediatric Inpatient Music Therapy Assessment Form (PIMTAF)	Descriptive and prescriptive	Behavior checklist	6	None provided	None	None
Layman, Hussey, & Laing (2002)	Beech Brook Music Therapy Assessment	Evaluation of children with emotional disorders	Systematic observation	4	Suggests age-appropriate live music with a variety of instruments	−2 to +2	Strong interrater reliability
Adler (2001)	Musical Assessment of Gerontologic Needs and Treatment (MAGNET)	Descriptive and prescriptive; designed to complement the Minimum Data Set	Behavior checklist	13	Model session provided	None	None
Hintz (2000)	Geriatric Music Therapy Clinical Assessment	Descriptive, prescriptive, evaluative	Behavior checklist	5	None provided	0–3 for each domain	None
Loewy (2000)	Music Psychotherapy Assessment	Reveal themes to serve as baseline for treatment	Descriptive analysis	13 areas of inquiry	Components of the session are described; case examples given	None	None
Wolfe (2000)	Music Therapy Services,	Prescriptive, evaluative	Client survey	7	None provided	None	None

84

	Purpose	Method	Number	Format	Scoring	Reliability/Validity
Relaxation, and Stress Management Assessment						
Bruscia (2000) GIM Responsiveness Scale (GIMR)	Systematically observe a traveler's experience	Systematic observation	5	Standard GIM protocol	1–5	Strong interrater reliability; good content validity; limited construct-related validity (Meadows, 2000)
Brunk & Coleman (1999) Special Education Music Therapy Assessment Process (SEMTAP)	Determine usefulness of MT in meeting IEP objectives	Not a tool but a process	Determined by child's IEP	MT session format based on child's IEP objectives	None	None
Lipe (1995) Music-Based Evaluation of Cognitive Functioning (MBECF)	Evaluate cognitive functioning in older adults with dementia	Systematic observation	1	19 specific singing, verbal, melodic, and rhythm tasks	0–3 for each task	Strong test–retest reliability and internal consistency; strong known-groups and criterion validity (Lipe, 1995); strong construct validity (Lipe, York, & Jensen, 2007)
York (1994) Residual Music Skills Test (RMST)	Evaluate residual music skills in people with Alzheimer's disease	Systematic observation	6	11 specific singing, verbal, rhythm, and movement tasks	0–31; varies by task	Strong interrater reliability and criterion validity (York, 1994); strong test–retest reliability (York, 2000) and construct validity (Lipe, York, & Jensen, 2007)

Note. DD, dual diagnosis; MT, music therapy; TBI, traumatic brain injury.

Development of Music Therapy Assessment Instruments/ Procedures

Given the information provided above, how should the music therapist proceed if it is necessary to develop an assessment for his or her own clinical use? The steps listed below are taken from my own experience and from guidelines suggested by Benson and Clark (1982).

• *Step 1: Specify the purpose of the assessment.* Be as specific as possible. Isenberg-Grzeda (1988) suggests five parameters that might be helpful in assessment design: the music, the population, institutional requirements, and the therapist's treatment philosophy and personal skill set. Focus on one or two domains that are most frequently addressed in your setting.

• *Step 2: Content validation phase.* Review the literature to see what is already being used. Focus on music therapy techniques and approaches that have been successful in meeting the treatment objectives most pertinent to your clinical setting. Solicit suggestions from colleagues: What approaches have been successful in their practice? Also review standardized tools used by other treatment team members in your setting. Consider how information on responses to music might add additional or unique information to a client's profile. Begin to develop an item format (e.g., behavior checklist, systematic observation) and consider how the items might be scored. Decide on the music tasks that should be included and whether several types of tasks are appropriate or whether one approach is preferred (e.g., rhythm tasks, improvisational tasks). Once a draft has been developed, share it with colleagues and solicit their feedback: Do the items reflect current practice? Are directions clear? Is the scoring sufficient to reflect the diversity of client response? Pilot test the tool with small groups of clients and make necessary revisions.

• *Step 3: Quantitative evaluation.* The first phase of psychometric testing typically involves measuring the instrument's reliability, as described above. This step may include an item analysis to determine the degree to which the information obtained on each item contributes to the total assessment and whether or not each item yields useful variations between client responses.

• *Step 4: Validation phase.* The second phase of psychometric testing usually involves determining the instrument's validity, as described above. In psychometric research, steps 3 and 4 are repeated numerous times by many researchers to ensure that the tools are doing what they are intended to do. If quantitative evaluation seems particularly daunting, seek out the expertise of colleagues who have research knowledge and experience; assessment development is an ongoing, evolutionary (but exciting and creative) process!

Toward Evidence-Based Assessment in Music Therapy

There is a strong emphasis in music therapy on *evidence-based practice* (EBP). The AMTA Board of Directors adopted a definition of evidence-based practice in music therapy that combines "the best available research, the music therapists' expertise, and the needs, values and preferences of the individual(s) served" (AMTA, 2013). Although there is some discussion among music therapy practitioners regarding what constitutes acceptable evidence (Abrams, 2010; Kern, 2010; Wigram & Gold, 2012), evidence hierarchies drawn from medicine and psychology continue to shape practice in many settings in which music therapists are employed. Jensen-Doss (2011) notes that in order to provide high- quality services, attention also needs to focus on *evidence-based assessments* (EBAs). She indicates that EBAs have the potential to ensure that all necessary information is consistently gathered in order to more effectively target *evidence-based treatment* (EBT). Challenges to developing EBAs involve the variability of assessment methods among practitioners, the relevance of standardized tools to clinical practice, as well as time and cost concerns (Jensen-Doss, 2011). Hunsley and Mash (2008) note that "as the identification of evidence-based treatments rests entirely on the data provided by assessment tools, ignoring the quality of these tools places the whole evidence-based enterprise in jeopardy" (p. 3). They offer rating criteria for evaluating assessment tools along a continuum from adequate to excellent in the areas of norms, reliability, validity, treatment sensitivity, and clinical utility.

Clearly, many assessment approaches and instruments are available to the practicing music therapist. The choice comes down to the approach that is most likely to provide the best information that will lead to the establishment of the most accurate treatment goals and objectives for a given client, and that can provide a way to evaluate the effectiveness of treatment. Although it is important to select the best option for one's own clinical situation, it also is important to consider the development of the profession. What approaches most consistently lead to best-practice decisions? Clinicians and researchers who are providing the psychometric evidence that will move the profession toward standardized assessments are paving the path to EBA. Assessment research also demonstrates that music therapists can negotiate both artistic and scientific domains with considerable skill. Much remains to be done, yet a solid foundation is in place to successfully move the profession forward.

ACKNOWLEDGMENTS

I gratefully acknowledge Jane Creagan and AMTA staff for providing access to the AMTA library, to Joy Schneck and CBMT staff for supplying copies of historical documents, and to numerous colleagues who quickly responded to e-mail questions with helpful guidance and information.

REFERENCES

Abrams, B. (2010). Evidence-based music therapy practice: An integral understanding. *Journal of Music Therapy, 47*(4), 351–379.

Adler, R. (2001). *Musical Assessment of Gerontologic Needs and Treatment: The MAGNET survey*. St. Louis, MO: MMB Music.

American Music Therapy Association (AMTA). (2010). *Definition: Evidence-based music therapy practice*. Retrieved from *www.musictherapy.org/research/strategic_priority_on_research/evidence-based_practice*.

American Music Therapy Association (AMTA). (2013). *AMTA standards of practice*. Retrieved from *www.musictherapy.org/about/standards*.

Baxter, H. T., Berghofer, J. A., MacEwan, L., Nelson, J., Peters, K., & Roberts, P. (2007). *The Individualized Music Therapy Assessment Profile*. London: Jessica Kingsley.

Benson, J., & Clark, F. (1982). A guide for instrument development and validation. *American Journal of Occupational Therapy, 36*(12), 789–801.

Betz, S., & Held, J. (2013a). *Betz–Held Strengths Inventory for Children with Disabilities*. Walnut Creek, CA: Walnut Creek Music Therapy.

Betz, S., & Held, J. (2013b). *Betz–Held Strengths Inventory for Infants and Toddlers: Assessing child development through early strengths finding*. Walnut Creek, CA: Walnut Creek Music Therapy.

Boyle, J. D., & Radocy, R. E. (1987). *Measurement and evaluation of musical experiences*. New York: Schirmer Books.

Bradfield, C., Carlenius, J., Gold, C., & White, M. (2014, April). *Music Therapy Special Education Assessment Scale: A scored assessment model*. A continuing music therapy education session conducted at the meeting of the American Music Therapy Association, Mid-Atlantic Region, Buffalo, New York.

Brunk, B. K., & Coleman, K. A. (1999). *Special Education Music Therapy Assessment Process handbook*. Grapevine, TX: Prelude Music Therapy.

Bruscia, K. E. (1987). *Improvisational models of music therapy*. Springfield, IL: Charles C Thomas.

Bruscia, K. E. (1988). Standards for clinical assessment in the arts therapies. *Arts in Psychotherapy, 15*, 5–10.

Bruscia, K. E. (1998). *Defining music therapy* (2nd ed.). Gilsum, NH: Barcelona.

Bruscia, K. E. (2000). A scale for assessing responsiveness to guided imagery and music. *Journal of the Association for Music and Imagery, 7,* 1–7.

Carpente, J. (2013). *The Individual Music-Centered Assessment Profile for Neurodevelopmental Disorders (IMCAP-ND): A clinical manual.* Baldwin, NY: Regina.

Cassity, M. D., & Cassity, J. E. (1994). Psychiatric music therapy assessment and treatment in clinical training facilities with adults, adolescents, and children. *Journal of Music Therapy, 31*(1), 2–30.

Chase, K. M. (2004). Music therapy assessment for children with developmental disabilities: A survey study. *Journal of Music Therapy, 41*(1), 28–54.

Codding, P. A. (2002). A comprehensive survey of music therapists practicing in correctional psychiatry: Demographics, conditions of employment, service provision, assessment, therapeutic objectives, and related values of the therapist. *Music Therapy Perspectives, 20*(2), 56–68.

Crocker, L., & Algina, J. (1986). *Introduction to classical and modern test theory.* Fort Worth, TX: Holt, Rinehart & Winston.

Darrow, A.-A. (1987). An investigative study: The effect of hearing impairment on musical aptitude. *Journal of Music Therapy, 24*(2), 88–96.

Darrow, A.-A. (1989). Music therapy in the treatment of the hearing-impaired. *Music Therapy Perspectives, 6,* 61–70.

Daveson, B. A., Magee, W. L., Crewe, L., Beaumont, G., & Kenealy, P. (2007). The Music Therapy Assessment Tool for Low Awareness States. *International Journal of Therapy and Rehabilitation, 14*(12), 545–549.

Douglass, E. T. (2006). The development of a music therapy assessment tool for hospitalized children. *Music Therapy Perspectives, 24*(2), 73–79.

Feder, B., & Feder, F. (1988). *The art and science of evaluation in the arts therapies.* Springfield, IL: Charles C Thomas.

Folstein, M. F., Folstein, S. E., & McHugh, P. R. (1975). "Mini-Mental State": A practical method for grading the cognitive state of patients for the clinician. *Journal of Psychiatric Research, 12,* 189–198.

Gfeller, K., & Lansing, C. (1992). Musical perception of cochlear implant users as measured by the Primary Measures of Music Audiation: An item analysis. *Journal of Music Therapy, 29*(1), 18–39.

Gibbons, A. C. (1983a). Primary Measures of Music Audiation scores in an institutionalized elderly population. *Journal of Music Therapy, 20*(1), 21–29.

Gibbons, A. C. (1983b). Item analysis of the Primary Measures of Music Audiation in elderly care home residents. *Journal of Music Therapy, 20*(4), 201–210.

Groen, K. M. (2007). Pain assessment and management in end of life care: A survey of assessment and treatment practices of hospice music therapy. *Journal of Music Therapy, 44*(2), 90–112.

Hanser, S. (1987). *Music therapist's handbook.* St. Louis, MO: Warren H. Green.

Hintz, M. (2000). Geriatric Music Therapy Clinical Assessment: Assessment of music skills and related behaviors. *Music Therapy Perspectives, 18*(1), 31–37.

Hobson, M. R. (2006). The collaboration of music therapy and speech–language pathology in the treatment of neurogenic communication disorders: Part I. Diagnosis, therapist roles, and rationale for music. *Music Therapy Perspectives, 24*(2), 58–67.

Hunsley, J., & Mash, E. J. (2008). Developing criteria for evidence-based assessment: An introduction to assessments that work. In J. Hunsley & E. J. Mash (Eds.), *A guide to assessments that work* (pp. 3–14). New York: Oxford University Press.

Isenberg-Grzeda, C. (1988). Music therapy assessment: A reflection of professional identity. *Journal of Music Therapy, 25*(3), 156–169.

Jensen-Doss, A. (2011). Practice involves more than treatment: How can evidence-based assessment catch up to evidence-based treatment? *Clinical Psychology Science and Practice, 18*(2), 173–177.

Jeong, E. (2013). Psychometric validation of a music-based attention assessment: Revised for patients with traumatic brain injury. *Journal of Music Therapy, 50*(2), 66–92.

Jeong, E., & Lesiuk, T. L. (2011). Development and preliminary evaluation of a music-based attention assessment for patients with traumatic brain injury. *Journal of Music Therapy, 48*(4), 551–572.

Kern, P. (2010). Evidence-based practice in early childhood music therapy: A decision-making process. *Music Therapy Perspectives, 28*(2), 116–123.

Langan, D. (2009). A music therapy assessment tool for special education: Incorporating education outcomes. *Australian Journal of Music Therapy, 20,* 78–98.

Layman, D. L., Hussey, D. L., & Laing, S. J. (2002). Music therapy assessment for severely emotionally disturbed children: A pilot study. *Journal of Music Therapy, 39*(3), 164–187.

Lipe, A. (1995). The use of music performance tasks in the assessment of cognitive functioning among older adults with dementia. *Journal of Music Therapy, 32*(3), 137–151.

Lipe, A., York, E., & Jensen, E. (2007). Construct validation of two music-based assessments for people with dementia. *Journal of Music Therapy, 44*(4), 369–387.

Loewy, J. (2000). Music psychotherapy assessment. *Music Therapy Perspectives, 18*(1), 47–58.

Madsen, C. K., & Darrow, A.-A. (1989). The relationship between music aptitude and sound conceptualization of the visually impaired. *Journal of Music Therapy, 26*(2), 71–78.

Magee, W. L. (2007). Development of a music therapy assessment tool for patients in low awareness states. *NeuroRehabilitation, 22*(4), 319–324.

Magee, W. L., Siegert, R. J., Daveson, B. A., Lenton-Smith, G., & Taylor, S. M. (2013). Music Therapy Assessment Tool for Awareness in Disorders of Consciousness (MATADOC): Standardisation of the principal subscale to assess awareness in patients with disorders of consciousness. *Neuropsychological Rehabilitation: An International Journal, 24*(1), 101–124.

Mahoney, J. (2010). Interrater agreement on the Nordoff–Robbins Evaluation Scale: I. Client–Therapist Relationship in Musical Activity. *Music and Medicine, 2*(1), 23–28.

Maue-Johnson, E. L., & Tanguay, C. L. (2006). Assessing the unique needs of hospice patients: A tool for music therapists. *Music Therapy Perspectives, 24*(1), 13–21.

Meadows, A. (2000). The validity and reliability of the Guided Imagery and Music Responsiveness Scale. *Journal of the Association for Music and Imagery, 7*, 8–33.

Meadows, A., Wheeler, B. L., Shultis, C. L., & Polen, D. W. (2005). Client assessment. In B. L. Wheeler, C. L. Shultis, & D. W. Polen (Eds.), *Clinical training guide for the student music therapist* (pp. 27–55). Gilsum, NH: Barcelona.

Moon, S., & Ko, B. (2014). The validity and reliability of the Korean version of the Music-Based Evaluation of Cognitive Functioning. *Korean Journal of Music Therapy, 16*(1), 49–63.

Nordoff, P., & Robbins, C. (1977). *Creative Music Therapy*. New York: John Day.

Nordoff, P., & Robbins, C. (2007). *Creative Music Therapy: A guide to fostering clinical musicianship* (2nd ed.). Gilsum, NH: Barcelona.

Norman, R. (2012). Music therapy assessment of older adults in nursing homes. *Music Therapy Perspectives, 30*(1), 8–16.

O'Kelly, J. W., & Magee, W. L. (2013). The complementary role of music therapy in the detection of awareness in disorders of consciousness: An audit of concurrent SMART and MATADOC assessments. *Neuropsychological Rehabilitation, 23*(2), 287–298.

Radocy, R. E., & Boyle, J. D. (1988). *Psychological foundations of musical behavior* (2nd ed.). Springfield, IL: Charles C Thomas.

Radocy, R. E., & Boyle, J. D. (1997). *Psychological foundations of musical behavior* (3rd ed.). Springfield, IL: Charles C Thomas.

Reisberg, B., Schneck, M. K., Ferris, S. H., Schwartz, G. E., & DeLeon, E. D. (1983). The Brief Cognitive Rating Sale (BCRS): Findings in primary degenerative dementia (PDD). *Psychopharmacology Bulletin, 139*, 1136–1139.

Rohrbacher, M. (2007). *Functions of music therapy for persons with Alzheimer's disease and related disorders: Model demonstration program in adult day healthcare* (Grant No. 90AM2638). Washington, DC: Administration on Aging, Department of Health and Human Services.

Saxton, J., & Swihart, A. (1989). Neuropsychological assessment of the severely impaired elderly patient. *Clinics in Geriatric Medicine, 5*(3), 531–543.

Silverman, M. (2007). Evaluating current trends in psychiatric music therapy: A descriptive analysis. *Journal of Music Therapy, 44*(4), 388–414.

Snow, S. (2009). The development of a music therapy assessment tool: A pilot study. In S. Snow & M. D'Amico (Eds.), *Assessment in the creative arts therapies* (pp. 47–98). Springfield, IL: Charles C Thomas.

Solomon, A. L. (1985). A historical study of the National Association for Music Therapy, 1960–1980 (Doctoral dissertation, University of Kansas, 1984). *Dissertation Abstracts International, 46*, 2957-A.

Wechsler, D. (1975, February). Intelligence defined and undefined: A relativistic appraisal. *American Psychologist, 30*, 135–139.

Weller, C. M., & Baker, F. A. (2011). The role of music therapy in physical rehabilitation: A systematic literature review. *Nordic Journal of Music Therapy, 14*(1), 15–32.

Wheeler, B. L. (2013). Music therapy assessment. In R. Cruz & B. Feder (Eds.), *Feder's the art and science of evaluation in the arts therapies* (2nd ed., pp. 344–382). Springfield, IL: Charles C Thomas.

Wigram, T., & Gold, C. (2012). The religion of evidence-based practice: Helpful or harmful to health and wellbeing? In R. Macdonald, G. Kreutz, & L. Mitchell (Eds.), *Music, health and wellbeing* (pp. 164–182). Oxford, UK: Oxford University Press.

Wilson, B. L., & Smith, D. S. (2000). Music therapy assessment in school settings: A preliminary investigation. *Journal of Music Therapy, 37*(2), 95–117.

Wolfe, D. (2000). Group music therapy in acute mental health care: Meeting the demands of effectiveness and efficiency. In D. S. Smith (Ed.), *Effectiveness of music therapy procedures: Documentation of research and clinical practice* (3rd ed.,

pp. 265–296). Silver Spring, MD: American Music Therapy Association.

York, E. (1994). The development of a quantitative music skills test for patients with Alzheimer's disease. *Journal of Music Therapy, 31*(4), 280–296.

York, E. (2000). A test–retest reliability study of the Residual Music Skills Test. *Psychology of Music, 28*, 174–180.

CHAPTER 8

Music Therapy Research

Debra S. Burns
Anthony Meadows

Research plays multiple roles within the profession of music therapy, including documenting the historical developments and events within the field, describing what is currently happening within clinical practice, and exploring the processes and outcomes of interventions. In clinical practice, research is important because it (1) assists in the identification of music-based interventions that have data justifying their use, (2) describes or analyzes therapeutic processes that deepen our understanding, (3) helps us understand therapists' and clients' experiences of music and music therapy, (4) enriches our understanding of the theories underpinning clinical practice, and (5) propels the field forward by generating new questions for further investigation. The combination of knowledge from different research methods provides music therapists and consumers with information about why and how music therapy can be used to encourage growth and development and decrease suffering.

Professional organizations advocating for music therapists (e.g., National Association for Music Therapy [NAMT], American Association for Music Therapy [AAMT], American Music Therapy Association [AMTA], World Federation of Music Therapy [WFMT]) have long placed a strong emphasis on research as a way to illustrate the benefits of music therapy, define standards of clinical practice, and create a body of evidence that defines the practice and effectiveness of music therapy. The research process typically follows a series of systematic steps, undertaken according to the stance of the researcher and phenomenon of interest, including (1) identifying a problem/phenomenon of interest, (2) formulating hypotheses or research questions, (3) denoting a methodology derived from the hypotheses or research questions, (4) collecting data, (5) analyzing the data, and (6) disseminating the findings. This process helps to ensure that results or conclusions from the study provide information to clinicians and stakeholders in a way that maintains methodological integrity.

Defining Research Perspectives and Methodologies

Music therapy researchers use systematic processes and strategies developed from disciplines such as psychology, education, and medicine, along with designs indigenous to the arts (Hillecke, Nickel, & Bolay, 2005; Ledger & Edwards, 2011). Two basic methodologies, quantitative and qualitative, and newer mixed methodologies flow from paradigmatic viewpoints that guide research methods and strategies. *Quantitative* research methods and strategies flow from a *postpostivistic* worldview that emphasizes the use of variables based on a theory. Deductively derived variables are measured with numbers and analyzed with statistical procedures in order to confirm theory, predict relationships, and generalize results to a larger population (Creswell, 2009). The second broad umbrella, *qualitative* research, can be understood as "the study of things in their natural settings, attempting to make sense, or interpret phenomena in terms of the meanings people bring to them" (Denzin & Lincoln, 2011, p. 3). Finally, mixed methods (a combination of both qualitative and quantitative strategies within a single study) follow a *pragmatic* worldview that is not restricted to any one perspective but combines the strengths and assumptions of various worldviews when designing and conducting research (Creswell, 2009; Teddlie & Tashakkori, 2009).

Research Questions in Music Therapy

Within the context of broad paradigmatic viewpoints, researchers usually begin with a question that, over time, evolves into a systematic research process that includes a focus area (e.g., examining the impact of a music therapy intervention on social skills development for children with autism), a method for collecting information (e.g., a checklist identifying the presence of social skills), and a method of analyzing the data gathered (e.g., a statistical analysis). These kinds of questions, called *research questions*, can be categorized according to foundational, discipline-specific, and professional foci (Bruscia, 2005b).

Foundational research, also called *preclinical* or *basic/bench research*, involves gathering information to develop an in-depth understanding about a problem or phenomenon (Sidani & Braden, 2011). Foundational research may not be music therapy research, for example, but from a closely related field. Foundational questions can evolve into several different methodologies and can be formulated and answered inductively or deductively, but the main focus is developing an understanding of the problem or phenomenon. An example would be exploring the relationships between psychophysical properties of music, preference, and familiarity on relaxation (Tan, Yowler, Super, & Fratianne, 2012), or how familiarity with specific music pieces is related to neural correlates of music appreciation (Pereira et al., 2011). Although not specific to music therapy, findings from foundational studies have clinical relevance, serving as a foundation for clinical practice and future research.

Discipline-specific research includes studies examining music therapy clinical practice, such as understanding and defining a problem or phenomenon (assessment), theoretical framework (intervention development), and ultimately the evaluation of interventions (evaluation) (Bruscia, 2005b; Sidani & Braden, 2011). Research questions examining clinical practice can be descriptive or predictive. An example is developing a grounded theory describing the benefits experienced by health care providers who witness patient-focused music therapy (O'Callaghan & Magill, 2009). Randomized controlled trials (RCTs) can be included within this category of research, because RCTs focus on the outcome of therapy. RCT questions or hypotheses (predictive statements) focus on whether or not an intervention is beneficial.

Profession-specific research "includes all those studies that deal with music therapists and what they do collectively to establish and promote music therapy as a healthcare service" (Bruscia, 2005b, p. 81).

Research on the profession covers a broad spectrum of topical areas that includes employment practices, profiles of student and professional music therapists, academic and curricular requirements related to education and training, professional standards, legislation, and the history and culture of the discipline and/or profession of music therapy (Bruscia). An example is a study examining music therapy students' perceptions of a short-term music therapy process group, focusing on their developing understanding of therapy and the resulting implications for education and training (Jackson & Gardstrom, 2012). Such studies fall under the category of professional education and training because of the focus on the relevance of personal therapy in an educational curriculum.

The Researcher's Perspective and Experience

Deciding on a research question or concept does not occur in a vacuum. Researchers are almost always focused on areas/topics that are of interest to them, drawing upon their personal experiences and curiosities; education and training; and philosophies of music, therapy, and therapeutic change. Researchers' life experiences can have a marked effect on the areas of research in which they choose to focus. For example, Anthony Meadows's explorations of his role and experiences as a male music therapist informed his decision to examine how male and female clients are viewed by their male and female therapists, and the kinds of constructs these therapists use when thinking about their clients (Meadows, 2002).

Similarly, the ways in which researchers develop methodological frameworks are influenced by their beliefs about how research should be conducted as much as they are by education and research training. Further, training in psychotherapy, cognitive-behavioral therapy, humanism, the psychology of music, human develop-

ment, and so forth, adds more layers or lenses through which researchers develop their research questions. These multiple sources of influence can lead to a single study, motivated by a specific question, or a whole research program, in which a researcher uses one study to inform a series of studies, all related to one another in the process of developing a complex view of a phenomenon (Burns, Robb, & Haase, 2009; Burns, Robb, Phillips-Salimi, & Haase, 2010; Robb, 2003).

Thus, music therapy research draws together several different elements, all of which influence the decisions the researcher makes at each step of the research process. These elements include the researcher's perspective and methodological frame, life and clinical experiences, and his or her education and training.

Research as Process

It is also important to understand that research is as much a process as a product. A novice researcher may begin with a question related to his or her clinical work, and under the supervision of an academic supervisor or mentor, design and complete the project. More experienced researchers—usually those with advanced research training or experience—may develop a multistage study that involves several different clinical sites and numerous co-researchers.

Finally, researchers can use the research process to ask questions and explore concepts or phenomena that provides a deeper understanding of the phenomena and to demonstrate development in their theoretical and methodological thinking. Thus, developing a research program allows the researcher to deepen his or her understanding of the phenomena under study, as well as expanding his or her knowledge of the research process. Further, like all forms of knowledge, the researcher's perspective can evolve and shift. For example, a researcher may begin by exploring a phenomenon using quantitative procedures, then shift to qualitative, and finally to mixed methods, developing breadth and depth of knowledge in doing so.

Research Designs and Methodologies

Once a researcher has settled on a research question or questions, the next stage is to develop a strategy for examining the question. Such a strategy would include participant recruitment, data collection, and analytic procedures, commonly called the *research method*. There are a wide variety of methods for conducting research, falling into three broad categories: quantitative, qualitative, and mixed methods approaches. In the following sections, each of these approaches is described and an example of music therapy research is provided. Multiple resources can be accessed to gain a comprehensive review of these methods (Creswell & Plano Clark, 2011; Tashakkori & Teddlie, 2010; Wheeler, 2005).

Quantitative Approaches

Quantitative research methods include the numerical measurement of predetermined variables based on a theoretical framework. Sometimes a researcher chooses to do a pilot study at this point to test the variables and be sure that they have been defined as well as possible. The collected data are then tested statistically to determine relationships, predictions, and differences. The results from the statistical tests are interpreted in light of research questions, hypotheses, and previous studies. Quantitative designs can be categorized by the number of contacts (cross-sectional, pretest/posttest, longitudinal), reference period (prospective, retrospective), or the nature of the investigation (experimental, nonexperimental, quasi-experimental) (Kumar, 2005).

Descriptive Research Designs

Sometimes, in the beginning of a research program or when a researcher is starting to explore a new area of interest, the most prudent designs/methodologies involve exploring what is currently known about a given topic, including theoretical frameworks, current practices, and so forth. Descriptive, correlational, and survey research methods are approaches that can answer questions such as, What is currently happening?, How is *this* related to *that* (or, are there any relationships)?, and How are music therapists currently practicing?

Descriptive studies (observational and survey approaches) seek to describe a phenomenon, group of people, program, or service (Kelley, Clark, Brown, & Sitzia, 2003; Kumar, 2005). Descriptive studies can be one shot or cross-sectional (considering a moment of time), or they can take place over a period of time (longitudinal). The main purpose of such studies is to describe what is common within the context of an issue or problem under study. With the development of web-based engines (e.g., Survey Monkey), surveys have become very popular in music therapy. Surveys have several advantages, including the collection of empirical data, and, depending upon the sampling plan, the data can be representative of a larger population and thus the results can be generalized. Surveys can also produce a large amount of data in a relatively short period of time, making the method more economical and efficient than experimental studies (Kelley et al.). Tanguay (2008) used survey methodology to explore common supervision practices and attitudes in music therapy internships from the perspective of internship directors. Procedures included questionnaire development (including feedback from the target population), distribution of the questionnaire (including reminders), and analysis of compiled data to describe the profiles of current internship directors, their supervisory practices, and attitudes about supervision.

Retrospective or ex post facto designs, although rare in music therapy, take advantage of data that have been collected in the past to characterize clinical practice or relationships between available variables. In health services research, retrospective designs are used to describe the delivery of services, compare outcomes for those receiving various services, and compare costs associated with program delivery. Hilliard (2004) used an ex post facto design to explore the benefits of music therapy for nursing home residents receiving music therapy as part of hospice care. Procedures included randomly selecting patients from electronic medical records and grouping individuals based on the receipt of music therapy services. Outcomes for the study were formulated in terms of length of life, time of death in relation to last social worker or music therapy visit, and number of visits and minutes in direct care. This type of analysis has several benefits, including cost efficiency, the relevance of real clinical practice as opposed to controlled trials, and sometimes easier board (i.e., ethics review board) approval for the use of human subjects.

Experimental Designs

Experimental designs are often used in music therapy to determine the influence of a music intervention on targeted therapeutic outcomes. Six characteristics are shared across experimental designs: (1) the equivalence of research participants in different groups, which is accomplished by random assignment; (2) the comparison of two or more groups or conditions; (3) the direct manipulation of at least one independent or treatment variable; (4) measurement of each dependent variable or outcome; (5) the use of inferential statistics; and (6) use of a design that provides maximum control over extraneous variables (McMillan & Schumacher, 1989). The specific char-

acteristics of experimental designs have been detailed elsewhere, including associated threats to internal and external validity (Shadish, Cook, & Campbell, 2002). Experimental procedures assist researchers in ensuring that they can validly infer the causal relationships between music therapy and changes in targeted outcomes. Several design options are available to structure a project in a way that increases the researcher's ability to infer causality.

Common experimental designs are the pretest–posttest control group design, posttest-only control group design, factorial design, and the within-subjects (or repeated measures) design (Bradt, 2012; Shadish et al., 2002). Perhaps the most common experimental design is the parallel group pretest–posttest designs wherein individuals are randomly assigned to two or more groups. There are many examples of the pretest–posttest design throughout the music therapy literature (e.g., Burns et al., 2009; Goldbeck & Ellerkamp, 2012). Bradt (2012) details important decision points and design possibilities of randomized trials to test the efficacy or effectiveness of a music therapy intervention.

The posttest-only control group design is useful when randomization of individuals is difficult. For example, Silverman (2013) used a posttest-only design to determine the effects of a psychoeducational songwriting group, a psychoeducational group (no music), and a recreational music therapy group. Although session content was randomly assigned, group equivalence was determined by comparing the results of important demographic information, thereby reducing the need for randomization at the individual patient level (Silverman). The decision to not randomize individuals to groups was necessary based on the typical routine of the psychiatric hospital environment—it would have been very difficult to randomize individuals to different groups without disrupting the milieu of the unit. This design may have been more feasible than a traditional RCT, given the daily schedule of the patients and the requirement to attend other group therapy sessions.

Factorial designs are more complex experimental designs that test the effect of more than one independent variable. For example, McKinney, Tims, Kumar, and Kumar (1997) were interested in the synergistic effects of music and imagery on beta-endorphin levels. Because of previous research demonstrating the beneficial effects of music listening and imagery individually on beta-endorphin levels, they chose a 2 × 2 factorial design to isolate the effects of music and imagery combined. This design included three treatment groups (music, music plus imagery, and imagery) and a control group. The interpretation of the data analysis confirmed the hypothesis: The music imagery group scored significantly lower on measures of peripheral beta-endorphin than the other three groups, and there appeared to be a synergistic effect of the combination of music and imagery (McKinney et al.). This design could have also answered questions about which aspect of an intervention was most important (music, imagery, or the combination).

Another type of design used in music therapy research is the *within-subjects design* (also referred to as *repeated measures* or as *using subjects as own controls*; Elefant, Baker, Lotan, Lagesen, & Skeie, 2012). This design may or may not include randomization, but either way, all subjects are introduced to all levels of the independent variable (i.e., the treatment). Within-subjects designs are advantageous under several conditions. They are useful when withholding a useful treatment from a group of individuals would be unethical and when it is not feasible to randomize individuals or groups to treatment/ no-treatment groups (e.g., classrooms, intact therapy groups). Robb and colleagues (2008) used a within-subjects design to explore the benefits of active music engagement toward increasing coping-related behavior in children with cancer. The dif-

ferent experimental conditions were used to isolate the influence of structure, autonomy support, and relatedness, and each child participated in each condition. Having each child participate in each condition reduces the variability in the measurement, which subsequently increases power.

Qualitative Approaches

Qualitative researchers ask a variety of research questions that generally involve a focus on (1) events, actions, and interactions: focusing on anything observable that happens within a defined, real-world context (e.g., examining the ways music therapists interact with clients during clinical improvisation); (2) experiences: how people (e.g., clients, therapists, family members) apprehend, perceive, feel, and think about things (e.g., how a client feels after a music therapy session); (3) written and spoken language: how people communicate and act upon one another through verbal and written means (e.g., analyzing the transcript of a verbal exchange between client and therapist discussing a musical life review); (4) art works: a focus on the materials that result from music therapy sessions, such as music and art (e.g., a musical analysis of client improvisations); and (5) persons: a focus on understanding an individual, group, community, or culture, within a defined setting or context (e.g., interviewing music therapists about their experiences of *being present* to clients) (Bruscia, 2005a).

The purposes of asking these kinds of questions can vary considerably. Drawing upon his experiences as a researcher, clinician, and educator, Bruscia (2005a) identified the following kinds of purposes: (1) holistic description: provides a comprehensive picture of a phenomenon, with a minimum of interpretation (e.g., holistically describing what happens in a music therapy session with a group of children with autism); (2) definition of essence: identifies the essential, defining properties of a phenomenon (e.g., interviewing therapists to understand

and define what it means to *be there* for a client); (3) analysis: identifies regularities, themes, relationships, and patterns in data, and, based upon these, offers meaningful explanations of the phenomenon (e.g., analyzing the ways music therapists engage nonverbal clients in vocal play to develop a set of guidelines for future clinical work); (4) theory building: formulates constructs, principles, laws, and conceptual schemes that explain a phenomenon in some way (e.g., analyzing the musical and verbal processes that unfold during clinical improvisation with adults to develop a theory of how clients change during this process); (5) interpretation: researcher's tacit knowledge of a phenomenon, in conjunction with relevant theories (or interpretations by others), is used to derive meaning out of data (e.g., using psychodynamic theory to interpret the clinical process of a group of patients with psychiatric problems in long-term therapy); and (6) self-reflection: researcher examines his or her own actions, interactions, experience, language, to deepen self-awareness (e.g., a therapist examines how he or she interprets the musical and nonmusical behaviors of children with severe and multiple disabilities during music therapy, to understand the mechanisms he or uses in this interpretation process and the implications of doing so).

Qualitative researchers utilize a range of approaches to data collection and analysis (e.g., grounded theory or phenomenology) in seeking to answer these questions and fulfill these purposes. Although varied, these researchers share a number of characteristics that provide a frame for understanding qualitative research processes. Creswell (2009, pp. 175–176) identifies these characteristics:

1. Qualitative researchers tend to examine phenomena in natural settings. Data collection occurs in the field rather than in a controlled setting and is linked to the specific context of the data.

2. Researchers are the key instrument in the research process, collecting data themselves, whether through interview, observation, or some other form of data collection. They tend not to use standardized questionnaires.

3. Multiple data sources are favored, such as the combination of interviews, observations, and documents.

4. Inductive data analysis is common. Qualitative researchers tend to build data analysis from the bottom up—building patterns, categories, and themes directly from the data and not according to predetermined templates.

5. Participants' meanings are valued and often included. Although the researcher may interpret the data, there is usually a strong focus on learning the meaning the participants hold about the problem or issue, not the meaning that the researcher brings to the process.

6. In general, the design for the qualitative research is an emergent one. All phases of the process are subject to change in response to the specific context and/or setting in which the research is undertaken. The key concept is the researcher's ability to capture the phenomenon under investigation in a comprehensive and trustworthy manner; thus design and data collection reflect the phenomenon, not the other way around.

7. Theoretical lenses are valued and acknowledged. Qualitative researchers often use a specific lens through which to frame their research (e.g., culture, gender, race, class) and/or may organize it around a specific social, political, or historical context.

8. Interpretation is central. Qualitative researchers use various forms of interpretation to understand what they see and hear. Their interpretations cannot be separated from their own backgrounds, history, contexts, and prior understandings. Inherent in the research process is an understanding that the researcher, and often the participants, make interpretations of the phenomenon under

investigation. The research is therefore inextricably context-bound and ideographic.

9. Holistic accounts are valued and commonly sought. Qualitative researchers seek to develop a complex understanding of a phenomenon by holistically gathering, interpreting, and reporting from multiple perspectives. Through this process, a larger picture of the phenomenon emerges.

Within these broad guidelines, specific methods of data collection and analysis have been developed, each for a different purpose. For example, the data collection and analysis methods associated with phenomenological inquiry are concerned with studying lived human experiences as unified wholes (Forinash & Grocke, 2005). In contrast, grounded theory is primarily concerned with using a systematic, comparative analytic process to generate an inductive theory from a phenomenon of interested (O'Callaghan, 2012). The next section describes two examples of qualitative methods of data collection and analysis.

Phenomenological Inquiry

Phenomenologists examine what is called the *lived experience* (Forinash & Grocke, 2005). As such, they are concerned with how we, as humans, experience places, people, and events. For example, phenomenological researchers may focus on the experience of being in a music therapy session, the experience of sadness while singing, or the experience of anger while improvising. They might also focus on therapists' experiences. For example, studies of the experience of therapist intuition (Brescia, 2005) and music therapists' experiences of adults in pain (Kwan, 2010) both used principles and procedures of phenomenology to collect and analyze data.

In terms of methodology, phenomenology involves a systematic sequence for collecting, transcribing, analyzing, and defin-

ing the essence of an experience. Several approaches have been developed (e.g., Colaizzi, 1978; Moustakas, 1994). As an example, Muller (2008) sought to understand how music therapists experienced *being present* for their clients. He began with two research questions: (1) How does the music therapist's experience of being present unfold?, and (2) What defines being present as a music therapist? Muller interviewed eight experienced music therapists, beginning with the following question: "Can you recall a particularly strong experience when you worked with a client and you felt connected or present to the client, or that you were there for the client, or that you deeply heard or understood the client?" The ensuing interview expanded upon the experience of the music therapist, allowing the researcher and the music therapist to describe, moment by moment, this experience.

Data analysis unfolded over five stages: In stage 1, each interview was transcribed, read as whole, and culled to omit the researcher's questions and any dialogue unrelated to the purpose. In stage 2, transcripts were condensed and segmented into meaning units, revealing 33 preliminary data codes (8 client, 12 therapist, and 13 music). In stage 3, Muller returned to the uncondensed interviews to ground the codes—that is, to verify the extent to which the codes represented the clinicians' experiences. In so doing, the original codes were redefined, merged, and clarified, resulting in final codes. In stage 4, each interview was culled again to form a flowing synopsis of each therapist's experience. Finally, in stage 5, major themes were developed to represent the experience of being present. The result was a holistic description of the characteristics of being present, as experienced by the therapists he interviewed.

Grounded Theory

Grounded theory methodologies generate and verify a theory from qualitative data through a predominantly inductive process. O'Callaghan (2012) explains: "Grounded theory involves taking comparisons from data and reaching up to construct abstractions [while] simultaneously reaching down to tie these abstractions to data" (p. 237). Grounded theory has a long and prominent history in qualitative music therapy research, focusing on a range of experiences and phenomena, including moments of insight (Amir, 1996), music and identity (Ruud, 1997), and the boundaries and identity of community music therapy practice (O'Grady & McFerran, 2007).

In terms of methodology, grounded theory moves through a series of steps to collect, analyze, and code data. Amir (1996) provides an excellent example of grounded theory methods. In seeking to understand how music therapists and clients experienced meaningful moments in music therapy, Amir interviewed four music therapists and four clients to develop a grounded theory of 15 meaningful moments, conditions under which these moments occur, and the contribution of these moments to participants' lives. Interviews were transcribed and analyzed using a nine-stage process, outlined as follows: In stages 1 and 2 interviews were transcribed verbatim, with researcher comments, thoughts, and feelings added, and initial organization of the data was completed. In stages 3 and 4 transcripts were reread and further (axial) coded, with core categories and subcategories developed. Additional categories were also developed. For example, client's spiritual, emotional, and physical reactions were organized into different categories, along with various categories related to the therapists' experiences (e.g., perceptions of client readiness, client–therapist relationship, trust). In stages 5 and 6 individual participant profiles were created and a cross-analysis of the therapists' profiles and of the clients' profiles was completed, so that common experiences were combined and overarching constructs enhanced. In stages 7 and 8 a cross-analysis of common elements (e.g., therapists' and clients' emotional experiences) was undertaken to develop core constructs that subsume both kinds of experience. In stage 9 all data were synthesized and an overarching theory of the experience of meaningful moments was presented.

Additional Qualitative Methods

Phenomenology and grounded theory are but two qualitative methods used by music therapists. A rich and varied tradition of qualitative research is woven into music therapy research literature and includes *naturalistic inquiry* (the study of people, events, and experiences in their natural setting); *first-person research* (in which the researcher gathers data on him- or herself, using introspection and self-inquiry to enrich self-awareness); *participatory action research* (in which the researcher and research participants co-participate in all or some aspects of the research process to develop shared knowledge); and *narrative inquiry* (in which texts are analyzed to enrich understanding of the textual materials). See Wheeler (2005) for additional information on these methods.

Mixed Methods

The combination of quantitative and qualitative research methods, either concurrently or sequentially, has expanded exponentially in social and health science literature (Plano Clark, 2010). Several recent research studies have utilized mixed methods (Barry, O'Callaghan, Wheeler, & Grocke, 2010; Carr et al., 2012), wherein one data source provides additional, contrasting, complementary, or explanatory information for the other. For example, Barry et al. (2010) examined the benefits of a music therapy intervention involving the creation of a CD on the distress and coping abilities of pediatric oncology patients during their first radiation therapy treatment. Using concurrent triangulation, parallel qualitative and quantitative data were collected from questionnaires, interviews (of participants and their parents), and a reflective journal (of the music therapy clinicians). Quantitative and qualitative data were analyzed separately and then integrated, allowing the strengths of each method to be captured in the initial analysis phase and then integrated in later comparisons.

Standards of Research Integrity

Music therapy research follows the same standards of integrity that other professions use in their research activities. In addition to requiring informed consent and approval for using human subjects, qualitative and quantitative methodologies have standards of rigor. For instance, qualitative researchers are interested in establishing trustworthiness, whereas quantitative researchers are concerned with internal and external validity and reliability. Mixed methods research requires rigor in both qualitative and quantitative methods, and also has its own standards of rigor for data integration and presentation.

Conclusions

Music therapists have long valued research to provide the best possible care for patients and families receiving their services. Although music therapy is a relatively small profession, its body of knowledge provides a foundation that guides practice in various clinical settings. As the use of music therapy continues to increase and health care needs and funding become even more challenging, the need for larger, more rigorous studies will be imperative. Music therapists and colleagues in related disciplines have many opportunities to build the current state of the science.

REFERENCES

Amir, D. (1996). Experiencing music therapy: Meaningful moments in the music therapy process. In M. Langenberg & K. Aigen (Eds.), *Qualitative music therapy research: Beginning dialogues* (pp. 109–130). Gilsum, NH: Barcelona.

Barry, P., O'Callaghan, C., Wheeler, G., & Grocke, D. (2010). Music therapy CD creation for initial pediatric radiation therapy: A mixed methods analysis. *Journal of Music Therapy, 47*(3), 233–263.

Bradt, J. (2012). Randomized controlled trials in music therapy: Guidelines for design and implementation. *Journal of Music Therapy, 49*(2), 120–149.

Brescia, T. (2005). A qualitative study of intuition as experienced and used by music therapists. *Qualitative Inquiries in Music Therapy, 2,* 62–112.

Bruscia, K. E. (2005a). Designing qualitative research. In B. L. Wheeler (Ed.), *Music therapy research* (2nd ed., pp. 129–137). Gilsum, NH: Barcelona.

Bruscia, K. E. (2005b). Research topics and questions in music therapy. In B. L. Wheeler (Ed.), *Music therapy research* (2nd ed., pp. 81–93). Gilsum, NH: Barcelona.

Burns, D. S., Robb, S. L., & Haase, J. E. (2009). Exploring the feasibility of a therapeutic music video intervention in adolescents and young adults during stem-cell transplantation. *Cancer Nursing: An International Journal of Cancer Care, 32*(5), E8–E16.

Burns, D. S., Robb, S. L., Phillips-Salimi, C., & Haase, J. E. (2010). Parental perspectives of an adolescent/young adult stem cell transplant and a music video intervention. *Cancer Nursing: An International Journal of Cancer Care, 33*(4), E20–E27.

Carr, C., d'Ardenne, P., Sloboda, A., Scott, C., Wang, D., & Priebe, S. (2012). Group music therapy for patients with persistent post-traumatic stress disorder: An exploratory randomized controlled trial with mixed methods evaluation. *Psychology and Psychotherapy: Theory, Research, and Practice, 85*(2), 179–202.

Colaizzi, P. F. (1978). Psychological research as the phenomenologist views it. In R. S. Valle & M. King (Eds.), *Existential–phenomenological alternatives for psychology* (pp. 48–71). New York: Oxford University Press.

Creswell, J. W. (2009). *Research design: Qualitative, quantitative, and mixed methods approaches* (3rd ed.). Thousand Oaks, CA: Sage.

Creswell, J. W., & Plano Clark, V. L. (2011). *Designing and conducting mixed methods research* (3rd ed.). Thousand Oaks, CA: Sage.

Denzin, N. K., & Lincoln, Y. S. (Eds.). (2011). *The Sage handbook of qualitative research* (4th ed.). Thousand Oaks, CA: Sage.

Elefant, C., Baker, F. A., Lotan, M., Lagesen, S. K., & Skeie, G. O. (2012). The effect of group music therapy on mood, speech, and singing in individuals with Parkinson's disease: A feasibility study. *Journal of Music Therapy, 49*(3), 278–302.

Forinash, M., & Grocke, D. (2005). Phenomenological inquiry. In B. L. Wheeler (Ed.), *Music therapy research* (2nd ed., pp. 321–334). Gilsum, NH: Barcelona.

Goldbeck, L., & Ellerkamp, T. (2012). A randomized controlled trial of multimodal music therapy for children with anxiety disorders. *Journal of Music Therapy, 49*(4), 395–413.

Hillecke, T., Nickel, A., & Bolay, H. V. (2005). Scientific perspectives on music therapy. *Annals of the New York Academy of Sciences, 1060*, 271–282.

Hilliard, R. E. (2004). A post-hoc analysis of music therapy services for residents in nursing homes receiving hospice care. *Journal of Music Therapy, 41*(4), 266–281.

Jackson, N. A., & Gardstrom, S. C. (2012). Undergraduate music therapy students' experiences as clients in short-term group music therapy. *Music Therapy Perspectives, 30*(1), 65–82.

Kelley, K., Clark, B., Brown, V., & Sitzia, J. (2003). Good practice in the conduct and reporting of survey research. *International Journal for Quality in Health Care, 15*(3), 261–266.

Kumar, R. (2005). *Research methodology: A step-by-step guide for beginners* (2nd ed.). Thousand Oaks, CA: Sage.

Kwan, M. (2010). Music therapists' experiences with adults in pain: Implications for clinical practice. *Qualitative Inquiries in Music Therapy, 5*, 43–85.

Ledger, A., & Edwards, J. (2011). Arts-based research practices in music therapy research: Existing and potential developments. *Arts in Psychotherapy, 38*(5), 312–317.

McKinney, C. H., Tims, F. C., Kumar, A. M., & Kumar, M. (1997). The effect of selected classical music and spontaneous imagery on plasma beta-endorphin. *Journal of Behavioral Medicine, 20*(1), 85–99.

McMillan, J. H., & Schumacher, S. (1989). *Research in education: A conceptual introduction* (2nd ed.). Glenview, IL: Scott Foresman.

Meadows, A. T. (2002). Gender implications in therapists' constructs of their clients. *Nordic Journal of Music Therapy, 11*(2), 127–141.

Moustakas, C. (1994). *Phenomenological research methods*. Thousand Oaks, CA: Sage.

Muller, B. (2008). Phenomenological investigation of the music therapist's experience of being present to clients. *Qualitative Inquiries in Music Therapy, 4*, 69–112.

O'Callaghan, C. (2012). Grounded theory in music therapy research. *Journal of Music Therapy, 49*(3), 236–277.

O'Callaghan, C., & Magill, L. (2009). Effect of music therapy on oncologic staff bystanders: A substantive grounded theory. *Palliative and Supportive Care, 7*(2), 219–228.

O'Grady, L., & McFerran, K. (2007). Community Music Therapy and its relationship to community music: Where does it end? *Nordic Journal of Music Therapy, 16*(1), 14–26.

Pereira, C. S., Teixeira, J., Figueiredo, P., Xavier, J., Castro, S. L., & Brattico, E. (2011). Music and emotions in the brain: Familiarity matters. *PLoS One, 6*(11).

Plano Clark, V. L. (2010). The adoption and practice of mixed methods: U.S. trends in federally funded health-related research. *Qualitative Inquiry, 16*(6), 428–440.

Robb, S. L. (2003). Designing music therapy interventions for hospitalized children and adolescents using a contextual support model of music therapy. *Music Therapy Perspectives, 21*, 27–40.

Robb, S. L., Clair, A. A., Watanabe, M., Monahan, P. O., Azzouz, F., Stouffer, J. W., et al. (2008). A non-randomized [corrected] controlled trial of the active music engagement (AME) intervention on children with cancer. *Psycho-Oncology, 17*(7), 699–708. [Erratum appears in *Psycho-Oncology*, 2008, *17*(9), 957.]

Ruud, E. (1997). Music and identity. *Nordic Journal of Music Therapy, 6*, 3–13.

Shadish, W. R., Cook, T. D., & Campbell, D. T. (2002). *Experimental and quasi-experimental designs for generlized causal inference*. Belmont, CA: Wadsworth, Cengage Learning.

Sidani, S., & Braden, C. J. (2011). *Design, evaluation, and translation of nursing interventions*. Chichester, UK: Wiley-Blackwell.

Silverman, M. J. (2013). Effects of group songwriting on depression and quality of life in acute psychiatric inpatients: A randomized three-group effectiveness study. *Nordic Journal of Music Therapy, 22*, 131–148.

Tan, X. L., Yowler, C. J., Super, D. M., & Fratianne, R. B. (2012). The interplay of preference, familiarity and psychophysical properties in defining relaxation music. *Journal of Music Therapy, 49*(2), 150–179.

Tanguay, C. L. (2008). Supervising music therapy interns: A survey of AMTA national roster internship directors. *Journal of Music Therapy, 45*(1), 52–74.

Tashakkori, A., & Teddlie, C. (2010). *Sage handbook of mixed methods in social and behavioral research* (2nd ed.). Thousand Oaks, CA: Sage.

Teddlie, C., & Tashakkori, A. (2009). *Foundations of mixed methods research: Integrating quantitative and qualitative approaches in the social and behavioral sciences.* Thousand Oaks, CA: Sage.

Wheeler, B. L. (Ed.). (2005). *Music therapy research* (2nd ed.). Gilsum, NH: Barcelona.

CHAPTER 9

Evidence-Based Practice in Music Therapy

Felicity A. Baker

When music therapy practitioners meet with clients, before they can commence therapy practitioners must assess and decide the most appropriate therapy plan for each client. Over the past two decades, evidence-based practice (EBP) has emerged as the preferred clinical decision-making method in the health care environment. As music therapists are often part of a multidisciplinary team, they too must engage in EBP to inform their clinical decisions. This chapter aims to provide an overview of EBP; a description of what constitutes levels of evidence, including current debates around this issue; and an outline of the steps involved in EBP methods. This chapter summarizes the evidence available for music therapy.

What Is Evidence-Based Practice?

In EBP the practitioner systematically locates and appraises the most current and valid research findings and uses these as the basis for clinical decisions. Prior to the EBP movement, clinical experience, expert opinion, and intuition were highly regarded and underpinned many health care practices (e.g., the Heimlich maneuver; Howick, 2011). This was especially the case in music therapy, which has emerged through the experiences and practices of pioneers in the field. Indeed, much of my own practice as a clinician in the 1990s in neurorehabilitation evolved by drawing on methods taught to me during my music therapy training and adapting these to fit the specialized needs of adults with traumatic brain injury (Baker & Tamplin, 2006). As noted in the Cochrane review by Bradt, Magee, Dileo, Wheeler, and McGilloway (2010), there are no experimental or quasi-experimental music therapy studies addressing traumatic brain injury that meet Cochrane criteria prior to 1995, and only few case studies existed on which I could draw as I developed my practice with this clinical group.

EBP introduced a paradigm shift in health care that downgrades intuition and unsystematic clinical experience, suggesting they are inadequate for clinical decision making. Instead, evidence-based practice emphasizes that evidence from clinical research should inform decision making and is essential for ethical and efficacious practice (Howick, 2011). The most widely cited definition states that evidence-based practice is "the conscientious, explicit and judicious use of current best evidence in making decisions about the care of individual patients" (Sackett, Rosenberg, Gray, & Richardson, 1996, p. 71). EBP questions, finds, and appraises the relevant data and then draws on the information generated to inform the clinician's practice.

The EBP Process

In the EBP decision-making process, the clinician needs to complete six steps:

1. *Posing the question.* In this step, the clinician thoroughly assesses the client, and through his or her interaction with the client, it becomes apparent that there is a clinical problem or question that needs consideration. Questions might concern which intervention method to select (e.g., active vs. receptive methods, improvisation vs. songwriting); which context (e.g., group vs. individual vs. family therapy, institution vs. community vs. home-based care): which clinical orientation (e.g., cognitive-behavioral vs. psychodynamic vs neurologic music therapy); or what dose (e.g., single session vs. short programs vs. longer programs). From here, the clinician constructs a clinical question that relates to the client's context. For example, "How many music therapy sessions are needed to reduce depressive symptoms in this adult with a severe mental disorder?" The question can then be used to guide a thorough search for the available evidence that will answer the question.

2. *Locating relevant research knowledge.* In this step, the clinician aims to efficiently locate the research literature that will assist in answering the clinical question. Sackett, Richardson, Rosenberg, and Haynes (1997)

proposed a clinical question model to assist the clinician in determining what information to search for:

a. "What are the characteristics of a group of clients very similar to my client?"

b. "What intervention do I wish to learn about?"

c. "What are the main alternatives to this intervention?"

d. "What outcomes do I and the client hope for? How will outcomes be determined?"

e. "What type of intervention question am I asking? Treatment, diagnosis, prevention, etiology, or prognosis?"

Considerations as to which sources should be searched are important here. The clinician should set the boundaries for collecting the evidence so that the client's specific context is most closely matched with the sources retrieved. For example, if searching for evidence about which music therapy interventions enhance joint attention of children with autism, the boundaries of the searching should be specific enough so that studies of adults with autism are excluded, children with other developmental disabilities are excluded, studies that address other challenges associated with autism are excluded, and studies that are not about music therapy are excluded. At the same time, if the search fails to locate any matches, loosening the criteria may be necessary so that some data from a related area may assist in informing the clinical decisions: for example, widening the criteria so that adults with autism are included in the search. Following the guidelines for systematic literature reviews can be useful to ensure identification of the most relevant literature and to prevent unnecessary time and energy expenditures sifting through large numbers of articles to locate the relevant ones (Bradt & Dileo, 2005).

3. *Critically appraising the quality and applicability of located knowledge.* The next step in the EBP review is to appraise the evi-

dence by assessing the validity (closeness of fit to the clinical issue being considered), and, importantly, applicability (usefulness in clinical practice) of the selected research. So what makes evidence valid and applicable? There has been much debate in the literature about what constitutes good evidence, or more specifically, the best evidence. Research tells us that reviewing studies on a subject can result in conflicting findings even when the same variables are being measured. When there are conflicting findings, it is even more essential that the clinician carefully appraise the literature so that the *best* evidence is identified for the clinical issue of concern.

Early definitions of EBP were very rigid in that *good evidence* was ranked according to hierarchies, with randomized controlled trials (RCTs) and meta-analyses/systematic reviews of RCTs constituting the best evidence (Howick, 2011). More recently, the Oxford University Centre for Evidence-Based Medicine (2009) established a hierarchy of seven levels (Table 9.1). Note that there is no mention of qualitative studies in this hierarchy whatsoever, a point Else and Wheeler (2010) note and that I address below.

Only studies ranked level 1 allow us to reliably conclude a cause-and-effect relationship in intervention trials. However, one should not discount what is found in studies at levels 3a and 3b. We know that research often begins with exploratory studies and case studies that investigate the effect of the intervention on a specific individual or small group of people. Such research assists us in determining what constitutes a treatment approach. Descriptive and correlational studies also help to clarify what other attributes may exacerbate or diminish the impact of the treatment (Drisko & Grady, 2012).

Another problem associated with the controlled trials in the level 1 hierarchy is that they are often designed to examine the effect of just one variable. The highly controlled nature of the trials often leads to the

TABLE 9.1. Hierarchies of Evidence

Level	Therapy outcomes
1a	Systematic reviews of several experimental research studies showing homogeneity of results
1b	Individual RCTs with narrow confidence interval that show that results of treatment are better than no treatment
2a	Systematic reviews of several quasi-experimental or cohort studies where there is no control group or retrospective control group and where results show homogeneity
2b	Single cohort study, including low-quality RCT
2c	Outcomes research or observational studies based on retrospective matching of clients; lacks random assignment
3a	Systematic review with homogeneity of results of case–control studies
3b	Single case–control study
4	Case series, poor-quality cohort, and case–control studies
5	Expert opinion

Note. Based on Oxford University Centre for Evidence-Based Medicine's Levels of Evidence (2009). RCTs, randomized clinical trials.

inclusion of participants with a very specific set of diagnoses (efficacy studies) and to the exclusion of individuals with multiple, comorbid disorders that are based on real-world conditions (effectiveness studies). Although including people with comorbid conditions and varied circumstances reduces the internal validity of the studies, they may have more value to the clinician who is working with real-world clients who of have comorbid disorders (Drisko & Grady, 2012). Further, applicability may be threatened when controlled studies have overly circumscribed sociocultural criteria. For example, when studies contain partici-

pants from a narrow socioeconomic, sociocultural, or religious group, the effects of
the treatment may not be generalizable to
other groups.

Many RCTs may report good outcomes,
but their protocols and contexts may be
vastly different from those of the clinician
and his or her client. For example, in a systematic review and meta-analysis of music
therapy for people with serious mental disorders, Gold, Solli, Krüger, and Lie (2009)
found that there was a dose–response relationship (i.e., the size of the effect is related
to the number of sessions provided), with
the largest effects emerging when 16–51
sessions were conducted. However, for a clinician servicing a community of people for
whom short, acute hospital stays are more
typical, the applicability of the evidence
may be limited. In summary, the specific
context will determine the degree of applicability for each study considered. It is
important to recognize that the EBP process of investigating evidence may not lead
to just one answer to the question posed
but to a range of options. Here, the clinician needs to consider several factors that
may be influenced by the client's preferences, cultural or religious considerations,
or practical considerations such as length
of stay in a facility, frequency with which
the music therapist can visit the client, facility constraints, and resources. In other
words, the clinician needs to take into consideration how the research findings can be
understood within the unique situation of
the client, and how much of the evidence is
relevant to the client based on the client's
unique presentation and the context in
which treatment takes place.

4. *Discussing the research results with the
client and assessing the fit of effective options
with the client's values and goals*. After synthesizing and summarizing the findings,
treatment options should be communicated to the client. Discussion allows clients
to communicate their views and interests
and to report what they know and expect

from treatment based on their own understandings. Sometimes treatment options
are refused, despite a strong evidence base,
because they conflict with cultural expectations or religious beliefs or more practical challenges such as transportation to
the music therapy clinic (Drisko & Grady,
2012).

5. *Collaboratively developing a plan of intervention*. Once the client's perspectives on
the treatment options have been explored,
a final treatment plan should be developed.
This plan should include the goals of the
treatment approach and the expected outcomes. Including a discussion of expected
outcomes is important, because different
treatment approaches may result in different outcomes. For example, music therapy
practiced within a cognitive-behavioral
therapy model will generate different outcomes from psychodynamically oriented
music therapy.

6. *Implementing the intervention*. The final
step in the EBP process is to implement
the intervention, documenting the client's
progress or regression.

What Evidence Do We Have for Music Therapy?

If music therapy EBP should be informed
by the hierarchies of evidence proposed by
the Oxford University Centre for Evidence-
Based Medicine (2009), then what evidence
do we have for music therapy? A thorough
search of the literature for systematic reviews generated a number of studies. Table
9.2 outlines 26 systematic reviews and their
main findings. Bradt and Dileo (2005) performed a substantial meta-analysis of 183
studies. Because of the sheer size of this
meta-analysis, Table 9.2 includes only the
statistically significant findings, so that the
reader may gain a sense of what evidence
we do have, rather than what evidence we
do not.

TABLE 9.2. Meta-Analyses and Systematic Reviews in Music Therapy

Authors	Clinical populations	No. of studies	Main findings
Bradt & Dileo (2005) (selected results)[a]	Surgery	51	Music listening effective in decreasing heart rate, positively affecting respiration rate, moderating blood pressure and arterial pressure, reducing need for analgesic or sedative drugs, reducing nausea/vomiting, reducing anxiety.
	Cardiology/ICU	14	Music listening effective in decreasing heart rate, positively affecting respiration rate, reducing anxiety.
	Cancer/terminal illness/HIV	18	Music listening may reduce nausea/vomiting.
	Neonatology	17	Music listening effective in heart rate normalization, reducing the length of hospital stay, reducing distress behaviors.
	Rehabilitation	18	Active music therapy effective in normalizing gait.
	Alzheimer's disease	26	Active music therapy may improve in-seat behavior, reduce agitation and aggression, improve social interaction, and enhance verbal communication.
	General findings (non-population-specific)		Music listening is effective in increasing oxygen saturation levels and may improve immune functioning; music therapy may be effective in decreasing depression or enhancing mood in medical patients and may improve patient well-being and life satisfaction.
Weller & Baker (2011)	Physical rehabilitation	15	Music therapy effective in gait, fine motor and gross motor rehabilitation; music therapy is functional, goal directed, interesting, repetitive, and progressive in complexity.
Bradt et al. (2010)[a]	Mechanically ventilated	8	Listening to recorded music produced relaxation response and reduced heart rate and respiratory rate. Weak evidence for improved oxygen saturation and reduced blood pressure. No evidence of improved quality of life (QoL), postdischarge outcomes, mortality, or cost-effectiveness.
Bradt & Dileo (2009)[a]	Coronary heart disease	23	Main intervention—listening to recorded music: moderate effect on anxiety, but results inconsistent across studies. No evidence for reduction of psychological distress. Music listening reduced heart rate, respiratory rate, and blood pressure. Studies that included two or more music sessions led to small and consistent pain-reducing effect.
de Dreu et al. (2012)[a]	Parkinson's disease	6	Music-based movement significantly effective in improving balance, gait, and stride length. No significant effects for Unified Parkinson's Disease Rating Scale—motor score, freezing of gait, and QoL.
Wilson et al. (2008)[a]	Colonoscopy	8	Listening to music is effective in reducing procedure time, anxiety, and amount of sedation.

(continued)

TABLE 9.2. *(continued)*

Authors	Clinical populations	No. of studies	Main findings
Bechtold et al. (2009)[a]	Colonoscopy	8	Music played improved patients' experiences. Music varied from classical to patient-directed; timing of music inconsistent across studies; endoscopist not blinded in most studies.
Bradt et al. (2010)[a]	Brain injury	7	Rhythmic auditory stimulation (RAS) may help improve gait parameters in stroke patients. Insufficient data to examine effects of music therapy on upper extremity function, communication, mood/emotions, social skills, pain, behavioral outcomes, activities of daily living (ADLs), and adverse events.
Hurkmans et al. (2012)	Brain injury rehabilitation	15	Improvements reported in all studies, but methodological quality low. Melodic intonation therapy (MIT) method most commonly used.
Vink et al. (2011)[a]	Dementia	10	Methodological quality poor; study results could not be validated or pooled for further analysis.
Standley (2002)[a]	Premature infants	10	Recorded lullabies effective to pacify, increase oxygen saturation, and reduce stress, from 28 weeks corrected gestational age. Dose: 20- to 30-minute intervals at beginning of sleep times and immediately after stressful medical/care procedures. Sung lullabies help sustain homeostasis during multimodal stimulation, from 32 weeks. Recorded female lullaby effective reinforcement of non-nutritive sucking.
Klassen et al. (2008)	Children undergoing procedures	19	Overall methodological quality poor. Meta-analysis (nine studies) showed music therapy significant in reducing pain and anxiety. Passive as effective as active music therapy. Most affected were girls, very sick children, and children with low pain thresholds. Multifaceted interventions that include music are more effective than music alone.
Mrázová et al. (2010)	Pediatric patients (broad range)	28	Mostly poor-quality studies, heterogeneous interventions, diagnoses, control groups, duration, and outcome parameters. Most revealed positive results.
Treurnicht et al. (2011)	Children (broad range)	17	Meta-analysis not possible due to heterogeneous interventions, outcomes, and measurement tools. Poor methodological quality. Mixed results in studies of children with learning/developmental disorders; promising trends in children undergoing stressful life events or acute and/or chronic illness; no evidence that music therapy is effective with adolescents with mood disorders or other psychopathology.

(continued)

TABLE 9.2. *(continued)*

Authors	Clinical populations	No. of studies	Main findings
Whipple (2004)[a]	Autism spectrum disorder	9	All use of music highly effective, regardless of treatment design, age, music used, treatment methodology, or profession of music provider.
Gold et al. (2010)[a]	Autism spectrum disorder	3	Music therapy superior to placebo for verbal and gestural communication skills; effects not significant for behavioral outcomes. Studies encouraging, but limited applicability to practice.
Bradt et al. (2011)[a]	Cancer	30	13 trials used active music therapy; 17 used recorded music: both formats reduced anxiety, had positive impact on mood, but no change to depression. Small reductions in heart rate, respiratory rate, and blood pressure. Moderate pain-reducing effect. Pooled test of two trials suggested QoL improvement.
Bradt & Dileo (2011)[a]	End of life	5	Weak evidence for music therapy reducing pain or anxiety. A limited number of studies suggest that music therapy may benefit QoL, but these results are from studies with high risk of bias.
Mössler et al. (2011)[a]	Schizophrenia (and similar)	8	Music therapy plus standard care superior to standard care for global state; good effects on negative symptoms, general mental state, depression, anxiety, and social functioning. Music therapy had positive effects on cognitive function and behavior. Better effects found when "sufficient" number of music therapy sessions provided by qualified music therapists.
Gold et al. (2009)[a]	Serious mental disorders	15	Music therapy plus standard care result in significant effects on global state, general symptoms, negative symptoms, depression, anxiety, and functioning. Effects not dependent on diagnosis or study design, but on dosage. Between 16 sessions (depressive symptoms) and 51 sessions (functioning) needed for large effects.
Silverman (2003)[a]	Psychosis	19	Music therapy effective in suppressing and combating symptoms of psychosis; no difference between recorded and live music; no difference between structured groups and passive listening, nor between preferred or therapist-selected music; classical music not as effective as nonclassical.
Maratos et al. (2009)[a]	Depression	5	Meta-analysis not appropriate (heterogeneous in interventions and populations). Four RCTs reported greater symptom reduction for music therapy participants.

(continued)

TABLE 9.2. *(continued)*

Authors	Clinical populations	No. of studies	Main findings
Chan et al. (2011)	Depression	17	Music listening: Meta-analysis not possible (heterogeneous listening interventions, duration, frequency, and type). Music listening (particularly patient-preferred) over 2–3 weeks helped reduce depressive symptoms in adults; multiple sessions more effective than single.
de Niet et al. (2009)[a]	Sleep	5	Music-assisted relaxation had moderate effect on sleep quality of patients with sleep complaints; no side effects.
Pelletier (2004)[a]	Stress	22	Music alone and music-assisted relaxation significantly decreased arousal. Degree of stress reduction differed with age, type of stress, musical preference, previous music experience, and type of intervention.
Mays et al. (2008)	Substance abuse	19	No consensus regarding effectiveness of music therapy plus standard care.
Clark et al. (2012)[a]	Older adults in rehabilitation	12	Low- to moderate-quality studies; within-session differences did not increase physical activity, but there were cumulative benefits following programs with music over several weeks.

Note. I wish to thank Wendy Chatterton for her assistance in organizing the data presented in this table. RCTs, randomized clinical trials.
[a] Studies that are Cochrane reviews or meta-analyses published elsewhere.

A few trends emerge from the evidence presented in Table 9.2. First, music listening reduces heart rate and respiration in surgical, coronary heart disease, medically ventilated, and cancer, HIV, and terminally ill patients, suggesting that the effects are generalizable across several different clinical populations. Similarly, blood pressure is reduced in surgical, medically ventilated, and coronary heart disease patients. Cross-population evidence suggests that music listening and music therapy reduce anxiety (to varying degrees) as measured in surgical, coronary heart disease, colonoscopy, cancer, and HIV patients and in those with terminal illness and serious mental illness, including schizophrenia. Symptoms of depression are alleviated through music therapy and music listening interventions during admissions to surgery; in people with cancer, HIV, or serious mental illness; in those with a primary diagnosis of depression; and in those who are terminally ill. Music listening contributes to improved oxygen saturation levels in neonates and those who are medically ventilated. Pain reduction was found for children undergoing surgery, people with cancer, and those who are facing the end of life, and music listening tended to reduce the need for analgesic or sedative medications in patients undergoing surgery and colonoscopy.

There were encouraging and consistent findings across reviews and meta-analyses in the field of rehabilitation, particularly in relation to the effects of active music therapy on gait (in general rehabilitation interventions, for those with Parkinson's disease, and for those who have had strokes). Other effects of music therapy were strong but confined to specific populations. For example, active music therapy improved social interaction and functioning in people with Alzheimer's disease or schizophrenia. Similarly, verbal communication was improved in those with Alzheimer's disease or autism spectrum disorder.

The Role of Qualitative Research in EBP

Although the hierarchy levels 1–3 in Table 9.1 may constitute the *best* forms of evidence and enable us to make cause-and-effect claims, other types of research and inquiry nonetheless contribute to our knowledge base. The upper levels of the hierarchy do not enable us to explore situations in which treatment approaches are ineffective or how new treatment models would be created. Qualitative research can enhance EBP by assisting clinicians in understanding how and why music therapy interventions work, clarifying unexpected results from the quantitative studies, and understanding what a client's experience of treatment in music therapy is like (Drisko & Grady, 2012). For example, in an RCT utilizing mixed methods, Schwantes (2011) implemented a music therapy program with Mexican migrant farmworkers, focusing her outcomes on decreasing levels of depression and anxiety and reducing social isolation. She conducted focus group interviews, the analysis of which revealed important information about how the music therapist's role facilitated the development of relationships among the participants. From the perspectives of those involved in the treatment, this type of evidence cannot be understood by considering the quantitative outcome measures used in the study.

Abrams (2010) raises the issue that because of the limited (although growing) body of literature on music therapy practice, theory, and research, an "inclusive understanding" of what constitutes evidence and an "integral understanding" of how different forms of evidence can inform music therapy are necessary (pp. 351–352). He

suggests that there are multiple epistemological domains of evidence and proposes a definition of evidence that is more inclusive than that provided by the accepted hierarchy: Evidence includes "indications, manifestations, and/or signs that serve as sufficient grounds for beliefs, judgments, formation of conclusions, or proof about a given phenomenon, by bearing witness to, and making plain or clear, certain aspects of that phenomenon" (p. 352). Drawing on Wilber's (2001) integral model which identifies different epistemological perspectives of ways of knowing reality, Abrams suggests that evidence can be observed from the outside (exterior) or experienced from the inside (interior); can be understood at the micro (individual) or macro (collective) level; and can be viewed as subjective, objective, intersubjective, or interobjective. Abrams also argues that music therapists are not only scientists but also artists, for whom subjectivity, aesthetics, creativity, and individuality are core elements of practice. With this broad view of evidence in mind, qualitative research can be seen as providing possibilities for understanding the individual or collective music therapy experiences of research participants, because their inner worlds and individual responses to music therapy practice are forms of evidence, albeit within their specific contexts.

What Abrams (2010) proposes is not about hierarchies of evidence but rather different *forms* of evidence, all with specific roles to play, depending upon one's epistemology. According to the four main quadrants in Wilber's (2001) model, Abrams (p. 364) identified different forms of evidence to support the objective, interobjective, subjective, and intersubjective categories of experience:

1. Objective/individual forms of evidence exist when outcomes from interventions can be verified or disconfirmed and are observable and measurable using valid, reliable instruments.
2. Interobjective/collective forms of evi-

dence exist when outcomes from interventions can be verified or disconfirmed via observable demonstrations of the workings of dynamical systems.

3. Subjective/individual evidence involves the affirmation or disaffirmation of how artistically, substantively, and meaningfully therapeutic opportunities are created as well-informed and trustworthy constructions for individual change, via personal witness and appraisal. Evidence is constructed by the researcher and may comprise triangulation (sourcing data in multiple forms) and member checking (asking participants to comment on the researcher's constructions).

4. Intersubjective/collective forms of evidence exist when there is intersubjective agreement or disagreement on how meaningfully therapeutic opportunities are co-constructed for contextually informed individual and communal change, via shared witness and appraisal.

There are several approaches to evaluating qualitative studies as a means of building evidence, many of which are described in detail in by Burns and Meadows (Chapter 8, this volume). Two that are gaining recognition in the field of health, particularly nursing, are meta-synthesis (Kent, Fineout-Overhold, 2008; Zimmer, 2006) and narrative synthesis approaches (Rodgers et al., 2006). A *meta-synthesis* is a form of qualitative research whereby the researcher or clinician collects a series of qualitative studies on a specific topic and uses the findings of each study to determine links among them. According to Zimmer, meta-syntheses are not just integrated reviews of the studies, but rather the researcher interprets the findings of the original studies and then synthesizes these into the review. From this process, new interpretations may be made. The challenge for the researcher is to ensure that he or she remains true to "the philosophical, theoretical, and conceptual frameworks associated with the original re-

search designs" (Kent & Fineout-Overhold, 2008, p. 160).

A *narrative synthesis* intends to synthesize qualitative papers to determine what is known about a subject area. Unlike meta-syntheses, narrative syntheses may include both quantitative and qualitative studies. As the term *narrative* implies, narrative synthesis is a systematic review that uses words to describe and explain the findings of the synthesizing process; it aims to tell the story of the findings (Rodgers et al., 2006).

Meta-syntheses can be particularly useful in music therapy research because increased numbers of qualitative studies are being published. Large, sufficiently powered RCTs are expensive to implement, whereas many qualitative studies may not require a large budget. Individually, the findings of these qualitative studies may not be generalizable, but if a researcher can pull these studies together and compare, translate, and analyze the original findings to produce new interpretations, such evidence may carry more weight (Kent & Fineout-Overhold, 2008; Zimmer, 2006). However, this approach is not without its challenges. The researcher may confront numerous studies that differ in participants' and researchers' perspectives. How does the researcher allow for these differences and still produce a synthesized report?

The approach to undertaking a meta-synthesis has some similarities with systematic reviews and meta-analyses. The process begins with the formulation of the clinical question to be answered. The question might focus on issues of effectiveness, efficacy, feasibility of implementation, or appropriateness of intervention in relation to clients' needs (Rodgers et al., 2009). The question guides the second stage: the search and retrieval of the relevant articles for review. Once the articles have been collected, the third stage involves a process of deciding which articles to include and which to exclude (Walsh & Downe, 2005) based on inclusion and exclusion criteria.

The fourth stage involves appraising the studies for methodological quality. At this point, additional studies may be excluded if they are not methodologically sound (Rodgers et al.). The fifth stage involves analyzing the studies. In meta-syntheses this analysis includes the researcher's interpretations of individual article findings. In narrative synthesis, this involves writing textual descriptions, grouping and clustering the studies, constructing a common rubric (transforming the data), or analyzing the content thematically (translating the data; Rodgers et al.). The sixth and final stage in the process is to explore the relationships within and between studies.

As a means of generating an evidence base, meta-syntheses and narrative syntheses have not yet been applied in the music therapy field, but their utilization is imminent. A recent *descriptive* review (a variation of narrative synthesis) of music therapy with people who have disabilities was undertaken by McFerran, Lee, Steele, and Bialocerkowski (2009). What is important here is not what the authors found, but that they have now introduced this approach to evidence-based practice to the field of music therapy.

Final Thoughts

This chapter has presented a growing body of evidence that can inform the clinical approaches that practitioners employ when seeking to alleviate negative symptoms or enhance the well-being of a range of clientele. Further, these evidence-based findings can be used to argue for the utilization of music therapy services in various medical, education, and community settings; to apply for national registration (a current area of interest in the European countries and Australia); or to make a case for clients being reimbursed for music therapy services through their private health insurance. Still missing from our evidence base are systematic reviews of qualitative stud-

ies, wherein rigorous appraisal of studies provide evidence of what our clients experience and value from their participation in music therapy. This missing component will assist us in understanding the bigger picture of the treatment experience and enable us to tweak our treatment approaches and strategies to ensure not only observable improvements in clients' well-being, but also that we tailor treatment and respond sensitively and appropriately to ensure that the experience of treatment is meaningful for our clients.

REFERENCES

Abrams, B. (2010). Evidence-based music therapy practice: An integral understanding. *Journal of Music Therapy, 47*(4), 351–379.

Baker, F., & Tamplin, J. (2006). *Music therapy in neurorehabilitation: A clinician's manual.* London, UK: Jessica Kingsley.

Bechtold, M. L., Puli, S. R., Othman, M. O., Bartalos, C. R., Marshall, J. B., & Roy, P. K. (2009). Effect of music on patients undergoing colonoscopy: A meta-analysis of randomized controlled trials. *Digestive Diseases and Sciences, 54*(1), 19–24.

Bradt, J., & Dileo, C. (2005). *Medical music therapy: A meta-analysis and agenda for future research.* Cherry Hill, NJ: Jeffrey Books.

Bradt, J., & Dileo, C. (2009). Music for stress and anxiety reduction in coronary heart disease patients. *Cochrane Database of Systematic Reviews, 2009*(2), CD006577.

Bradt, J., & Dileo, C. (2010). Music therapy for end-of-life care. *Cochrane Database of Systematic Reviews, 2010*(1), CD007169.

Bradt, J., Dileo, C., & Grocke, D. (2010). Music interventions for mechanically ventilated patients. *Cochrane Database of Systematic Reviews, 2010*(12), CD006902.

Bradt, J., Dileo, C., Grocke, D., & Magill, L. (2011). Music interventions for improving psychological and physical outcomes in cancer patients. *Cochrane Database of Systematic Reviews, 2011*(8), CD006911.

Bradt, J., Magee, W. L., Dileo, C., Wheeler, B. L., & McGilloway, E. (2010). Music therapy for acquired brain injury. *Cochrane Database of Systematic Reviews, 2010*(7), CD006787.

Chan, M. F., Wong, Z. Y., & Thayala, N. V. (2011). The effectiveness of music listening in reducing depressive symptoms in adults: A systematic review. *Complementary Therapies in Medicine, 19*(6), 332–348.

Clark, I. N., Taylor, N. F., & Baker, F. (2012). Music interventions and habitual physical activity in older adults: A systematic literature review and meta-analysis. *Journal of Rehabilitation Medicine, 44,* 710–719.

de Dreu, M. J., van der Wilk, A. S. D., Poppe, E., Kwakkel, G., & van Wegen, E. E. H. (2012). Rehabilitation, exercise therapy and music in patients with Parkinson's disease: A meta-analysis of the effects of music-based movement therapy on walking ability, balance and quality of life. *Parkinsonism and Related Disorders, 18*(Suppl. 1), S114–S119.

de Niet, G., Tiemens, B., Lendemeijer, B., & Hutschemaekers, G. (2009). Music-assisted relaxation to improve sleep quality: Meta-analysis. *Journal of Advanced Nursing, 65*(7), 1356.

Drisko, J., & Grady, M. (2012). *Evidence-based practice in clinical social work.* New York: Springer-Verlag.

Else, B., & Wheeler, B. (2010). Music therapy practice: Relative perspectives in evidence-based reviews. *Nordic Journal of Music Therapy, 19*(1), 29–50.

Gold, C., Solli, H. P., Krüger, V., & Lie, S. A. (2009). Dose–response relationship in music therapy for people with serious mental disorders: Systematic review and meta-analysis. *Clinical Psychology Review, 29*(3), 193–207.

Gold, C., Wigram, T., & Elefant, C. (2010). Music therapy for autistic spectrum disorder. *Cochrane Database of Systematic Reviews, 2010*(2), CD004381.

Howick, J. (2011). *The philosophy of evidence-based medicine.* Oxford, UK: Blackwell-Wiley.

Hurkmans, J., de Bruijn, M., Boonstra, A., Jonkers, R., Bastiaanse, R., Arendzen, H., et al. (2012). Music in the treatment of neurological language and speech disorders: A systematic review. *Aphasiology, 26*(1), 1–19.

Kent, B., & Fineout-Overhold, E. (2008). Using meta-synthesis to facilitate evidence-based practice. *Worldviews on Evidence-Based Nursing, 5,* 160–162.

Klassen, T. P., Klassen, J. A., Liang, Y., Tjosvold, L., & Hartling, L. (2008). Music for pain and anxiety in children undergoing medical procedures: A systematic review of randomized controlled trials. *Acute Pain, 10*(2), 106–106.

Maratos, A. S., Gold, C., Wang, X., & Crawford, M. J. (2009). Music therapy for depression. *Cochrane Database of Systematic Reviews, 2009*(1), CD004517.

Mays, K. L., Clark, D. L., & Gordon, A. J. (2008). Treating addiction with tunes: A systematic review of music therapy for the treatment of patients with addictions. *Substance Abuse, 29*(4), 51–59.

McFerran, K., Lee, J. Y., Steele, M., & Bialocerkowski, A. (2009). A descriptive review of the literature (1990–2006) addressing music therapy with people who have disabilities. *Musica Humana, 1*(1), 45–80.

Mössler, K., Chen, X., Heldal, T. O., & Gold, C. (2011). Music therapy for people with schizophrenia and schizophrenia-like disorders. *Cochrane Database of Systematic Reviews, 2011*(12), CD004025.

Mrázová, M., & Celec, P. (2010). A systematic review of randomized controlled trials using music therapy for children. *Journal of Alternative and Complementary Medicine, 16*(10), 1089–1095.

Oxford University Centre for Evidence-Based Medicine. (2009, March). *Levels of evidence.* Retrieved from *www.cebm.net/index.aspx?o=1025.*

Pelletier, C. L. (2004). The effect of music on decreasing arousal due to stress: A meta-analysis. *Journal of Music Therapy, 41*(3), 192–214.

Rodgers, M., Sowden, A., Petticrew, M., Arai, L., Roberts, H., Britten, N., et al. (2009). Testing methodological guidance on the conduct of narrative synthesis in systematic reviews: Effectiveness of interventions to promote smoke alarm ownership and function. *Evaluation, 15,* 49–73.

Sackett, D. L., Richardson, W. S., Rosenberg, W., & Haynes, R. B. (1997). *Evidence-based medicine: How to practice and teach EBM.* New York: Churchill Livingstone.

Sackett, D. L., Rosenberg, W. M. C., Gray, J. A. M., & Richardson, W. S. (1996). Evidence based medicine: What it is and what it isn't. *British Medical Journal, 312,* 71–72.

Schwantes, M. (2011). *Music therapy's effects on Mexican migrant farmworkers' levels of depression, anxiety, and social isolation: A mixed methods randomized control trial utilizing participatory action research.* Aalborg University, Aalborg, Denmark.

Silverman, M. J. (2003). The influence of music on the symptoms of psychosis: A meta-analysis. *Journal of Music Therapy, 40*(1), 27–40.

Standley, J. M. (2002). A meta-analysis of the efficacy of music therapy for premature infants. *Journal of Pediatric Nursing, 17*(2), 107–113.

Treurnicht Naylor, K., Kingsnorth, S., Lamont, A., McKeever, P., & Macarthur, C. (2011). The effectiveness of music in pediatric healthcare: A systematic review of randomized controlled trials. *Evidence-Based Complementary and Alternative Medicine,* Article ID 464759, 1–18.

Vink, A. C., Bruinsma, M. S., & Scholten, R. J. P. M. (2011). Music therapy for people with dementia. *Cochrane Database of Systematic Reviews, 2003*(4), CD003477.

Walsh, D., & Downe, S. (2005). Meta-synthesis method for qualitative research: A literature review. *Journal of Advanced Nursing, 50*(2), 204–211.

Weller, C. M., & Baker, F. A. (2011). The role of music therapy in physical rehabilitation: A systematic literature review. *Nordic Journal of Music Therapy, 20*(1), 43–61.

Whipple, J. (2004). Music in intervention for children and adolescents with autism: A meta-analysis. *Journal of Music Therapy, 41*(2), 90–106.

Wilber, K. E. (2001). *A theory of everything.* Boston: Shambhala.

Wilson, T. W. S., Wong, E. L. Y., & Twinn, S. F. (2008). Effect of music on procedure time and sedation during colonoscopy: A meta-analysis. *World Journal of Gastroenterology, 14*(34), 5336–5343.

Zimmer, L. (2006). Qualitative meta-synthesis: A question of dialoguing with texts. *Journal of Advanced Nursing, 53*(3), 311–318.

CHAPTER 10

Music Therapy Methods

Susan Gardstrom
Suzanne Sorel

From time to time, a music therapist is asked what she *does* with a client in a music therapy session. Does she select a program of recorded music for the client so that he can experience profound relaxation? Does she teach the client to play an adapted musical instrument? Does she help the client to write a song or to express his immediate feelings on a drum? Perhaps you already know that the answer is yes, yes, yes, and yes! Music therapists do all of these things and many more.

Simply put, the therapist arranges for the client to have various types of music experiences that have been selected or designed to meet the client's identified needs. These experiences are called music therapy *methods*. Bruscia (2014) identifies four distinct methods, which he terms receptive (or listening), composition, improvisation, and re-creative (or performance). The methods describe what the client (not the therapist) is doing in relationship to music. In song discussion, for instance, in which the therapist guides the client to listen to and discuss the meaning and relevance of a song, it is the client's role as a listener that defines the experience as *receptive*.

Within each of the four methods are multiple *variations*, or what some call *experiences, interventions,* or even *applications*. Song discussion is one variation of a receptive method. Imaginal listening is another variation. Music anesthesia is yet another. Each of these variations is unique in many regards, and yet all three are bound together in the sense that the client comes to and responds within the music experience as a listener. One clear advantage of using music-oriented nomenclature to describe what music therapists do is that it is neither clientele-specific nor rooted in any one particular approach to clinical practice: Variations of the four methods are used with all types of clientele by music therapists (1) with both entry-level and advanced training, (2) who espouse all types of theoretical and philosophical perspectives, and (3) who practice at supportive, reeducative, or reconstructive levels of therapy (see Wheeler, 1983).

A *method* is different from a procedure and a technique. Briefly, a *procedure* is a set of sequential actions or steps taken by the therapist as she facilitates a particular experience. A *technique*, on the other hand, can be thought of as a single, in-the-moment verbal, gestural, or musical action or interaction of the therapist during a specific procedural step that serves to elicit a desired response or deepen the client's experience or satisfaction within the experience. Let's put the terms all together in one example: Song discussion is one variation of a receptive method. It involves sequential action steps, or procedures, undertaken by the therapist, such as (1) selecting a song based on group needs; (2) describing the purpose and process of song discussion for the clients; (3) playing the song with careful attention to the clients' responses; and (4) facilitating a discussion about the clients' responses to the song. During step 4 in this example, the therapist may use verbal techniques, such as probing or self-disclosure, to elicit a response from a particularly withdrawn client.

Consider that each particular method—that is, each way of being in relationship to music—offers inherent and unique challenges and opportunities for the client. The experience of listening to music is different from the experience of composing music, which is different from the experience of spontaneous music making, and so forth. It is precisely the distinctive challenges and opportunities afforded by each of these experiences that make certain music therapy methods particularly suited to a client's individualized clinical needs and treatment plan.

In this chapter, we introduce you to the essence of each of the four music therapy methods. We also highlight a few of the many unique variations within each method, discuss therapeutic aims that can be addressed with these variations, and provide a few actual clinical examples to illustrate some of the challenges and opportunities afforded by each.[1]

---

[1] For a comprehensive listing of variations, please see Bruscia's (2014) seminal book, *Defining Music Therapy*.

Receptive Methods

As suggested above, receptive methods are those in which the client assumes the role of a listener in the music experience. Contrary to what you might think, however, this is not a passive role. Although the client is not making music, he is called upon to actively respond to what he hears, in overt and covert ways. His overt responses are external and observable and might include movement to the pulse or verbalizations about what he hears. His covert responses are internal and largely unobservable, and might include his associations and memories or a physiological relaxation response. These types of responses may occur with the other methods, too; the distinction is that receptive experiences are selected or designed intentionally to elicit these various overt and covert responses. Although the inherent challenges placed upon the client are unique to the variation used, all receptive experiences presume that a client can hear and respond to what he hears.

There are more identified receptive variations than any other method. Some frequently employed examples have already been cited above. Others that are commonly used include song (music) communication, eurhythmic listening, and music-assisted relaxation.

Song discussion (Bruscia, 2014), used with verbal clients, essentially involves the client and therapist listening to a song together and finding its meaning and relevance to the client's life. In the case of group therapy, song discussion often functions as supportive therapy—helping clients to experience meaningful connections and a decreased sense of isolation as they communicate with others. As a reeducative tool (see Wheeler, 1983), song discussion can help clients develop insight through the identification, exploration, and communication of thoughts and emotions evoked by their encounter with a selected song, as follows.

CLINICAL EXAMPLE:
Group Song Discussion

At 19, Emily was the youngest resident of the women's unit at the addictions treatment facility where my students and I (Susan Gardstrom) were working. She had attended two prior music therapy sessions but had not uttered a single word (other than her name) or played any instruments, seemingly intimidated by the music-making process or by the presence of the other women, many of whom were twice her age. On this particular day, my cotherapist and I bring in a recording of "Addicted" by Kelly Clarkson and ask the women to take a deep breath and simply allow the words and sounds to enter their consciousness. Emily sits with her head down and her arms folded across her chest, as if for self-protection. The recording begins with the singer's low, breathy voice exposed against a sparse accompaniment of minor harmonies and hollow, percussive sounds. Clarkson's voice increases in intensity but somehow retains its desperate, vulnerable quality as she nears the chorus. Here, she jumps up an octave and delivers an angry message, the potency of which is emphasized by a thick texture of "screaming" guitars and driving drumbeats that can be felt in the chest.

Emily looks up and her eyes are filled with tears. Carla, one of the older and more seasoned members sitting next to Emily, hands her a tissue. As soon as the last sound fades away, Emily speaks about the recent heroin overdose that nearly killed her and that had led to her placement at the facility. As she speaks, it is if the armor melts away, and she gains a new awareness of her own desperate need for help. This disclosure opens the door for verbal sharing from the other women— stories about their own trajectories to and through addiction and all of its attendant emotions. Emily and Carla leave the session arm in arm.

Emily identified closely with the singer and her message. The lyrics of the song— supported by congruous and highly evocative, emotionally rendered music— functioned to bring to the surface critical feelings that could no longer be denied. Tears led to personal storytelling, which led to self-insight and compassionate support from others. (For a detailed account of the mechanisms of song discussion, see Gardstrom & Hiller, 2010.)

A related intervention is called *song (music) communication* or *song sharing*. The essence of this variation is that the client and/or therapist chooses a song to share with others as a way to express or disclose something about self or about the therapeutic relationship or process (Bruscia, 2014). I (Susan Gardstrom) have used song communication in initial sessions with runaway teens as a way "to gently initiate the process of personal sharing in a music therapy group, to learn about the clients and assess their musical proclivities, and to convey interest in the teens' musical offerings as a way to build rapport" (Gardstrom, 2013, p. 632).

Imaginal listening, as the name implies, refers to the use of music with individuals or groups to stimulate imagery. The term *imagery* most often connotes visual images (i.e., mental pictures), but imagery evoked by music may take the form of imagined sounds, smells, bodily sensations, and myriad other incarnations. Imaginal listening has been used to promote increased self-awareness toward "psychological and physical relaxation" (Houghton et al., 2005, p. 206) and well-being (Short, 2007); expand consciousness, support creativity, and assist in the integration of various aspects of the self (Association for Music and Imagery, 2012); deepen spiritual understanding (Maack & Nolan, 1999); manage pain and nausea (Sahler, Hunter, & Liesveld, 2003); and control performance anxiety (Kim, 2008), among other aims.

There are several different types of music-based imagery experiences, such as *music imagery* and the *Bonny Method of Guided Imagery and Music*. These types can be differentiated according to clinical aims, therapist training and role (e.g., level of directiveness), client developmental stage and age, type and length of music selections presented, and level of alertness of the client while listening. *Music imagery* is used within supportive or reeducative levels of clinical practice (see Wheeler, 1983) and can be defined as "directive verbally guided imagery supported by carefully chosen music" (Goldberg & Dimiceli-Mitran, 2012, n. p.). A clinical focus for the experience is predetermined by the therapist and/or the client. The client sits upright (sometimes with eyes closed) and is in a highly relaxed state while listening and imaging. Instrumental recorded music is used most often for music imagery. The selections are brief and contained—that is, they have a simple, repetitive form and minimal variability and tension in all musical elements. The therapist verbally guides the client into the agreed-upon focus by talking over portions of the music; the client then opens his eyes (if closed) and continues imaging—sometimes through drawing or writing—as the music continues to play. Verbal processing typically follows.

The *Bonny Method of Guided Imagery and Music* (BMGIM or GIM; Bonny, 1975) is a reconstructive method (see Wheeler, 1983) used to expand consciousness and bring awareness of inner resources and strengths. In GIM, the adult client (1) reclines and undergoes a brief *induction* by the therapist to promote an altered state of consciousness, (2) *travels* in the imagination while listening to recorded Western classical music and dialogues about the resulting imagery with the therapist, then (3) returns to an alert state to process the imagery and its significance. The music often triggers and supports dynamic imagery. The images revealed are thought to be indicative of unconscious psychological issues that seek resolution (e.g., memories, conflicts, repressed emotions). The client interprets his own imagery with the therapist's guidance. The therapist must have supervised, postgraduate training in order to practice

GIM, as this method often elicits complex unconscious material that requires immediate, sensitive, and skillful attention, as in the following example.

CLINICAL EXAMPLE:
Individual GIM Session

Elisha, 54 years old, sought therapy from Marge, a GIM-trained therapist, to gain some clarity about and relief from nagging regret connected to her mother's dementia. After an assessment period, Marge selected three pieces of symphonic music that have been found to be particularly evocative of emotion, including Barber's "Adagio for Strings." She invited Elisha to lie down, close her eyes, and become conscious of her breathing. To help Elisha fully relax and go inward, Marge asked her to imagine the earth's healing energy traveling progressively upward through her body. This induction concluded with the statement, "Now, full of positive energy, let the music take you where you need to go."

As the initial piece began, Elisha immediately began to see the sprawling backyard of her childhood home, with two stately elm trees standing against a perfect summer sky. She was 8 years old. Elisha's two younger brothers appeared in the scene. As the three children played tag in the green grass, Elisha reported, "I can't see anyone else there, but someone is watching over us, protecting us from threat." When the music selection changed, Elisha again saw her younger self, but this time she was sitting alone in a dark and unfamiliar wooded area. Again, she had the sense that someone protective was in her midst. She stated, "I'm alone, but I can be in this scary place and not feel afraid." As the music increased in dynamics and harmonic tension, Elisha imagined herself walking along an emerging path, without knowing where she was headed. She encountered several mythical creatures and, although some were grotesque and seemed to have malevolent intentions, still Elisha felt no fear. As the Barber selection came to a close, Elisha was sitting peacefully on the path, holding a locket that had been given to her by her grandmother. The therapist helped Elisha gradually return to a fully conscious state and invited her to draw a mandala (circle draw-ing) to depict any aspect of her journey. Elisha drew the two elm trees from the first scene. When asked to look at her drawing from a distance, Elisha realized that the trees repre-sented her mother and grandmother, both of whom had shielded her as a child from the verbal and physical abuse that her father had perpetrated on her brothers.

In that moment Elisha understood that her recent regret stemmed from the fact that she had not expressed her debt of gratitude and never could: Her grandmother was deceased and her mother had forgotten much of what had occurred during Elisha's childhood. She began to weep, unable to speak for several minutes. Marge sat in attentive, compassion-ate silence. Elisha requested to hear some comforting music; Marge selected a short piece from Kobialka's *Timeless Motion* CD. The music "held" Elisha until her crying subsided and her breathing steadied. She and Marge then discussed Elisha's newfound awareness and made a tentative plan for a second GIM session to begin exploring her feelings about the abuse in her family of origin.

Music anesthesia is a receptive application that can be conceptualized as the use of music listening to reduce the client's per-ception of pain and anxiety related to pain, whether chronic or associated with specific medical procedures or surgeries. Music therapy for pain management involves a broad range of music interventions, all of which are individualized in relation to cli-ent need (as determined through assess-ment) and presented within the context of a therapeutic relationship (Kirby, Oliva, & Sahler, 2010). Music therapists have studied and employed music anesthesia with a host of diagnostic groups within both pediatric and adult medical settings (Dileo & Bradt, 2005; Standley & Whipple, 2003).

Procedural support is an important appli-cation of music anesthesia. In this applica-tion the therapist—espousing the broadly accepted gate control theory of pain (Mel-zack & Wall, 1965)—uses live or recorded music stimuli to flood the client's neural pathways, thereby competitively blocking pain messages that would otherwise be perceived in the brain (Kirby et al., 2010; Krout, 2007). For instance, a therapist might engage a child undergoing a medi-cally invasive and painful procedure such as an injection through action listening, evoking a specific movement or verbal re-sponse with carefully selected song mate-rial. In this way the therapist uses music stimuli to redirect the child's attention to lessen his perception of pain.

Eurhythmic listening uses music listening as a way to help clients coordinate some type of motor activity. Various sorts of music can be used, and presentation may be live or recorded, depending on the situation. Examples include pieces with a strong pulse to support rhythmic chore-ography (e.g., dance or aerobic exercise), free-flowing instrumental selections to elicit creative/expressive movements (e.g., moving freely in response to the charac-ter of the music), and music for repetitive or complex movement patterns within a physical rehabilitation protocol (e.g., gait retraining after a stroke). Eurhythmic lis-tening can help individuals or client groups release emotions through an active modal-ity, improve body image, improve physical functioning, and learn movement concepts. Movement can also address clients' needs for increased cardiovascular exercise aimed at weight control. The following example il-lustrates the use eurhythmic listening in an academic setting.

CLINICAL EXAMPLE: High School Boys' Dance Group

Three 16-year-old boys from a self-contained classroom for students diagnosed with intel-lectual disabilities were referred to music therapy by the physical education (PE) in-structor at their high school. All three boys had Down syndrome but were verbal and ambulatory. Two of the three, Brian and Thomas, exhibited behaviors common dur-ing adolescence: rapid mood swings and occasional defiance of authority. The third boy, Jonah, was emotionally stable and cooperative; he had a secondary diagnosis of cerebral palsy, causing weakness on the right side of his body. All three had been having difficulties of one sort or another in their PE course. The PE instructor thought that music therapy might assist the boys in developing the gross motor skills outlined in their individualized educational programs (IEPs).

The music therapist read the students' IEPs, observed all three boys in their PE courses in order to get a sense of the movement expectations and their current capabilities, and talked to the boys about their popular music preferences. The music therapist selected a Linkin Park song that was suitable for rhythmic movement. She choreographed the selected song with modified street dance movement sequences, which the students were able to learn in their music therapy sessions over the course of several weeks. Because the song was preferred and the dance steps perceived as "cool," all three boys were motivated to practice.

In the process of learning the steps, the boys demonstrated achievement of several annual IEP objectives, including (1) maintaining kneeling and standing balance; (2) speeding up, slowing down, or changing direction of movement; (3) jumping with a preparatory movement that includes flexion of both knees with arms extended behind the body; and (4) crossing the midline with upper extremities. The boys also demonstrated social/interpersonal growth as they followed established rules, discovered ways to negotiate differences of opinion, and asked for help from the therapist and each other in a positive manner. In an unprecedented show of compassion, Thomas was able to gently encourage Jonah, who became frustrated with his inability to complete a specific maneuver in the desired tempo.

Music relaxation or *music-assisted relaxation* (MAR) is the use of music to support the client's physiological, physical, or psychological relaxation. Although musical stimuli yield highly individualized responses (Scartelli, 1987), it is believed that certain music experiences, carefully designed and

skillfully facilitated, can produce a palpable calming effect. Music listening, in particular, can be used to mask unwanted environmental sounds (e.g., hospital sounds), serve as a diversion from stressful stimuli, or, as noted above, act as "competing stimuli for other peripheral nerve impulses" such as pain (Krout, 2007, p. 135). Additionally, certain cognitive processes that occur as a result of music listening, such as imagery and attention to relaxation narratives, may positively influence brain structures associated with relaxation (Krout).

Robb (2000) notes that music therapists use MAR for both situational (transient) and chronic (persistent) stress conditions. MAR may be indicated "when clients self-report or are observed to have distressing or intrusive levels of anxiety" (Gardstrom, 2013, p. 633), or when they could benefit from learning relaxation techniques toward self-care. MAR also can be used to induce a relaxed state for imagery, promote sleep, and, as noted above, reduce the perception of pain, which is linked to anxiety. MAR is most effective with clients who have strong receptive language skills and the ability to sit still or lie down for extended periods of time without becoming distracted. In this regard, very young children are not good candidates for MAR.

Two basic types of MAR appear in the music therapy literature: *autogenic relaxation* (AR) and *progressive muscle relaxation* (PMR). AR involves "passive concentration of bodily perceptions (e.g., heaviness and warmth of arms, legs, and abdomen; rhythm of breath; and heartbeat) that are facilitated by self-suggestions" (Stetter & Kupper, 2002, p. 45). PMR involves alternately tensing and releasing various muscle groups toward physical relaxation, which may, in turn, lead to increased psychological comfort (Jacobsen, 1938). In both cases, music can be live or recorded, will likely be instrumental, and will have a stable, consistent character, as variability of musical elements may heighten, rather than lower, the physiological and emotional reactivity of the listener. With PMR, tempo and phrasing of the music are selected for their ability to support periodic tensing and releasing of muscle groups.

Compositional Methods

Compositional methods are different from receptive methods in that they involve a different type of participation on the part of the client. A client who is involved in the process of composition—whether individually or as part of a group experience—is called upon to generate and refine personal opinions, ideas, fantasies, and so forth, and to put them into a workable musical and/ or lyrical structure. Clients' abilities to organize, problem-solve, take responsibility, and communicate can be targeted via compositional processes and products (Bruscia, 2014). Therapeutic themes may emerge and be addressed.

Although variations of this method include instrumental composition and music collage (e.g., music audiobiography), *songwriting* is used more frequently than any other type of composition. Because of the centrality of popular song in American culture—it is omnipresent on radio, television, and the Internet—clients of all ages seem to embrace song as an accessible creative form (Baker & Wigram, 2005). Individually and in groups, clients may write a song from scratch or engage in *song transformation* (Bruscia, 2014), in which they personalize a preexisting song structure by rewriting lyrics and/or altering the musical elements accordingly. The therapist's role is to provide varying levels of technical assistance and interpersonal and emotional support during the compositional process. In a group, the therapist serves as a facilitator or mediator, helping the members to recognize and pursue their common aim and reconcile differences that may arise in the creative process.

Improvisational Methods

The word *improvisation* might conjure images of sitting in a dark, smoke-filled jazz club, listening to a trumpeter taking a solo with his trio. This is one way to characterize improvisation—as music that is invented, composed, or created with minimal preparation, often in a performance venue (*Free Dictionary*, 2012). As a music therapy method, improvisation has some of the same characteristics as an improvisational performance, but there are distinct differences in how and why the music is created and played.

Improvisation in music therapy includes any experiences in which the client actively participates in spontaneous music making with the therapist and/or other clients—playing instruments, vocalizing, or sounding their bodies or other objects (Bruscia, 2014). Improvisation that is centered on meeting clinical goals is often referred to as *clinical improvisation*. The creation of extemporaneous music helps clients organize their physical movements in space, initiate new ideas, have an aesthetic experience, develop a relationship with another person, and identify and explore feelings (Bruscia, 2014; Nordoff & Robbins, 2007; Wigram, 2004). The immediacy of improvisation to meet a variety of emotional states and physical needs is a hallmark of this method and the reason that it is used often and successfully across different settings and clientele. Clients in individual therapy can improvise alone or with the therapist; clients in group therapy can also improvise alone or with the therapist, but often improvise with other group members.

The music itself can take a variety of forms, depending upon the media used to produce sound. As noted above, musical instruments and the voice can be used. Clients also can use their bodies to make sounds through stomping, clapping, or can make a combination of sounds with instruments, vocalizations, and the body. The therapist and client have a range of elements with which to work, including rhythmic, tonal, and expressive (e.g., dynamics, articulation, phrasing), to name a few. The client and therapist develop the improvisation by combining these media and elements in unique ways. The character of the improvisation is reflective of the current emotional and physical state of the client and the potential goal areas.

Improvisations can be either nonreferential or referential. A *nonreferential improvisation* is organized solely around, and derives its meaning from, the music and sounds, without representing or referring to something outside of itself (Bruscia, 1987). A *referential improvisation*, on the other hand, is thematic; it is created "in reference to something other than the music itself," such as an "image, title, story, feeling or work of art" (Gardstrom, 2007, p. 16). Following is an example of a referential improvisation in which the music depicts a planetary theme.

CLINICAL EXAMPLE: Individual Vocal and Instrumental Improvisation

Reva is a 4-year-old girl diagnosed with autism spectrum disorder (ASD). She is verbal, articulate, and bright, yet can be demanding and controlling, requiring a certain sameness and ritual often associated with children with ASD. Ten minutes into her first music therapy session, she moves to the cymbal and begins to spin it. "The sun," she says, quietly. "The planets move around the sun," she continues. It sounds as though she is repeating something she has heard on television or in a movie. I (Suzanne Sorel) listen to her verbal idea and sing a melodic line incorporating her words: "The planets circle around the sun, yes they do." I repeat this descending melody, as Reva begins to move the xylophone, hand drums, and a small conga drum in a circle around the "sun"—the cymbal. I sing the phrase again, and Reva sings it back sweetly, matching pitch and looking over at me briefly, with a hint of a smile on her face. She then declares, with more energy, "There's Venus!", and I musically reflect her statement.

Reva improvises an ascending melodic line, "There's Earth," while striking the drum one definitive time. I sing back her phrase, reflecting the tonal and timbral quality.

This exchange continues as we sing about most of the planets together, with Reva in a floaty and high-pitched sing–speak manner. The musical event comes to a climax with a rocket ship ride to Venus, complete with my improvised support during a countdown to blast off. My music of the sun and planets is lilting, with a steady rhythmic ground that provides a musical structure for her fantasy and musical play. The "blast off" music is energetic and mysterious, with diminished chords and ascending chromatic lines to reflect the anticipation of the flight. Reva's "script," which in other settings she would likely recite in a robotic, noninteractive way, has been transformed into a dynamic, joint musical relationship in which she begins to explore a more natural way of communicating through verbalizing, singing, and drumming—all expressing her creativity. The client develops trust in me as she realizes that her scripted words are taking on new meaning and are validated and developed through the forms that are created. She is more apt to share stories and work through crises in future sessions because of the groundwork laid during this improvisational exchange.

Sometimes clients and therapists improvise melodies and lyrics that develop into song forms during the course of the sessions. These songs can be reflective of anything that is related to the client. Clients can also create an improvisation by conducting others who are playing or singing, thus engaging in another kind of improvisatory experience.

Nordoff–Robbins Music Therapy (NRMT), also called *Creative Music Therapy*, is an improvisational approach that requires advanced training. Developed in 1959 by Paul Nordoff and Clive Robbins, the approach involves the improvisational use of music to evoke responses; develop relationships; and address emotional, cognitive, social, and musical goal areas (Nordoff & Robbins, 2007; Sorel, 2010). Many NRMT-trained therapists work in teams: The primary therapist improvises the music related to the immediate needs and goals of the client, and the cotherapist facilitates the client's relationship to the music through vocalizing, physical and vocal prompting, and movement experiences. The training is humanistic and music-centered, including comprehensive experiential components focused on developing a wide array of improvisatory skills on either piano or guitar. In NRMT the music acts as the primary agent of change (Aigen, 2005), as opposed to functioning as a means to an end or solely as a vehicle for reaching nonmusical goals (Sorel, 2013). The following case exemplifies the Nordoff–Robbins approach.

CLINICAL EXAMPLE: Individual Vocal and Instrumental Improvisation

Ari is a tall, lanky, 16-year-old adolescent with autism. He is primarily nonverbal and often has his hand over his ear in a defensive position. He has a history of self-abuse, such as banging his head and pulling out his hair. He also has had some violent outbursts toward his caregivers, particularly when he becomes overstimulated by sound.

Ari enters his first Nordoff–Robbins Music Therapy session escorted by the cotherapist, Jenny. As the primary therapist, I (Suzanne Sorel) immediately notice the pace of Ari's gait, his solemn facial expression, and the way he grabs the drum mallet and begins to beat in a deliberate way. I join Ari's slow and loud playing by creating a theme on the piano based upon closely textured intervals of fourths and fifths. I am thinking that these intervals may create a sense of grounding and openness. A musical theme is not yet established, as we all get to know each other musically, exploring sounds that are not derivative of any particular musical key. The music has both a holding quality, due to the harmonic intervals, and a sense of forward movement, with the use of certain rhythmic patterns and articulations.

Ari continues to cover his right ear with his hand as he beats loudly with the other. Jenny and I sing a melody that is related to the intervals being played. As the theme develops and we sing out more strongly, Ari hums, lifts his head, and begins to play with alternating hands more assertively. I create, and then repeat, a particular melodic rhythm, and Ari immediately incorporates my idea into his playing, exhibiting his innate musicality by punctuating the phrase with a flourish on the cymbal. Although Ari does not repeat this phrase again, he begins to make vocal sounds and stands up straighter, more fully involved and engaged, demonstrating his acute listening. Ari, who tends to be isolated, obsessed with routines, and unable to form meaningful relationships, immerses himself in this musically creative improvisational experience with these two new people. His sustained attention and involvement through and with the music are notable.

Because improvisation is associated with freedom and thought to be formless (and possibly chaotic), you might think that a therapist and a client just start playing whatever comes to mind. On the contrary, clinical improvisation generally has some kind of underlying structure, guided by the therapist's clinical responsibility and sensitivities. Thus, the therapist must develop skills in initiating, shaping, and guiding the music that is being created.

Re-Creative Methods

Re-creative methods involve the client's reproduction of precomposed musical material, much of which therapists may find in the public domain. Clients can re-create music vocally, instrumentally, through participation in musical productions and games involving music, and by conducting music using a musical score (Bruscia, 2014). On the surface, re-creative experiences may look just like a performance, a recreational sing-along, or even a music lesson. However, in re-creative music therapy—even when performance for others is involved—the focus is on specific clinical aims, a few of which Bruscia (2014) lists as "Develop sensorimotor skills; Improve attention and reality orientation; Develop memory skills; Improve interactional and group skills" (p. 132). Clients may also experience feelings of self-worth and achievement through performance of a song or participation in a musical production.

As with the other music therapy methods, music therapists who use re-creative experiences first identify the needs of their clients and then choose or arrange compatible music experiences—experiences that will challenge the client in a particular way or provide a unique opportunity for growth and development. Sometimes these challenges and opportunities are best presented in the *process* of re-creating music, and sometimes they are best presented via the re-created musical *product*; sometimes the focus of a single experience or session shifts between process and product, because both have value for a particular client or client group.

In the selection and arrangement of musical material, music therapists consider the musical elements, formal structure, lyrical content, and emotional tone, among other factors. The therapist's facilitation may involve modeling, teaching (with or without adaptive or traditional notation), and coordinating rehearsals and performances. The therapist can also support clients' musical offerings through listening, providing feedback, accompanying, and joining.

Vocal re-creation involves using the voice to re-create precomposed material, as in the following example.

CLINICAL EXAMPLE: Vocal Re-Creation

Rosalie, an 80-year-old woman with middle-stage Alzheimer's disease, spends most of her time disoriented and anxious, unable to recognize many close friends and family members, and unaware of her immediate surroundings. When the music therapist begins to play and sing the song "I Could Write a Book," from the musical *My Pal Joey*, Rosalie immediately begins to sing most of the lyrics,

smiles, and plays the basic beat on a tambourine. The memory of the song is vivid and intact, and she is immediately brought into the present moment emotionally and musically, as demonstrated by her playing, singing, smiling, and relating to the music therapist. Despite her inability to have a conversation, Rosalie's ability to respond meaningfully within this re-creative experience illustrates the benefits of using familiar music from her past. Hours after the music therapy session, nurses in her assisted living center comment that, despite her inability to remember the actual music therapy session, Rosalie is smiling and her emotional state remains placid and content.

Singing songs with live accompaniment is just one example of vocal re-creation; clients can also engage in vocal work, chanting, rapping, and singing along with recordings.

With *instrumental re-creation*, clients rehearse and perform certain parts in a piece of music. Learning and reading notation may be part of this endeavor, as well as playing along with a recording (Bruscia, 2014). Some music therapists use musical games and activities, such as "Name That Tune" or "Musical Chairs." In certain clinical situations, clients conduct peers, guiding a group as "dictated by a score or other notational plan" (Bruscia, p. 133).

With *musical productions*, clients are involved in the planning, rehearsing, and performance of a show, musical, or other kind of performance (Bruscia, 2014). The rehearsals that precede the performance can serve as a time to focus on numerous domains of functioning, including communication, sensorimotor, cognitive, social, and emotional domains. Most cultures, communities, and societies regard music as something to be shared with others. The benefits for the individual involved in the production can relate directly to clinical goals. The following vignette illustrates the re-creative method of musical productions.

CLINICAL EXAMPLE:
Creation and Performance of *Holiday*
***on Wheels* by Adult Group**

Eight adults with cerebral palsy and physical, emotional, and cognitive deficits write and perform their own musical as part of the music therapy program at their adult day treatment center. Goals for this project are addressed in multiple ways within the writing, rehearsing, planning, and, finally, performing of the production. I (Suzanne Sorel) initially meet with the group to discuss ideas regarding the production. Ryan, one of the clients, wants the show to relate to the upcoming winter holidays, but he also wants to use the performance to demonstrate his capabilities. All other clients in the group agree: The setting of the musical centers on the holidays, and the characters in the story should overcome some kind of challenge or obstacle to reach a goal. Jill, who likes to write poetry, begins to write lyrics to a song titled "Holiday on Wheels," which relates to the challenges of mobility when living in a wheelchair. Over many weeks, through improvisation and songwriting, the production begins to take shape. Each client explores feelings, both musically and verbally, regarding his or her unique role in the play and how the story regarding the characters should unfold. When the performance day finally arrives, the clients are excited and nervous. They perform the songs and recite their lines to the roar of applause. *Process* and *product* are equally valued in this experience, and the clients are active agents in a distinctive, creative endeavor.

Conclusions

Music is a unique and powerful medium, used throughout the ages to promote health, healing, learning, emotional expression, and community. In music therapy the needs of clients in individual and group sessions are always carefully assessed, and a therapeutic plan is designed to address those needs. The four music therapy methods and their variations highlight the myriad ways that music can target identified aims, within the context of a strong therapeutic relationship.

It is clear that the range of possible experiences is broad, thus requiring extensive clinical and musical skills set on the part of the practitioner. Listening to, composing, improvising, and performing music can be complex endeavors; when choosing how to proceed with her clients, the therapist must carefully consider the inherent challenges and opportunities afforded by these methods. Finally, knowledge of the *how-to*'s of each music experience must be united with a fervent belief in music's potency and a commitment to meeting and treating the individual person.

REFERENCES

Aigen, K. (2005). *Music-centered music therapy*. Gilsum, NH: Barcelona.

Association for Music and Imagery. (2012). Retrieved from *http://ami-bonnymethod.org*.

Baker, F., & Wigram, T. (2005). *Songwriting: Methods, techniques and clinical applications for music therapy clinicians, educators and students*. London: Jessica Kingsley.

Bonny, H. L. (1975). Music and consciousness. *Journal of Music Therapy, 12*(3), 121–135.

Bruscia, K. (1987). *Improvisational models of music therapy*. Springfield, IL: Charles C Thomas.

Bruscia, K. (2014). *Defining music therapy* (2nd ed.). Gilsum, NH: Barcelona.

Dileo, C., & Bradt, J. (2005). *Medical music therapy: A meta-analysis and agenda for future research*. Cherry Hill, NJ: Jeffrey Books.

Free Dictionary, The. (2012). *Improvisation*. Retrieved from *www.thefreedictionary.com/improvisation*.

Gardstrom, S. (2007). *Music therapy improvisation for groups: Essential leadership competencies*. Gilsum, NH: Barcelona.

Gardstrom, S. (2013). Adjudicated adolescents. In L. Eyre (Ed.), *Guidelines for music therapy practice: Mental health of adolescents and adults* (pp. 622–657). Gilsum, NH: Barcelona.

Gardstrom, S., & Hiller, J. (2010). Song discussion as music psychotherapy. *Music Therapy Perspectives, 28*(2), 147–156.

Goldberg, F., & Dimiceli-Mitran, L. (2012). *Guided imagery and music–level I training* [handout]. St. Charles, IL: Conference of the American Music Therapy Association.

Houghton, B. A., Scovel, M. A., Smeltekop, R. A., Thaut, M. H., Unkefer, R. F., & Wilson, B. L. (2005). Taxonomy of clinical music therapy programs and techniques. In R. F. Unkefer & M. H. Thaut (Eds.), *Music therapy in the treatment of adults with mental disorders* (pp. 181–206). Gilsum, NH: Barcelona.

Jacobsen, E. (1938). *Progressive relaxation.* Chicago: University of Chicago Press.

Kim, Y. (2008). The effect of improvisation-assisted desensitization and music-assisted progressive muscle relaxation and imagery on reducing pianists' music performance anxiety. *Journal of Music Therapy, 45*(2), 165–191.

Kirby, L. A., Oliva, R., & Sahler, O. J. Z. (2010). Music therapy and pain management in pediatric patients undergoing painful procedures: A review of the literature and a call for research. *Journal of Alternative Medicine Research, 2*(1), 7–16.

Krout, R. (2007). Music listening to facilitate relaxation and promote wellness: Integrated aspects of our neurophysiological responses to music. *Arts in Psychotherapy, 34,* 134–141.

Maack, C., & Nolan, P. (1999). The effects of guided imagery and music therapy on reported change in normal adults. *Journal of Music Therapy, 36*(1), 39–55.

Melzack, R., & Wall, P. (1965). Pain mechanisms: A new theory. *Science, 150*(3699), 971–979.

Nordoff, P., & Robbins, C. (2007). *Creative music therapy: A guide to fostering clinical musicianship.* Gilsum, NH: Barcelona.

Robb, S. L. (2000). Music assisted progressive muscle relaxation, progressive muscle relaxation, music listening, and silence: A comparison of relaxation techniques. *Journal of Music Therapy, 37*(1), 2–21.

Sahler, O. J., Hunter, B. C., & Liesveld, J. L. (2003). The effect of using music therapy with relaxation imagery in the management of patients undergoing bone marrow transplantation: A pilot feasibility study. *Alternative Therapies in Health and Medicine, 9*(6), 70–74.

Scartelli, J. P. (1987). *Music and self-management methods: A physiological model.* St. Louis, MO: MMB Music.

Short, A. (2007). Theme and variations on quietness: Relaxation focused music and imagery in aged care. *Australian Journal of Music Therapy, 18,* 39–61.

Sorel, S. (2010). Presenting Carly and Elliot: Exploring roles and relationships in a mother–son dyad in Nordoff–Robbins Music Therapy. *Qualitative Inquiries in Music Therapy, 5,* 173–238.

Sorel, S. (2013). Musicing as therapy in Nordoff–Robbins training. In K. Bruscia (Ed.), *Self-experience in music therapy training* (pp. 315–338). Gilsum, NH: Barcelona.

Standley, J. M., & Whipple, J. (2003). Music therapy with pediatric patients: A meta-analysis. In S. Robb (Ed.), *Music therapy in pediatric healthcare: Research and evidence-based practice* (pp. 1–18). Silver Spring, MD: American Music Therapy Association.

Stetter, F., & Kupper, S. (2002). Autogenic training: A meta-analysis of clinical outcome studies. *Applied Psychophysiology and Biofeedback, 27*(1), 45–98.

Wheeler, B. (1983). A psychotherapeutic classification of music therapy practices: A continuum of procedures. *Music Therapy Perspectives, 1*(2), 8–12.

Wigram, T. (2004). *Improvisation: Methods and techniques for music therapy clinicians, educators and students.* London: Jessica Kingsley.

PART II

ORIENTATIONS
AND APPROACHES

INTRODUCTION

Many music therapists incorporate elements of various approaches in their work, whereas others follow a particular model of music therapy. Approaches can be taken from a psychotherapeutic system such as psychodynamic, humanistic, or cognitive-behavioral. Some models, including Nordoff–Robbins or Creative Music Therapy, the Bonny Method of Guided Imagery and Music, Analytical Music Therapy, and Neurologic Music Therapy, have been developed specifically for music therapy. This part includes both approaches to psychotherapy as they have influenced music therapy and models of music therapy practice.

The first three chapters in Part II describe psychotherapeutic orientations that can provide foundations for music therapy. Other orientations, such as existential or biomedical, could have been included. Applications to music therapy form an important part of each chapter.

Chapter 11, "Psychodynamic Approaches," describes music therapy as informed by psychodynamic theory, from its origins in Freudian theory through its development in ego psychology, object relations theory, and self psychology. The author suggests ways in which psychodynamic music therapy is congruent with psychodynamic psychotherapy, with instrumental improvisation, for example, being the counterpart of free association, and the patient–therapist relationship in both music and psychotherapy understood to unfold through the transference and countertransference.

Humanistic approaches to music therapy (Chapter 12) are guided by the tenets of humanism, which posit that all persons have innate capacities for actualizing their own unique potentials for health and well-being, given adequate opportunities for change. Therapists adopting these approaches can employ virtually any specific methods, provided the work is understood according to humanistic principles and precepts. This chapter elaborates upon applying this understanding to music therapy.

Cognitive-behavioral approaches are discussed in Chapter 13, beginning with the history of behaviorism and cognitive therapy. The chapter presents both behavioral music therapy, with its long tradition in music therapy, and newer work using cognitive-behavioral techniques. Both have numerous music therapy adaptations, which are presented with examples from mental health, medical, and chemical dependency settings.

Chapter 14, "Developmental Approaches," presents developmental models related to early childhood tasks of developing a sense of self and building attachment with others, as well as models of musical skill development. Many of the same biological components that underlie music—rhythm, timbre, pitch, dynamics, phrasing, and relationship—are at the core of contemporary models of how humans learn to attach, attune, and communicate. The focus of the chapter is on how models of human development and research regarding models of child development and music can inform music therapy practice.

The next chapters introduce important models of and orientations to music therapy. These models were developed by music therapy pioneers and continue their development with current practitioners.

Chapter 15 describes Creative Music Therapy, also known as *Nordoff–Robbins Music Therapy*, which traces its origins to the work begun by Paul Nordoff and Clive Robbins in the 1960s. It features the use of spontaneously improvised, client-inspired, clinically effective music that can also be brought back in structured forms, such as greeting and activity songs, at any point in the course of therapy. The responses that Nordoff and Robbins observed in children with special needs led them to hypothesize the existence of a *music child*, an inborn nexus of musical ability and responsiveness that exists in everyone and can be engaged to initiate or resume the process of personal development.

The "Bonny Method of Guided Imagery and Music" (Chapter 16), also called *Guided Imagery and Music* (GIM), was developed by Helen Bonny beginning in the 1970s. The client or traveler in GIM is helped to focus awareness in order to achieve an altered state of consciousness. Specially selected classical music is then used to support the traveler's self-exploration, with the assistance of the therapist or guide. In its traditional form, GIM is conducted in an individual session, but group sessions and music imaging approaches have also been developed.

Analytical Music Therapy (AMT), the focus of Chapter 17, is based on the work of British music therapist Mary Priestley. AMT uses free improvisation to facilitate the client's personal growth and become aware of and work with issues that are unconscious or with which the client is reluctant to deal. The improvisation allows the material to become conscious so that the person can process it verbally. The author provides information on training for AMT, as well as research and adaptations of the method by several practitioners.

Neurologic Music Therapy (NMT), the topic of Chapter 18, is a research-based system of standardized clinical techniques that uses music for sensorimotor, speech and language, and cognitive training. The transformational design model is a clinical model intended to guide the thought process of the NMT clinician in selecting the best therapeutic music intervention, based on the client's functional assessment needs and goals. Therapeutic goals and interventions address rehabilitation, development, and maintenance of functional behaviors. Because the clinical applications in NMT are based on current basic science and clinical research, NMT techniques result in consistent and functional results.

In Chapter 19 "Community Music Therapy (CoMT) is distinguished from traditional music therapy by its participatory, ecological, and sometimes also activist orientation. The focus on how music therapy can function outside of normal boundaries, often in nontraditional ways in the community, implies that social change, not only individual change, is part of the agenda. The author says that CoMT "encourages musical participation and social inclusion, equitable access to resources, and collaborative efforts for health and well-being in contemporary societies." Because sensitivity to context is highly valued in CoMT, it is practiced in diverse ways around the world.

Chapter 20, "Music Therapy in Expressive Arts," presents a multimodal approach that combines the visual arts, music, dance/movement, drama, photo/filmmaking, writing, literary art, and other creative processes in psychotherapy, social services, and community work. The author describes an approach called *music-centered expressive arts therapy*. A common basis for this work is the interplay of experiences, emotions, behavior, and physical health that characterizes a mind–body connection.

Other important music therapy models could also be included. Rolando Benenzon's (1981) model, very influential in Latin America and parts of southern Europe, is one. Carolyn Kenny's (1989) *The Field of Play* and *Music and Life in the Field of Play* (2006), written to provide theoretical underpinnings for music therapy and the many positive things that she witnessed, are additional examples. Several chapter authors refer to The Field of Play. Another important treatment method is Diane Austin's (2009) Vocal Psychotherapy.

A number of other orientations could also be included. Aigen (2014) suggests that these orientations are "tendencies of thought," not models, and that they "offer a mode of experiencing, describing, and explaining the value of existing music therapy practices" (p. 223). He distinguishes them from models because they do not include "specific interventions, procedures and goals" (p. 223). These orientations include Biomedical Music Therapy (Taylor, 2010), Culture-Centered Music Therapy (Stige, 2002), Aesthetic Music Therapy (Lee, 2003), Complexity-Based Music Therapy (Crowe, 2004), Music-Centered Music Therapy (Aigen, 2005), Analogy-Based Music Therapy (Smeijsters, 2005), Feminist Music Therapy (Hadley, 2006; see also Curtis, 2000; Chapter 33, this volume), Dialogical Music Therapy (Garred, 2006), and Resource-Oriented Music Therapy (Rolvsjord, 2010). Some of these will prove more important over time than others and would therefore be covered in an entire chapter in a future book. Readers who desire more information on any of these orientations should, of course, consult the original source.

As can be seen, Part II provides the basis for much of what is included in other parts as well as much of what music therapists do. Its contents will enrich both reading about and carrying out clinically oriented music therapy work.

REFERENCES

Aigen, K. (2005). *Music-centered music therapy*. Gilsum, NH: Barcelona.

Aigen, K. S. (2014). *The study of music therapy: Current issues and concepts*. New York: Routledge.

Austin, D. (2009). *The theory and practice of vocal psychotherapy: Songs of the self*. London: Jessica Kingsley.

Benenzon, R. O. (1981). *Music therapy manual*. Springfield, IL: Charles C Thomas.

Crowe, B. (2004). *Music and soulmaking: Toward a new theory of music therapy*. Lanham, MD: Scarecrow Press.

Curtis, S. L. (2000). Singing subversion, singing soul: Women's voices in feminist music therapy (Doctoral dissertation, Concordia University, 1997). *Dissertation Abstracts International, 60*, (12-A), 4240.

Garred, R. (2006). *Music as therapy: A dialogical perspective*. Gilsum, NH: Barcelona.

Hadley, S. (Ed.). (2006). *Feminist perspectives in music therapy*. Gilsum, NH: Barcelona.

Kenny, C. B. (1989). *The Field of Play: A guide for the theory and practice of music therapy*. Atascadero, CA: Ridgeview.

Kenny, C. B. (2006). *Music and life in the Field of Play: An anthology*. Gilsum, NH: Barcelona.

Lee, C. (2003). *The architecture of music therapy*. Gilsum, NH: Barcelona.

Rolvsjord, R. (2010). *Resource-oriented music therapy*. Gilsum, NH: Barcelona.

Smeijsters, H. (2005). *Sounding the self: Analogy in improvisational music therapy*. Gilsum, NH: Barcelona.

Stige, B. (2002). *Culture-centered music therapy*. Gilsum, NH: Barcelona.

Taylor, D. B. (2010). *Biomedical foundations of music as therapy* (2nd ed.). Eau Claire, WI: Barton.

CHAPTER 11

Psychodynamic Approaches

Connie Isenberg

"The talking cure": With the use of this phrase at the end of the 19th century, the age of psychoanalysis was ushered in. Although often attributed to Sigmund Freud, the expression was, in fact, first used by Josef Breuer's patient, Bertha Pappenheim (pseudonym *Anna O.*), who was the subject of the first case study on hysteria written by Breuer and Freud (1893–1895/2001). Since psychodynamic therapies are derived from Freudian psychoanalysis, this term plunges us right into the hub of ongoing controversy within the field of music psychotherapy in general and, more specifically, Psychodynamic Music Therapy.

Whereas earlier questions (e.g., Schneider, Unkefer, & Gaston, 1968) focused on whether the music psychotherapeutic process unfolds through the musical engagement or through the relationship between the therapist and the patient, current questions focus more specifically on the relative importance of music versus words (e.g., Ahonen & Lee, 2011; Erkkilä, 2004; Sekeles, 2011). After all, if psychoanalysis is the *talking cure* and psychodynamic therapies are derived from it, how do we reconcile the use of nonverbal modalities such as music with verbally based psychodynamic theories? This issue begs the question of whether music therapy should depend upon extant theories or on independent music therapeutic theories, which has also been a subject of controversy within the music therapy literature.

Isenberg, Goldberg, and Dvorkin (2008) elaborated upon, but did not resolve, the question of whether music therapy should rely exclusively on theories specific to music therapy. The authors referred to Ruud (1980) and Wheeler (1981), both of whom advocated reliance upon psychological theories, with Ruud at the same time identifying music and the relationship between human beings and music as the main contributors to the unique nature of music therapy. Wheeler suggested that relying on psychotherapeutic theories had the advantage of providing a conceptual map for clinical work, while also serving to enhance the status of the profession within the mental health community.

The present chapter focuses on elucidating Psychodynamic Music Therapy. This is not a straightforward topic. The complexities of it were recently revealed when Silverman (2007) found that, although 49.2% of psychiatric music therapists who responded to a survey reported *using* a psychodynamic approach, only 5.7% listed psychodynamic theory as their primary philosophical orientation. Reconciling these seemingly contradictory responses is not the object of this chapter. It is clear, though, that it is timely to address Psychodynamic Music Therapy from metapsychological and disciplinary historical perspectives. This chapter aims to do both.

History and Theoretical Tenets

A historical review of the development of psychodynamic theory precedes that of Psychodynamic Music Therapy. Associated conceptual terms are also presented. In this section, the development of psychodynamic psychotherapy is traced from its origins in Freudian drive theory through its developments in ego psychology, object relations theory, self psychology, and more recently, intersubjective theory. Although Carl Jung is frequently cited in music therapy literature, Jung's Analytical Psychology diverged sufficiently from Freudian theory as to not be included among the psychodynamic theories. For the purposes of this chapter, the various terms used to describe therapy based on psychodynamic theory—*psychoanalytic psychotherapy, psychodynamic psychotherapy,* and *insight-oriented psychotherapy*—are not distinguished from each other.

Freudian Theory (Drive/Conflict Theory)

Freudian theory is a metapsychology, that is, a comprehensive theoretical framework for understanding mental functioning and development. It provides us with a model that encompasses both normal and pathological mental functioning and with the tools for exploring the human mind. In this way, Freud laid a foundation for theoretical, technical, and clinical aspects of psy-

choanalysis. Given the vastness of Freudian theory, I focus here on a select number of theoretical constructs.

Two of the central hypotheses of Freudian theory (Brenner, 2006) are those of psychic determinism and the prevalence of unconscious mental processes. *Psychic determinism* means that there is causality in psychic function; that is, psychic events are influenced by previous ones and are meaningful, rather than random and meaningless. The clinical implication of this belief in causality is that the analyst attempts to understand *all* psychic phenomena, even when seemingly trivial. Who, in everyday life, has not experienced slips of the tongue or misplaced an object? Rather than viewing these as mere accidents, the principle of psychic determinism engages the analyst in a quest for meaning, seeking the wishes or hidden intentions that might have led to these phenomena. Dreams, too, are seen as meaningful rather than as a sequence of random psychic events. The relationships among and between dream images and other psychic events render the dream meaningful. We can extrapolate from these everyday occurrences to psychopathological states. Symptoms, for example, can also be perceived as having a meaning. We can say that, in a way, they are a language, although often, similar to a foreign language, they can be hard to decipher.

The examples of psychic determinism presented above are at the same time illustrative of the importance of *unconscious mental processes*. If the causal links to slips of the tongue, to dreams, and to symptoms seem elusive, it is precisely because they are connected to unconscious rather than conscious mental processes. Uncovering the unconscious wish behind a dream, for example, may reveal its meaning. Unconscious processes cannot, however, be observed directly but must be studied indirectly. Psychoanalysis, the method developed by Freud, allows unconscious processes to be detected.

The concept of *drives* is basic to Freudian theory. Freud believed that humans are at the mercy of drives, sexual and aggressive in nature, which, when opposed to each other create conflict. The struggle of opposing forces that Freud saw as an integral part of the human being, defines Freudian theory as a *conflict theory*. What defines psychodynamic theory is the *unconscious* nature of internal conflict.

Freud conceptualized two major models of psychic organization. The first, the *topographic* model, described the psychic mechanism in relation to systems of consciousness—the *conscious*, the *preconscious*, and the *unconscious*—whereas the second, the *structural*, grouped functionally related mental processes into three structures—the id, the ego, and the superego. The *id* is comprised of psychic representatives of the drives, *ego* functions deal with our relationship to the environment, and the *superego* comprises our moral functions as well as our aspirations toward an ideal. From a developmental perspective, the ego and the superego gradually differentiate themselves from the id over time, with the *reality principle* slowly supplanting the *pleasure principle* and the ego gradually taming id impulses and taking the conditions of the external world into consideration. The ego functions to achieve a balance between the impulsive demands of the id, the moral pressures of the superego, and the demands of reality.

The goal of therapy in this classical model is to resolve unconscious conflicts. To bring the unconscious to consciousness, the patient engages in *free association*, that is, speaks freely without censoring his or her thoughts, and also reports dreams. In a complementary fashion, the analyst maintains an attitude of *neutrality*—listens freely and openly from a nonjudgmental stance. Free associations, dreams, and *defense mechanisms* are analyzed. Defense mechanisms—unconscious coping mechanisms that aim at reducing anxiety—may serve as *resistance*, obstructing the therapeutic process. Resistance, too, needs to be analyzed.

The patient's attitudes toward the analyst contain projections and displacements from significant others in the patient's past. This process is called *transference* and is a hallmark of psychoanalysis and psychodynamic psychotherapy. "The transference is acknowledged to be the terrain on which all the basic problems of a given analysis play themselves out: the establishment, modalities, interpretation and resolution of the transference are in fact what define the cure" (Laplanche & Pontalis, 1967/1973, p. 455). The goal of therapy in the Freudian model can now be restated in terms of resolving *unconscious conflicts as they are expressed through the transference* to the analyst. The analyst, in turn, has transference reactions to the patient, known as the *countertransference*. Originally considered by Freud to impede analytic work and to be something to overcome, the conceptualization of countertransference evolved and is now recognized as a therapeutic tool that can enhance understanding of the patient.

In summary, Freudian theory espouses the prevalence of the unconscious and of psychic conflicts; that the past influences the present, most often unconsciously; that present behavior can be best understood in relation to early life experiences; and that early relationships are influenced by sexual and aggressive impulses and wishes in the infant and young child.

Ego Psychology

Ego psychology is one of the major schools of psychoanalytic thought derived from classical Freudian theory, specifically from structural theory, which describes the three agencies of the mind: the ego, the id, and the superego. In distinction to drive theory, which focuses more on the id and the superego and on ego functions as related to conflict among the agencies, ego psychology focuses primarily on the ego itself and its adaptive functions. The name that is most closely associated with ego psychology is that of Heinz Hartmann who, along with colleagues such as Kris and Lowenstein, followed by Arlow and Brenner, developed this predominantly American school of thought.

As we have seen above, the clinical focus in drive theory is on internal conflicts and wishes and, as we shall see below, in object relations theory it is on internal relationships. In ego psychology, the focus is on reality testing, defenses, and adaptation, with the ego as the agent of adaptation. Hartmann (1939/1958) posited the existence of a *conflict-free sphere*, believing that ego functions must have autonomy from the drives in order to be successful. Ego functions such as memory and perception are seen as necessary for adaptation to the environment and as having their own energy *not* derived from instinctual drive. *Ego interests* such as a desire for wealth, status, and professional success are also seen as autonomous motivations.

Whereas in drive theory the emphasis is on the individual's psychic reality, Hartmann emphasized the importance of the environment, per se. His term, the *average expectable environment*, refers to the environmental requirements such as sustenance, nurturance, and protection from physical and psychological danger sufficient for physical and psychic development. Guntrip (1973) describes adaptation using Hartmann's words: "We call a man well-adapted if his productivity, his ability to enjoy life, and his mental equilibrium are undisturbed. . . . But degree of adaptiveness can only be determined with reference to environmental conditions" (p. 105).

From a clinical perspective, ego psychology focuses attention on the ego and its functions, including defenses. The goal of analysis in the ego psychology model is to achieve as harmonious a relationship as possible among the id, ego, and superego, that is, the agencies of the mind and the outside world. As in drive theory, interpretation is the primary tool of the analyst.

Object Relations Theory

Object relations theory is another of the major schools of thought derived from classical Freudian drive theory and is generally associated with the British School of object relations, from Melanie Klein (whose adherents formed a distinct Kleinian school of psychoanalytic thought) to Donald Winnicott, including Fairbairn and Guntrip, among others. American object relations theorists include Jacobson, Mahler, and Kernberg.

From the perspective of object relations theory, the primary human motivation is to establish relationships. In distinction to Freudian theory, humans are seen as predominantly object—rather than pleasure—seeking, with the basic unit of experience being an *object relation*. Fairbairn (1943) coined the term *object relations theory*, but the conceptualization of the object as an internalized one is largely derived from Klein's work and is fundamental to understanding this theory. In other words, object relations do not refer to interpersonal interactions but to internalized *self- and object-representations* and representations of the interaction between the self and the object.

Klein introduced several concepts that have taken hold within the wider mental health community, including the concept of *part objects*—that is, in the infant's mind the object exists in relation to its functions, so the *good breast* is the one that feeds the hungry infant, whereas the *bad breast* is the one that withholds. This process of *splitting* is not restricted to the object but also applies to the self. A child or adult can project a part of him- or herself that is too painful or anxiety provoking into another, thereby reducing his or her own pain. Alternatively, the child may see him- or herself as the bad one, taking on the blame, for example, in the case of abuse. This splitting allows the child to hope for better treatment, protects him or her from excessive pain and hopelessness, and allows for the maintenance of an attachment in an otherwise impossible situation.

Winnicott is a British object relations theorist frequently cited by music therapists. His emphasis on play and on the importance of the creative process for both development and therapeutic treatment renders his work very relevant to the creative arts therapies. Winnicott's (1958) theory is a quintessential *relational* theory. "There is no such thing as a baby," he stated. "If you show me a baby you certainly show me also someone caring for the baby. . . . One sees a 'nursing couple'" (p. 99). For Winnicott, the psychic development of the infant is dependent upon the quality of care provided by the caretaker, that is, the mother. The *good-enough mother* provides a *holding environment* for the infant's primitive, unintegrated psychic state. Her responsiveness to the infant's needs results in a *moment of illusion*, as the infant feels that he or she has actually created the mother to fulfill his or her needs. This illusion strengthens the infant's ego and results in the formation of a *true self*. In contrast, when the mother is unable to adapt to her infant's needs, with her own taking precedence, the infant's omnipotence is not supported, "the infant gets seduced into a compliance" (Winnicott, 1965, p. 146), and a *false self* is developed.

A goal of object relations therapy is to increase the patient's awareness of the repetition of internalized object relations in current interpersonal relationships, particularly those fraught with difficulties. Interpretations place great emphasis on the relationship between the analyst and the patient. For Winnicott, it is not the analyst's interpretive function, per se, that leads to cure, but rather the capacity of the analytic setting to meet early developmental needs in such a way as to allow the emergence of the patient's *self*. Acknowledging parental failures in adaptation, the analyst's reliable presence with, attentiveness to, and *mirroring* of the patient provide *holding* and *containment* for the patient's emotional expression. In a fashion parallel to that of the good-enough mother, the analyst's capacity to survive the patient's destructiveness is crucial.

In recent years, interest in and attention given to the writings of Wilfred Bion, a prolific theorist analyzed by Klein, have grown rapidly. He is a very original psychoanalytic thinker who provides a new language to describe the development of the capacity to think built upon early emotional experience. I briefly review a few selected concepts.

Bion's is a *theory of thinking*. In a paper bearing that name (Bion, 1967), he posits that thoughts exist prior to the development of an apparatus for thinking, thereby necessitating the presence of another mind for psychic survival. The infant, terrified by his or her own raw, unmetabolized, unbearable affect, referred to by Bion as *beta-elements*, needs the mother to deal with his or her feelings through the *alpha-function*, and return the feelings to him in a less toxic form, that is, as *alpha-elements*. In other words, the mother, in a state of *maternal reverie*, serves as the *container* for the infant's unbearable projections and processes, digests, and returns them to the infant in a tolerable and accessible form (1962/1984).

In parallel fashion the analyst performs the containing function, receiving the patient's most disturbing projections and processing them, without retaliation or reassurance, and returns them in a form accessible to thought and dreams. The analyst recognizes that the patient's psychic reality is contextualized within external reality (Oliner, 2013).

Self Psychology

Self psychology, a distinct psychoanalytic theory associated with Heinz Kohut, can be seen as a further development of object relations theory (Bacal & Newman, 1990), although Kohut, himself, did not, given his focus on the development of the self and on the relationship between the self and selfobjects. According to Kohut (1971), psychopathology is the result of flaws in the self—that is, defects in the structure of the self, distortion of the self, or weakness of the self. The flawed self, in whichever form, results from failures in early childhood self-selfobject relationships with significant others. The term *selfobject* refers to the fact that, from the infant's perspective, significant others are viewed as parts of the self, not as autonomous objects.

Kohut identified three major selfobject needs that, if met, would lead to the development of a cohesive self. These are a need for *mirroring*, for *idealization*, and for *twinship*. A mirroring selfobject can satisfy children's need to be acknowledged for their innate qualities and their accomplishments by providing an affirming responsiveness, recognition, and confirmation of their competence and value. This affirmation leads to feeling pride in oneself. Children also need to idealize their significant others, to admire them, and to see within them admirable qualities with which to identify. The child can then experience merging with the idealized selfobject, leading the child to feel more secure and to set high goals. A third need that children have is to feel similar to a parent, to belong, and to be involved in a relationship. In Kohutian terms, this is a twinship selfobject need. If this need is satisfied, children will feel more connected, be more empathic, have better social skills, and engage in relationships. When selfobject needs are met, the child develops a more cohesive sense of self; becomes better at, and less dependent on others, for self-regulation; and does not require the other to fulfill selfobject functions. This process of *transmuting internalization* leads to a more self-reliant stance.

Kohut (1984) describes three steps in the curative analytic process, the first consisting of defense analysis and the second, the un-folding of the transference. The third and defining step in self psychology allows for "the establishment of empathic in-tuneness between self and selfobject on mature adult levels" (p. 66). The analyst's empathic failures disrupt the patient's transference and result in a retreat to earlier archaic selfobject relationships. By interpreting the dynamics of the patient's retreat subsequent to the analyst's empathic failure, the analyst restores the flow of empathy.

In summary, both object relations theory and self psychology can be categorized as relational psychoanalysis, that is, as a form of psychoanalysis that bridges interpersonal relations and object relations (Greenberg & Mitchell, 1983).

To complete our historical review, we will mention one more relational theory. *Intersubjective theory*, in contrast to the analytic neutrality espoused in Freudian theory, acknowledges the subjectivity of the analyst that is influenced by, and in turn influences, the patient's subjectivity (Stolorow, Brandschaft, & Atwood, 1987). From this perspective, the change process is conceptualized as one that occurs within an intersubjective matrix that is codetermined by both patient and analyst. The real reactions to the patient move into the foreground of the analyst's awareness.

Psychodynamic Music Therapy

Having traced the development of psychodynamic psychotherapy from its Freudian roots to the present, we now turn our attention to Psychodynamic Music Therapy, which can be defined as a music therapy orientation that is informed by psychodynamic theory. We have seen, however, that there are many models of psychodynamic theory, each having different theoretical and clinical emphases. We might ask, Are there some underlying beliefs inherent to Psychodynamic Music Therapy practice that are held by a majority of psychodynamic music therapists? I would suggest that Psychodynamic Music Therapy is a depth therapy in which the music therapist:

- Focuses on process while acknowledging the importance of technique.
- Addresses questions of meaning.
- Recognizes the impact of the patient's past experiences on the present.
- Believes in the tremendous power that the unconscious exerts over behaviors, thoughts, and feelings for both patient and therapist.
- Believes in the centrality of transference and countertransference within the therapeutic context and uses both to increase understanding of the patient and to work through impediments to change, however they are conceptualized.
- Is aware that, although patients strive to change, the therapeutic process engenders resistances that must be overcome before change can occur.
- Although solidly anchored in a psychodynamic theoretical/conceptual framework, engages the patient in a music-centered therapeutic process through the accomplished and skillful use of music in its many varied forms.

Having listed characteristics of Psychodynamic Music Therapy, there are further questions that present themselves, the first being, What is it about music that lends itself to use within a psychodynamic orientation? It is of note that music has long attracted the interest of psychoanalysts and psychiatrists. This interest is addressed in a literature that, to some degree, predates that of psychodynamically oriented music therapists—a literature that may, without this intention, support and validate the development of Psychodynamic Music Therapy. Let us consider this literature briefly.

Pinchas Noy (1966, 1967a, 1967b, 1967c, 1967d), an Israeli psychoanalyst, wrote a five-part series titled "The Psychodynamic Meaning of Music," published in the *Journal of Music Therapy*. In his historical overview of psychoanalysts' understanding of the psy-

chological functions of music, Noy included references to the ability of music to weaken censors, thereby facilitating the expression of unconscious fantasies, and to be perceived as nonthreatening, thereby facilitating involvement in the therapeutic process. Ira Altshuler (1953), a psychiatrist, referred to effects of music "upon the Id, the Ego, and Superego, and their inter-relationship" (p. 4). Prior to developing self psychology, Heinz Kohut wrote about music in the clinical setting. He explored the sources of pleasure derived from listening to music (Kohut & Levarie, 1950) as well as the psychological functions of music, recognizing the potential importance of music as a medium that could be used to work through conflict (Kohut, 1957). He examined music's facilitation of "emotional catharsis for repressed wishes, playful mastery of the threats of trauma, and enjoyable submission to rules" (p. 406). The trauma to which he referred is the tension created within the listener by musical dissonance, which triggers an early fear response to chaotic and threatening sounds that could overwhelm the primitive ego of the infant. The formalized intelligibility of music engenders a sense of relief and mastery as the disorganized preverbal state of dissonance returns to consonance, neutralizing anxiety.

Music remains a subject of much interest to psychoanalysts to this day. Abella (2010), for example, examines the psychic functions of music, and Rusbridger (2008) examines music through a psychoanalytic lens. This literature, although psychodynamic, does not fall directly within the purview of Psychodynamic Music Therapy. It falls upon music therapists to explicate and elaborate upon the use of music within a Psychodynamic Music Therapeutic context. Bridging the interests of psychoanalysts in the therapeutic uses of music and the interests of music therapists in Psychodynamic Music Therapy, there are music therapists who have also shown interest in examining the psychic functions of music. For example, music therapist and psychoanalyst

Edith Lecourt (2004) considers musical structure as a psychic organizer, with the vertical structure reflecting and expressing the group dimension of the psyche, whereas Lehtonen (1997) describes music as a "psychic integration process" (p. 49) that "externalizes the internal" (p. 50) and underlines the psychic similarities between dreams and music. Erkkilä (2004) examines improvisational music as a preverbal, presymbolic language—that is, a language without words but not without meaning.

Having arrived at a general understanding of Psychodynamic Music Therapy and having reviewed some of the psychic functions of music as elaborated by both psychoanalysts and music therapists, let us now return to the different psychodynamic theories presented above and see in which specific ways they have informed Psychodynamic Music Therapy thought and practice. Each of the theories outlined above evolved from an earlier theory (e.g., Freudian or Kleinian), and in the process new theoretical constructs were developed. It is the specificity of the psychodynamic concepts upon which we will reflect. To do so, we will highlight those theorists who are more commonly cited in the music therapy literature, beginning with Freud.

The centrality of free association as a technique within the Freudian psychoanalytic model was described above. Music therapy techniques such as instrumental improvisation (Ahonen & Lee, 2011) and free associative singing (Austin, 2008) readily lend themselves to use as musical counterparts of free association, in parallel fashion allowing for the expression of the patient's unconscious material. References to the concepts of transference and countertransference, cornerstones of Freudian theory that help to explicate the relationship between the analyst and the patient, abound in the music therapy literature. For example, Gardstrom and Hiller (2010) focus on the potentially harmful effects of the therapist's countertransference in the selection and discussion of songs, and

Isenberg-Grzeda (1998) elaborates upon transference resistances. Underlining the importance of these concepts, Bruscia (1998) devotes an entire book to the elucidation of transference and countertransference within the context of Psychodynamic Music Therapy. (Although Klein has also had a great influence on Psychodynamic Music Therapy, her theoretical formulations are considered in the section below on Analytical Music Therapy.)

Winnicott, a representative of the object relations model, is perhaps the most cited psychodynamic theorist within the music therapy literature (e.g., Ahonen-Eerikäinen, 2007; De Backer & Van Camp, 2003; Dvorkin, 2013; Sutton, 2011). The following quote might clarify why creative arts therapists, in general, and music therapists, specifically, identify so much with his theories. Winnicott (1971) states:

> The general principle seems to me to be valid that *psychotherapy is done in the overlap of the two play areas, that of the patient and that of the therapist*. If the therapist cannot play, then he is not suitable for the work. If the patient cannot play, then something needs to be done to enable the patient to become able to play, after which psychotherapy may begin. The reason why playing is essential is that it is in playing that the patient is being creative. . . . It is in playing and only in playing that the individual child or adult is able to be creative and to use the whole personality, and it is only in being creative that the individual discovers the self. (p. 63, emphasis in original)

This theoretical formulation gets to the heart of the essential nature of music therapy as the engagement of the patient by the therapist in a musical interaction that taps into the patient's core creativity, personality, and unconscious inner self. The play area described by Winnicott is a *potential space* that is neither internal psychic reality nor the external world, although it is outside the individual. He describes the playing child as in a preoccupied state of near withdrawal that resembles an adult state of deep concentration. Just as instincts can threaten the capacity to play, with excessive levels of excitement and unbearable levels of anxiety disrupting the play, anxiety can also disrupt the analytic process. Winnicott's (1971) concept of a *transitional object*, an antidote to anxiety, is also of particular interest to music therapists. This term refers to a process in which an inanimate object substitutes for the soothing effect of the caretaker, thereby facilitating separation from him or her. Dvorkin (2013) describes how a song can be used as a transitional object, serving as a self-soothing device.

Bion's theory is based on the infant's earliest development—that is, on the preverbal stage of development. This might be one of the reasons that his general theory is of particular interest to those music therapists who focus on music as a nonverbal language and form of communication (Ahonen-Eerikäinen, 2007; Robarts, 2003; Sutton, 2011). In addition, Bion emphasizes the importance of the analyst maintaining a link with the analysand, in the moment—a task that the patient might attempt to derail. He cautions the analyst to not be subverted by either memory, which would move his or her attention from the present to the past, or by desire, which would move his or her attention from the present to the future, but to maintain the link with the patient. I suggest that this concept resonates with the music therapist's focus on being "experience-near" with the patient; that is, in the here and now through musical interaction.

Kohut, who developed self psychology, is another psychoanalytic theorist often cited by music therapists (e.g., Ahonen-Eerikäinen, 2007; Nirensztein, 2003). Music therapists' affinity for him may be explained in two ways. Firstly, Kohut uses a language that is well suited to music therapy. Two of the concepts that are integral to his theory, mirroring and empathy, are equally integral to music therapeutic treatment, with both concepts applying to musical improvisation and the latter also to

Receptive Music Therapy. Improvisational techniques allow the therapist to mirror the patient's musical expression, in an externalized form; that is, to mirror the patient's internal world as expressed musically. In this context mirroring is an empathic response. Within the context of receptive music (i.e., listening to music), a sensitive musical selection can constitute an empathic response on the therapist's part. A poor selection, on the other hand, could be construed as an empathic failure. In the former case, the patient will feel understood; in the latter, misunderstood.

The second source of affinity for Kohut is his own interest in and understanding of the therapeutic benefits of music (1957), as expressed in part by his recognition of the potential importance of music as a medium that could be used to work through conflict. The importance of a highly respected psychoanalyst as an object of identification for music therapists cannot be overestimated.

Let us now consider more closely some specific Psychodynamic Music Therapy models. From a historical perspective it is not so long ago that few names sprang to mind when invoking the term *Psychodynamic Music Therapy*. Florence Tyson in the United States and Juliette Alvin and Mary Priestley in England were early proponents of Psychodynamic Music Therapy, either describing a clinical application—psychiatry in the case of Tyson—or elaborating a model of music therapy—Analytical Music Therapy (AMT) in the case of Priestley. AMT has evolved over the years and currently flourishes throughout Europe and North America. It is a method based on improvisational techniques that allows for the symbolic expression of unconscious thoughts and feelings. Priestley (1975, 1994) describes the relationship between the therapist and patient as unfolding through the transference and countertransference. AMT is derived from Kleinian theory, but Priestley did insist on the difference between AMT and psychoanalysis (Priestley & Eschen, 2002): The shared experience of playing together in the former provides real gratification of the patient's wish for closeness, in contradistinction to the analyst's abstinence. According to Priestley, the music therapist is more open to the patient and more disclosing of his or her own personhood in the musical engagement, as contrasted with the verbal.

As we consider the session structure and techniques used as they unfold within the context of the relationship with the therapist, we can also see the way in which AMT is informed by psychodynamic theory. In a typical AMT session, the patient begins by talking about how he or she is feeling, and the music therapist listens in such a way as to "be in touch with the music that is behind the words" (Priestley, 1994, p. 10). Once something that can be explored musically together is identified, the therapist and patient go to the instruments. Whereas the patient can choose from a wide-ranging instrumentarium, the therapist will often use the piano. Sometimes the patient will select the theme of the improvisation, but often the therapist will make the selection from the patient's material. Priestley describes the therapist's dual function during the improvisation as containing the patient's emotions and using the countertransference to identify and musically reproduce the patient's unconscious feelings. After the improvisation, the patient may talk about the experience and the therapist may also share verbally. The improvisations are recorded and after the initial verbal processing, the tape is played back and listened to. This can be followed by further verbal processing of the musical experience.

Many AMT techniques can be used for the musical improvisation. According to Priestley (1975), a picture of the patient's internal state develops in the mind of the therapist as the patient talks. It is this picture that leads the therapist toward a choice of technique. For example, the *holding* or *containing* technique promotes the patient's full emotional expression while being held musically by the therapist in a symbolic safe container. The *splitting* technique can be useful when the patient projects part of him- or herself on to another, or splits two people, seeing one as *good* and the other as *bad*. The therapist and patient are able to play both sides of the split, facilitating the reintegration of the patient's projected emotion and resolving the split. Musical improvisations also allow for an exploration of the transference. The patient can improvise in the role of the therapist while the therapist plays the patient. In this way, expression of the patient's feelings and fantasies toward the therapist are invited. For some patients who have trouble accessing their own internal world, techniques employing images can be used; for example, watching the mouth of a cave or ascending a mountain.

The use of imagery is a defining characteristic of another popular music therapy method, Guided Imagery and Music (GIM). Although originally conceptualized by Helen Bonny as a humanistic/transpersonal model, in more recent years, some students of her method have approached GIM from a psychodynamic perspective (e.g., Bruscia, 1998; Isenberg-Grzeda, 1998). A description of GIM can further deepen our understanding of what it means to be a psychodynamic music therapist.

GIM is a music psychotherapy method that consists of the use of classical music to evoke imagery that will allow the patient, in an altered state of consciousness, to arrive at greater self-understanding, conflict resolution, transformation, and change. Although Bonny originally derived her theoretical language from, among others, Assagioli's method of psychosynthesis, the theoretical bases for this work have since been vastly expanded to include psychodynamic thinking. From a structural–technical perspective, GIM sessions are divided into four parts: the prelude, the relaxation/induction, the music listening/guiding, and the postlude. The prelude consists of a verbal exchange, often indistinguishable from verbal psychotherapy, followed by a process of relaxation and mental induction that serves to render the patient receptive to the music listening that is to follow. The patient, lying down with eyes closed and in an altered state of consciousness, then listens to music selected by the therapist from musical sequences developed by Bonny and shares with the therapist all aspects of the experience as it evolves. This part resembles free association as it occurs in psychoanalytic treatment. The musically evoked imagery can then be processed with the therapist, verbally or through an art form, with ensuing insights then related to the patient's presenting problems.

If we recall the earlier definition of psychodynamic music therapy as a depth therapy, the first two elements were (1) the focus on process while acknowledging technique and (2) addressing questions of meaning. What are the implications of this definition for our understanding of GIM? As a music therapist, I am interested in the selection of the music and its impact on the patient (Isenberg-Grzeda, 1996), the use of verbal interventions and their impact on the patient, the nature of the imagery evoked, and so forth. And the questions raised from this perspective are important. However, if I think of myself as a psychodynamic music therapist who is interested in process and meaning, my focus shifts. The questions I ask, of necessity, also change. I now turn my attention from technical questions, that is, part processes, to the metaprocess (Isenberg-Grzeda, 1998).

Whereas it remains important to explore the relationship between the music selected, the patient's affect, and the imagery evoked, this exploration becomes the content in a metainteraction that involves the therapist offering music to the patient. What does it mean to the patient that the therapist is offering music? What does it mean when the music is withheld? What does it mean to the therapist to offer or withhold music? What does this metaprocess evoke in both patient and therapist? Just as my adherence to a psychoanalytic theoretical framework leads me to focus on the underlying process and questions of meaning, my focus on the underlying process leads me back to a psychodynamic framework. Language and belief systems become inextricably intertwined.

So what are some of the relevant concepts for us to consider? Let us begin with the concept of empathy. The music therapist selects music on the basis of his or her understanding of the patient's needs at that moment, the selection thereby reflecting the degree of empathy. The patient may experience an accurate musical choice as an empathic response, whereas a selection that doesn't quite fit may be felt as an empathic failure with all its attendant disappointments. We might ask if the actual provision, itself, of music could be experienced as a source of nourishment, and the withholding of music as a source of frustration (Isenberg-Grzeda, 1996).

One patient, over a series of GIM sessions, talked about the organizing principles of the music and the mapping out of internal experience. Her belief was that the music created a map of sorts that resulted in more cohesion between images and affective states. In turn, this cohesion facilitated linking, which allowed for a spatial structuring of internal process and of affect, thereby creating an affective–imaginal map. Although we can imagine the benefits of this organizing function, we might also ask if there are times when it is useful to sit with internal confusion and chaos. What is the impact of this perceived mapping process on the patient's growth process? Could this mapping be construed as transference of dependency needs from the therapist to the music? Can the mapping concept be used as a resistance to allow for wish fulfillment, rather than having to deal with the frustration and pain of the absence of the internal map and thereby obviating the need to find a way to map, the inside for oneself? Can functions that are generally internalized from interactions with a person early in life be internalized from the music?

What happens to silence and the notion of being alone in the presence of another? Winnicott (1965) stresses the importance of learning to be alone by being alone in the presence of another, a state in which external factors do not impinge on the individual. If the music is playing, it is impinging upon the patient, stimulating, evoking reactions, and obviating the possibility of waiting for stimulation to arise from within. Will this intervention, of necessity, preclude the development of the capacity to be alone?

The questions that can be raised are numerous. Further questions related to the containing function and to the splitting of transference have been dealt with elsewhere (Isenberg-Grzeda, 1998). We have seen how the conceptual shift away from technique has plunged us into a deeper examination of unconscious intra- and interpsychic phenomena.

Although the practice of psychoanalysis is not as popular today as it was in the 1950s and 1960s, the music therapy literature is replete with psychodynamic terminology. Concepts such as transference and countertransference have become common currency within the music therapy community. There also seem to be more books devoted exclusively to a psychodynamic approach. For example, Bruscia's (1998) book, *The Dynamics of Music Psychotherapy*, highlights transference and countertransference phenomena within the music psychotherapeutic relationship; Hadley (2003) provides a collection of case studies in Psychodynamic Music Therapy; and Ahonen-Eerikäinen (2007) describes a psychodynamic group music process titled *Group Analytic Music Therapy*. Psychodynamic Music Therapy is also well represented in a recent book that provides an overview of current music therapy practice (Meadows, 2011) and another that focuses on music therapy in mental health settings (Eyre, 2013). It is the conceptual framework rather than the actual music therapy approach that determines the therapist's clinical thinking—that is,

the way in which the therapist understands the therapeutic process and therapeutic change. Music therapy approaches abound and are used by both psychodynamic and other music therapists, with vocal and instrumental improvisation techniques, songwriting, and music listening techniques not falling under the aegis of any one conceptual framework. Nonpsychodynamic music therapists may use approaches strongly associated with psychodynamic thought, such as AMT or GIM. But does this usage render them psychodynamic music therapists? I think not. This possibility might explain, in part, Silverman's (2007) finding that many more music therapists describe themselves as using psychodynamic *approaches* than as adhering to a psychodynamic *theoretical orientation*.

Psychoanalytic theory provides a theoretical framework that addresses questions of meaning. Rather than ask what we must do, we ask: What is the impact of what we do on the patient? How does what we do allow us to understand the patient's internal world? How does it influence the therapeutic process as it unfolds within the context of interpsychic and interpersonal relationships between the therapist and the patient? How do the patient's behavior, thoughts, and feelings impact upon us? And so on.

Conclusions

As music therapy has matured as a discipline, we have witnessed a considerable increase in the literature devoted to Psychodynamic Music Therapy. Although differences abound among authors, there are also shared beliefs that underlie Psychodynamic Music Therapy. It is commonly accepted that past experiences influence the present and that the unconscious exerts tremendous control over behaviors, thoughts, and feelings. The concepts of transference and countertransference are universally accepted as the hallmarks of psychodynamic theory, and it is recognized that the working through of the transference is central to therapeutic change. The commonly accepted belief in the ubiquity of defenses and resistance, and the therapist's role in helping to overcome resistance, requires of the music therapist the understanding that music making may serve resistance just as much as the refusal to engage musically.

A major goal of therapy is to work through the obstacles, in whatever form, to maximize functioning in the present. Although the explanatory model for pathology and symptoms may differ, there is a commonly held belief that an explanation can be found, and that elucidating it and working it through will effect change. Although there might be a dispute as to whether it should be verbally or musically mediated, most psychodynamic music therapists would agree that the acquisition of insight is important.

The question of the relative importance of music and words is far from resolved. As recently as 2011, Sekeles asks if it is possible to do therapy without words: "Music may be the language of therapy, but can we conduct therapy without words?" (p. 314). Pavlicevic (1997), addressing the complexity of this question, suggests that there is no single answer, with times when it is better to remain solely with the musical experience and others when verbal exchanges can enrich the therapeutic experience. She cautions against associating the use of the word with a psychodynamic approach.

Perhaps in relation to Psychodynamic Music Therapy, we need to ask if the music therapist is a psychodynamically *oriented* therapist and hence a psychodynamically *trained* therapist. Priestley (1994) and Bonny (2002) did not espouse training in psychotherapy, but rather both prescribed a personal therapeutic process in their respective models as a prerequisite for practice. This personal therapy comprises an obligatory component of the training programs and allows the trainee to explore his or her internal world using the method in which he or she is training.

This model of learning how to do therapy from the inside out is derived from psychoanalysis: Freud held the analyst responsible "to make himself capable, by a deep-going analysis of his own, of the unprejudiced reception of the analytic material" (1926/2001, p. 220). A training analysis is one of the requirements of analytic training. I believe that Psychodynamic Music Therapy is a depth therapy and, as such, is complex. Its practice requires a high level of skill that can be acquired only by pursuing advanced training in both musical and verbal psychotherapeutic skills.

REFERENCES

Abella, A. (2010). Contemporary art and Hanna Segal's thinking on aesthetics. *International Journal of Psychoanalysis, 91,* 163–181.

Ahonen, H., & Lee, C. A. (2011). The meta-musical experiences of a professional string quartet in music-centered psychotherapy. In A. Meadows (Ed.), *Developments in music therapy practice: Case study perspectives* (pp. 518–541). Gilsum, NH: Barcelona.

Ahonen-Eerikäinen, H. (2007). *Group analytic music therapy.* Gilsum, NH: Barcelona.

Altshuler, I. M. (1953). Music therapy: Retrospect and perspective. In E. G. Gilliland (Ed.), *Music therapy 1952* (pp. 3–18). Lawrence, KS: National Association for Music Therapy.

Austin, D. (2008). *The theory and practice of vocal psychotherapy: Songs of the self.* London: Jessica Kingsley.

Bacal, H. A., & Newman, K. M. (1990). *Theories of object relations: Bridges to self psychology.* New York: Columbia University Press.

Bion, W. (1967). *Second thoughts.* London: Jason Aronson.

Bion, W. (1984). *Learning from experience.* London: Karnac Books. (Original work published 1962)

Bonny, H. (2002). Guided imagery and music (GIM): Mirror of consciousness. In H. Bonny & L. Summer (Eds.), *Music and consciousness: The evolution of guided imagery and music* (pp. 93–102). Gilsum, NH: Barcelona.

Brenner, I. (2006). *Psychoanalysis or mind and meaning.* New York: Psychoanalytic Quarterly.

Breuer, J., & Freud, S. (2001). Studies on hysteria. In J. Strachey (Ed. & Trans.), *The standard edition of the complete psychological works of Sigmund*

Freud (Vol. 2, pp. 20–47). London: Hogarth Press. (Original work published 1893–1895)

Bruscia, K. (Ed.). (1998). *The dynamics of music psychotherapy*. Gilsum, NH: Barcelona.

De Backer, J., & Van Camp, J. (2003). The case of Marianne: Repetition and musical form in psychosis. In S. Hadley (Ed.), *Psychodynamic music therapy: Case studies* (pp. 273–297). Gilsum, NH: Barcelona.

Dvorkin, J. (2013). Adults and adolescents with borderline personality disorder. In L. Eyre (Ed.), *Guidelines for music therapy practice in mental health* (pp. 511–541). University Park, IL: Barcelona.

Erkkilä, J. (2004). From signs to symbols, from symbols to words: About the relationship between music and language, music therapy and psychotherapy. *Voices: A World Forum for Music Therapy, 4*(2). Available online at *https://voices.no/index.php/voices/article/view/176*.

Eyre, L. (Ed.). (2013). *Guidelines for music therapy practice in mental health*. University Park, IL: Barcelona.

Fairbairn, W. R. D. (1943). The repression and the return of bad objects. In *Psychoanalytic studies of the personality* (pp. 59–81). London: Routledge & Kegan Paul.

Freud, S. (2001). The question of lay analysis. In J. Strachey (Ed. & Trans.), *The standard edition of the complete psychological works of Sigmund Freud* (Vol. 20, pp. 177–250). London: Hogarth Press. (Original work published 1926)

Gardstrom, S. C., & Hiller, J. (2010). Song discussion as music psychotherapy. *Music Therapy Perspectives, 28*, 147–156.

Greenberg, J. R., & Mitchell, S. A. (1983). *Object relations in psychoanalytic theory*. Cambridge, MA: Harvard University Press.

Guntrip, H. (1973). *Psychoanalytic theory, therapy, and the self*. New York: Basic Books.

Hadley, S. (Ed.). (2003). *Psychodynamic music therapy: Case studies*. Gilsum, NH: Barcelona.

Hartmann, H. (1958). *Ego psychology and the problem of adaptation* (D. Rapaport, Trans.). New York: International Universities Press. (Original work published 1939)

Isenberg, C., Goldberg, F., & Dvorkin, J. (2008). Psychodynamic approach to music therapy. In A.-A. Darrow (Ed.), *Introduction to approaches in music therapy* (2nd ed., pp. 79–104). Silver Spring, MD: American Music Therapy Association.

Isenberg-Grzeda, C. (1996, July). *Transference and transference resistance in guided imagery and music training*. Paper presented at the meeting of the International Congress of the World Federation of Music Therapy, Hamburg, Germany.

Isenberg-Grzeda, C. (1998). Transference structures in guided imagery and music. In K. Bruscia (Ed.), *The dynamics of music psychotherapy* (pp. 461–479). Gilsum, NH: Barcelona.

Kohut, H. (1957). Observations on the psychological functions of music. *Journal of the American Psychoanalytic Association, 5*, 389–407.

Kohut, H. (1971). *The analysis of the self*. New York: International Universities Press.

Kohut, H. (1984). *How does analysis cure?* Chicago: University of Chicago Press.

Kohut, H., & Levarie, S. (1950). On the enjoyment of listening to music. *Psychoanalytic Quarterly, 19*, 64–87.

Laplanche, J., & Pontalis, J. B. (1973). *The language of psycho-analysis* (D. Nicholson-Smith, Trans.). London: Hogarth Press. (Original work published 1967)

Lecourt, E. (2004). The psychic functions of music. *Nordic Journal of Music Therapy, 13*, 154–160.

Lehtonen, K. (1997). Is there correspondence between the structures of music and the psyche? *Nordic Journal of Music Therapy, 6*, 43–52.

Meadows, A. (Ed.). (2011). *Developments in music therapy practice: Case study perspectives*. Gilsum, NH: Barcelona.

Nirensztein, S. (2003). The knight inside the armor: Music therapy with a deprived teenager. In S. Hadley (Ed.), *Psychodynamic music therapy: Case studies* (pp. 225–240). Gilsum, NH: Barcelona.

Noy, P. (1966). The psychodynamic meaning of music: Part I. A critical review of the psychoanalytic and related literature. *Journal of Music Therapy, 3*, 126–135.

Noy, P. (1967a). The psychodynamic meaning of music: Part II. A critical review of the psychoanalytic and related literature. *Journal of Music Therapy, 4*, 7–23.

Noy, P. (1967b). The psychodynamic meaning of music: Part III. A critical review of the psychoanalytic and related literature. *Journal of Music Therapy, 4*, 45–51.

Noy, P. (1967c). The psychodynamic meaning of music: Part IV. A critical review of the psychoanalytic and related literature. *Journal of Music Therapy, 4*, 85–94.

Noy, P. (1967d). The psychodynamic meaning of music: Part V. A critical review of the psychoanalytic and related literature. *Journal of Music Therapy, 4*, 117–125.

Oliner, M. (2013). An essay on Bion's beta function. *Psychoanalytic Review, 100*, 167–183.

Pavlicevic, M. (1997). *Music therapy in context: Music, meaning and relationship.* London: Jessica Kingsley.

Priestley, M. (1975). *Music therapy in action.* London: Constable.

Priestley, M. (1994). *Essays on analytical music therapy.* Gilsum, NH: Barcelona.

Priestley, M., & Eschen, J. T. (2002). Analytical music therapy: Origin and development. In J. T. Eschen (Ed.), *Analytical music therapy* (pp. 11–16). London: Jessica Kingsley.

Robarts, J. (2003). The healing function of improvised songs in music therapy with a child survivor of early trauma and sexual abuse. In S. Hadley (Ed.), *Psychodynamic music therapy: Case studies* (pp. 141–182). Gilsum, NH: Barcelona.

Rusbridger, R. (2008). The internal world of *Don Giovanni. International Journal of Psychoanalysis, 89,* 181–194.

Ruud, E. (1980). *Music therapy and its relationship to current treatment theories.* Gilsum, NH: Barcelona.

Schneider, E. H., Unkefer, R., & Gaston, E. T. (1968). Introduction. In E. T. Gaston (Ed.), *Music in therapy* (pp. 1–4). New York: Macmillan.

Sekeles, C. (2011). From the highest height to the lowest depth: Music therapy with a paraplegic soldier. In A. Meadows (Ed.), *Developments in music therapy practice: Case study perspectives* (pp. 315–333). Gilsum, NH: Barcelona.

Silverman, M. J. (2007). Evaluating current trends in psychiatric music therapy: A descriptive analysis. *Journal of Music Therapy, 44,* 388–414.

Stolorow, R., Atwood, G., & Brandshaft, B. (Eds.). (1987). *Psychoanalytic treatment: An intersubjective approach.* Hillsdale, NJ: Analytic Press.

Sutton, J. (2011). A flash of the obvious: Music therapy and trauma. In A. Meadows (Ed.), *Developments in music therapy practice: Case study perspectives* (pp. 368–384). Gilsum, NH: Barcelona.

Wheeler, B. (1981). The relationship between music therapy and theories of psychotherapy. *Music Therapy, 1,* 9–16.

Winnicott, D. W. (1958). Anxiety associated with insecurity. In *Collected papers: Through paediatrics to psycho-analysis* (pp. 97–100). London: Tavistock.

Winnicott, D. W. (1965a). Ego distortion in terms of true and false self. In *The maturational processes and the facilitating environment* (pp. 140–152). London: Hogarth Press.

Winnicott, D. W. (1965b). The capacity to be alone. In *The maturational processes and the facilitating environment* (pp. 29–36). London: Hogarth Press.

Winnicott, D. W. (1971). *Playing and reality.* New York: Penguin Books.

CHAPTER 12

Humanistic Approaches

Brian Abrams

In *humanistic* approaches to music therapy, the components and processes of the work are understood according the tenets of *humanism*, which posits that all persons have innate capacities for actualizing their own unique potentials for health and well-being, given conditions that can serve adequately as opportunities for change. Music therapists working within a humanistic orientation can employ a wide variety of methods, provided they are ultimately guided by humanistic precepts and principles. This chapter elaborates on (1) the history of humanism and its manifestations in the development of music therapy; (2) theoretical tenets of humanistic music therapy; and (3) applications of humanistic music therapy, consisting of a summary of sources from the music therapy literature, as well as a detailed synopsis of one case example.

History

Humanism

Humanism has ancient roots in the Buddhism, Taoism, and Confucianism of Asia; the Zoroastrianism of the Middle East; and the pre-Socratic, Ionian philosophies of Greece. In the Western, European world, the 14th century was a significant period in the development of humanism, marked by rediscovery of knowledge from Classical Greek and Roman Antiquity, accompanied by key advances in science, technology, and the arts. A key progenitor of humanism who lived during this period was the poet/ lyricist, scholar, and diplomat Francesco Petrarca (1304–1374), also known as Petrarch. Petrarch's work emphasized individual identity, personhood, and humanness (Highet, 1949; Pfeiffer, 1976), and helped propel European society toward the Renaissance, following the lengthy phase of human disenfranchisement in the West known as the *Dark Ages*—a term credited to Petrach (Mommsen, 1942). Through the Renaissance and the centuries following, the expanding influence of humanism prompted numerous shifts in social and political ideals, including the 18th-century revolutionary thought of Jean-Jacques Rousseau (1712–1778) and Thomas Paine (1737–1809), and the 19th-century transcendentalism of Ralph Waldo Emerson (1803–1882) and Henry David Thoreau (1817–1862).

In the 20th century, beginning in the late 1930s, humanism made a pivotal impact upon the field of psychology when there emerged a growing interest in theoretical and clinical perspectives that departed radically from both the prevailing psycho-analytic orientation established in the late 19th century (by Freud and others) and the growing popularity of the behavioral orientation (originating with figures such as John Watson and, eventually, B. F. Skinner). Unlike the emphasis these orientations placed upon primitive, physiological drives or behavioral conditioning, this emerging humanistic orientation acknowledged those uniquely human constructs that primarily concern human meaning and value, such as being, selfhood, hope, self-esteem, love, creativity, individuality, and authenticity, all considered integral to human well-being, and all capacities that persons are innately equipped to pursue (Schneider & Krug, 2010).

One pioneer of humanistic psychology was Carl Rogers (1902–1987). In his first book, Rogers (1939) articulated the early foundations of what would eventually come to be known as *client-centered* therapy (Rogers, 1951) and, later still, as *person-centered* therapy. In place of treating a client's psychological disorders in a manner analogous to medical treatment of disease, client-centered work involved the therapist establishing an intrinsically healing, therapeutic relationship and environment characterized by empathy (experiencing life from the client's perspective), unconditional positive regard (nonjudgmental and respectful acceptance), and congruence (transparency and trustworthiness) (Corey, 2009; Corsini & Wedding, 1995).

Another pioneer of humanistic psychology was Abraham Maslow (1908–1970). Maslow (1943) advanced the theoretical dimensions of humanistic psychology via his hierarchy of human motives, ranging from primal motives for basic survival to the metamotive for self-actualization, a level of uniquely human well-being that surpasses mere normalcy and absence of disorder, as was the conventional understanding of psychological health at that time. Carl Jung (1875–1961), psychoanalytic scholar and clinician (and something of a protégé and close colleague of Freud, for a number of years during Jung's early professional career), also contributed significantly to humanistic currents in psychology, through transcendent concepts of the psyche and psychological well-being (Jung, 1963/1989). The work of the various progenitors of humanistic psychology eventually led to the establishment of the Association for Humanistic Psychology and its scholarly periodical, the *Journal of Humanistic Psychology*, both in the early 1960s. These developments, in turn, contributed to the general emergence of a broad *human potential movement* that informed areas such as education and parenting during the 1960s and 1970s (Leonard, 1987).

Contributing significantly to the development of humanistic psychology were certain 20th-century philosophies, such as the phenomenology of Edmund Husserl and Maurice Merleau-Ponty, and the existentialism of Søren Kierkegaard, Friedrich Nietzsche, Martin Heidegger, Jean-Paul Sartre, Karl Jaspers, and Martin Buber. During the 1950s and 1960s, paralleling the ascendance of humanistic psychology and the human potential movement, psychology scholars and practitioners such as Rollo May, Ludwig Binswanger, Viktor Frankl, R. D. Laing, and Irvin Yalom established psychological theory and clinical work specifically rooted in existential thought (Schneider & Krug, 2010). Due to the many relationships and similarities between existential and humanistic psychologies, many began to use the hyphenated term *existential-humanistic* (Schneider & Krug) to denote a single, larger orientation. Areas of theory and practice emerging from both existential and humanistic psychologies include *positive psychology*, concerned with emphasizing existing strengths and healthy tendencies (Seligman & Csikszentmihalyi,

2000); *transpersonal psychology*, concerned with spirituality, transcendence of individual sense of self, and nonordinary states of consciousness (Walsh & Vaughan, 1993); and *person-centered expressive art therapy*, developed by Natalie Rogers, daughter of Carl Rogers, based upon the role of creativity and expressive media in facilitating human transformation (Rogers, 1993; Sommers-Flanagan, 2007).

Humanism in Music Therapy

Music therapy formally emerged as a profession in the 1950s, during the apex of the popularity of behavioral psychology, yet prior to widespread acceptance of humanistic psychology. Music therapy, since its inception, had already been addressing a wide spectrum of person-centered needs through the uniquely human phenomenon of music—thus, it was, in a sense, "ahead of the curve" in developing a humanistic therapy orientation. In fact, humanistic values had advanced the roles of music in medical and psychiatric care long before the formal emergence of music therapy (Bunt, 1994).

The work of numerous pioneers in the field of music therapy has embodied humanistic ideals. One such pioneer was British music therapist Juliette Alvin (1897–1982). Although Alvin's work is commonly associated with psychoanalytic theory, many dimensions of it embodied principles of humanism. Alvin was the innovator of free improvisation therapy, which targeted such outcomes as self-liberation; positive relationships; and physical, intellectual, and social–emotional development—all by allowing the client to find his or her own musical way without fixed rules, structures, or themes (Bruscia, 1988). Two other important pioneers were Paul Nordoff (1909–1977) and Clive Robbins (1927–2011), who developed a model known as *Creative Music Therapy*, in which a music-centered relationship (primarily improvisational) helps clients transcend disabling conditions through musical support and challenges that mobilize creative resources for well-

being, expressed directly through actualization of their music potential (Kim, 2004). Yet another pioneer was Helen Lindquist Bonny (1921–2010), a music therapist whose participation in certain humanistically informed studies at the Maryland Psychiatric Research Center eventually prompted her to develop the Bonny Method of Guided Imagery and Music, in which the client experiences images in response to sequences of recorded classical music while dialoguing interactively with a guide (i.e., the therapist; Clark, 2002).

By the 1980s, definitions of humanistic music therapy began to emerge in the literature. For example, Wheeler (1981), in the context of discussing music therapy in terms of theories of psychotherapy, provided the following description of humanistic (and, more specifically, person-centered/Rogerian) approaches to music therapy: "A relationship in which the client is free to grow, with the therapist helping to clarify awareness of inner experiences. This philosophy can be applied to a variety of music therapy situations. The therapist would first accept whichever musical—or nonmusical—endeavor the client chooses and then help the client to musically and verbally express his or her inner experiences" (p. 12).

Polit (1993) later offered the following definition: "Humanistic Music Therapy refers to the psychotherapeutic space wherein the personal and transpersonal development of the person through sound and music is facilitated, using an approach emphasizing respect, acceptance, empathy and congruence" (p. 366).

Theoretical Tenets

Humanistic Music Therapy is largely informed by the general tenets of humanistic psychology. According to Bugental (1964), the following five core principles, or postulates, guide therapeutic practices based upon humanistic psychology (paraphrased here): Human beings (1) supersede the sum of their parts and cannot be reduced to components; (2) exist in a uniquely human context; (3) are conscious and aware of being conscious, both in the context of others (i.e., relationally); (4) have both choice and responsibility; and (5) are intentional; have goals; are aware that they play a role in future events; and seek meaning, value, and creativity.

Although related to these general tenets of humanistic psychology, the tenets of Humanistic Music Therapy have their own unique character and configuration, based upon that which is indigenous to the nature of music therapy practice (e.g., a working medium that transcends verbal communication; work with clients who may not be cognitively aware in a conventional sense, etc.). Thus, here, four essential components of music therapy have been selected as a foundation for explicating Humanistic Music Therapy: (1) clients, (2) music, (3) therapy goals, and (4) therapy processes. In turn, each of these components is discussed in terms of four core humanistic constructs: (1) being, (2) holism, (3) agency, and (4) relationship.

Clients

In humanistic approaches to music therapy, clients are regarded first as persons and, hence, as beings. A being is not a reified biological or psychological *thing*, nor an inanimate fact of science with a concrete reality located in measurable space and time. Rather, a *being* is a particular *way* of existing (Abrams, 2012), located in humanity, uniquely distinguished by an identity and, as is typically part of that identity, a name. Humanistically oriented music therapy is, therefore, more about ways of existing than it is about things (objects) and is far more concerned about the *who* than the *what* of client needs.

From a humanistic standpoint, music therapy clients are considered irreducible, indivisible *whole* persons, transcending aggregate biopsychological parts or traits (Bugental, 1964), such as brains, neurologi-

cal processes, thoughts, and feelings. Likewise, from this perspective, a person is not a person by virtue of specific physiological or psychological criteria, such as number of body parts, neurological activity, or cognition. All clients, therefore, retain their personhood and, hence, their ethical rights to basic dignity and respect, regardless of biobehavioral status.

From a Humanistic Music Therapy perspective, all clients retain basic *agency*, or "the capacity, condition, or state of acting or of exerting power" (*Webster's Ninth New Collegiate Dictionary*, 1990). "Exerting power" in its most basic, human sense means the power to exist as a person. As Kant (1785/1996) asserted, persons are never objects to be acted upon but rather *subjects who act*, a concept supported by Ruud (1998) and others, specifically in the context of music therapy. Agency is not merely conscious intention or a cognitive act of will or choice; rather, a client's agency is always acknowledged at a fundamental level of the client's humanity, regardless of mental status. Moreover, agency is not beholden to forces of cause-and-effect determinism, as would be consistent with the disciplines of physics, chemistry, biology, and behavioristic psychology. Although determinism may apply to the parts (or the *what*) of a person, it does not apply to the whole (or the *who*) of a person, where agency is located. As Frankl (1984) wrote in the context of describing his existential model of psychotherapy, known as *logotherapy*, "A human being is not one thing among others; *things* determine each other, but *man* is ultimately self-determining" (p. 135).

Also from a Humanistic Music Therapy perspective, a client's very existence as a person is *relational*, meaning that it is situated within the client's interpersonal, sociocultural, and historical contexts. In relational contexts, a person remains a person, independently of physiological and psychological conditions. By the same token, outside of relational contexts, even the most *highly functioning* person would be merely a biophysical object, without personhood.

As Heidegger (1962) articulated, a *being* (*Da-Sein*) is fundamentally a *being-with* (*Mit-Sein*), relationally situated within humanity. This implies that, from a humanistic perspective, any client can *be with* others (e.g., the therapist) on a human level, and has the potential to benefit from therapy through treatment of the client's *humanity* (whether or not the client is ever overtly aware of this benefit). Thus, to treat a client is to treat the client's humanity (and, on some level, humanity itself) in relational context.

Music

From a humanistic perspective, like a person, music is not an object or a thing but a *way of being*. Specifically, at its core, music can be considered a way of being aesthetic, in time (Abrams, 2011). Physical sound may serve as a medium through which music is expressed, but music is not located in sound, any more than a story is located in the physical (or electronic) medium in which it is written. Music, like personhood, is located in humanity. Hence, from a Humanistic Music Therapy orientation, any reified understanding of music is considered problematic (Garred, 2006; Ruud, 1998, 2010).

Like persons, music is a *whole* that transcends the aggregate of its parts. None of the individual elements of music (rhythm, melody, harmony, etc.) exists independently *as* music. Moreover, as music unfolds experientially in time (whether precomposed or improvised), it simultaneously builds upon that which has already been heard while implying some sort of direction about where it is going (Zuckerkandl, 1956). Any given excerpt or moment of music derives all of its meaning and value from its place and role within the larger, whole musical experience. Therefore, just as humanistic music therapists do not work with clients as disembodied parts, they do not work with music as superficial sound characteristics (e.g., 60-beats-per-minute music) or as isolated moments (i.e., sound bites) without

an understanding of their place within the whole musical art form.

From a humanistic standpoint, music is also an embodiment of human *agency* and is often understood in a way consistent with its verb form, *musicing* (Elliott, 1995), as the expression of a person's aesthetic agency in action. From this perspective, music is not something to use because *it* works or has some deterministic effect; rather, music is a way for clients and therapists to work together (i.e., a way *we* work) in the interest of addressing therapy goals. To reify music is to deny its agency and, hence, its humanity—essentially, subtle forms of both art desecration and dehumanization.

In humanistic approaches to music therapy, music is understood as intrinsically *relational*. Music, as art, has no fixed meaning independently of (1) how its various elements relate to one another; (2) how the whole work relates to other works; (3) its significance within the life of a given composer, performer, improviser, or listener; and (4) its significance within community, society, culture, and history. In music therapy, these various relational dimensions of music contribute to a client's unique *musical identity* (Ruud, 1998) and constitute the basis of music as contextually situated within humanity. Moreover, music involves a *dialogical* process, in which all of its contextual factors dynamically interact, negotiate, and reconfigure through client and therapist participation in the music experience (Garred, 2006). Thus, from a Humanistic Music Therapy perspective, the notion of generalized or stereotyped *uses* of music based upon presumptive, abstracted meanings and values (e.g., good genres for a given health condition, music that is intrinsically relaxing or happy, etc.) is considered absurd.

Therapy Goals

In Humanistic Music Therapy, goals centrally address the client's ongoing, evolving pursuit of *self-actualization*, or the maximal expression of human potential (Rogers, 1961). Whereas persons may share certain health needs in common with all biological entities, self-actualization is a distinctly human construct concerning the client's way of being.

Self-actualization goals are based upon an understanding of clients as *whole*, contextually situated persons, as noted above. In the client's pursuit of self-actualization, the presenting symptom, which may be considered the main issue from a biobehavioral perspective, is not always humanistically relevant. A goal involving improvement of a client's range of motion in one arm, for example, would not simply be about a corrective intervention for the client's arm as an end in itself, but rather about how the range of motion is relevant to the client's actualized humanity. At times, self-actualizing serves as a basis for a client's own management of basic life challenges outside of therapy, encouraging self-sufficiency and independence (Frankl, 1984; Yalom, 1983)—a valued outcome in humanistic therapies (Scovel & Gardstrom, 2005). Sorel (2011) has presented this understanding of music therapy goals, across specific health domains, as ultimately pertaining to the whole person.

Self-actualization often involves mobilizing one's greatest potentials for expressing human *agency*. As part of honoring the client's agency, his or her active participation in the goal formulation process is important. As a distinctive feature of music therapy, expressions of agency can include musical freedom, maximization of expressive musical options, engagement in moments of aesthetic depth, and so forth. Because music-based self-actualization can be considered a more healthful way of being in itself, music in Humanistic Music Therapy need not always be considered a means to nonmusical ends (Abrams, 2011; Aigen, 2005). A good example is the phenomenon of *play* in music. The capacity for play and playfulness is not merely a means to achieving greater well-being, but is *itself*, already,

an expression of greater well-being and of human agency. Moreover, musical goals can be met without ever concretely generalizing them outside of the therapy setting, because they already signify the actualization of agency that represents a fundamental shift in being, even after only one occurrence in a single session.

Self-actualization, as an inherently human goal, is also relational. The client relationship to (and with) other persons, community, society, and humanity itself is an inherent part of the client's self-actualization. Music (musicing) creates possibilities for being with others, in relationship-developing ways, supporting goals pertaining to self-actualization. For example, the experience of preparing and participating in a community music performance can, by virtue of relationship to the members of the community, contribute to a client's possibilities for self-esteem, while challenging the client's capacity to accept responsibility for the quality of the public aesthetic product (Scovel & Gardstrom, 2005).

Therapy Processes

In Humanistic Music Therapy the client and therapist engage in various ways of *being*, musically, to support self-actualization. Although techniques do not define this sort of process, it is important to acknowledge that they can be helpful, even within a humanistic orientation (Frankl, 1967). Any technique can be valid, provided it ultimately serves a humanistic purpose (Scovel & Gardstrom, 2005). For example, as Dimaio (2010) has illustrated, a mechanism such as entrainment (i.e., the tendency toward synchronization between two cyclical or periodic phenomena in nature) can be meaningfully employed as a musical basis for self-actualization by encouraging greater alignment between the individual and the healthful, creative properties of music.

In Humanistic Music Therapy processes, interventions are never understood as isolated techniques that accomplish isolated results; rather, they are understood within the larger context of the client's whole being. Specific properties of music—for example, the physiological benefits as a sound stimulus—can be a part of this context, but ultimately, they must be assessed according to their relevance to the client's whole, human identity.

From a humanistic perspective, interventions in the music therapy process are not technical manipulations with deterministic outcomes that can be predicted in the same way that a medication exerts a statistically predictable effect upon a medical condition. Rather, interventions are best understood as opportunities upon which a client may act, using his or her agency, to promote his or her self-actualization. For Rolvsjord (2010), drawing upon the music sociology theories of DeNora (2000, 2003) and others, the music in music therapy can be understood as a resource in the form of social capital, or affordance, that clients (via their agency) can appropriate in the interest of actualizing their human potentials. Within this sort of framework, evidence-based music therapy practice is not based upon cause–effect mechanisms (or any sort of precise dose–response predictions), but is rather about understanding the best ways to support clients in actualizing their agency, given certain musical opportunities, in the context of who they are (Abrams, 2010).

In Humanistic Music Therapy work, the process of therapy is also relational. The value of a given therapy process is less about what the client does in response to an intervention and more about what the therapy affords the client in mitigating the social and/or environmental contexts that can help the client to deepen his or her own humanization (e.g., more empowered, more dignified, more meaningful). Also in humanistic work, relationship is not just a factor or component in therapy—it *is* the therapy and is the basis of change. For Rogers (1951), the therapist's relational disposition, characterized by congruence/genuineness,

unconditional positive regard/nonjudgmental acceptance, and empathy, is the sine qua non of the humanistic therapy process. Garred (2006) articulates the importance of a humanistic disposition, specifically in music therapy, drawing upon Buber's (2004) understanding of human encounters as the meeting of mutual, whole, contextually situated, acting subjects, wherein oneself is understood as *I* and another person is understood as *thou* (and vice versa, from the other person's perspective), with neither party ever being construed as an *it*. Garred adds the concept of the music as yet another I or thou within a triangular, relational configuration constituting the music therapy process.

Music Therapy Applications

Humanistic frameworks have been applied to music therapy assessment (Scovel & Gardstrom, 2005; Wigram, 1999) as well as to treatment (Bruscia, 1991a; Meadows, 2011). Currently, the richest source of documented Humanistic Music Therapy applications is the case study literature. A diverse array of cases, across a wide range of orientations and approaches, is found in the collections of Bruscia (1991a) and Meadows (2011). In spite of 20 years separating the publication dates of these two volumes, both include numerous manifestations of Humanistic Music Therapy work. A summary of these cases follows (with publication dates identifying the source volume; refer to Table 12.1 for a guide to source citations). Cases identified as examples of Humanistic Music Therapy practices have featured clients at various stages of their lives, have addressed a wide range of presenting client needs and conditions, and have employed an array of music experiences, as can be seen from the listings in Table 12.1.

It is notable that the theoretical underpinnings of the work described in some of these cases are based upon the humanistic psychology literature—for example, Yalom

TABLE 12.1. Case Studies Featuring Humanistic Approaches to Music Therapy

Developmental life stages	Client needs and conditions	Types of music experiences
• *Childhood*: Aigen (1991); Burke (1991); Carpente (2011); Robbins & Robbins (1991a); Salas & Gonzalez (1991)	• *Sensory disabilities*: Salas & Gonzalez (1991)	• *Music listening and imaging*: Bruscia (1991b); Bunt (2011); Clark (1991); Pickett (1991); Summer (2011)
• *Adolescence*: McFerran (2011); Robbins & Robbins (1991b)	• *Brain damage*: Robbins & Robbins (1991b)	• *Song recreation and/or compilation*: Martin (1991); Stige (2011); Wittall (1991)
• *Adulthood*: Bruscia (1991b); Bunt (2011); Clark (1991); Martin (1991); Pickett (1991); Stige (2011); Summer (2011); Trondalen (2011); Van Den Hurk & Smeijsters (1991); Wittall (1991)	• *Multiple disabilities*: Robbins & Robbins (1991a)	• *Improvisation*: Aigen (1991); Carpente (2011); McFerran (2011); Robbins & Robbins (1991a, 1991b); Salas & Gonzalez (1991); Stige (2011); Trondalen (2011); Van Den Hurk & Smeijsters (1991)
• *Older adulthood*: Hilliard & Justice (2011)	• *Autism*: Carpente (2011) • *Behavioral issues*: Aigen (1991) • *Major psychiatric diagnoses*: Pickett (1991); Stige (2011); Summer (2011) • *Anxiety and panic disorders*: Bruscia (1991b); Van Den Hurk & Smeijsters (1991) • *Chemical dependency*: McFerran (2011); Pickett (1991) • *Eating disorders*: Pickett (1991); Trondalen (2011) • *Emotional trauma and/or grief*: Bruscia (1991b); Bunt (2011); Burke (1991); Clark (1991) • *Life-threatening illness and/or other end-of-life issues*: Bruscia (1991b); Hilliard & Justice (2011); Martin (1991); Wittall (1991)	• *Song composition*: Burke (1991); Hilliard & Justice (2011); McFerran (2011)

Note. Sources are Bruscia (1991a) and Meadows (2011).

(Trondalen, 2011), Rogers (Stige, 2011), and Maslow (McFerran, 2011). Likewise, the work described in certain cases was informed specifically by models found in the humanistically oriented music therapy literature, such as Bonny's Model of Guided Imagery and Music (e.g., Bruscia, 1991b; Bunt, 2011; Clark, 1991; Pickett, 1991; Summer, 2011) or Nordoff and Robbins's model of Creative Music Therapy (e.g., Carpente, 2011; Robbins & Robbins, 1991a, 1991b).

Abrams (partially summarized in Abrams & Kasayka, 2005[1]) presented a case study involving the application of the Bonny Method of Guided Imagery and Music (GIM) with Lisa, a woman with life-threatening, metastatic breast cancer, receiving services at the cancer treatment center where the therapist was employed at the time. A brief account of this case follows, shared from the first-person perspective of the author (Abrams).

CLINICAL EXAMPLE

When I first met Lisa at the cancer center where I practiced music therapy, I encountered a very down-to-earth woman in her 40s. She had undergone a double mastectomy and invasive implantation of a central line for infusion of caustic chemotherapy medications that would otherwise be damaging to her vascular tissue. In spite of this, her manner was energetic and enthusiastic, and she wore her "battle scars," including her very short hair, proudly. In her somewhat pressured conversational style, I immediately sensed a certain defensiveness—a wall around a most understandable experience of supreme vulnerability. I knew right away that I would need to tread lightly, and to prepare myself for what it would take to join her empathically in her pain and trauma.

Lisa shared with me that she was in a medical profession, and that this had represented a deeply valued part of her identity. Now, this aspect of her life was severely disrupted. At the same time, her professional training rendered her all too familiar with what was happening to her on a medical level, and seemed to do little to mitigate the impact of what she considered to be the objectifying and dehumanizing dimensions of the treatment.

On a more personal level, Lisa also disclosed that, over the years pre-dating her initial diagnosis, she had also experienced estrangement from family, particularly her son—something that was now having a significant impact, given her new levels of vulnerability and need for love and support. At different points during the progression of her illness, Lisa had been hospitalized, placed in various nursing care facilities, and sent home to take care of herself, alone, all contributing to a sense of "wandering" without a safe, stable, place of belonging. Although a self-identified "fighter" under challenging circumstances, Lisa was now experiencing a general sense of being "trapped" within life's heavy darkness, leaving her with a sense of isolation, powerlessness, and being a victim of numerous internal and external forces beyond her control. Lisa openly shared all of this with me—and how it was, for her, due to all of these factors that she chose to pursue music therapy with me at the cancer center—specifically, through GIM as a means of identifying inner resources she desperately needed.

Consistent with the tenets of Humanistic Music Therapy, as the therapist (guide), I began by validating Lisa's experiences, primarily through listening, reflecting, and being present to her as supportively as possible. Once she and I were able to establish a sense of trust—and, along with it, an initial rapport and working relationship—we engaged in a therapy assessment process. This took the form of Lisa exploring various "ways of being" through creative imaging to the classical masterworks in the GIM recording, and by drawing upon the humanity embodied in the music's aesthetic depths. Through this initial process, Lisa and I collaboratively formulated goals targeting her cultivation of emotional strength, identification of inner resources for coping, and managing relationship issues concerning those in her family (such as her son) and others.

Lisa then began working with me in a series of weekly GIM sessions. Through the rigors of her process, Lisa struggled to engage the opportunities in the music as imaginatively

---

[1] Used with permission of Jeffrey Books.

as possible, often finding herself "stuck" and "weighed down" in numerous ways. As guide, I experienced myself struggling right along with her, and sought supervision whenever I myself felt likewise immobilized and burdened by the existential weight of her struggles that I often "took on" in ways that may have impacted my capacity for effective presence and support. Several recurring symbols in Lisa's images included a friendly black bird (with whom she experienced a sense of identification), a bent tree with unusual "tractor" forces that it used to drag Lisa toward itself (which Lisa and I both found somewhat menacing), and a glowing gold box that imparted a sense of comfort and strength. Rather than emphasizing a psychodynamic interpretation of these symbols, Lisa and I worked with the symbols as expressions of potential resources that Lisa could utilize or appropriate in the interest of achieving greater liberation of her humanity under her particularly challenging circumstances, as this was the most relevant approach to addressing Lisa's needs.

In her tenth and final session of the series, Lisa encountered several of her familiar symbols again, but now in a new context. The music we used in this particular excerpt of the session was Richard Strauss's "Im Abendrot" ("At Sunset")—one of his *Vier Letzte Lieder* (*Four Last Songs*), performed by Jessye Norman. In Lisa's imagery, she found herself walking, carrying her glowing gold box. As she walked, she encountered a mountain, where her friendly bird joined her, flying overhead. After taking a moment to appreciate the fresh aroma of pine (as an affirmation of health and life), she began ascending. At a certain point, she began to struggle more intensely as the mountainside became increasingly steep. I asked Lisa if she could find something to help her. She located a "funny, curvy walking stick," reminiscent of the sinister, bent tree, but in this form, as something helpful—that propelled her in the direction her will was already moving (as a subject), as opposed to dragging her against her will (as an object). In fact, during this session, she began to experience her entire body, and entire being, as lighter—almost floating—and I, as therapist, experienced this sense of lightness along with her. As she neared the top, her gold box began to glow more brightly, until it

emanated brilliant white at the summit. Lisa's bird circled above her several times (as if to say "goodbye") and then departed. As the sun set, the box's glow lit up the night. I asked her if she needed anything at that moment. She indicated that the light was enough, that she did not need anything more, and that she was OK.

Although Lisa's cancer remained in an advanced stage during her work in music therapy, she nonetheless discovered a new way of being through her engagement with the music. For her, this was a new *lightness* of being, both in the sense of physical buoyancy and of visual and emotional brightness. Her bird, a symbolic resource, served as an inner guide that helped her find her way to where (and how) she needed to be. She imaginatively transformed her tree image from something manipulating and threatening into something with forces she was able harness and incorporate into the power of her own human agency. The image of reaching the apex of the mountain, surrounded in her own light even as evening fell was, both literally and figuratively, a *peak experience* (Maslow, 1964) and a marker of her own self-actualization. Regardless of whatever was to come next for her, this new dimension of her being would remain, mitigating how she could now experience, confront, cope with, and embrace life.

Conclusions

Humanistic approaches to music therapy are documented across a wide range of models, methods, and practices within the field, and have been evident from the earliest stages of the field's development. Although there is no single example of an approach that necessarily incorporates all of the tenets of the humanistic orientation, per se, these tenets can be found throughout the theoretical and clinical literature, in various forms, serving clients in various ways. In spite of this existing literature, the value of continuing to develop resources on Humanistic Music Therapy theory, practices, and research remains.

REFERENCES

Abrams, B. (2010). Evidence-based music therapy practice: An integral understanding. *Journal of Music Therapy, 47*(4), 351–379.

Abrams, B. (2011). Understanding music as a temporal–aesthetic way of being: Implications for a general theory of music therapy. *Arts in Psychotherapy, 38*(2), 114–119.

Abrams, B. (2012). A relationship-based theory of music therapy: Understanding processes and goals as being-together-musically. In K. E. Bruscia (Ed.), *Readings in music therapy theory* (pp. 58–76). Gilsum, NH: Barcelona.

Abrams, B., & Kasayka, R. (2005). Music imaging for persons at the end of life. In C. Dileo & J. V. Loewy (Eds.), *Music therapy at the end of life* (pp. 159–170). Cherry Hill, NJ: Jeffrey Books.

Aigen, K. (1991). Creative fantasy, music and lyric improvisation with a gifted, acting-out boy. In K. E. Bruscia (Ed.), *Case studies in music therapy* (pp. 109–126). Gilsum, NH: Barcelona.

Aigen, K. (2005). *Music-centered music therapy.* Gilsum, NH: Barcelona.

Bruscia, K. E. (1988). A survey of treatment procedures in improvisational music therapy. *Psychology of Music, 16*, 10–24.

Bruscia, K. E. (Ed.). (1991a). *Case studies in music therapy.* Gilsum, NH: Barcelona.

Bruscia, K. E. (1991b). Embracing life with AIDS: Psychotherapy through Guided Imagery and Music (GIM). In K. E. Bruscia (Ed.), *Case studies in music therapy* (pp. 581–602). Gilsum, NH: Barcelona.

Buber, M. (2004). *I and thou.* London: Continuum International.

Bugental, J. (1964). The third force in psychology. *Journal of Humanistic Psychology, 4*(1), 19–26.

Bunt, L. (1994). *Music therapy: An art beyond words.* London: Routledge.

Bunt, L. (2011). Bringing light into darkness: Guided Imagery and Music, bereavement, loss, and working through trauma. In A. Meadows (Ed.), *Developments in music therapy practice: Case study perspectives* (pp. 501–517). Gilsum, NH: Barcelona.

Burke, K. (1991). Music therapy in working through a preschooler's grief: Expressing rage and confusion. In K. E. Bruscia (Ed.), *Case stud-ies in music therapy* (pp. 127–135). Gilsum, NH: Barcelona.

Carpente, J. A. (2011). Addressing core features of autism: Integrating Nordoff–Robbins music therapy within the Developmental, Individual-Difference, Relationship-Based (DIR)®/ Floortime™ model. In A. Meadows (Ed.), *Developments in music therapy practice: Case study perspectives* (pp. 134–149). Gilsum, NH: Barcelona.

Clark, M. F. (1991). Emergence of the adult self in Guided Imagery and Music (GIM) therapy. In K. E. Bruscia (Ed.), *Case studies in music therapy* (pp. 321–331). Gilsum, NH: Barcelona.

Clark, M. F. (2002). The evolution of the Bonny Method of Guided Imagery and Music (BMGIM). In K. E. Bruscia & D. E. Grocke (Eds.), *Guided imagery and music: The Bonny method and beyond* (pp. 5–27). Gilsum, NH: Barcelona.

Corey, G. (2009). *Theory and practice of counseling and psychotherapy* (8th ed.). Belmont, CA: Thomson/Brooks/Cole.

Corsini, R. J., & Wedding, D. (1995). *Current psychotherapies* (5th ed.). Itasca, IL: F. E. Peacock.

DeNora, T. (2000). *Music in everyday life.* Cambridge, UK: Cambridge University Press.

DeNora, T. (2003). *After Adorno: Rethinking music sociology.* Cambridge, UK: Cambridge University Press.

Dimaio, L. (2010). Music therapy entrainment: A humanistic music therapist's perspective of using music therapy entrainment with hospice clients experiencing pain. *Music Therapy Perspectives, 28*(2), 106–115.

Elliott, D. J. (1995). *Music matters: A new philosophy of music education.* New York: Oxford University Press.

Frankl, V. E. (1967). *Psychotherapy and existentialism.* New York: Washington Square Press.

Frankl, V. E. (1984). *Man's search for meaning: An introduction to logotherapy* (3rd ed.). New York: Washington Square Press.

Garred, R. (2006). *Music as therapy: A dialogical perspective.* Gilsum, NH: Barcelona.

Heidegger, M. (1962). *Being and time* (rev. ed.). New York: Harper & Row.

Highet, G. (1949). *The classical tradition: Greek and Roman influences on Western literature.* New York: Oxford University Press.

Hilliard, R., & Justice, J. (2011). Songs of faith in end of life care. In A. Meadows (Ed.), *Developments in music therapy practice: Case study perspectives* (pp. 582–594). Gilsum, NH: Barcelona.

Jung, C. G. (1989). *Memories, dreams, reflections* (A. Jaffe, Ed.; C. Winston & R. Winston, Trans.). New York: Vintage Books. (Original work published 1963)

Kant, I. (1996). *The metaphysics of morals* (M. Gregor, Trans.). Cambridge, UK: Cambridge University Press. (Original work published 1785)

Kim, Y. (2004). The early beginnings of Nordoff–Robbins music therapy. *Journal of Music Therapy, 41*(4), 321–339.

Leonard, G. B. (1987). *The transformation: A guide to the inevitable changes in humankind.* New York: J. P. Tarcher.

Martin, J. A. (1991). Music therapy at the end of a life. In K. E. Bruscia (Ed.), *Case studies in music therapy* (pp. 617–632). Gilsum, NH: Barcelona.

Maslow, A. H. (1943). A theory of human motivation. *Psychological Review, 50*(4), 370–396.

Maslow, A. H. (1964). *Religion, values and peak experiences.* New York: Viking.

McFerran, K. (2011). Moving out of your comfort zone: Group music therapy with adolescents who have misused drugs. In A. Meadows (Ed.), *Developments in music therapy practice: Case study perspectives* (pp. 248–267). Gilsum, NH: Barcelona.

Meadows, A. (Ed.). (2011). *Developments in music therapy practice: Case study perspectives.* Gilsum, NH: Barcelona.

Mommsen, T. E. (1942). Petrarch's conception of the "Dark Ages." *Speculum, 17*(2), 226–242.

Pfeiffer, R. (1976). *History of classical scholarship: From 1300 to 1850.* New York: Oxford University Press.

Pickett, E. (1991). Guided imagery and music (BMGIM) with a dually diagnosed woman having multiple addictions. In K. E. Bruscia (Ed.), *Case studies in music therapy* (pp. 497–512). Gilsum, NH: Barcelona.

Polit, V. (1993). Music therapy in Mexico. In C. Dileo Maranto (Ed.), *Music therapy: International perspectives* (pp. 365–383). Pipersville, PA: Jeffrey Books.

Robbins, C., & Robbins, C. (1991a). Self-communications in creative music therapy. In K. E. Bruscia (Ed.), *Case studies in music therapy* (pp. 55–72). Gilsum, NH: Barcelona.

Robbins, C., & Robbins, C. (1991b). Creative music therapy in bringing order, change and communicativeness to the life of a brain-injured adolescent. In K. E. Bruscia (Ed.), *Case studies in music therapy* (pp. 231–249). Gilsum, NH: Barcelona.

Rogers, C. (1939). *The clinical treatment of the problem child.* Boston: Houghton Mifflin.

Rogers, C. (1951). *Client-centered therapy: Its current practice, implications and theory.* London: Constable.

Rogers, C. (1961). *On becoming a person.* Boston: Houghton Mifflin.

Rogers, N. (1993). *The creative connection: Expressive arts as healing.* Palo Alto, CA: Science & Behavior Books.

Rolvsjord, R. (2010). *Resource-oriented music therapy in mental health care.* Gilsum, NH: Barcelona.

Ruud, E. (1998). *Music therapy: Improvisation, communication, and culture.* Gilsum, NH: Barcelona.

Ruud, E. (2010). *Music therapy: A perspective from the humanities.* Gilsum, NH: Barcelona.

Salas, J., & Gonzalez, D. (1991). Like singing with a bird: Improvisational Music Therapy with a blind four-year-old. In K. E. Bruscia (Ed.), *Case studies in music therapy* (pp. 17–28). Gilsum, NH: Barcelona.

Schneider, K. J., & Krug, O. T. (2010). *Existential-humanistic therapy.* Washington, DC: American Psychological Association.

Scovel, M., & Gardstrom, S. (2005). Music therapy within the context of psychotherapeutic models. In R. Unkefer & M. Thaut (Eds.), *Music therapy in the treatment of adults with mental disorders: Theoretical bases and clinical applications* (2nd ed., pp. 117–132). Gilsum, NH: Barcelona.

Seligman, M. E. P., & Csikszentmihalyi, M. (2000). Positive psychology: An introduction. *American Psychologist, 55*(1), 5–14.

Sommers-Flanagan, J. (2007). Development and evolution of person-centered expressive art therapy: A conversation with Natalie Rogers. *Journal of Counseling and Development, 85*(1), 120–125.

Sorel, S. (2011, November 17). *Writing humanistic music therapy goals in an evidenced-based world.* Continuing Music Therapy Education Course presented at the annual meeting of the American Music Therapy Association, Atlanta, GA.

Stige, B. (2011). The doors and windows of the dressing room: Culture-centered music therapy in a mental health setting. In A. Meadows (Ed.), *Developments in music therapy practice: Case study perspectives* (pp. 416–433). Gilsum, NH: Barcelona.

Summer, L. (2011). Music therapy and depression: Uncovering resources in music and imagery In A. Meadows (Ed.), *Developments in music therapy practice: Case study perspectives* (pp. 486–500). Gilsum, NH: Barcelona.

Trondalen, G. (2011). Music therapy is about feelings: Music therapy with a young man suffering from anorexia nervosa. In A. Meadows (Ed.), *Developments in music therapy practice: Case study perspectives* (pp. 434–452). Gilsum, NH: Barcelona.

Van Den Hurk, J., & Smeijsters, H. (1991). Musical improvisation in the treatment of a man with obsessive–compulsive personality disorder. In

K. E. Bruscia (Ed.), *Case studies in music therapy* (pp. 387–402). Gilsum, NH: Barcelona.

Walsh, R., & Vaughan, F. (1993). On transpersonal definitions. *Journal of Transpersonal Psychology, 25*(2), 125–182.

Webster's Ninth New Collegiate Dictionary. (1990). Agency. Springfield, MA: Merriam-Webster.

Wheeler, B. (1981). The relationship between music therapy and theories of psychotherapy. *Music Therapy, 1*(1), 9–16.

Wigram, T. (1999). Assessment methods in music therapy: A humanistic or natural science framework? *Nordic Journal of Music Therapy, 8*(1), 6–24.

Wittall, J. (1991). Songs in palliative care: A spouse's last gift. In K. E. Bruscia (Ed.), *Case studies in music therapy* (pp. 603–610). Gilsum, NH: Barcelona.

Yalom, I. D. (1983). *Inpatient group psychotherapy*. New York: Basic Books.

Zuckerkandl, V. (1956). *Sound and symbol*. New York: Pantheon Books.

CHAPTER 13

Cognitive-Behavioral Approaches

Suzanne Hanser

Cogito ergo sum [I think, therefore I am]
—RENÉ DESCARTES (1637/1910)

Cognitive-behavioral therapy (CBT) is a contemporary approach to psychotherapy that recognizes and values the basic premises of both cognitive therapy and behavior therapy: that thoughts, ideas, feelings, and behaviors are inextricably linked and that these elements arc under our personal control. Although the merger of these two established modern psychotherapies is relatively recent, the origins of the signature techniques of CBT are rooted in ancient teachings and early philosophy. Indeed, the contemplative wisdom traditions related to Buddhist, shamanic, Vedic, Jewish kabbalistic, Chinese medicinal, and a multitude of ancient practices too numerous to list emphasize methods of thought control such as meditation, mindfulness, and mantra/prayer. These methods, which aided yogis and God-seekers of many religious persuasions in their search for enlightenment, have now entered the psychological lingo of a contemporary society that is seeking help to deal with stimulus overload and stress as a part of daily existence.

Variants of meditation, mindfulness, and mantra are part and parcel of CBT today, with a contemporary slant and new vocabulary. Furthermore, the field of integrative medicine is welcoming Eastern thinking into the practice of Western medicine and promoting the amalgamation of ancient therapies with conventional, standard care. So, the growing prevalence of these nontraditional approaches among traditional ones has made it possible for these methods to be accepted more readily by potential clients in the 21st century. As a function of this openness, music therapy, too, thrives within this integrative model of care.

Music therapy has benefited greatly from the evolution of CBT, as music is easily integrated into many of the old and new cognitive-behavioral methodologies and applications. In addition, just as behavioral and cognitive approaches were becoming firmly embedded in mid-20th-century psychotherapeutic practices, the profession of music therapy was establishing itself in the United States during this same time.

History

In the Beginning

What are now known as principles of CBT have appeared and reappeared in various forms throughout history. During the Golden Age of Greece (500–300 B.C.E.), philosophers tended to refer to their treatises as *meditations*, and Roman stoicism developed as a school of philosophy that dealt with the art of living. Among the stoics, Epictetus (1877) is particularly cognitive-behavioral in orientation. He stated, "Men are disturbed not by things which happen, but by the opinions about the things" (p. 381), and "On the occasion of every accident (event) that befalls you, remember to turn to yourself and inquire what power you have for turning it to use" (p. 383). Stoic philosophers were also proponents of self-dialogue, attention to the here and now, active self-inquiry, reflection on daily challenges, and Socratic questioning—all of which are part of current CBT practice. The stoics emphasized the virtues of human beings, as did Confucius, and they advocated for the rehearsal of certain dogmas, much like the mantras of Indian tradition. Of course, these practices proved to be the precursors of self-talk, positive affirmations, and autosuggestion—tools of the trade for cognitive-behavioral therapists everywhere (Robertson, 2010).

The sophists were a group of philosophers in 450–400 B.C.E., of which Protagoras was one of the first. Generally, the sophists were intellectuals who charged people for divulging their wisdom (although Socrates offered his teachings freely) and were known for using rhetoric in their convincing arguments. Rhetoric was also used to address conflict by having the debating parties use persuasion to defend their positions. The sophists' rhetoric and logic have also framed some present-day cognitive therapy practices, particularly in group therapy, where participants engage in competitive games and debates.

History of Behaviorism

Ivan Pavlov's famous classical conditioning experiments of salivation in dogs, occurring after the ring of a bell previously paired with food, were not actually the first behavioral experiments, and Pavlov was not even a psychologist, although he is perhaps best known as one of the founders of behavioral theory (Pavlov, 1927). Many decades earlier, in the 1860s, another Russian physiologist named Ivan—Ivan Sechenov—studied external factors in determining mental life and behavior and went on to study what he identified as reflexes, signals, and central inhibition (Sechenov, 1863/1965). His seminal work became more fully developed in classical conditioning theories of behaviorism and in psychoneuroimmunology (Greenwood, 2009). Then, by the close of the 19th century, another early behaviorist, Edward L. Thorndike, was developing theories of operant conditioning that would have significant impact on the emerging systems of behaviorism. Thorndike observed the behavior of kittens, dogs, and chicks in a series of experiments that led him to formulate the *law of effect*, a notion that a behavior that produces a pleasurable or desirable outcome—a payoff of sorts—will be repeated, and one that fails to produce such an effect will diminish in frequency and strength. He was one of the first to use the vocabulary of behavior modification, publishing a monograph on animal intelligence (Thorndike, 1898). John B. Watson (1913) translated some of these ideas into theories of human behavior and provided insights into the human response to changes in the surrounding environment.

Perhaps the most well-known leader in behaviorism is Burrhus Frederic Skinner, the man whose radical behaviorism combined emerging theories of analytical, methodological, and psychological behaviorism. His first major treatise presented the operant conditioning model, detailing how the contingencies of behavior—that is, the antecedents and consequences of a behavior—determine the strength and frequency of that behavior (Skinner, 1938). In his prolific writings and lectures, he revealed a science of human behavior that focused on the ways in which behavioral change could be manifested through an experimental analysis of behavior. He characterized thinking as mental behavior and translated internal workings of the mind as private events that could be understood in the same way as other more clearly observable behavior. He developed a vocabulary and paradigm that has achieved significant longevity in psychology and the behavioral sciences (Skinner, 1957).

In England, Hans Eysenck (1967) drew on Pavlov's work involving the nervous system and Hull's (1943) learning theory to devise a system relating the brain to behavior. He contributed greatly to the understanding of the human personality through his explorations of the interrelationships among personality and cognition, emotion, behavior, and environment. Eysenck was a champion in England for behavioral alternatives to the popular psychoanalytic treatments of the time.

Applied behavior analysis was a movement that sprang from these many behavioral theories and utilized various techniques—for example, the manipulation of discriminative, conditioned, and reinforcing stimuli; positive and negative reinforcement/punishment; functional analysis; contingency management; and other behavioral principles—as part of therapy and education. Meanwhile, in South Africa, Joseph Wolpe extended the compendium of behavioral clinical techniques for psychotherapists who were treating anxiety disorders (Wolpe & Lazarus, 1966). Wolpe's development of a strategy called *reciprocal inhibition* proved to be effective in reducing anxiety with the introduction of an incompatible, calming stimulus. *Systematic desensitization* became another important clinical tool perfected by Wolpe and Lazarus to deal with fears and phobias.

History of Cognitive Therapy

As the field of psychotherapy advanced through the 20th century, Alfred Adler (1931) was the first of Freud's followers to break away from the strictures of traditional psychoanalysis. The accessibility of his ideas to the general public, including his emphasis on thoughts of inferiority and superiority and his optimistic view of humankind, contributed to the formation of a new school of psychotherapy, named in his honor. Adlerian psychotherapy, particularly the techniques that examine schemas and their influence on different personality types, as well as emphasis on the here and now, deeply influenced Albert Ellis, whose rational emotive behavior therapy (REBT; formerly rational therapy, then rational emotive therapy) was a forerunner of cognitive therapy (Ellis, 1962). REBT is a very active approach that directs the client to dispute the beliefs that are sandwiched in between an activating event and its emotional reaction. Ellis's ABCD model of therapy involves identifying an "A," Activating event or Adversity; the "B," Beliefs or automatic and evaluative thoughts generated by A; the "C," emotional or behavioral Consequences of the experience; and, finally, "D," Disputation of the beliefs. Disputing involves learning a variety of techniques that identify and challenge irrational or destructive thinking, as well as develop functional alternatives.

One of the primary proponents of classical cognitive therapy, as it evolved in the 1960s, is Aaron Beck, psychiatrist and creator of the concept of *automatic thoughts*, whose innovations include techniques to challenge negative thoughts and dysfunctional assumptions through examining ideas, behaviors, attitudes, judgments, and beliefs. Beck also introduced the term *collaborative empiricism* to describe a working therapeutic alliance between therapist and client(s) that calls upon insights from the client as well as the therapist. His problem-solving approach is short-term, goal-directed, and focused on the thought patterns that lead to detrimental emotional consequences and dysfunctional behavior (Beck, 2005).

The Advent of CBT

Over time, the intercorrelations among thinking, feeling, and acting were recognized in the growing varieties of cognitive and behavioral therapies. Some of the more recent terminology includes *clinical behavior analysis* (CBA; Kohlenberg, Tsai, & Dougher, 1993), which provides a conceptual framework for the integration of multiple approaches, including more behaviorally based dialectical behavior therapy, behavioral activation therapy, functional analytic psychotherapy, acceptance and commitment therapy (ACT), integrative behavioral couples therapy and traditional behavioral marriage therapy, behavioral pediatrics, and community reinforcement and family training, among others. On the cognitive side, metacognitive therapy and mindfulness-based cognitive therapy comprise two of the more popular treatment modalities. Known now as the third wave of CBT, the respectability of these treatments is significant, owing largely to the extensive evidence that supports their efficacy with a long list of clinical problems and diagnoses.

Current Status

In the 2000s, the third generation of therapists and treatments came under scrutiny. Currently, the disparate forms of CBT have been well researched and highly valued. Over 500 outcome studies identify an extensive list of successful applications of cognitive-behavioral interventions (Chambliss & Ollendick, 2001). The National Institute for Health and Care Excellence in the United Kingdom recommends CBT as an effective treatment option for many mental health problems (Department of Health, 1999). This institute reports that it is particularly indicated for people with depression, anxiety, obsessive–compulsive disorder

(OCD), and posttraumatic stress disorder (PTSD), and cites benefits, such as reducing (1) the requirement for antidepressant medications, (2) referrals to secondary care services, (3) severity and exacerbation of symptoms, and (4) suicide risk (National Institute for Health and Care Excellence in the United Kingdom, 2008). In the United States, the National Institute of Mental Health (2012) details the positive impact of CBT for depression and anxiety disorders, bipolar disorder, eating disorders, schizophrenia, and trauma-related disorders in children and adolescents.

In 2008, Ost conducted a meta-analysis of the efficacy of the third wave of CBT interventions and found strong evidence for each of the therapies. Kahl, Winter, and Schweiger (2012) updated and extended this review to include randomized controlled trials since 2007. They confirmed that these modern approaches are, indeed, empirically supported through a substantial body of research. The authors conclude:

> The third wave of behavioral psychotherapies is an important arena of modern psychotherapy development. It has added considerably to the spectrum of empirically supported treatments for mental disorders. The presented methods include a diversity of new techniques and open up possibilities for patient groups such as borderline personality disorder, chronic depression or generalized anxiety disorder that had received only little specific attention in the past. (p. 527)

History of Cognitive-Behavioral Music Therapy

Jeffrey (1955) was perhaps the first to publish work on the contingent use of music with children, as referenced in the journal *Science*. This article highlighted a new and potentially effective form of reinforcement, namely music, and touted its more naturally and educationally satisfying side effects, when compared with candy or toys. In 1970, brothers Clifford K. Madsen and Charles H. Madsen, Jr., collaborated on two important texts (1970a, 1970b), and their conceptual articles and research have influenced generations of music therapists in clinical practice and research. Remarks by Madsen and colleagues 45 years ago are prescient of the evolution of behavioral music therapy:

> Our basic concern should be for experimentation based upon control and manipulations of the behaviors and instruments involved. After this experimentation, applications of music therapy which prove successful can be incorporated into a more extensive body of behavioral techniques. It will then be possible to proceed with more scientifically formulated information. Such experimentation might include the use of music for desensitization, music for hypnosis, music for specific conditioning, music as a reward for appropriate behaviors and the contingent use of music for shaping all aspects of desirable behaviors. These remain in the foreseeable future. We may find that music is capable of much more than we previously considered possible. (Madsen, Cotter, & Madsen, 1968, p. 71)

In a landmark analysis of the extant literature on music as a reinforcer, Standley (1996) examined 208 variables in 98 studies that applied music as a contingency, perhaps the most obvious application of the operant conditioning paradigm. Contingent music revealed an effect size of 2.90, meaning that the benefits were nearly three standard deviations beyond baseline conditions or compared to a control group. Standley indicated that music served as a very effective means of reinforcement, while providing educational benefits as a source of content for learning. In addition, she found that academic and social behaviors that occurred in the context of the reinforced behaviors improved. Music served as a powerful motivator, with no evidence of negative impact.

Gregory (2002) conducted a content analysis of the 607 articles published in the *Journal of Music Therapy* between 1964 and 1999 to determine the prevalence of behavioral research designs in the music therapy litera-

ture. The number of articles that met criteria for a behavioral research approach (96, or 15.8% of the total) increased over this time period, with a much greater variety of clinical populations being represented in the last 20 years of the sample.

In addition to the robust representation of behavioral music therapy in a plethora of clinical populations, and usage of behavioral research designs, a recent survey of music therapists in psychiatric practice (Silverman, 2007) revealed that behavioral approaches were used by 83.1% of the respondents. Music therapists identified their primary philosophical orientation, in a single forced choice, as eclectic (39.3%), followed by cognitive-behavioral (21.3%), behavioral (16.3%), and humanistic (14.2%), with fewer responding as psychodynamic, cognitive, and biomedical therapists.

Silverman is a champion of the use of Cognitive-Behavioral Music Therapy (CBMT) in the psychiatric setting, having authored thorough conceptual papers and rigorous research studies on the subject. He has not only enabled fellow music therapists to benefit from his analyses of clinical cases and research, but also delineated a research agenda, based on the best practices of cognitive-behavioral trials (Silverman, 2008).

Theoretical Tenets

The purpose of CBT is to offer more adaptive learning experiences and behaviors, while undoing dysfunctional learning and thought patterns. Elements of classical CBT include (1) a strong therapeutic alliance with active participation by clients and collaboration between therapists and clients; (2) an individual conceptualization of each client's problems, in a constantly evolving formulation; (3) goal- and problem-oriented focus; (4) attention on the present; (5) an educative philosophy, with the ultimate aim of teaching clients to be their own therapists; (6) relapse prevention; (7)

short-term and time-limited process; (8) structured therapeutic sessions; (9) clients who identify, evaluate, and challenge their dysfunctional or irrational thoughts and beliefs; (10) techniques that change thinking, mood, and behavior; and (11) a Socratic method of questioning.

The treatment process emphasizes the positive aspects of a person's adaptability, while working through structured sessions that identify and respond to dysfunctional thoughts and behaviors. Homework assignments help to facilitate cognitive and behavioral change between sessions. Therapeutic content is centered each person's core beliefs (rules, attitudes, and assumptions); the situations that bring up automatic thinking; and the emotional, behavioral, and physiological reactions or consequences.

A typical session might start with a mood check, then move toward problem identification and goal setting. Guided discovery and discussion would ensue, as clients and therapists work together to identify the ABCDs—antecedents, beliefs, consequences, and potential disputes—relative to each problem. Beliefs would be detailed so that irrational or dysfunctional thinking could be identified. Behavioral activation and experiments might be part of the process, with homework assignments providing a chance for clients to try out different ways of responding to an emotionally packed antecedent. Clients would be asked to record data on their daily activities and to chart their response to pleasant events, or complete their own ABCD, when a distressing emotional consequence is encountered. Clients might use imagery to create problematic situations in their minds and observe themselves working out the issues in a more constructive manner, or approaching an aversive situation in a calmer state of mind.

A more classical dialectical behavior therapy model (Linehan & Koerner, 2012) adds a collection of other techniques to the process. In order to better tolerate distress, radical acceptance in the form of coping statements—for example, "I can only control

the present moment" or "The past cannot be changed, but I can change my reaction"—is introduced as new vocabulary to substitute for more dysfunctional reactions to a stressor. Mindfulness exercises provide an opportunity to stay in the present moment, avoid worries about the past or future, and observe behavior nonjudgmentally without attempting to change it. Emotion regulation focuses on observing feelings without overreacting or becoming overwhelmed. Clients also learn tools to improve interpersonal effectiveness by practicing the setting of limits, expressing themselves, or negotiating solutions to problems. Another technique involves noticing the body language that accompanies an emotion, selecting an opposite action, and trying it out.

The approaches outlined here are commonly observed in cognitive-behavioral practices, but CBT is by no means limited to these techniques. A multiplicity of strategies and frameworks is consistent with the major tenets of CBT and will undoubtedly evolve into a fourth wave of implementation.

Music Therapy Applications

Music therapy is a natural partner to CBT (Luce, 2001). As an inherently positive approach to living, music therapy emphasizes one's abilities and talents. Participation in musical experiences offers a metaphor for actions outside of the music therapy setting and provides a safe opportunity to try out new ways of acting and reacting. The impact of various forms of music and music activities as a form of positive reinforcement, the ability of music to serve as a stimulus for new behavior to be developed, its accessibility as a pleasant event, and its ability to evoke mood change, make music a valuable resource. Music therapists have applied music to enhance CBT techniques, developed specific music therapy techniques that are consistent with the CBT approach, and investigated their impact through rigorous research.

CBMT practitioners utilize music therapy activities such as songwriting, lyric substitution, and improvisation that are commonly employed by music therapists of other persuasions. However, for cognitive-behavioral music therapists, their intentions for presenting these activities and the manner in which the activities are implemented represent the specific values of cognitive and behavioral ideologies. The clinical music therapy applications described here illustrate some of the prevailing CBMT strategies that have been supported by clinical and scientific evidence.

Mental Health

Stoudenmire (1975) was one of the first to document the idea of complementing muscle relaxation training with music in the treatment of anxiety. Progressive muscle relaxation (PMR), a widespread application and vital part of the systematic desensitization of anxiety and phobias, can be enhanced by the accompaniment of calming music (Scheufele, 2000). When combined with guided imagery, the music can even influence re-entrainment of circadian rhythms and release of adrenal corticosteroids, a type of stress hormone (Rider, Floyd, & Kirkpatrick, 1985). Yet Robb (2000) provides evidence that PMR alone, PMR plus music, music listening, and silence may each be equally effective in reducing stress. She cautions that individual preferences are an important factor in determining efficacy, and that direct instruction may be necessary to enhance a music listening experience. Music is successful in eliciting two distinctive states of relaxation, the alert and the sedate, and the selected intervention must suit the particular needs of the client for one versus the other.

Several research studies by me and my colleague, Susan Mandel, support a variety of evidence-based techniques to condition a relaxation response, as presented in our text and CD, *Manage Your Stress and Pain through Music* (Hanser & Mandel, 2010).

These strategies include listening to a wide variety of musical selections along with gentle exercise, facial massage, PMR, and guided imagery to promote a relaxed body and a relaxed mind. We recommend that individuals identify music that has special meaning, associations, or memories, and play it when they need it most. We offer suggestions for creating one's personal "jingle" that asserts a positive affirmation: for example, singing "I can do it" or "I can be who I want to be" silently or aloud when feeling ineffective or unsuccessful. We emphasize how learning a new musical instrument, joining a musical ensemble, or composing a song can empower a person to change how he or she feels by spending more time engaging in enjoyable musical activities. Silence is also indicated at times, as is music-facilitated meditation.

Kerr, Walsh, and Marshall (2001) utilize music-assisted reframing as a cognitive strategy for dealing with anxiety. Group members are asked to visualize an anxiety-provoking scenario and to focus on the surrounding thoughts, sensations, and feelings. The therapists then play excerpts of "Barcarolle" from *The Tales of Hoffman* by Offenbach, music designed to match an anxious mood, followed by "Morning" from *Peer Gynt* by Grieg, designed to evoke a more optimistic mood. They conclude with visualizations of more positive scenes to neutralize the experience and introduce more encouraging sensations. In this strategy, "music served the function of stimulating emotion schemes already within the subject's repertoire. These schemes, integrating affect and cognition, then became synthesized and reorganized in consciousness to form new (affective and cognitive) experiences and understandings of the anxiety-provoking situation" (Kerr et al., p. 206).

CBMT has been used effectively with women who have eating disorders. Hilliard (2001b) demonstrates how music facilitates stress reduction when it accompanies progressive relaxation, breathing techniques, movement, and imagery. During meals, listening to music (and, in some cases, singing) helps to improve focus while also decreasing the anxiety that surrounds eating for these individuals. Immediately after meals, musical games, sing-alongs, and songwriting serve as cognitive divergence and provide a functional activity that is incompatible with the physical and emotional distress that often occurs at this time. Lyric analysis of songs with themes that resonate with participants' experiences can also be very useful—for example, "Running on Empty" by Jackson Browne can validate feelings, and "Don't Quit" by Caron Wheeler can instill hope. The contemporary song literature is replete with all sorts of emotional themes that can stimulate a genuine sharing process about the feelings underlying an eating disorder. Finally, writing songs and raps is a pleasurable and sometimes humorous way to express both the insights gained throughout treatment and a sense of optimism about the future, especially when these compositions include rousing choruses filled with empowering words and beautiful melodies. Hilliard (2001a) uses similar techniques with bereaved children, accompanied by songs and music adapted for children on themes of death, loss, and grief.

Dileo Maranto (1996) advocates for the use of improvisation within a cognitive-behavioral framework because musical improvisation allows for the release of cognitions and feelings that may not be easily accessible or responsive to talk therapies. Its versatility is such that improvisation can be executed individually, in dyads, or an entire group, and it can be free-form or theme-based. In any of these modalities, it is capable of providing a safe container for the examination of existing core beliefs and the reconstruction of new ones. Improvising can, then, serve as the experience to be analyzed within a standard CBT model.

In Slotoroff's (1994) work with survivors of trauma, improvisation on drums is geared to manage anger. As rapport builds between therapist and client and the cli-

ent identifies anger or assertiveness as a personal goal, the therapist explains that this technique is designed to evoke anger so that it can be understood and ultimately controlled. Introducing the activity, the therapist gives the client control over when the therapist can begin and end playing the drum, and the therapist must always ask permission to play. Through highly interactive, structured drumming exercises, the process is analyzed. As an example, the therapist plays a rhythm that is highly disruptive to the pattern initiated by the client and then questions the client, for example, as to how it felt, when those feelings began, and what it was that bothered the client. Drumming provides the context for a thorough cognitive analysis of the generation of anger, its progression, and its potential control. Lessons on assertiveness are similarly learned through the drumming.

Silverman (2011) has developed a rather different assertiveness training program that is implemented in a single session. Bob Marley's "Get Up, Stand Up" is the focus for this approach that involves lyric analysis, singing, and a *rock opera* created by the group. In this latter expressive format, group members have the opportunity to act assertively in role-played situations, interspersed with the group's singing of the chorus from Bob Marley's song. The musical segments are rounded out by group discussion, therapist coaching, positive reinforcement for appropriate assertive behavior, constructive feedback from the group, and verbal processing of the experience.

Maultsby (1977) describes how arousal of emotions through music can be explored through an investigation of the ideas and conditions surrounding this experience, as in the REBT model of CBT. Lyrics carrying personal meaning can be sung repeatedly to condition the connection between the music and the thinking process inherent in the lyrics. Lyrics can also reflect the messages of REBT and reinforce the process. In fact, Ellis (1987) himself composed some humorous songs to teach people about the therapeutic process. Bryant (1987) worked

with a perfectionistic flutist through Ellis's ABCD model. Playing the flute for an
audience (A) elicited some dysfunctional
thoughts: "I must play the flute well" and
"I should continue to play the flute" (B).
These thoughts led to anxiety and nervous-
ness (C) and allowed the music therapist to
present alternatives to the *must* and *should*
statements that she made (D).

Cheek, Bradley, Parr, and Lam (2003)
tackled the issue of teacher burnout with
a brief CBMT intervention. The investiga-
tors asked teachers to select music that was
meaningful and relevant to the aspects of
burnout that were introduced in the first
session. They shared their music with the
group and discussed the impact of music
listening at home. Cognitive restructuring
and relaxation techniques were used to facilitate discussions.

Medical Settings

Individuals with medical conditions must
deal with the psychological distress surrounding illness in addition to coping with
symptoms and painful treatments. Ghetti
(2013) integrated emotion approach coping (EAC) into a music therapy protocol
for patients who were about to undergo
cardiac catheterization. Similar to other
cognitive-behavioral techniques, this stress
management strategy requires individuals
to acknowledge, express, and investigate
the emotions that they are carrying. In a
randomized controlled trial of 37 patients,
Ghetti found that music therapy plus EAC
was more effective than both talk therapy
plus EAC and a control group in improving
positive affect. Although not statistically
significant, those in the music therapy condition required less anxiolytic medication
and less time for the procedure.

Chemical Dependency

Lyric analysis and songwriting appear to
be interventions of choice in group music
therapy for those with chemical dependency. In one detoxification facility, Jones

(2005) used "Victim of the Game" by Garth
Brooks to draw the group together around
common emotions. A songwriting exercise that turned the words of "Yesterday"
by John Lennon into "Today" and "Tomorrow" gave group members the opportunity
to define the present and future in a original and inventive manner. The outcome
was significant emotional change, with
three-quarters of the participants stating
that music therapy proved to be a significant tool in their recovery.

Lyric analysis and songwriting are integral to a program for Substance Abuse and
Mental Illness (SA/MI) at the Cleveland
Music School Settlement in Ohio. This
community agency has a strong history of
using behavioral techniques and research
designs for a vast array of clinical music
therapy services (Steele, 1977), and CBMT
is an effective model for those who are dually diagnosed (Gallagher & Steele, 2002).
In their work, groups play instruments together and also partake in music-assisted
relaxation, music games, and producing
videos.

In their CBMT program in a detoxification and acute-phase treatment facility,
Dingle, Gleadhill, and Baker (2008) focus
on the issues being addressed in concurrent cognitive-behavioral counseling and
therapy: problem solving; communication
styles; exploring emotions; planning the
day; exploring depression, anger, and anxiety; and improving self-esteem and developing self-identity. Participants contribute
their favorite recordings for lyric analysis,
song parody, and singing/listening. Popular choices include "Imagine" by John Lennon, "Best of You" by the Foo Fighters, and
"Better Man" by Pearl Jam. Outcomes of
their research include high levels of engagement, motivation to participate, and enjoyment.

Cevasco, Kennedy, and Generally (2005)
used music to augment a group sophistry
intervention. As the name implies, this approach harkens back to the Greek sophists and Zimpfer's (1992) adaptation. Here,
clients engage in competitive games that

require them to react to song lyrics where hidden reasons for action are embedded. One team explicates the rationale for these hidden reasons and the other speaks against them. The debriefing among group members helps to clarify emotional states triggered by the experience, as well as to understand the hidden reasons for their behavior.

Conclusions

CBMT is well founded, researched, and applied in a wide variety of clinical settings. The vast supportive literature is excerpted here in an effort to introduce the wide scope and varied practices of this evolving evidence-based approach.

REFERENCES

Adler, A. (1931). *What life could mean to you*. Center City, MN: Hazelden.

Beck, A. T. (2005). The current state of cognitive therapy: A 40-year retrospective. *Archives of General Psychiatry, 62*, 953–959.

Bryant, D. R. (1987). A cognitive approach to therapy through music. *Journal of Music Therapy, 24*(1), 27–34.

Cevasco, A., Kennedy, R., & Generally, N. R. (2005). Comparison of movement-to-music, rhythmic activities, and competitive games on depression, stress, anxiety, and anger of females in substance abuse rehabilitation. *Journal of Music Therapy, 42*(1), 64–80.

Chambliss, D., & Ollendick, T. H. (2001). Empirically supported psychological interventions. *Annual Review of Psychology, 52*, 685–716.

Cheek, J. R., Bradley, L. J., Parr, G., & Lam, W. (2003). Using music therapy techniques to treat teacher burnout. *Journal of Mental Health Counseling, 25*(3), 204–217.

Department of Health, National Health Service Executive. (1999). *National service framework for mental health*. Wetherhy, UK: Author.

Descartes, R. (1910). *Discourse on the method of rightly conducting the reason and seeking of the truth in the sciences*. In C. W. Eliot (Ed.), *The Harvard classics* (Vol. 34, Pt. 1). New York: Collier. (Original work published 1637)

Dileo Maranto, C. (1996). A cognitive model of music in medicine. In R. R. Pratt & R. Spintge (Eds.), *Music medicine* (Vol. 2, pp. 327–332). St. Louis, MO: MMB Music.

Dingle, G. A., Gleadhill, L., & Baker, F. A. (2008). Can music therapy engage patients in group cognitive behaviour therapy for substance abuse treatment? *Drug and Alcohol Review, 27*(2), 190–196.

Ellis, A. (1962). *Reason and emotion in psychotherapy*. Oxford, UK: Lyle Stuart.

Ellis, A. (1987). The use of rational humorous songs in psychotherapy. In W. F. Fry, Jr., & W. A. Salameh (Eds.), *Handbook of humor and psychotherapy* (pp. 265–285). Sarasota, FL: Professional Resource Exchange.

Epictetus. (1877). *The discourses of Epictetus: Encheiridion and fragments* (G. Long, Trans.). London: George Bell.

Eysenck, H. J. (1967). *The biological basis of personality*. Springfield, IL: Charles C Thomas.

Gallagher, L. M., & Steele, A. L. (2002). Music therapy with offenders in a substance abuse/mental illness treatment program. *Music Therapy Perspectives, 20*(2), 117–122.

Ghetti, C. M. (2013). Effect of music therapy with emotional-approach coping on preprocedural anxiety in cardiac catheterization: A randomized controlled trial. *Journal of Music Therapy, 50*(2), 93–122.

Greenwood, J. D. (2009). *A conceptual history of psychology*. New York: McGraw-Hill Higher Education.

Gregory, D. (2002). Four decades of music therapy behavioral research designs: A content analysis of *Journal of Music Therapy* articles. *Journal of Music Therapy, 39*(1), 56–71.

Hanser, S. B., & Mandel, S. E. (2010). *Manage your stress and pain through music*. Boston: Berklee Press.

Hilliard, R. E. (2001a). The effects of music therapy-based bereavement groups on mood and behavior of grieving children: A pilot study. *Journal of Music Therapy, 38*(4), 291–306.

Hilliard, R. E. (2001b). The use of cognitive-behavioral music therapy in the treatment of women with eating disorders. *Music Therapy Perspectives, 19*(2), 109–113.

Hull, C. L. (1943). *Principles of behavior: An introduction to behavior theory*. Oxford, UK: Appleton-Century.

Jeffrey, W. E. (1955). New technique for motivating and reinforcing children. *Science, 121*(3141), 371.

Jones, J. D. (2005). A comparison of songwriting and lyric analysis techniques to evoke emotional change in a single session with people who are chemically dependent. *Journal of Music Therapy, 42*(2), 94–110.

Kahl, K. G., Winter, L., & Schweiger, U. (2012). The third wave of cognitive behavioural therapies. *Current Opinion in Psychiatry, 25*(6), 522–528.

Kerr, T., Walsh, J., & Marshall, A. (2001). Emotional change processes in music-assisted reframing. *Journal of Music Therapy, 38*(3), 193–211.

Kohlenberg, R. J., Tsai, M., & Dougher, M. J. (1993). The dimensions of clinical behavior analysis. *Behavior Analyst, 16*(2), 271–282.

Linehan, M. M., & Koerner, K. (2012). *Doing dialectical behavior therapy*. New York: Guilford Press.

Luce, D. W. (2001). Cognitive therapy and music therapy. *Music Therapy Perspectives, 19*(2), 96–103.

Madsen, C. K., Cotter, V., & Madsen, C. H. (1968). A behavioral approach to music therapy. *Journal of Music Therapy, 5*(3), 69–71.

Madsen, C. H., & Madsen, C. K. (1970a). *Teaching/discipline: Behavioral principles toward a positive approach*. Boston: Allyn & Bacon.

Madsen, C. K., & Madsen, C. H. (1970b). *Experimental research in music: Workbook in design and statistical tests*. Princeton, NJ: Prentice Hall.

Maultsby, M. (1977). Combining music therapy and rational behavior therapy. *Journal of Music Therapy, 14*(1), 89–97.

National Institute for Health and Care Excellence. (2008). *Cognitive behavioural therapy for the management of common mental health problems*. Retrieved from *www.nice.org.uk/media/878/f7/cbtcommissioningguide.pdf*.

National Institute of Mental Health. (2012). *Psychotherapies*. Retrieved from *www.nimh.nih.gov/health/topics/psychotherapies/index.shtml*.

Ost, L. G. (2008). Efficacy of the third wave of behavioral therapies: A systematic review and meta-analysis. *Behavioral Research and Therapy, 46*, 296–321.

Pavlov, I. P. (1927). *Conditioned reflexes*. London: Oxford University Press.

Rider, M. B., Floyd, J. W., & Kirkpatrick, J. (1985). The effect of music, imagery, and relaxation on adrenal corticosteroids and the re-entrainment of circadian rhythms. *Journal of Music Therapy, 22*(2), 46–58.

Robb, S. (2000). Music assisted progressive muscle relaxation, progressive muscle relaxation, music listening, and silence: A comparison of relaxation techniques. *Journal of Music Therapy, 37*(1), 2–21.

Robertson, D. (2010). *The philosophy of cognitive-behavioural therapy (CBT): Stoic philosophy as ra-tional and cognitive psychotherapy*. London: Karnac Books.

Scheufele, P. M. (2000). Effects of progressive relaxation and classical music on measurements of attention, relaxation, and stress responses. *Journal of Behavioral Medicine, 23*, 207–228.

Sechenov, I. M. (1965). *Reflexes of the brain*. Cambridge, MA: MIT Press. (Original work published 1863)

Silverman, M. J. (2007). Evaluating current trends in psychiatric music therapy: A descriptive analysis. *Journal of Music Therapy, 41*(4), 388–414.

Silverman, M. J. (2008). Quantitative comparison of cognitive behavioral therapy and music therapy research: A methodological best-practices analysis to guide future investigation for adult psychiatric patients. *Journal of Music Therapy, 45*(4), 457–506.

Silverman, M. J. (2011). Effects of a single-session assertiveness music therapy role playing protocol for psychiatric inpatients. *Journal of Music Therapy, 48*(3), 370–394.

Skinner, B. F. (1938). *The behavior of organisms: An experimental analysis*. Oxford, UK: Appleton-Century.

Skinner, B. F. (1957). *Verbal behavior*. Cambridge, MA: Prentice Hall.

Slotoroff, C. (1994). Drumming technique for assertiveness and anger management in the short-term psychiatric setting for adult and adolescent survivors of trauma. *Music Therapy Perspectives, 12*(2), 111–116.

Standley, J. M. (1996). A meta-analysis on the effects of music as reinforcement for education/therapy objectives. *Journal of Research in Music Education, 44*(2), 105–133.

Steele, A. L. (1977). The application of behavioral research techniques to community music therapy. *Journal of Music Therapy, 14*(3), 102–115.

Stoudenmire, J. (1975). A comparison of muscle relaxation training and music in the reduction of state and trait anxiety. *Journal of Clinical Psychology, 3*, 490–492.

Thorndike, E. L. (1898). Animal intelligence: An experimental study of the associative processes in animals (*Psychological Review*, Monograph Supplements, No. 8). New York: Macmillan.

Watson, J. B. (1913). Psychology as the behaviorist views it. *Psychological Review, 20*, 158–177.

Wolpe, J., & Lazarus. A. (1966). *Behavior therapy techniques*. Oxford, UK: Pergamon Press.

Zimpfer, D. G. (1992). Group work with adult offenders: An overview. *Journal for Specialists in Group Work, 17*, 54–61.

CHAPTER 14

Developmental Approaches

Cynthia A. Briggs

When a music therapist begins working with a client of any age, one of the first questions the therapist should ask in relation to assessment and treatment planning is, "At what developmental level is the client currently functioning?" Music therapists need to have knowledge of models of how typical development unfolds physiologically and psychologically. Music therapists also need to understand how and when music skills are developed, and the relationship between developmental stages and age-related music skills.

The ability of the music therapist to assess a client developmentally is also part of the contribution the music therapist makes as a member of a treatment team. Whereas the physical therapist can speak about a client with regard to physical skills and needs, or the art therapist in terms of art development, the music therapist needs to assist the team in understanding where the client's music skills place the client developmentally. Musical development may also give clues to nonmusical developmental levels that may not be directly observable. Human development is often uneven, especially when an individual has a developmen-

tal disorder. Accurate assessment assists in identifying an individual's current level, determining goal areas, and identifying areas of strength for a client.

Barbara Wheeler and Sylvia Stultz (2008) illustrated the value of knowing typical infant development in understanding children with developmental disabilities. Studying videotaped sessions with typically developing children and children with developmental disabilities, they used Stanley Greenspan's model of psychosocial development (Greenspan & Weider, 1998) to discuss how his developmental framework could inform their understanding of where an individual is functioning developmentally, regardless of chronological age, and then guide the therapist in facilitating his or her progress.

This chapter explores developmental models related to the early childhood tasks of developing a sense of self and building attachment with others, as well as models of musical skill development. Contemporary models of how humans learn to attach, attune, and communicate have, at their core, many of the same biological components that underlie music: rhythm, timbre, pitch, dynamics, phrasing, and relationship. There is music in relatedness, and there is relatedness in music. Developmental music therapy models are also reviewed. The chapter focuses on how models of human development and research regarding models of child development and music can inform music therapy practice.

Human Development

Many models address components of human development across the lifespan. Models have traditionally focused on cognitive, psychological, social, or physical development, and traditional models are usually linked to chronological development. Some contemporary models include a focus on the impact the sociocultural environment may have on development. Many developmental models are also structured around stages that are determined by the transitions that occur in an individual's ability to act, move, or process information in new ways. Examples include the cognitive models of Jean Piaget (Beins, 2012) and Robert Kegan (1982) and the psychological model of Erik Erikson (1968). Although a solid grounding in these models provides a structured way to think about human development, it is essential to also remember that our knowledge of development is constantly changing as research continues to inform us as to how development unfolds.

A biopsychosocial framework is one way of gathering developmental information across the biological, psychological, and sociocultural domains. Developmental information pertaining to each of the three domains informs the other two, so that it is understood within a context that addresses the full human being. Development may be dramatically influenced by events related to a specific domain, changing the developmental process of an individual temporarily or permanently (Bronfenbrenner, 1989).

Models that consider the full lifespan, such as those of Erikson (1968) and Matilda

Riley (1979), view development as changing across an individual's life. In the biopsychosocial framework, to understand development we must know what came before or after each developmental event, with aging and time being key variables in understanding development. Development is also impacted temporally, in that our knowledge, morals, and perspectives change over time, so that the same behavior may be viewed differently at different stages in life.

Our knowledge of neurological development has changed enormously in the last 20 years because of technology that allows us to study the brain directly—a dramatic change from earlier reliance solely on behavioral observation for the study of neurology. This ability to study brain functioning has greatly increased our knowledge of infant and child development and, more specifically, musical development, which has moved music to the foreground in neuroscience research. Neuroscience technology has also allowed us to better understand the neurology of human relationship and attachment, as well as how these skills develop and change (Schore, 2003; Stern, 2010a). We must always be willing to think of development within new contexts. As new knowledge informs how we understand development, we have to be willing to learn and embrace evolving models.

Attachment, Attunement, and the Developing Sense of Self

CLINICAL EXAMPLE: Assessing the Musical Development of a Young Boy with a Visual Impairment

Robbie is a busy 2½-year-old boy who participates in an infant and parent program for children with visual impairments, ages birth to 3 years old. Robbie was born blind due to prenatal injury to the organ of the eyes; he has no vision. It takes only a few minutes to realize that, even without formal testing, Robbie is a bright, alert boy who processes information quickly and who is fearless in his explorations of space and sound. He enjoys the other children in the group, but, typical of children his age, he sticks close to his mother for most of the session. Robbie is eager to grab a small drum, and he beats along to the rhythm of the lyrics. He can sing any song he has heard a few times, singing most of the lyrics and the contour of the musical phrases with steadily increasing accuracy. He appears to recognize final cadences and ends with a drumming flourish. Since many of the group's songs are done in the same order each session, he anticipates what is next by naming a portion of the next song or trying to say the first line. His task focus throughout the 30-minute group is excellent, with only a few prompts needed from his mother to remain on task.

Robbie is a young child with a sensory deficit, yet he is typically developing cognitively and is advanced in his musical development. How were these characteristics determined, and of what use is this information? Formal cognitive testing, medical evaluations, and other types of evaluations may be available to the music therapist who works with Robbie. But the music therapist's knowledge regarding typical development in music, and where musical developmental milestones fit in relation to other models of child development, is important in assessing his current level of functioning. Knowing where a child is performing developmentally informs the music therapist regarding what skills the child has and where to begin. Developmental assessment provides a context for the child's skills that allows the music therapist to determine which skills come next and therefore what goals and objectives are developmentally appropriate.

It is not a coincidence that Robbie's group is for young children and their parents. Margaret Mahler and her colleagues (Mahler, Pine, & Bergman, 1975) referred to the first 3 years of life as comprising the *separation–individuation process* that heralds the psychological birth of a young child. A child's powerful connection to parents and his or her later ability to individuate—to

move to a sense of self as well connected to parents yet able to view the world with a sense of autonomy—were viewed by Mahler as the major psychological tasks for the child under 3.

John Bowlby and Mary Ainsworth were contemporaries of Mahler. Their separate and shared work in the area of infant–parent attachment pioneered the field of *attachment theory* (Bretherton, 1992). From the beginning, researchers in the field of human attachment patterns recognized that vocalizations were a part of the early sound repertoire and interactive communication between infants and parents or caregivers. Beginning with cries and coos, babies learn early to communicate their wants and needs with those around them by vocalizing. Mahler et al. (1975) identified types of vocalizations used by parents and children to stay connected physically and emotionally. Bowlby's and Ainsworth's infant–parent studies (Bretherton, 1992) showed that infants signaled first indiscriminately but later with increasing focus on primary care figures, using cries and calls that they honed to express anxiety, pleasure, unhappiness, affection, and other emotions.

Robbie clearly enjoys music, but he stays near his mother and turns to her often for reassurance. Because of his visual impairment, she gives him vocal or tactile reassurance while urging him to participate.

Daniel Stern and his colleagues' study of the vocalizations between mothers and infants suggest that mothers and infants have two modes of vocalizing with each other: unions and alternations (Stern, Jaffe, Beebe, & Bennett, 1974). These two modes differ both structurally and functionally. Stern, Spieker, and MacKain (1982) also studied both the child's and the mother's vocalizations for patterns. They identified five common pitch contours used by mothers: bell, sinusoidal, bell-right, rise, and fall. Their study demonstrated that maternal vocal signals are most likely arranged by context, so that the infant can learn to respond to intonational contours, and that intonational structures might be among the earliest, most basic forms of interpersonal signaling in the auditory domain. Young children and caregivers rely on finely honed, nonverbal communication rooted in the building blocks of music: rhythm, phrasing, intonation, and intensity.

Stern (1985) introduced a major change in the understanding of how attachment and separation unfold in the young child in his text *The Interpersonal World of the Infant*. Stating that he did not think there was a symbiotic-like phase, as Mahler and her contemporaries had suggested, Stern instead proposed that each stage is a foundation for the stages that develop later, and that each stage exists across the lifespan. In the first sense of self, the *emergent self*, the infant in the first 2 months of life begins to develop a sense of organization regarding how people relate to one another. Between the second and sixth month, the child beings to develop what Stern named the *core self*, whereby the experiential sense of self and self-and-others emerges. The *subjective self* develops between the seventh and 15th month, adding the possibility of intersubjective relatedness: the beginning of understanding and sharing the affective experiences of others. Stern's final domain is the *verbal self*, when language begins to develop and information is conveyed verbally with others, leading to shared meaning and the ability to begin to self-reflect. Some self-domains exist prior to the development of language and the ability to self-reflect, yet are ongoing across a lifetime. Each developing sense of the self continues to grow, with successive phases becoming simultaneous domains of self-experience.

CLINICAL EXAMPLE: Helping a Child Experience Her Actions and Emotions

Maggie is a 2-year-old in Robbie's group. She begins moving to a song without awareness.

When the music therapist says, "Maggie is dancing!", she looks at herself, realizes she is dancing, and smiles as she continues to dance, enjoying having an audience.

Antonio Damasio (1999, 2012) writes that the *sense of self* is basic to understanding emotions. Without the sense of self, an individual is not able to create and understand the emotion being experienced. In presenting the neurology of the development of a sense of self, Damasio discusses how emotions are felt as well as how we recognize that we are feeling a specific emotion. Later in development, children acquire the ability to recognize the emotions of others.

A sense of self is a basic underpinning to understanding emotion and is needed to make the signals that constitute the feeling of emotion known to the individual who is having the emotion. Understanding the neural underpinnings of the self helps us to understand the very different biological impact of three distinct, though closely related, phenomena: an emotion, the feeling of that emotion, and knowing that we are feeling that emotion (Damasio, 1999).

Consciousness and emotion cannot be separated. Different brain systems are connected to different emotions. Our ability to develop an understanding of emotions grows over time. Damasio (1999) suggests that we develop three selves over our lifetimes: a protoself, a core self, and an autobiographical self. He refers to the *protoself* as the nonconscious state prior to the development of a *core consciousness*. The brain's protoself structures lie below the level of the cerebral cortex and are attached to the parts of the body that constantly provide signals to the brain (i.e., respiration, pulse). The protoself maintains our body states, running always in the background as we develop higher levels of consciousness. Originating at the brainstem level, the protoself creates primordial feelings that reflect the current state of the body.

The *core self* is action oriented as the individual and an object come into relationship. *Core consciousness* marks the beginning of our sense of self in the moment. The brain has to acquire subjectivity to move to core consciousness. Subjectivity allows us to think about our self as we experience the events and sensations around us. In infancy we see the protoself as the baby responds primarily to body sensations. It is in relatedness with caregivers that the core self begins to emerge. The baby develops a sense of subjectivity, of him- or herself in the moment or in relationship. The caregivers also enhance the baby's experiences through affect attunement and sensory engagement.

Our emotional experiences move us to an *autobiographical self*, whereby feeling what happens as we see, hear, or touch an object becomes a part of making images that, when organized and remembered, direct our sense of self. The autobiographical self is our organized memory; it includes the past and the anticipated future. Each type of consciousness is ongoing for a lifetime. The autobiographical self begins as the child begins to organize memory beyond the present moment. Language development enhances the development of an autobiographical self, as does an increased ability to make meaning of the sensations and images experienced so that the child can recognize, label, and organize the feelings he or she is experiencing. All three selves continue to influence us, informing each other and creating the complex emotional experiences that we process every day.

CLINICAL EXAMPLE: Sharing an Affective State between Mother and Child

Jason, a 15-month-old boy, is playing with toys on the floor. He spots a new toy and immediately crawls to it. As he picks it up, he gurgles, then shrieks and smiles. His mother smiles, raises her eyebrows and hands, and says, with excitement in her voice, "*Weeeee!*"

Stern (1985) suggests that the ongoing sense of self is built on a growing under-

standing of relatedness. Two of his important constructs that are part of the developing sense of self relate closely to musical elements. The first construct is that of *vitality affects*, the felt quality of an experience such as *rushing, bursting,* or *surging.* Though not emotions, these words best describe the vitality of an affect. Vitality affects are rooted in human movement, our most fundamental experience, and express a subjective inner state. These exaggerated expressions help regulate an infant's arousal and, later in development, communicate the dynamics of an affect.

The second construct is *affect attunement,* defined by Stern (1985) as "the performance of behaviors that express the quality of feeling of a shared affect state without imitating the exact behavioral expression of the inner state" (p. 142). Attunement is often expressed vocally with vocal glides or squeals, crescendo or decrescendo, a change in intensity by getting louder or softer, or a rhythmic alteration or pattern. Affect attunement is based on matching forms of vitality across different modes of expression and is a basic building block in intersubjective relatedness, such as connecting with another and communicating and understanding his or her underlying affective state. Affect attunement includes the components of intensity, timing, and shape to express the perceived feeling of another person. Vitality affects are often the affect upon which an attunement expression is built. Jason's mother attuned to Jason's joy over the toy by responding with an animated "*Weeeee.*"

In more recent work, Stern (2004, 2010a, 2010b) expands on the importance of vitality affects, referring to them as the dynamic markings of affect communication. In music, whereas notation tells us what note to play, it is the crescendo, staccato, or legato markings that convey the expression or affect of the note. Vitality affects are an essential component of communicating emotionally with others. They precede language and stay with us as an important way to communicate affect. Dynamic forms, or forms of vitality, are created and organized by movement, force, space, intention, and time. As we move in space to gesture and put force behind our movement or gesture, organizing it across time, we express ourselves nonverbally. These forms of vitality serve as the basis of all nonverbal communication. As infants, we first move through space. Later we understand how to move with force and intention to emphasize what we are doing, and all of these actions become organized by time. Some of our understanding of the use of vitality affects comes from the attunement with others that has helped us understand how to use vitality affects to communicate feelings as well as to understand the feelings of others.

Maggie's mother says, "Time to go home." Maggie wrinkles her forehead, shakes her head "no," and kicks her feet a little. Her mother responds, "I know you would like to stay. Music is fun."

Alan Schore (1994) has published extensive work on the neurobiology of emotional development as well. His research focuses on the importance of socioaffective stimulation from caregivers in the development of the infant's ability to regulate affect (Schore, 1994, 2001). Stating that "the vast majority of the development of axons, dendrites, and synaptic connections that underlie all behavior is known to take place in early and late human infancy" (2001, p. 12), Schore views the end of the first year of life as a critical period in the development of affect regulation. If this critical period passes for a child without the attunement and attachment to a caregiver, important skills may go undeveloped.

Musical Development

Extensive research helps us understand how infants and young children respond to music and the elements of music. Infants are sensitive to contour (Trehub, Bull, & Thorpe, 1984), consonance and dissonance (Trainor & Heinmiller, 1998), and pitch changes (Trehub, 1993). Maternal singing regulates infant arousal (Shenfield, Trehub, & Nakata, 2003), and lullabies can be found throughout the world. Lullabies may function as a natural prototype, containing elements that communicate biologically determined affective meaning regardless of cultural context (Trehub & Unyk, 1991, p. 79). Infants were more self-focused when listening to lullabies and more externally focused when listening to play songs (Rock, Trainor, & Addison, 1999).

De L'Etoile (2006) summarized the literature related to music skills in infancy as they relate to infant-directed singing. She concluded that infant-directed singing serves four important functions: attracting and maintaining infant attention, conveying emotional information through singing, helping infants regulate their affective state, and coordinating emotions between infant and mother to create a bond.

Gooding and Standley (2011) completed an extensive review of the literature to develop charts that detail specific music skill development and learning characteristics by age range. The charts begin with pre-birth knowledge and follow the literature to detail music skill information through the age of 20 years. Their material is organized into eight tables:

1. Responses to sound/auditory learning characteristics
2. Responses to music
3. Pitch, tonality, and harmony skills
4. Rhythm skills
5. Movement abilities
6. Singing skills
7. Instrument performance skills
8. Other musical skills and/or factors to consider

The authors' charts provide an extensive summary of the information documented in the research literature related to the development of musical skills.

Early Developmentally Based Models of Music Therapy

In their landmark text, *Creative Music Therapy* (1977), Paul Nordoff and Clive Robbins described their work with children with developmental disabilities as "creating a musical setting with form and mood: a musical–emotional environment with which [the child] may feel some affinity" (p. 93). In responding to the child's expression, movements, and mood, the music therapist communicates to the child "as he [or she] is" (p. 93). The authors created two evaluation scales—Scale I: Child–Therapist Relationship in Musical Activity, and Scale II: Musical Communicativeness—to assess the child's ongoing level of connection and engagement with the therapists and the music. Scale I evaluates a child for relatedness on a 10-point scale that starts with *total obliviousness* at level 1 and ends at level 10 with *establishment of functional independence in group work* (p. 182). Similarly, Scale II uses a 10-point scale that begins with *no communicative responsiveness* at level 1 and ends with *commitment to musical objectives in group work* at level 10. The newborn is only marginally engaged and communicative, though perhaps not as severely detached as the children Nordoff and Robbins were treating, but through their developmental sequence, the end point is a child who can participate in music in an active, focused, and autonomous manner.

Juliette Alvin framed her work with children with autism in a developmental context (Alvin & Warwick, 1991). Alvin conceptualized her work with each child in a developmental framework related to the child's ability to develop relatedness and, later, musical independence. Alvin's focus for the first stage or step in music therapy was on creating a safe space. By assisting each child to create a nonverbal relationship with the music and the music environment, the child became more open to relating to the therapist. Alvin first emphasized awareness of sound and later on, relating different sounds together. During the first period, no cognitive demands were made upon a child.

The second stage was characterized by the child's beginning acceptance of the music therapist and his or her use of voice for self-expression. Musical creations became more structured in this stage, and there was pleasure in the act of playing music. Some children progressed further than others, but Alvin's goal was always social integration. For each developmental step, Alvin considered the developmental components of rhythm and melody and how to use those musical components to facilitate a child's therapeutic progress.

Briggs (1991) contributed a model that integrates the research on musical skill development in children with cognitive and psychological frameworks of child development. Briggs' framework for musical development divides childhood musical development into four stages: reflex, ages 0–9 months; intention, ages 9–18 months; control, ages 18–36 months; and integration, ages 36–72 months (Briggs & Bruscia, 1985). The stages reflect what is occurring in the developing child across cognitive, psychological, and musical development, and musical skill development is organized by auditory, vocal/tonal, rhythmic, and later cognitive musical ability. The Briggs–Bruscia model provided music therapists with an integrated developmental framework that could be applied to many client groups.

Bruscia (1991, 2012) integrates musical development with models of human development, focusing on the musical elements that are part of each developmental stage. Starting with an amniotic period, before a child is born, Bruscia integrates musical components and developmental components across the lifespan, ending with the transpersonal stage. He also discusses pathologies that originate in specified developmental periods, articulating how the integration of developmental models can assist music therapists in facilitating development, remediating developmental disorders, and returning a client to a developmental problem to facilitate resolution.

Schwartz (2008) constructed a developmental model as an outgrowth of the Briggs–Bruscia model. Based on her work with young children with developmental disorders, Schwartz expanded her model to five developmental levels: awareness, trust, independence, control, and responsibility. For each developmental level, Schwartz organized the research to identify which musical skills develop when. She emphasizes setting goals and creating interventions for children functioning at each level. For a child at the awareness level, the goal might be to "turn eye gaze toward source of sound" or to "calm to familiar melodies." For each level, the acquisition of targeted skills and behaviors through music therapy is addressed. Schwartz also considered the impact of disability on the acquisition of specific level-related skills and how these needs might be addressed.

Elmer (2011) constructed a theory regarding the development of singing skills in children and summarized the current knowledge about singing to conceptualize seven stages:

Stage 1. *Beginning co-evolution of innate expressive predispositions with the social environment*: Characterized by infant's and caregiver's uses of vocalization for communication and dialogue.

Stage 2. *Deferred imitation, emergent rituals, and extended vocal play*: Characterized by reciprocal imitation of vocal patterns, use of established rules and rituals, vocal patterns, and beginning dialogue.

Stage 3. *Intentions to produce singing-like or speech-like vocalizations*: Characterized by the intention to produce singing-like or speech-like vocalizations using identifiable and consistent melodic and rhythmic patterns and movements.

Stage 4. *Sensorimotor strategy: Auditory–vocal coordination to produce song fragments or entire songs*: Characterized by the child's imitation of melody fragments or entire songs with accuracy. The child adapts pitches, syllables, and timing to another person's singing. Deviation from conventional rules is not of concern, and mental concepts do not connect with conventional rules. Imitative performance is typical, as is creating a variety of sound patterns.

Stage 5. *Generalizing examples, idiosyncratic song repertoire, and idiosyncratic singing rules*: Characterized by the child's combining of sensorimotor strategies from the previous stage with an adoption of acquired patterns. The child uses idiosyncratic and inconsistent rules with some emergence of stable and generalized patterns, such as phrase repetition or ending on tonic.

Stage 6. *Conventional rules on song singing are implicitly integrated*: Characterized by a growing repertoire of songs and the emergence of general rules that can be applied to various contexts, including invented songs. The child starts to understand that singing is a socially shared activity, and there is growing self-control that inhibits spontaneous singing. Preferences influenced by social groups contribute to personal and social identity.

Stage 7. *Beginning reflection of actions, means, symbols, and concepts*: Characterized by previous implicit structural knowledge becoming subject to conscious reflection. Postconventional thinking, beyond cultural rules, begins. The child recognizes generalized affective patterns, and singing is used for intra- and interpersonal affective states. Cultural symbols are increasingly used.

Elmer's model reflects both the developmental concepts of attachment and those related to steadily growing autonomy. The increasing ability to organize and think about music in a more abstract way characterizes her later stages.

CLINICAL EXAMPLE: Assessing the Musical Development of a Young Man with Developmental Disabilities

Sean is a 28-year-old man who lives in a group home with three other young adults with significant developmental disabilities. On cognitive evaluations, Sean scores in the moderately cognitively impaired range of ability. He is emotionally labile, with unpredictable mood swings to which he is very reactive. As his moods shift, so do his behaviors. When he is distressed, Sean becomes very difficult to engage. Sean has been in the glee club music therapy program for 3 years, meeting weekly with a group of peers. The group interventions focus on developing positive social skills and increasing impulse control. Sean enjoys the group and is actively engaged during the session most of the time. Musically, Sean cannot match pitch, maintain a tonal center, or maintain a simple rhythmic beat pattern. He can recognize familiar songs, but his recall of lyrics is limited. Sean has only one level of vocal intensity: loud. His affect is usually flat, even when his motor behavior indicates that he is excited.

For the music therapist Sean presents an example of how a developmental disorder impacts cognitive ability, musical skill, and behavior. Sean's skills are those of a younger child. He has not acquired a tonal center, pitch matching, or rhythmic pulse, and his social skills are also far younger than his chronological age. By assessing Sean developmentally, his music therapist can determine which skills and stages to target when setting music therapy goals for Sean.

Combining Developmental Models to Inform Practice

Pearce and Rohrmeier (2012) present a well-documented argument that music cognition needs to be seen as part of the cognitive sciences rather than a separate and unique area of study, stating:

> From the perspective of studying the human mind, the cognitive processing of music simultaneously engages most of the perceptual, cognitive, and emotional processes that we (as cognitive scientists and neuroscientists) are interested in rendering it an ideal object for the study of domain-general temporal and emotional processing, as well as motor activity and interaction. (p. 470)

CLINICAL CASE EXAMPLE: Using Music Therapy to Build Attachment and Relatedness

Andre is an 11-year-old boy who was adopted when he was 2 years old. Prior to his adoption, he lived with two foster families. Andre was able to make the transition to his adoptive family without any significant problems, but his adoptive parents report that he was very distant when they first took him home, and his affect was flat much of the time. They were pleased to report that they saw steady improvement in his ability to engage with them and to be more expressive of his feelings. Andre has a younger sister who was adopted at birth, when he was 4 years old. He was very jealous of the new baby when she first joined the family, but the parents were able to help him, and he only occasionally seems jealous when she is receiving more attention than he is.

Andre is in sixth grade in a middle school near his home. He has struggled with making friends at school. His teachers report that he often competes with peers for attention, even when it isn't necessary. Andre's behavior is mildly immature compared to his peers, and his peers sometimes tease him.

The social worker who worked with the family during the adoptions recently recommended that Andre's parents consider music therapy for him to help him work on socialization and relationship-building skills. Andre liked the idea of learning to play guitar and singing popular songs, and, after the initial session, he told his parents that he liked music therapy because the music therapist liked him, and he would be the only one in the session with his therapist.

Andre's opportunity to develop attachment to his parents was delayed. The affect attunement and sense of self that would enable him to understand his emotions as well as the emotions of others were disrupted by a changing family situation during his first 2 years. Some of the impact of this delay can be seen later when he struggles to express his emotions to his family and friends and when he tries to understand what his peers may be feeling, such that he appears immature compared to classmates.

For Andre, music therapy offers the opportunity to build those skills using the elements of music. Tonality, rhythm, phrasing, accent—the elements that organize music and make it expressive—are the same expressive components of our emotional lives. Further, the lyrics and emotion of musical expression provide Andre with the opportunity to experience and express his feelings and to begin to understand the feelings of others. Music therapy also provides a setting for him to practice attachment skills through the therapeutic relationship he builds with his music therapist.

Conclusions

An in-depth understanding of models of human and musical development can enhance multiple areas of music therapy. A full understanding of the client within a biopsychosocial model that illuminates the individual across multiple developmental aspects, assists the music therapist in seeing the different components and influences that are part of the client's development. Developmental assessment also helps the therapist to place the behaviors assessed and observed into a context that identifies where a client's abilities fall within a developmental sequence. This same knowledge can assist in setting an appropriate sequence of goals and objectives that unfolds along developmental lines.

The music therapist's understanding of multiple developmental perspectives also helps to integrate music therapy with other disciplines. In articulating where music skills and processes fit within broader developmental sequences, other professions are helped to see how music therapy interventions may be used to facilitate specific therapeutic goals and objectives. As Stern (2008) points out, models of development have shifted from a one-person psychology to a two-or-more-person psychology. This shift has had a profound impact on how we understand cognitive and affective models of development. Whether the goal is developing early relationship or learning to recognize emotions, the musical and nonverbal nature of music therapy may be the most appropriate intervention for the development of these skills.

Finally, as we become better informed about the science of how we attach, attune, and learn to express our relatedness, we also learn the skills that contribute to being a skilled therapist. The skills of interrelatedness and intersubjectivity, of affect attunement and vitality affects, and of empathy are all part of being an effective, insightful therapist.

REFERENCES

Alvin, J., & Warwick, A. (1991). *Music therapy for the autistic child* (2nd ed.). Oxford, UK: Oxford University Press.

Beins, B. C. (2012). Jean Piaget. In W. E. Pickren, D. A. Dewsbury, & M. Wertheimer (Eds.), *Portraits of pioneers in developmental psychology* (pp. 89–107). New York: Psychology Press.

Bretherton, I. (1992). The origins of attachment theory: John Bowlby and Mary Ainsworth. *Developmental Psychology, 28*(5), 759–775.

Briggs, C. A. (1991). A model for understanding musical development. *Music Therapy, 10*(1), 1–21.

Briggs, C. A., & Bruscia, K. (1985, November). *Developmental models for understanding musical behavior.* Paper presented at the Joint Conference on the Creative Art Therapies, National Coalition of Arts Therapy Associations, New York.

Bronfenbrenner, U. (1989). Ecological systems theory. In R. Vasta (Ed.), *Annals of child development: Vol. 6. Six theories of child development:*

Revised formulations and current issues (pp. 187–250). Greenwich, CT: JAI Press.

Bruscia, K. E. (1991, May 1). *Musical origins: Developmental foundations for music therapy.* Paper presented at the annual conference of the Canadian Music Therapy Association, Regina, Saskatchewan, Canada.

Bruscia, K. E. (2012). Musical origins: Developmental foundations for music therapy. In K. E. Bruscia (Ed.), *Readings in music therapy theory* (Reading No. 8). Gilsum, NH: Barcelona.

Damasio, A. (1999). *The feeling of what happens.* New York: Harcourt.

Damasio, A. (2012). *Self comes to mind.* New York: Vintage Books.

De L'Etoile, S. (2006). Infant-directed singing: A theory for clinical intervention. *Music Therapy Perspectives, 24,* 22–29.

Elmer, S. (2011). Human singing: Towards a developmental theory. *Psychomusicology: Music, Mind and Brain, 21*(1–2), 13–30.

Erikson, E. H. (1968). *Identity: Youth and crisis.* New York: Norton.

Gooding, L., & Standley, J. (2011). Musical development and learning characteristics of students: A compilation of key points from the research literature organized by age. *Update: Applications of Research in Music Education.* Retrieved from *http://upd.sagepub.com/content/early/2011/09/01/8755123311418481.*

Greenspan, S. I., & Weider, S. (1998). *The child with special needs.* Reading, MA: Addison-Wesley.

Kegan, R. (1982). *The evolving self: Problem and process in human development.* Cambridge, MA: Harvard University Press.

Mahler, M. S., Pine, F., & Bergman, A. (1975). *The psychological birth of the human infant.* New York: Basic Books.

Nordoff, P., & Robbins, C. (1977). *Creative music therapy: Individualized treatment for the handicapped child.* New York: John Day.

Pearce, M., & Rohrmeier, M. (2012). Music cognition and the cognitive sciences. *Topics in Cognitive Science, 4,* 468–484.

Riley, M. W. (1979). Introduction. In M. W. Riley (Ed.), *Aging from birth to death: Interdisciplinary perspectives* (pp. 3–13). Boulder, CO: Westview.

Rock, A. M. L., Trainor, L. J., & Addison, T. L. (1999). Distinctive messages in infant-directed lullabies and play songs. *Developmental Psychology, 35,* 527–534.

Schore, A. N. (1994). *Affect regulation and the origin of the self.* Hillsdale, NJ: Erlbaum.

Schore, A. N. (2001). Effects of a secure attachment relationship on right brain development, affect regulation, and infant mental health. *Infant Mental Health Journal, 22*(1/2), 7–66.

Schore, A. N. (2003). *Affect regulation and the repair of the self.* New York: Norton.

Schwartz, E. (2008). *Music, therapy and early childhood: A developmental approach.* Gilsum, NH: Barcelona.

Shenfield, T., Trehub, S. E., & Nakata, T. (2003). Maternal singing modulates infant arousal. *Psychology of Music, 31,* 365–375.

Stern, D. N. (1985). *The interpersonal world of the infant.* New York: Basic Books.

Stern, D. N. (2004). *The present moment in psychotherapy and everyday life.* New York: Norton.

Stern, D. N. (2008). The clinical relevance of infancy: A progress report. *Infant Mental Health Journal, 29*(3), 177–188.

Stern, D. N. (2010a). *Forms of vitality.* Oxford, UK: Oxford University Press.

Stern, D. N. (2010b). The issue of vitality. *Nordic Journal of Music Therapy, 19*(2), 88–102.

Stern, D. N., Jaffe, J., Beebe, B., & Bennett, S. L. (1974). Vocalizing in unison and alternation: Two modes of communication within the mother–infant dyad. *Annals of the New York Academy of Science, 263,* 89–100.

Stern, D. N., Spieker, S., & MacKain, K. (1982). Intonation contours as signals in maternal speech to prelinguistic infants. *Developmental Psychology, 18*(5), 727–735.

Trainor, L. J., & Heinmiller, B. M. (1998). The development of evaluative responses to music: Infants prefer to listen to consonance over dissonance. *Infant Behavior and Development, 21,* 77–88.

Trehub, S. E. (1993). The music listening skills of infants and young children. In T. J. Tighe & W. J. Dowling (Eds.), *Psychology and music: The understanding of melody and rhythm* (pp. 161–176). Hillsdale, NJ: Erlbaum.

Trehub, S. E., Bull, D., & Thorpe, L. A. (1984). Infants' perception of timbre: Classification of complex tones by spectral nature. *Journal of Experimental Child Psychology, 49,* 300–313.

Trehub, S. E., & Unyk, A. M. (1991). Music prototypes in developmental perspective. *Psychomusicology, 10,* 73–87.

Wheeler, B., & Stultz, S. (2008). Using typical infant development to inform music therapy with children with disabilities. *Early Childhood Education Journal, 35,* 585–591.

CHAPTER 15

Nordoff–Robbins Music Therapy

Nina Guerrero
David Marcus
Alan Turry

As Nordoff–Robbins Music Therapy has expanded into a wide range of settings since its inception in 1959, it has maintained a consistent core of theoretical tenets rooted in the power of direct musical engagement to stimulate "the self-creating capacities of the human self" in various areas of functioning (Robbins, 2011, p. 65). The method has developed "through an inherent and ongoing process of *applied practical creativity*" in making music with different clients (p. 67, emphasis in original), rather than by conforming to any extrinsic therapy practice or theory. True to its spirit of creative flexibility, practitioners of Nordoff–Robbins Music Therapy have "evolved language for interdisciplinary communication and collaboration" in serving diverse populations; nevertheless, Robbins emphasizes, "the musical experience of self at the heart of this work" cannot be "fully or even adequately captured through ideas derived from non-musical modes of human expression and interaction" (p. 68). Any attempt to understand the processes and outcomes of this approach must recognize that its foundations "lie in the meanings of music-

making itself" (p. 66) and examine in depth the musical interactions through which therapeutic goals are pursued. This chapter illustrates the approach by exploring its history and presenting two cases: an example of Paul Nordoff and Clive Robbins's work with a child, and contemporary work with a self-referred adult client.

History

The early development of Nordoff–Robbins Music Therapy was significantly influenced by the philosophy of Rudolf Steiner (1861–1925), whose anthroposophical teachings encompassed a myriad of subjects relevant to the history and future of human consciousness (Steiner, 1977, 1998). In his lectures on "curative education" (Steiner, 1998) to a group of physicians and educators, Steiner suggested a variety of techniques for educating children with disabilities, whom he described as having "special needs of the soul" (p. vi). His emphasis on cultivating their developmental potential marked a significant departure from the assumptions and attitudes of mainstream culture.

Both Paul Nordoff in the United States and Clive Robbins in England lived with their wives and children in anthroposophical communities during the years before their initial encounter. A primary tenet of anthroposophy that resonated deeply with them was that working with children with disabilities yielded a wealth of implications for human development in general. The anthroposophical worldview inspired in them "an attitude of reverence for the meaningfulness of human destiny" and "a profound respect for the inner life of each child with whom they worked" (Robbins, 2011, p. 65). Throughout Nordoff's career as a pianist and composer—from his studies at the Philadelphia Conservatory of Music and Juilliard Graduate School, to his professorship at Bard College—he maintained a strong interest in the therapeutic use of music with children. On a sabbatical leave from Bard in 1958, he visited settings in Europe where music was being used interactively and creatively with children. Among these was Sunfield Children's Homes, an anthroposophical residence in Worcestershire, England.

Founding of the Partnership at Sunfield

During Nordoff's first visit to Sunfield, he briefly met Clive Robbins, who had worked there as an educator since 1954. The curriculum encompassed "music, eurythmy, painting, modeling, musical theater, puppet theater, handcrafts, and various extracurricular activities" (Robbins, 2011, p. 65). Proceeding on his journey to other anthroposophical settings in Europe, Nordoff was profoundly moved by the responses brought forth by music in children who were otherwise difficult to reach. Upon returning to the United States, he requested that his leave from Bard be extended to allow further investigation of this work. When his request was denied, he resigned his professorship—renouncing, in effect, his academic and performing career—to devote his full energies to the exploration of music therapy.

He returned to Sunfield and embarked upon a partnership with Clive Robbins. Robbins brought his years of experience and insight as a special educator to their collaboration, while Nordoff brought expertise in composition and improvisation. The distinct roles they played in sessions became an enduring model for teamwork in Nordoff–Robbins Music Therapy: One therapist provides the musical framework for a session on the piano or another harmonic instrument, consisting largely of spontaneously improvised music that is created to support and stimulate new developments within the client. The other therapist helps to facilitate the musical relationship by physically guiding the client's musical activity and interaction, becoming more or less active depending on the client's needs. In individual sessions, the therapist creating the musical framework is designated the primary therapist, while the other therapist serves as cotherapist; in group sessions, leadership is shared between the two therapists.

The environment of Sunfield not only nurtured the children but also embraced Nordoff and Robbins's creative approach to music as therapy. Beyond clear compassion for the children, all members of the Sunfield staff—physicians, educators, and assistants alike—demonstrated imagination, sensitivity, and joyful enthusiasm in their work. Each child was valued as a unique individual, and the challenge of disabling conditions was viewed as an opportunity for positive development. Nordoff and Robbins believed that the children's receptivity to their approach reflected the trust and confidence instilled in the children by the Sunfield community.

The children presented a wide variety of conditions: developmental delay, autism, emotional disturbance, learning disabilities, aphasia, visual and auditory impairments, severe physical challenges, and multiple disabilities. Nordoff and Robbins explored the potential of structural and expressive forces within music to address children's needs and strengths. In the first individual Nordoff–Robbins Music Therapy session at Sunfield, dramatic changes were observed in a child's emotional expression that seemed to be direct responses to improvised music alternating between two contrasting formulations of the pentatonic scale—between Chinese pentatonic as a starting point, and Japanese pentatonic with its altered tones creating dissonance. Subsequent individual courses of therapy expanded upon this seminal demonstration of the emotional potency contained within the musical elements.

The Philadelphia Project

After working together for a year at Sunfield, Nordoff and Robbins relocated to the United States, taking up a position at the Day-Care Unit for Psychotic Children within the Department of Psychiatry in the School of Medicine at the University of Pennsylvania. At the initiative of the principal investigator working with them, funding of $1 million (equivalent to approximately $7.68 million in 2012 dollars) was obtained in 1962 from the National Institute of Mental Health for a 5-year "Music Therapy Project for Psychotic Children under Seven," which encompassed treatment, training, and research. This was the first grant from the National Institutes of Health for the study of music therapy. Concurrently, Nordoff and Robbins developed music therapy programs for children with developmental disabilities in the Philadelphia public school district and at Devereux, a residential facility in a nearby suburb. Much of their work in the Philadelphia area became the basis for case studies used in teaching their music therapy approach (Aigen, 1998; Nordoff & Robbins, 1977/2007).

During these years, they published *Therapy in Music for Handicapped Children* (Nordoff & Robbins, 1971) and books of songs, plays, and instrumental activities (Nordoff & Robbins, 1962–1968, 1983), which continue to be valuable resources for therapy. They also gave many lectures and workshops in the United States. In 1977 they published *Creative Music Therapy* (Nordoff & Robbins, 1977/2007). Considered groundbreaking at the time for its audio excerpts and detailed documentation of music therapy sessions, it has recently been revised (2007) to include over 5 hours of clinical examples.

Further Expansion and Dissemination

In 1975, the Nordoff–Robbins Music Therapy Centre was established in London, and it was there that ongoing formal training in the method began. In the same year, Clive Robbins formed a new music therapy team with his wife, Carol. The Robbinses pioneered a music program for children with hearing loss at the New York State School for the Deaf (Robbins & Robbins, 1980) and also provided music therapy to children with multiple disabilities in Texas and Australia. In 1989, they founded the Nordoff–Robbins Center for Music Therapy at New York University, which became their professional home. Clinical work and training were also established in Germany, Australia, Scotland, and Korea. An organization dedicated to the study of Nordoff–Robbins Music Therapy was established in Japan, and courses in South Africa incorporated Nordoff–Robbins material. As Nordoff–Robbins practitioners found employment in a variety of clinical facilities, the approach was successfully applied to diverse populations, including medical and psychiatric clients, adolescents with emotional difficulties, and self-referred adults.

Theoretical Tenets

The Music Child

A central concept in Nordoff–Robbins Music Therapy is that of the *music child*: the capacity for musical perception and response inborn within every human being, whether child or adult, reflecting both the universal human heritage of "complex and subtle sensitivity to the ordering and relationship of tonal and rhythmic movement" and "the uniquely personal significance" of each individual's musical responsiveness (Nordoff & Robbins, 1977/2007, p. 3). The music child is considered to embody the healthy core potential for growth and development within an individual, irrespective of disabling conditions. Collaborative improvisation activates the music child within both the client and the therapist, allowing them to meet as equal partners in creative endeavor (Guerrero & Turry, 2012). Nordoff and Robbins found that musical encounters reached clients on a deep level, motivating them to take the next steps in their development, despite tremendous challenges. Working at clients' *developmental threshold* through spontaneous creative engagement—cultivating their "readiness to move out into new activities of increasing communicative significance, hopefully leading to positive and satisfying discoveries" (Robbins, 2008, p. 1)—remains a core principle of Nordoff–Robbins Music Therapy with various populations.

Clinical Musicianship: Musical Interactions as the Basis of Therapeutic Relationship

In this therapeutic approach, music serves as the essential medium of communication and interaction. In his preface to *Therapy in Music for Handicapped Children* (Nordoff & Robbins, 1971), composer Benjamin Britten observed that in contrast to the prevailing modernist aesthetic that questioned "the validity of communication in art," here was a musical approach "where the concentration is entirely on just this: on communication, pure and simple" (p. 9). Many of the children with whom Nordoff and Robbins worked had profound deficits in communication and interaction, as described here:

> There are . . . children who live so remotely that it is hard to gain insight into their experiencing and interpreting of life. These children are . . . unable to find significance in any usual life context, incapable of assimilating any of the forms, modes, or expressions of normal life. Their profound estrangement excludes them from the ensouling experience of communicable human emotion. Their prevailing emotional condition evokes the image of an inhospitable landscape in which they are fated to live. One may live amid tempestuous storms, another in an icy wasteland; another may walk alone in a bleak, comfortless desert. For such a child music can become something rare, evocative or consoling. It can become another landscape for him, one in which he will be able to find more than the limits of his own being. (Nordoff & Robbins, 1971, p. 55)

Nordoff and Robbins drew children into musical interaction that sparked their attention, active listening, and reciprocity. The children showed enhanced capacity and motivation to express themselves and withstand frustration. They developed an interest in relating to others and in sustaining a feeling of belonging.

Nordoff's ability to adjust his music responsively and artistically in a moment-to-moment fashion, along with Robbins's depth of experience in working with children, gave them the ability to attune quickly to each child's emotional state and expressive potential. They typically opened a session with improvised music that offered a musical–emotional environment to invite the child into creative exploration. By incorporating aspects of the child's self-presentation into the improvisation, they hoped to create a *musical portrait* of the child that would elicit recognition and response (Nordoff & Robbins, 1977/2007). Over the ensuing decades, therapists working in the Nordoff–Robbins approach have cultivated the breadth and depth of their own musicianship in order to enter into clients' internal landscapes and bring them to a new experience of themselves in the world.

Therapeutic Composition and Improvisation

Clinically focused composition and improvisation in a wide range of styles, utilizing specific aspects of musical form to address clients' goals, is a vital ingredient of Nordoff–Robbins Music Therapy. In precomposed instrumental pieces and songs, as well as in instrumental and vocal improvisation, musical forms are designed to elicit and to build upon the client's responses; in this way, the client makes an essential contribution to the music. Improvisation in this approach is often referred to as *compositional improvisation*, as it is structured by tonality, melodic themes, and phrasing that creates meter (Guerrero & Turry, 2012). Communicative interaction is emphasized through structural features such as turn taking and call-and-response.

Detailed Session Analysis

Nordoff and Robbins balanced the creative spontaneity of improvisational music making with careful study of the therapy process. To this end, they made high-quality audio recordings of each session for review prior to the next session. While reviewing a session, they frequently paused to examine significant events, noting the child's responses to therapeutic interventions and transcribing music they considered important to develop. Their intense focus upon the details of a session resonated with Goethe's principle of bringing love and devotion to the scientific investigation of an object (Ansdell & Pavlicevic, 2010). As the first editor of Goethe's scientific works, Steiner was strongly influenced by Goethe's philosophy of naturalistic inquiry (Ansdell, 2012). Close analysis of session recordings quickly became standard procedure in the Nordoff–Robbins approach, generating time-based *indexes* of significant events in each session for future reference. The recordings of early sessions were audio only; video recording was implemented as soon as the technology became readily available.

Music Therapy Applications

Historic Work with Children

The unfolding of the therapeutic relationship through musical interaction can be vividly heard in the audio recordings of Nordoff and Robbins's early cases. These cases illustrate the use of various musical elements, the spontaneous application of improvisational techniques, and ways of evoking and enhancing musical interaction. Particularly in children's spontaneous vocal exchanges with Nordoff, their mutual joy in connecting through music is clearly manifested. Among the studies selected by Nordoff and Robbins to teach the core principles of their method is the case of Edward.

CHILD CLINICAL EXAMPLE

The case of Edward is presented in detail in Chapter 2 of *Creative Music Therapy* (Nordoff & Robbins, 1977/2007, pp. 21–48), with accompanying audio excerpts. Here we review the case as it pertains to the principles of the approach we have discussed above, using some of the audio excerpts from *Creative Music Therapy* as well as a complete session recording that is not included in *Creative Music Therapy* (Session 9).[1]

At age 5½, Edward began to attend the Day-Care Unit for Psychotic Children at the medical center of the University of Pennsylvania where Nordoff and Robbins had been working for 4 years. Two weeks after enrolling in the Day-Care Unit, he began music therapy. Edward was diagnosed with emotional disturbance and cognitive delay, exhibiting

---

[1] Audio excerpts are reproduced with permission of Barcelona Publishers and the International Trust for Nordoff–Robbins Music Therapy. Rights to all recordings owned by the International Trust for Nordoff–Robbins Music Therapy and used by permission. Unauthorized duplication or reproduction is prohibited.

features of autism. The only person to whom he was able to relate was his mother. He had a history of panic reactions and was prone to prolonged rocking and head banging. He needed to be fed, washed, dressed, and toileted. In the day care program, his anxiety created disturbances. When upset, he would often cry, scream, run, jump, and finally roll on the floor. Such activities could become self-perpetuating and last indefinitely.

Session 1

• *Excerpt 1.*[2] The events described in this paragraph (until the End of Excerpt, below) are captured in Excerpt 1, taken from Edward's first session: Soft, fretful, tonal vocalization is heard from Edward as Paul Nordoff improvises on the piano. Clive Robbins shows Edward the drum and piano, and he explores the piano briefly. He paces the room, producing brief vocal phrases in synchrony with Paul's singing. His cries increase in intensity and pitch range, but remain related to the tonality of the music. He begins to jump while vocalizing; Paul accompanies his physical and vocal activity. [End of Excerpt.]

As the session continued, Edward's crying intensified further while remaining tonal, and he began to throw himself on the floor and roll. He was beginning to tantrum, but his engagement with the music prevented him from giving himself over to the tantrum entirely. The therapists cheered Edward's physical activities, conveying that they were with him emotionally and not distressed by his behavior. They were aware that despite his agitation, his crying involved no actual tears.

• *Excerpt 2.*[3] In the latter part of the first session, Edward expresses himself in unpitched screaming, tonal crying, and softer, more tonally defined vocalizations. Paul beats the drum and cymbal with his right hand while playing the piano with his left. Edward cries briefly in rhythm. The dynamics

---

[2]Audio recording available at *www.guilford.com/ wheeler-materials.*

[3]Audio recording available at *www.guilford.com/ wheeler-materials.*

of Edward's responses and Paul's playing are clearly related. [End of Excerpt.]

At this point, Clive attempted to end the session by leading Edward toward the door. Paul requested that he be brought back. Edward, who had become quiet in anticipation of leaving, resumed jumping and screaming. Paul musically accompanied this activity. The procedure of departure and return was repeated twice more. On his third return, Edward was brought to the piano. Each therapist took one of his hands and played clusters with him. Paul then put a mallet in his hand and beat hand over hand on the drum and cymbal, further incensing Edward. Finally, Edward was taken back to the unit. He was quiet as he left.

Much was communicated during this tempestuous first session, which lasted 11 minutes. Edward conveyed a highly sensitive musicality. His innate responsiveness to tonality, phrasing, and rhythm was evident to the therapists from the moment he arrived. Even his expressions of anger and frustration served to confirm the depth of his musical involvement with them. For their part, the therapists were trying to communicate to Edward a basic appreciation of his efforts at self-expression, whatever form they took, and to assure him that none of his actions—no matter how extreme or provocative—repelled or alienated them. They demonstrated that music could contain the whole range and intensity of his expression and make it a basis for interaction and communication. The events around his departure affirmed that the therapists were confidently guiding the course of the session, and that nothing he did could overwhelm them.

Session 2

This session, which occurred after a 4-week break, began with the introduction of a greeting song, "Good Morning to Edward, Good Morning." Edward sang in the tonality of the greeting song, responding to Paul's musical interventions. He initially resisted Clive's efforts to involve him in playing various instruments, but later he began to play of his own volition. The therapists complimented

Edward when he played independently on the piano. When the therapists took a pencil away from him, he protested vocally; the quality of this vocalization related strongly to the melodic and rhythmic aspects of Paul's singing in the greeting song.

After this brief musical interlude, Edward went to each therapist in turn and brought his nose close to the therapist's face. In order to preserve the positive mood, the session was ended at this point, just over 5 minutes after it began. Despite its brevity, the session confirmed that music reached Edward and enabled him to contain his anxiety. This confirmation indicated the possibility of creating a productive musical relationship that might foster the development of communication.

Session 3

Edward's next session occurred on schedule, a week after Session 2. He had been upset and crying prior to the session but was quiet upon entering. When Paul played energetic music from a past session, Edward sang in the tonality of the music. Then Paul began to play more quietly and simply. Edward positioned himself across the room, faced Paul, and sang in key with his crying voice, evidently vocalizing musical replies to the therapist.

• *Excerpt 3*.[4] A dramatic, rhythmically compelling motive is heard from the piano. Edward responds, seeming to wait for the ends of phrases and then sing between them intentionally. Paul joins him vocally, singing in ways that are not only musically imitative, but also emotionally responsive to Edward's expression. Edward follows Paul through various rhythmic developments, including silences, with uncanny anticipation. Therapist and child make compelling music together, each inspiring the other with the intensity of his personal expression. [End of Excerpt.]

The session lasted 7 minutes. The therapists observed that Edward's vocal–emotional expression was becoming more overtly musical—tonally, dynamically, and in its phras-

---

[4]Audio recording available at *www.guilford.com/ wheeler-materials*.

ing. They were also continually surprised at the degree of his musicality, particularly in light of the fact that he had never shown any interest in music on the unit. He never sang any children's songs or any recorded material that he might have heard. It had merely been observed that music "calmed him down."

Session 4

The fourth session began with the song "Good Morning to Edward," to which Edward was able to beat the drum with hand-over-hand assistance from Clive. Then Clive encouraged him to engage in his characteristic jumping. While Paul improvised the song "Jump, Edward," Clive joined Edward in jumping. They jumped together—holding hands—and apart, much to Edward's enjoyment.

After the jumping, Edward was brought to the drum, which he played very briefly. "Jump, Edward" was repeated and led naturally into "Dance, Edward," in which Clive, having observed his graceful, dance-like movements, invited Edward to dance freely with him.

The session ended after 6½ minutes. The therapists had deliberately taken the activities that Edward might engage in spontaneously and placed them in a musical context. The music reflected the active nature of his personality and responded to the dance-like nature of his movements.

Session 4 was the last session before the unit's summer break, during which Edward continued the process of settling into the unit, getting along better with others and becoming somewhat less fearful. His tantrums, however, remained frequent.

Session 5

Edward appeared genuinely pleased to see the therapists again, and came into the session willingly. He played the cymbal, danced, and once again responded to Paul's singing with tonal vocalization of his own.

Session 6

Upon entering the session, Edward seemed quietly intent upon making music. He used mallets to beat any number of objects, both musical and nonmusical. Paul accompanied this beating with familiar music. Halfway through the session Edward approached Clive, who was kneeling, put an arm around his neck, and looked closely into his face. There was a sense of emerging contact in this interaction. After a few minutes, the music became more active and stimulating, and Edward and Clive jumped and danced to the jumping song. Then Edward stopped jumping and approached Clive again in a friendly manner.

• *Excerpt 4.*[5] Paul plays a waltz version of "Good Morning to Edward, Good Morning." Clive beats to this music, resisting Edward's efforts to stop him. Edward takes Clive's mallets. Paul keeps playing the piano and Clive moves into a half-kneeling position. Edward approaches Clive and sits on his knee as Paul continues his accompaniment. Then Edward "speaks" to the therapists in a jargon that sounds conversational. Clive responds, using words and sounds to express agreement. [End of Excerpt.]

The conversational interaction between Edward and the therapists continued to the end of the session. He spoke in jargon once again, interacting with Clive. Paul played and sang, also in a form of jargon. In subsequently assessing the session, the therapists found that Edward appeared to be seeking closer contact with Clive, his approach becoming both bolder and more intimate.

Session 7

Shortly after the session began, Edward led Clive to a bench, climbed on it, and scrambled up into Clive's arms until he was upright, held against Clive's chest. He faced Paul over Clive's left shoulder. He maintained this position for the entire session, reestablishing it whenever Clive put him down. From this position, Edward vocalized in a variety of ways, mostly tonally.

• *Excerpt 5.*[6] Clive holds Edward high, moving to the music. From this position, Edward makes a variety of tonal, rhythmic vocalizations, including "'Awo!'" (approximating "Hello"). The therapists attempt interactive vocalization, with and without the piano. [End of Excerpt.]

As the session progressed, sporadic vocalizations followed. Clive continued to hold Edward high, and Paul continued to try to involve him in direct vocal interaction. The therapists noted Edward's efforts to further the development of closeness begun in Session 6. To some extent, they viewed his insistence upon being carried as a form of manipulation. His vocalizations had increased in number and variety; however, although most of them were musically responsive, few were truly interactive.

Session 8

Edward climbed upon Clive as soon as he entered the room, and made many vocalizations. Again, he approximated "Hello." After 7 minutes, Clive put Edward down, refusing to pick him up. Edward's response was intense physical activity that persisted when Paul played more slowly and in a minor key. Ultimately Edward began to cry (tonally), but did not want to leave the session when he was escorted out.

Upon reviewing this session, the therapists noted vocal sounds that were new for Edward. They realitzed that their musical perception had been overwhelmed during the session by the intensity of Edward's physical resistiveness. They decided to allow Edward to resume his climbing while they continued their work on vocalization.

Session 9

This session features over 16 minutes of continuously responsive vocal interplay; hence, it is considered a milestone of Edward's therapy, and is presented here in its entirety.

---

[5]Audio recording available at *www.guilford.com/ wheeler-materials.*

[6]Audio recording available at *www.guilford.com/ wheeler-materials.*

• *Excerpt 6: Complete session.*[7] Edward is already singing as he approaches the music room. On arrival, he immediately climbs upon Clive. He soon begins to repeat "hellos" antiphonally with Paul, initiating the kind of interactive vocalization that was lacking in the previous excerpt. He sings in the tonality of the music in this manner, and then begins to alter his singing to follow harmonic changes. He introduces a vocal game ("ee-ee-ee"), which becomes the basis of spontaneous rhythmic vocal interplay that grows increasingly melodic as it is repeated and developed (Nordoff & Robbins, 1977/2007, p. 38).

After the session, an additional 3-minute coda of antiphonal "goodbyes" occurred as Edward was escorted back to the unit.

Treatment Review: Sessions 1–9

In reviewing Edward's course of music therapy thus far, the therapists singled out two areas of significant development. The first of these was specifically musical: the ordering effects of music on his initially disorganized behavior. Over the course of nine sessions, Edward's inherent musicality—his innate sense of tone, rhythm, and phrase—was developed through participation in the various forms and types of specially improvised musical experiences that the therapists were able to provide. From the tonal crying of his first session, Edward moved through a process of development that culminated in the interresponsive, communicative singing of his ninth session. The ordering qualities of music—tonality in all its manifestations, such as pitch, scale, melody, and harmony; the whole spectrum of musical dynamics; the forces of rhythm and meter, regulating the flow of time—enabled Edward to engage directly with the therapists.

The second salient area of development was the cultivation of personal relationship. The manner in which the therapists related to Edward awakened in him the self-awareness that not only allowed him to express himself interresponsively, but also formed the content—the feelings, emotions, and sentiments—of

---

[7]Audio recording available at *www.guilford.com/ wheeler-materials.*

the communication that developed. This journey—from fear and anger at the beginning, through gradual approach and reassuring physical contact, to joyous, affirming vocal interaction—was made possible by the accepting, encouraging, yet firm stance of the therapists. In a very real sense, what Edward was expressing was the sheer joy of newfound human relationship.

Post-Session 9

After the interactive vocal play of Session 9, the therapists began to work toward speech by singing different words to Edward, with the hope that his natural musical responsiveness would inspire and enable him to sing them back. In Session 10, there were some imitative speech responses to words such as *nose* and *finger*, but for the most part Edward responded with syllables of his own creation. It was also noticed that after the epic Session 9, Edward became increasingly restless in sessions, perhaps in reaction to the sheer stimulation of the sessions and his own rapid progress into deeper and more intimate relationship (Nordoff & Robbins, 1977/2007, pp. 46-47). Nevertheless, it was observed that "a fundamental change was taking place in his attitude to spoken language" on the unit: "He imitated more sounds and words equally in all the circumstances of his daily life" (p. 46). Over the next year, he used 120 words, including verbs and short phrases (p. 47). Moreover, as his music therapy continued, Edward demonstrated a growing ability "to accept learning situations" (p. 47).

At the age of 7–1½ years after beginning music therapy—Edward's music therapy sessions were taken over by interns. At the age of 9, he was discharged from the Day-Care Unit for Psychotic Children and enrolled in a special education program.

Contemporary Work with Adults

The few adult clients with whom Nordoff and Robbins worked all had profound developmental disabilities. It was left to the next generation of Nordoff–Robbins practitioners to develop the approach with different adult populations, including those with medical issues and those seeking an alternative to traditional verbal psychotherapy. A body of clinical practice and research with such populations took place at the hospital associated with the Universitat in Witten-Herdecke, Germany. Pioneering applications of Nordoff–Robbins Music Therapy were incorporated into treatment plans at the hospital for patients with traumatic brain injury, coma, Parkinson's disease, Alzheimer's disease, and other forms of dementia (Aldridge, 1996, 1998, 2000, 2005). Similarly, the Nordoff–Robbins Music Therapy Centre in London began to provide therapy to a variety of adult clients, including those with HIV (Ansdell, 1995; Lee, 1996). More recently, a robust outreach program has successfully integrated Nordoff–Robbins Music Therapy into a variety of settings throughout England, including medical facilities, psychiatric units, and nursing homes. At the Nordoff–Robbins Center for Music Therapy at New York University (NYU) music therapists collaborate with occupational therapists from the Rusk Rehabilitation Institute at NYU Langone Medical Center to provide integrated rehabilitation therapy to stroke survivors in small groups, simultaneously addressing the physical, psychological, and social dimensions of well-being.

Self-referred adults who come for Nordoff–Robbins Music Therapy as an alternative to traditional psychotherapy have stimulated significant developments in the approach, as they bring the capacity to articulate verbally their needs, thoughts, feelings, and images. They present rich opportunities for therapists and researchers to understand the approach from clients' perspectives, as they can reflect upon the therapeutic relationship and the ways in which unconscious dynamics may affect them. This new population has required therapists to integrate psychodynamic understanding with musical awareness to a greater degree than was involved in the original Nordoff–Robbins work with chil-

dren, while maintaining their focus on careful listening and sensitive musical response to clients (Turry, 1998, 2009).

The palette of musical styles utilized by Nordoff–Robbins practitioners has expanded as jazz musicians and guitarists have pursued training in the approach. Particularly in working with adults, contemporary styles serve as a valuable resource for creating improvisations and compositions that are resonant with clients' musical preferences. In employing different musical genres, and in integrating psychodynamic and other theoretical influences, it is the therapist's authentic musical engagement with clients that is paramount. Next we present a case example of contemporary work with a self-referred adult client at NYU's Nordoff–Robbins Center for Music Therapy.

ADULT CLINICAL EXAMPLE

Maria has shared her experience of Nordoff–Robbins Music Therapy through publications, performances, and her personal website. In addition, several music therapists have discussed her case (e.g., Turry, 2009; Aigen, 2004, 2012; Stige & Aarø, 2012). The case description below includes links to improvised songs from sessions, which are posted on the therapist's website and on Maria's own website.[8] Like other clients who do not require a cotherapist's assistance to participate in musical interaction, Maria has worked alone with a primary therapist.

A successful single middle-aged woman living in New York City, Maria was diagnosed with stage 4 non-Hodgkin's lymphoma. At the outset of music therapy, Maria described herself as feeling hopeless and paralyzed, numb with fear, as she tried to grapple with her condition. She had undergone psychotherapy in the past, but a strong intuition led her to seek help through a different pathway at this juncture. The desperation triggered by the

---

[8]Rights to all recordings owned by the International Trust for Nordoff–Robbins Music Therapy and used by permission. Unauthorized duplication or reproduction is prohibited.

crisis fueled Maria to enter into the creative process of Nordoff–Robbins Music Therapy. Improvising sounds by playing a variety of instruments in her first session, she began to unfreeze from her self-described state of numbness. She laughed freely for the first time since her diagnosis 2½ months before. In subsequent sessions she explored the use of her voice, first nonverbally and then with words that became lyrics in improvised songs. As she describes,

> "I let out the fear in words and sounds. Alan encouraged me to make any sounds at all, loud guttural sounds, shrieking, moaning. I was not controlling my expression. It was pouring out of me. The words were simple, but the melodies expressed feelings for which I had no words." (in Logis, 2004, p. 25; listen to *www.alanturry. com*—"Tell the Truth")

Maria considered herself to be logical and organized when speaking with her friends, but in music therapy, "I felt my fear and anguish. The words in my mouth surprised me. I had not expressed this level of feeling to anyone" (in Logis, 2002, p. 5).

The coactive process between Maria and the therapist, though free associative, generated aesthetic musical forms. Maria shared that during moments of abject hopelessness, she would immerse herself in the piano music that the therapist was creating to attune to her emotional state and invite further expression. This triggered her own improvisation of melodic ideas to support her words. Even as Maria was experiencing sadness and despair, she also felt satisfaction in creating melodies. She described the melodies as giving her a sense of freedom and ameliorating the internal critical judgment that often impeded her self-expression.

Her self-critical tendency was one of many lifelong issues that she began to explore. Another was the sense of having no voice, of being stifled; only now could she directly address this long-standing psychological condition by improvising words and melodies in music therapy. The music comforted her, allowing her to feel emotionally understood; yet it also challenged her to persevere in exploring painful feelings (*www.alanturry.com*— "Oh My Child"). At times, she felt like giving up, but the music motivated her to continue.

Maria reflects on this process as a "journey deep into my underworld" from which "I have come back changed." She had long been aware of her psychological conflicts and had discussed them in verbal psychotherapy, but this was a different experience: one of immersing herself in the emotion and finding that the emotion was transformed through musical exploration. As she observes,

> "[The therapist] could hear my deep cry of sadness. He played music that didn't just respond to my words but pushed my emotional awareness and recognition into unexplored areas. Feelings of despair [*www.alanturry.com*—"Open Up My Arms," clip 1], silliness, fun [*www.alanturry. com*—"Scared and Paralyzed"], and fear [*www. alanturry.com*—"Uncharted Waters"] spewed out of me. Sometimes he answered me with big dissonant clusters, and at others he tuned in to my tears and sighing with lilting melodies. He played fabulous jazzy blues as I belted out words, and there were times when we entered into an eerie world with whole tone or atonal music." (in Logis, 2002, p. 7)

Maria's developmental threshold continually widened as she was able to delve ever more deeply into her emotional processes, perhaps because the music improvised by the therapist contained qualities that resonated with feelings that were not fully conscious within her. In this way the musical experience helped Maria to discover what she was feeling even as she was attempting to express herself. Repeated thematic material, often in song form, allowed her to reflect upon her emotional state.

Maria's feelings of helplessness subsided as she initiated her own musical ideas and began to trust herself. She felt strongly that this was a means to overcome her sense of having no self, which stemmed from her difficult relationship with her mother. Rather than remaining stifled and oppressed, constantly judging herself, she began to trust that she indeed had her own unique voice, which she could utilize for self-expression (*www.alanturry.com*—"Woman, Why Are You Weeping?").

Maria poetically describes the process by which spontaneous music making freed her to tap into her creative potentials:

> "The therapist creates a field of green grass and crocuses when he plays the piano, and I get to

run around in the field without shoes and socks. I wind up jumping, flying, walking, running and rolling on the grass, lyrics and melodies pouring out of me. I feel free and wild. I've come to see that I can't make a mistake." (in Logis, 2002, p. 8)

Improvising in song forms (*www.alanturry. com*—"All My Life") gave Maria the opportunity to feel a sense of pride in what was being created. She was motivated to learn the song improvisations and eventually perform them, first for close family and friends, then for a wider audience. In this respect, the work could be viewed within the lens of community music therapy (Aigen, 2004, 2012; Ansdell, 2010; Ansdell & DeNora, 2012; Stige & Aarø, 2012). Maria described her sense of completion when singing a song, and her feelings of strength when sharing her story and her music with a supportive community. She gained great satisfaction from inspiring others to feel hopeful in the face of difficult challenges.

Maria began to wonder what her mother, who was no longer alive, might think of her newfound immersion in music making, having staunchly resisted her mother's attempts to force piano lessons upon her as a child (*www.alanturry.com*—"Do I Dare Imagine?"). Would her mother forgive Maria for not listening to her? Could she imagine that her mother would be happy for her? Later in treatment, she improvised a song to thank her mother for the positive experiences they had shared. She sang that she forgave her mother for the obstacles she had created, at one point crying while singing, "Mamma, I love you." (*www.marialogis.com/video/watch/3 - Thank You, Mother*). In this way, Maria worked to heal her relationship with her mother years after her mother's death, while working to be more accepting and loving toward herself.

As Maria became more confident in using the medium of music for self-expression, she began to view herself as a creative artist—a new identity that expanded upon her previous one as an efficient corporate executive. She still struggled with internalized critical voices, but they were less intense and she was more satisfied with her involvement in life in general. She felt less isolated and more complete now that she was realizing her creative potential.

Conclusions

Considered together, the cases of Edward and Maria—a young boy just emerging into relationship and functional language, and an articulate, accomplished woman—illuminate core principles of Nordoff–Robbins Music Therapy. In both cases, the clients' strengths and needs are addressed through a creative partnership that engages both the clients' and the therapists' musical sensitivities. Therapeutic goals are pursued through "in-depth utilization of the structural and expressive elements of both improvised and pre-composed music" (Guerrero & Turry, 2012, p. 131). As Ansdell (1995) observes, this approach to music therapy "works in the way that music itself works" (p. 5).

For both preverbal and highly verbal clients, Nordoff–Robbins Music Therapy works to cultivate the interpersonal reciprocity and emotional expression that are fundamental to human communication. In order to use music effectively as a medium of communication, Nordoff–Robbins music therapists endeavor to draw upon a wide range of musical elements, tonalities, idioms, and styles with versatility and fluency. The application of these musical resources is creative rather than prescriptive, arising from the moment-to-moment interaction between client and therapist. Although the varieties of music, like verbal languages, derive from particular sociocultural and historical traditions of meaning, the meanings in music are ever newly generated because they are informed by the unique, unrepeatable circumstances under which music unfolds in time. Thus, *fluency* in musical communication resides in the emerging flow of relationship among participants in music making. Although there are specifiable forces that govern the structure of music in different styles and idioms, there is no lexicon of predetermined meanings in music; rather, clients and therapists create meaning together as they invest themselves in music and open themselves to its power.

REFERENCES

Aigen, K. (1998). *Paths of development in Nordoff–Robbins Music Therapy.* Gilsum, NH: Barcelona.

Aigen, K. (2004). Conversations on creating community. In M. Pavlicevic & G. Ansdell (Eds.), *Community music therapy* (pp. 186–213). London: Jessica Kingsley.

Aigen, K. (2012). Community music therapy. In G. E. McPherson & G. F. Welch (Eds.), *The Oxford handbook of music education* (Vol. 2, pp. 138–154). New York: Oxford University Press.

Aldridge, D. (1996). *Music therapy research and practice in medicine: From out of the silence.* London: Jessica Kingsley.

Aldridge, D. (Ed.). (1998). *Music therapy in palliative care: New voices.* London: Jessica Kingsley.

Aldridge, D. (Ed.). (2000). *Music therapy in dementia.* London: Jessica Kingsley.

Aldridge, D. (Ed.). (2005). *Music therapy and neurological rehabilitation: Performing healthy.* London: Jessica Kingsley.

Ansdell, G. (1995). *Music for life: Aspects of creative music therapy with adult clients.* London: Jessica Kingsley.

Ansdell, G. (2010). Where performing helps: Processes and affordances of performance in community music therapy. In B. Stige, G. Ansdell, C. Elefant, & M. Pavlicevic (Eds.), *Where music helps: Community music therapy in action and reflection* (pp. 161–186). Aldershot, UK: Ashgate.

Ansdell, G. (2012). Steps toward an ecology of music therapy: A readers' guide to various theoretical wanderings 1990–2011. In K. E. Bruscia (Ed.), *Readings in music therapy theory* (n. p., Reading No. 7). Gilsum, NH: Barcelona.

Ansdell, G., & DeNora, T. (2012). Musical flourishing: Community music therapy, controversy, and the cultivation of wellbeing. In R. MacDonald, G. Kreutz, & L. Mitchell (Eds.), *Music, health and wellbeing* (pp. 97–112). Oxford, UK: Oxford University Press.

Ansdell, G., & Pavlicevic, M. (2010). Practicing "gentle empiricism": The Nordoff–Robbins research heritage. *Music Therapy Perspectives, 28*(2), 131–138.

Guerrero, N., & Turry, A. (2012). Nordoff–Robbins music therapy: An expressive and dynamic approach for young children on the autism spectrum. In P. Kern & M. Humpal (Eds.), *Early childhood music therapy and autism spectrum disorders: Developing potential in young children and their families* (pp. 130–144). London: Jessica Kingsley.

Lee, C. (1996). *Music at the edge: The music therapy experience of a musician with AIDS.* London: Routledge.

Logis, M. (2002). *Maria's story.* Retrieved from *www.marialogis.com/media/pdf/Marias_Story.pdf.*

Logis, M. (2004). *Singing my way through it.* Unpublished manuscript, New York.

Nordoff, P., & Robbins, C. (1962–1968). *Children's play-songs: Books 1-5.* Bryn Mawr, PA: Theodore Presser.

Nordoff, P., & Robbins, C. (1971). *Therapy in music for handicapped children.* London: Victor Gollancz.

Nordoff, P., & Robbins, C. (1983). *Music therapy in special education* (2nd ed.). St. Louis, MO: MMB Music.

Nordoff, P., & Robbins, C. (2007). *Creative music therapy: A guide to fostering clinical musicianship* (2nd ed.). Gilsum, NH: Barcelona. (Original work published 1977)

Robbins, C. (2008). *Defining the developmental threshold.* Unpublished document, Nordoff–Robbins Center for Music Therapy, New York University, New York.

Robbins, C. (2011). On the connections between the Nordoff–Robbins practice of creative music therapy, Steiner's anthroposophy, Maslow's humanistic psychology, and other psychological and philosophical considerations. In Nordoff–Robbins Center Staff (Eds.), *Clinical improvisation: Expanding musical resources* (pp. 64–68). Unpublished document, Nordoff–Robbins Center for Music Therapy, New York University, New York.

Robbins, C., & Robbins, C. (1980). *Music for the hearing-impaired and other special groups.* St. Louis, MO: MMB Music.

Steiner, R. (1977). *Eurythmy as visible music* (2nd ed.). London: Rudolf Steiner Press.

Steiner, R. (1998). *Education for special needs: The curative education course–twelve lectures by Rudolf Steiner.* London: Rudolf Steiner Press.

Stige, B., & Aarø, L. E. (2012). *Invitation to community music therapy.* New York: Routledge.

Turry, A. (1998). Transference and countertransference in Nordoff–Robbins Music Therapy. In K. E. Bruscia (Ed.), *The dynamics of music psychotherapy* (pp. 161–212). Gilsum, NH: Barcelona.

Turry, A. (2009). Integrating musical and psychological thinking: The relationship between music and words in clinically improvised songs. *Music and Medicine, 1*(2), 106–116.

CHAPTER 16

The Bonny Method of Guided Imagery and Music

Madelaine Ventre
Cathy H. McKinney

The Bonny Method of Guided Imagery and Music (GIM) is an approach to self-exploration, psychotherapy, and spiritual growth. GIM, which is sometimes abbreviated as BMGIM or as the Bonny Method in the literature, combines the power of selected classical music and the human imagination. A trained therapist uses the music to help a client access and sustain an altered state of consciousness. The imagery that emerges during GIM sessions spans the reaches of human and transpersonal experience. The growing body of literature shows GIM to be an efficacious approach for effecting both psychological and physiological change in a variety of populations with diverse clinical needs.

History

GIM is a culmination of the life and work of Dr. Helen Bonny. She was born in 1921 to a mother who was a pianist and a father who was a minister. Music and spirituality were key influences early in Helen's life and would become the foundation for her pioneering work in music therapy. Through her school years, Helen excelled at violin and later graduated from Oberlin Conservatory of Music with a major in violin performance. She married a minister and began her life as a mother and minister's wife (Bonny, 2002a).

In 1948, Bonny went to a meeting in which Dr. Frank Laubach was to speak on prayer. That night, Dr. Laubach asked Helen to play the violin for the assembled group. This became a life-changing event. Helen later said that, during the performance, the music took on a life of its own. Indeed she played accurately and musically, yet the music that came from her violin was exquisite, magnificent, and not under her control. She felt as though the music had flowed through her and her violin. No matter what technique she used or did not use, the sounds coming from the violin were glorious. In response to Bonny's inquiry about how to hold onto this experience, Dr. Laubach suggested that she meditate daily and work with a prayer group (Bonny, 2002a).

Following his advice, Helen deepened her faith but also encountered some difficult personal material. She sought therapy with Dr. Kenneth Godfrey and, through hypnosis, was able to uncover, work through, and heal a childhood trauma (Bonny, 1995). She accomplished the work using the framework of internal imagery. When used this way, imagery includes experiences that engage all the senses: visual, auditory, olfactory, gustatory, physical, and kinesthetic. One moves beyond discussing a problem, issue, or memory to fully experience or re-experience it. The importance of imagery in therapy used during altered states of consciousness became another step along her path to GIM.

In 1960, at age 39, Bonny decided to further her education. She considered earning a master's degree in violin performance, but this would not support her desire to use music for therapeutic purposes. After hearing about the master's degree program in music therapy at the University of Kansas, she began her study there with Dr. E. Thayer Gaston. Under his tutelage, she learned the skills and value of research, especially as applied to music therapy. She had personally experienced imagery and its ability to support and encourage exploration in altered states of consciousness for therapeutic purposes. She also had felt the power of music to stimulate spiritual or transpersonal experiences. These came together in 1969 with an invitation to work at the Maryland Psychiatric Research Center, where researchers were doing pioneering work on the effects of mind-altering drugs, depth psychology, and altered states of consciousness. Bonny's job was to research and choose music for the LSD sessions that lasted between 8 and 10 hours. Prior to her joining the research staff, researchers had used various types of music throughout the session. Based on her observations, Bonny continued to use the client's preferred music before the drug took effect and as

it wore off; however, she found that classical music worked best in the heart of the session when the client's consciousness was most deeply altered (Bonny, 2002a). Combining careful observation with her broad knowledge of music and drawing from an extensive music library of vinyl records (LPs), she chose pieces with different properties to support different types of client experiences (Bonny, 1976, 1978/2002e).

In the early 1970s, the government withdrew funding for research on therapeutic uses of psychedelic drugs. Bonny already had begun exploring the effects of classical music on the psyche. With Louis Savary as coauthor, she published *Music and Your Mind* (Bonny & Savary, 1973), based on her research with diverse and relatively healthy groups, including staff from a drug rehabilitation program, college students, sisters from a religious order, and researchers at an international conference on consciousness. In response to inquiries and in order for the work to grow, she and Sr. Trinitas Bochini formed the Institute for Consciousness and Music, and Bonny began training others to facilitate GIM (Bonny, 1976). Shortly thereafter, she completed the PhD program at the Union Graduate School. Her dissertation described the process of GIM, including guidelines for facilitating individual sessions; outlined the role of music in GIM; and presented the first eight programs of classical music designed for the GIM method (Bonny, 1976).

Bonny's (1976) dissertation also included a report of the first randomized controlled trial of a series of individual GIM sessions, comparing the outcome to that of a series of brief intensive psychotherapy sessions in a sample of 24 adults with mild to moderate nonpsychotic mental disorders. She found that those in the GIM sessions required fewer hours of therapy to accomplish their goals. Moreover, a 6-month follow-up revealed that almost half of the verbal psychotherapy participants had reentered therapy, whereas none of the GIM participants had done so. Bonny published three monographs from her dissertation; they were republished in a collection of her writings (Bonny, 2002d).

By the time Bonny died in 2010, training in GIM had spread around the globe and evolved into 3 years of postgraduate study that included a series of personal GIM sessions in addition to training in the selection and use of music during altered states. Therapists also learned to facilitate the imagery and music processes, understand psychodynamic processes, and support transpersonal as well as personal GIM content through intensive seminars and supervised clinical work. Bonny had inspired many people to carry her transformative work to new applications.

Theoretical Tenets

Chief among the theoretical models that influenced the development of GIM are those from humanistic, Jungian, and transpersonal traditions. Bonny (1976, 1995, 2002a) found the work of Abraham Maslow, particularly his model of self-actualization and his concept of peak experience, to be congruent with her own philosophy and personal experience. She also acknowledged Carl Rogers's model of client-centered therapy as having greatly influenced the underlying principles of the GIM clinical relationship. The belief that there is a whole, wise, healthy part in every individual is fundamental to GIM therapy. From this viewpoint, the therapist can help clients discover that they have all the answers within themselves. Perhaps that wisdom has been clouded by a client's earlier history and events or his or her present-day situations. With the support and direction of the music, the client is empowered to explore the depths of his or her life experiences through imagery. As these unfold, that internal wisdom guides the client's ability to make healthier choices and reach a higher potential.

Bonny (1976, 2002a) acknowledged Carl Jung as aiding the development of GIM,

particularly his description of the collective unconscious, the technique of active imagination, and his opening the field of psychology to a consideration of transpersonal aspects of human existence. Subsequent GIM scholars have further explored GIM from a Jungian perspective (e.g., Ward, 2002).

Bonny (1976, 2002c) also credited the transpersonal model of Roberto Assagioli and the explorations of altered states of consciousness by Charles Tart for informing the early development of GIM. She agreed with Assagioli's assertion that contemporary psychological theories neglected higher aspects of human beings and that the view from the transpersonal self provided the opportunity to integrate and make conscious the total self (Bonny, 1976). More recently the transpersonal theories of Ken Wilber (Kasayka, 2002; Lewis, 1998–1999) and Frances Vaughan (1991) have contributed to our understanding of the transpersonal aspects of the GIM process.

GIM therapists have continued the development of the method. Additional theoretical perspectives include aspects of psychoanalytic theory (Bruscia, 1998), Gestalt approaches (Clarkson, 2002), and spiritual orientations (Kasayka, 2002).

Music Therapy Applications

GIM first emerged as a process for exploring and expanding consciousness (Bonny, 1976). Peak and transpersonal experiences were sought and believed to be healing, in and of themselves. As GIM-trained therapists have recognized the therapeutic potential of addressing psychological issues through the GIM process, the applications for GIM have expanded.

Session Format

A typical session consists of four parts (Bonny, 1976, 1978/2002b; Ventre, 2002): the prelude, induction, music, and postlude.

Prelude

In the beginning of the session, the client shares what has occurred since the last session as well as concerns that are present that day. The therapist reflects and helps the client focus on what is most important. The therapist makes decisions as to what induction and music would be most supportive to the work. This phase usually takes 20–30 minutes.

Induction

As the client assumes a comfortable position, the therapist offers suggestions to deepen the client's concentration and prepare him or her for the music. Depending on the client's needs, these suggestions may take a variety of forms, such as facilitation of relaxation or focus on the body or the breath, making sure to engage both the body and the mind. As a starting point, the therapist suggests an image, often drawn from the prelude, helping the client connect the different senses with that image. This process intensifies the client's focus, which helps to further shift attention inward and lessen the effect of external reality. The client, now in a more deeply altered state of awareness, is told that the music is beginning. The induction may be only seconds to a few minutes long.

Music

The music is the core of the session. The therapist chooses prerecorded music of the Western classical tradition, which may be one of the 35- to 45-minute programs designed by Helen Bonny (Grocke, 2002) or other trained GIM therapists (see Appendices B–I in Bruscia & Grocke, 2002). It may also be a sequence of pieces from the programs that the therapist chooses as the session unfolds to match the affect, energy, and emerging imagery of the client. As the session progresses and the client allows the unfolding of the story, he or she verbally relates the experience to the therapist. The therapist supports the client's process through a verbal dialogue. The client may share impressions from any of the senses, such as sights, sounds, or smells; bodily sensations, such as warmth, tingling, pressure, or discomfort; sensations of movement, such as flying or dancing; or any human emotion, from profound joy or awe to deep sadness or intense anger. The music supports and stimulates movement through the story, allowing the client to hear and take from the music what is needed. The music is programmed to allow for a natural beginning, middle, and end with opportunities for tension and release, conflict and resolution. The therapist assists the client's process and supports whatever the client needs to be or do. The therapist tells the client when the music has ended and facilitates the client's return into the more externally oriented reality. The music portion is approximately 35–50 minutes.

Postlude

As the client returns toward a more normal, externally oriented state of consciousness, the therapist follows the client's lead in reflecting on the experience. The client may have the opportunity to work with the material that has come up in the music. The postlude is a time for processing but not interpreting (Bonny, 1999/2002b). The images may be important to the client on many different levels, not all of which will be immediately apparent. Clients will find and integrate the interpretation that is most useful to them at this time in their process. The postlude typically lasts about 30 minutes. The whole GIM session takes around 2 hours, with each section flowing smoothly into the next.

CLINICAL EXAMPLE:
Finding Self-Expression and Self-Worth

J, a 40-year-old man, came to GIM to explore why he felt unable to live and express himself without feeling criticized, unworthy, and wrong. These excerpts are from three of his sessions.

During the prelude in an early session, J said that he had come to explore his early childhood. He had felt unsupported and unseen by his cold, critical parents, and he had let these feelings influence him all his life. To support the image of early childhood, the therapist offered an induction centered on a baby. The music chosen was a program that enables a person to explore the issues of nurturance. It contained simple structures and harmonies, repetition, little dissonance, and both male and female voices. J experienced the music as all that he did not receive as a baby. He felt that the music was giving him simultaneous but mixed messages to come and to disappear. At one point he felt like a baby rocking himself. In the postlude he noted that the music helped him express the pain he felt and the need to heal.

In a later session, working with the same issue, J explained that he was forced to play the piano when what he wanted to do was to dance. He was expected to be successful but was never good enough for his parents. They did not allow him to express his own personal needs. He was angry. He related that GIM allowed him to stop thinking so he could just feel. The induction centered on the rhythm of his breathing and how his body felt. The music chosen was strong, harmonically complex, and somewhat dense. The rhythms were insistent and powerful. During a piano concerto, he imagined playing the piano. As he played, he did not allow for any criticism of wrong notes. The intent was to freely make music. J experienced the notes of the piano as cold and hostile. He started to rebel against the image, his parents, and the music. He needed to be supported, to be heard in expressing his need. The therapist changed the music to a more supportive piece with gentler harmonies and rhythms. J responded by showing his parents what he needed from them. In the postlude, he admitted that he wanted the music changed but was afraid to ask, in fear that once again, he would not be heard. He felt it was a big step not to follow the music. It allowed him feel powerful, to fight for what he needed.

In this third example, J came to the prelude reporting that he was saying "no" more often; furthermore, it was not a childish "no," but one that was appropriately assertive and less fraught with anxiety. He was learning not to be perfect. The induction suggestion was to play as a child. The music chosen began with a piano piece, "Variations on a Nursery Theme," by Dohnányi. It is subtitled "For the enjoyment of humorous people and for the annoyance of others." Mozart also wrote variations on this same theme, "Twinkle, Twinkle Little Star." The client identified with the Mozart in his imagery, who was not playing the piano, just playing and laughing as a child and mocking the adults. An authority figure scolded J and told him to behave. The adult was furious. Still identifying with Mozart, J created a whole ballet, doing exactly as he wanted, allowing no one to control him. He then began to conduct the music. He ended the music portion of the session in the lap of a nurturing figure from his past, eating freshly baked cookies. In the postlude, with a big smile on his face, J said, "I really enjoyed that!"

Although this issue was not completely resolved, J had made much progress. He even fulfilled his wish to dance. The pain had lost its hold and the healing had begun.

Clinical Applications

The most common application for GIM is with healthy adults (McKinney, Antoni, Kumar, Tims, & McCabe, 1997) and those with nonpsychotic mental conditions such as mood or anxiety disorders (Körlin & Wrangsjö, 2002). Most people come to GIM to learn more productive and creative ways to live and to draw more fully and directly from an inner source of knowledge and inspiration. Others may come as a result of a situational crisis such as divorce, loss of a job, or loss of a loved one. Two experimental studies have demonstrated that GIM ameliorates depressed mood in healthy adults and normalizes levels of hormones associated with stress and disease (McKinney, Antoni, Kumar, & Kumar, 1995; McKinney et al., 1997).

CLINICAL EXAMPLE: Redefining Family-of-Origin Relationships

Laura was a professional woman in her early 30s who had married for the second time 2 months prior to the first session. Her parents had divorced when she was a child, and she had learned as an adult that her father was an alcoholic, a fact about which there continued to be substantial denial in the family. Her goals in GIM were to address issues related to her family of origin.

In her first session, to the music of Pierné's Concertstück for Harp and Orchestra, a small boy leads Laura through the woods. As they proceed, the path behind them disappears, and she feels sad. "It's something I've had to put behind me," she said. He leads her to a garden and communicates, without speaking, that he wants her to take care of it. "It's time, and you're the one," he silently tells her.

In the next session, she finds herself at her grandparents' house at Easter finding Easter eggs among the irises with the "Adagio" from Haydn's Cello Concerto in C. A heavy feeling comes to her chest. "It feels like a lump the size of a softball. Not hard, but heavy and gray." She describes the lump as "feeling alone, like I didn't matter, gray and abandoned." As she takes the music into the lump, she feels comforted and soothed. Later in the session she is at a cabin, when she becomes aware of someone approaching through the trees. At the same time, a pain, like a knot, is growing in her left shoulder. With the support of the "Largo ma non troppo" from Bach's Concerto for Two Violins, she notes that the pain "feels like responsibility, duty, or obligation. The more attention I give it, the tighter it gets. . . . It's like a jack with knobs and points."

At the time of her fourth session, Laura was apprehensive, anticipating a trip with her family of origin. As Bach's Passacaglia and Fugue in C Minor begins, Laura is at a point where two paths diverge. Her mother is with her and wants Laura to carry "some stuff" for her. She does not approve of Laura's plan to go down a different path. Laura describes the guilt she feels as a "yucky, brownish-green blob. It wraps itself around my shoulders and neck. . . . It feels heavy, stifling, thick, and opaque." She wants to rid herself of it, but does not know how.

As the fugue begins, it begins to rain, the blob slowly melts, and Laura initially feels sad for her mother, then angry that her mother wants to make her go her mother's way. Quickly, this anger changes to sympathy as she realizes, "She can't do it by herself." Laura is torn. She needs to go on her own path, yet feels the need to help her mother carry her load.

When the therapist asks, "Is there anything around that can help?" Laura becomes aware of a red wagon. To the slow, gentle strains of Stokowski's orchestration of Bach's chorale prelude, "Come, Sweet Death," she helps her mother load the "stuff" onto the wagon. Laura is ambivalent when her mother then wants to bring the wagon and come down Laura's path. "She doesn't want [the old pattern] to change," she says.

Laura acknowledges that she wants her mother to change, to be "grown up." As the "Adagio" from Brahms's Violin Concerto invites dialogue, she tells this to her mother, who cries, feeling shamed. Laura feels heaviness in her chest and tightness in her shoulders as she realizes that a bird is forming in her body. Its body is in her chest, and its wings spread across her shoulders.

As the "Largo ma no troppo" from Bach's Concerto for Two Violins begins, Laura says, "I know I have to let [the bird] go. It's going to carry away all desire to change my mother." As the bird takes flight, her attitude shifts. "I know I have to go on my path. If she wants to come along, she will; if she doesn't, she won't. I have to go on my own journey." As she starts down her path, Laura feels light, noticing emptiness in her chest, which begins to fill up with trees, stars, mountains, and sunsets. In the postlude to this session, Laura revealed that her desire for her mother to change was a new awareness gleaned from this session.

In only four sessions, Laura had gained insight into and begun to address issues arising from her relationships in her family of origin.

She had taken significant steps toward individuating from her mother and beginning to heal childhood wounds. She reported greater clarity about what was and was not her responsibility and increased assertiveness in responding to what she felt were unrealistic demands from her mother.

People in recovery from addiction or trauma are also reported to benefit from a series of individual GIM sessions. The creative process inherent in GIM allowed a woman with addictions to access and reconnect with lost aspects of herself (Pickett, 1991). Through the music, the client was able to explore her feelings of vulnerability, sadness, and low self-esteem. With hard work and sometimes painful honesty, she was able to remain drug free and begin to find new ways to deal with these emotions. She once again connected with and owned the gentle, positive parts of herself.

GIM has been shown to be a powerful method for addressing issues related to trauma. Several case studies have documented the effectiveness of GIM for resolving wounds stemming from childhood physical or sexual abuse (Bunt, 2011; Körlin, 2007–2008; Moffitt & Hall, 2003–2004; Ventre, 1994). In a study of 136 women receiving treatment with either GIM or psychodynamic imaginative trauma therapy, Maack (2012) found GIM to be highly effective in reducing dissociation and other symptoms of complex posttraumatic stress disorder (PTSD) in women in therapy for childhood abuse. Other therapists have reported that GIM is efficacious in recovering memories and alleviating symptoms resulting from war-induced PTSD (Blake & Bishop, 1994) and from traumatic brain injury (Pickett, 1996–1997).

CLINICAL EXAMPLE: Healing Wounds of Childhood Trauma

S, a woman in her 40s, came with a presenting issue of confusion about memories of sexual and physical abuse. Her stated goal was to gain access to those memories and feelings. She was aware of prolonged emotional and verbal abuse. She felt powerless, defensive, and untrusting. She had poor personal boundaries and difficulty maintaining relationships. Additional goals were to restore a sense of personal power, strength, and trust and to heal the wounds of the trauma.

S began to uncover, with startling clarity, long buried memories, including the physical and emotional feelings of early sexual abuse. She felt angry, sad, betrayed, and abandoned. S used the music to support her expression of these difficult feelings. She felt that the music was always there for her, never judging or abandoning her. She began, tentatively at first, to explore her body, her boundaries, her feelings, and eventually her sense of personal power.

This newfound strength and self-trust enabled S to explore and experience the memories and feelings that had brought her to GIM therapy. In early sessions, S experienced her sense of powerlessness, fear, and anger. In later sessions, she recovered memories of the verbal and emotional abuse and connected current physical symptoms with the sexual abuse.

Healing started to take place as S incorporated the trauma. During Vaughan Williams's "Fantasia on a Theme by Thomas Tallis," she encountered a girl whose body was deformed. In the following piece, Mahler's Symphony no. 4 ("Ruhevoll"), S was able to speak with the girl, who helped S understand what had really happened to her. In program notes that accompany the Mahler score, Redlich (1966) wrote, "The symphony's conceptual originality is based on the composer's successful identification with the soul of a child and its experience of seeking God and finding him at last" (p. 101).

In subsequent sessions, S learned to incorporate her "shadow," the darker elements of herself (Jung, von Franz, Henderson, Jacobi, & Jaffé, 1974). She cleansed the wounds from her past, acknowledged their effects, and moved on, stronger and more trusting in her own inner wisdom and ability to care for and nurture herself.

Several studies have documented the effectiveness of GIM for meeting the psychological needs of individuals with medical conditions. These studies have demonstrated that GIM not only affects the psychological status of individuals with health issues but may improve the physical state as well. These physical benefits include lowering both systolic and diastolic blood pressure in those with essential hypertension (McDonald, 1990), addressing the challenges of adjustment to pregnancy (Short, 1993), decreasing pain and number of affected joints and increasing walking speed in adults with rheumatoid arthritis (Jacobi & Eisenburg, 2001–2002), and improving quality of life in adults with cancer (Burns, 2001).

Individuals who have lost a loved one, as well as those who have received a terminal diagnosis, also have been found to benefit from GIM. Kirkland (2007–2008) found that GIM played a significant role in helping a mother transcend her sorrow by her *being with* the deceased child. Working with widowed persons, Creagh (2004) also found that GIM was effective in facilitating the mourning process. Other therapists have reported that GIM has assisted adults with terminal illness in resolving unfinished business, living fully while dying, and preparing for a peaceful death without fear (Cadrin, 2005–2006).

Modifications for Groups and Special Populations

GIM has been modified for a variety of situations, populations, and settings. Bonny (Bonny & Savary, 1973) described providing GIM experiences to groups of adults. Group sessions typically involve a shorter period of music, and group members engage in imagery in silence, sharing their experiences only after the music has ended. Others have modified the GIM procedure to meet the needs of children and adolescents (see Wesley, 2002, for a review),

people with various mental health issues (see numerous chapters in Eyre, 2013), and older adults in long-term care (Short, 2002). GIM can be modified to different venues and time frames, and may be called by a variety of names, such as group GIM or music and imagery, but the basic principles remain the same.

Conclusions

GIM evolved from the personal and scientific exploration of music and its ability to help people discover both the dark and the light, the depths and the heights of their psyches. It integrates the body, mind, and spirit through the wonder of music. It allows the healthiest, most creative, wisest part of individuals to expand and become the center from which they relate to themselves, to others, and to that which is beyond us all.

REFERENCES

Blake, R., & Bishop, S. R. (1994). The Bonny Method of Guided Imagery and Music (GIM) in the treatment of post-traumatic stress disorder (PTSD) with adults in the psychiatric setting. *Music Therapy Perspectives, 12,* 125–129.

Bonny, H. L. (1976). *Music and psychotherapy: A handbook and guide accompanied by eight music tapes to be used by practitioners of guided imagery and music.* Unpublished doctoral dissertation, Union Graduate School of the Union of Experimenting Colleges and Universities, Baltimore, MD.

Bonny, H. L. (1995). *The story of GIM: The beginnings of the Bonny method of guided imagery and music: As told by Helen L. Bonny* [Videorecording]. Blaine, WA: Association for Music and Imagery.

Bonny, H. L. (2002a). Autobiographical essay. In H. L. Bonny (L. Summer, Ed.), *Music and consciousness: The evolution of guided imagery and music* (pp. 1–18). Gilsum, NH: Barcelona.

Bonny, H. L. (2002b). Facilitating guided imagery and music (GIM) sessions. In H. L. Bonny (L. Summer, Ed.), *Music and consciousness: The evo-*

lution of guided imagery and music (pp. 269–297). Gilsum, NH: Barcelona. (Original work published 1978)

Bonny, H. L. (2002c). Guided imagery and music (GIM): Discovery of the method. In H. L. Bonny (L. Summer, Ed.) *Music and consciousness: The evolution of guided imagery and music* (pp. 42–52). Gilsum, NH: Barcelona.

Bonny, H. L. (2002d). *Music and consciousness: The evolution of guided imagery and music* (L. Summer, Ed.). Gilsum, NH: Barcelona.

Bonny, H. L. (2002e). The role of taped music programs in the guided imagery and music (GIM) process. In H. L. Bonny (L. Summer, Ed.), *Music and consciousness: The evolution of guided imagery and music* (pp. 299–324). Gilsum, NH: Barcelona. (Original work published 1978)

Bonny, H. L., & Savary, L. M. (1973). *Music and your mind: Listening with a new consciousness*. New York: Harper & Row.

Bruscia, K. E. (Ed.). (1998). *The dynamics of music psychotherapy*. Gilsum, NH: Barcelona.

Bruscia, K. E., & Grocke, D. E. (Eds.). (2002). *Guided imagery and music: The Bonny method and beyond*. Gilsum, NH: Barcelona.

Bunt, L. (2011). Bringing light into darkness: Guided imagery and music, bereavement, loss, and working through trauma. In A. Meadows (Ed.), *Developments in music therapy practice: Case perspectives* (pp. 501–517). Gilsum, NH: Barcelona.

Burns, D. (2001). The effect of the Bonny method of guided imagery and music on the mood and life quality of cancer patients. *Journal of Music Therapy, 38*, 51–65.

Cadrin, L. (2005–2006). Dying well: The Bonny method of guided imagery and music at the end of life. *Journal of the Association for Music and Imagery, 10*, 1–25.

Clarkson, G. (2002). Combining Gestalt dreamwork and the Bonny method. In K. E. Bruscia & D. E. Grocke (Eds.), *Guided imagery and music: The Bonny method and beyond* (pp. 245–256). Gilsum, NH: Barcelona.

Creagh, B. A. (2004). *Transformative mourning: The Bonny method of guided imagery and music for widowed persons*. Unpublished doctoral dissertation, Union Institute and University, Cincinnati, OH.

Eyre, L. (Ed.). (2013). *Guidelines for music therapy practice in mental health*. University Park, IL: Barcelona.

Grocke, D. E. (2002). The Bonny music programs. In K. E. Bruscia & D. E. Grocke (Eds.), *Guided imagery and music: The Bonny method and beyond* (pp. 99–133). Gilsum, NH: Barcelona.

Jacobi, E. M., & Eisenburg, G. M. (2001–2002). The efficacy of guided imagery and music (GIM) in the treatment of rheumatoid arthritis. *Journal of the Association for Music and Imagery, 8*, 57–74.

Jung, C. G., von Franz, M. L., Henderson, J. L., Jacobi, J., & Jaffé, A. (1974). *Man and his symbols*. New York: Dell.

Kasayka, R. (2002). A spiritual orientation to the Bonny method: To walk the mystical path on practical feet. In K. E. Bruscia & D. E. Grocke (Eds.), *Guided imagery and music: The Bonny method and beyond* (pp. 257–270). Gilsum, NH: Barcelona.

Kirkland, K. (2007–2008). Suffering and the sublime: A case study of music, metaphor, and meaning. *Journal of the Association for Music and Imagery, 11*, 17–38.

Körlin, D. (2007–2008). Music breathing: Breath grounding and modulation of the Bonny method of guided imagery and music (BMGIM): Theory, method, and consecutive cases. *Journal of the Association for Music and Imagery, 11*, 37–113.

Körlin, D., & Wrangsjö, B. (2002). Treatment effects in GIM. *Nordic Journal of Music Therapy, 11*(2), 3–12.

Lewis, K. (1998–1999). The Bonny method of GIM: Matrix for transpersonal experience. *Journal of the Association for Music and Imagery, 6*, 63–80.

Maack, C. (2012). *Outcomes and processes of the Bonny method of guided imagery and music (GIM) and its adaptations and psychodynamic imaginative trauma therapy (PITT) for women with complex PTSD*. Unpublished doctoral dissertation, Aalborg University, Aalborg, Denmark.

McDonald, R. G. (1990). *The efficacy of guided imagery and music as a strategy of self-concept and blood pressure change among adults with essential hypertension*. Unpublished doctoral dissertation, Walden University, Minneapolis, MN.

McKinney, C. H., Antoni, M. H., Kumar, A., & Kumar, M. (1995). The effects of guided imagery and music on depression and beta-endorphin levels. *Journal of the Association for Music and Imagery, 4*, 67–78.

McKinney, C. H., Antoni, M. H., Kumar, M., Tims, F. C., & McCabe, P. M. (1997). Effects of guided imagery and music (GIM) therapy on mood and cortisol in healthy adults. *Health Psychology, 16*, 1–12.

Moffitt, E., & Hall, A. (2003–2004). "New Grown with Pleasant Pain" (Keats): Recovering from sexual abuse with the use of the Bonny method of guided imagery and music and the use of poetry. *Journal of the Association for Music and Imagery, 9*, 59–77.

Pickett, E. (1991). Guided imagery and music (GIM) with a dually diagnosed woman having multiple addictions. In K. E. Bruscia (Ed.), *Case studies in music therapy* (pp. 497–512). Gilsum, NH: Barcelona.

Pickett, E. (1996–1997). Guided imagery and music in head trauma rehabilitation. *Journal of the Association for Music and Imagery, 5*, 51–59.

Redlich, H. (1966). *Program notes for G. Mahler, Symphony No. 4 (Ruhevoll)*. London: E. Eulenburg.

Short, A. E. (1993). GIM during pregnancy: Anticipation and resolution. *Journal of the Association for Music and Imagery, 2*, 73–86.

Short, A. E. (2002). Guided imagery and music in medical care. In K. E. Bruscia & D. E. Grocke (Eds.), *Guided imagery and music: The Bonny method and beyond* (pp. 151–170). Gilsum, NH: Barcelona.

Vaughan, F. (1991). Spiritual issues in psychotherapy. *Journal of Transpersonal Psychology, 23*(2), 105–119.

Ventre, M. E. (1994). Healing the wounds of childhood abuse: A guided imagery and music case study. *Music Therapy Perspectives, 12*, 98–104. [Errata in Vol. 13, p. 55]

Ventre, M. E. (2002). The individual form of the Bonny method of guided imagery and music. In K. E. Bruscia & D. E. Grocke (Eds.), *Guided imagery and music: The Bonny method and beyond* (pp. 29–35). Gilsum, NH: Barcelona.

Ward, K. M. (2002). A Jungian orientation to the Bonny method. In K. E. Bruscia & D. E. Grocke (Eds.), *Guided imagery and music: The Bonny method and beyond* (pp. 207–243). Gilsum, NH: Barcelona.

Wesley, S. B. (2002). Guided imagery and music with children and adolescents. In K. E. Bruscia & D. E. Grocke (Eds.), *Guided imagery and music: The Bonny method and beyond* (pp. 137–170). Gilsum, NH: Barcelona.

CHAPTER 17

Analytical Music Therapy

Benedikte B. Scheiby

Analytical Music Therapy (AMT) is an in-depth approach that combines music and psychoanalytic methods. The founder, Mary Priestley (1980), defines AMT as

> the symbolic use of improvised music by the therapist and client to explore the client's inner life and provide the proclivity for growth. Thus it does not aim directly at producing good experiences but rather at removing the blockages to further development, which may then allow them to happen in the way that best suits the client. (p. 18)

Priestley describes how, consciously or unconsciously, the client can use music to symbolize or connect with emotions, images, thoughts, or bodily sensations that cannot yet be verbalized. The music can symbolize or refer to something outside of itself. Symbols can create a bridge between the client's inner life and outer reality. Music can function to facilitate insight, to establish relationship, to maintain the flow of the session, and as a means of transformation for psychic material.

AMT is one of the major music therapy models currently taught worldwide. Music therapy clinicians, educators, and research-ers trained in AMT are working in Europe, the United States, Canada, Japan, and Israel.

History

AMT has been in use since the early 1970s. It was conceived and developed by Mary Priestley, Peter Wright, and Marjorie Wardle, three pioneers working as music therapy colleagues at St. Bernard's Hospital in London. They developed AMT through 96 self-experimentation sessions that they called *intertherapy*. Because Priestley took the leading role in describing the model in her book, *Music Therapy in Action* (1975), she is considered the founder of AMT.

Priestley was born in 1925 and is the daughter of the author J. B. Priestley. She studied violin, composition, and piano at the Royal College of Music (London) and the Geneva Conservatoire (Switzerland). In 1968 she began 10 years of Kleinian psychoanalysis with Dr. E. G. Wooster, to whom she attributes the greatest influence on her conceptualization of music therapy. In 1969, Priestley received her graduate music therapy degree (LGSM) from the Guildhall School of Music and Drama, London, with violin and piano as her main instruments. She then began working 2 days a week as a music therapist with individuals and groups with psychiatric problems at St. Bernard's Hospital in London. The rest of the week she had a private music therapy practice and conducted postgraduate AMT training for music therapists (I was one of her trainees). Priestley developed a specialized postgraduate AMT training program for music therapists based on her experiences in the intertherapy sessions with her colleagues and her work with patients. At the same time, she received Jungian analytical supervision for 11 years on her work with patients. She trained over 50 music therapists from 10 countries, many of whom are currently practicing and teaching her AMT approach.

Each music therapist undergoes individual AMT psychotherapy sessions, an important aspect of the AMT training program. Priestley believes that by directly experiencing the usefulness of the music therapy process, the trainee will be better able to understand the depth of the approach. Priestley was influenced by her experience with psychoanalytic training, where the psychoanalytic student is required to engage in psychoanalytic training for several years while learning clinical and theoretical fundamentals. Hadley (1998) quotes Priestley: "I thought that if they had to have their own analysis, then we should have our own music therapy, otherwise we don't understand the power of it. And I still think that way" (p. 27).

Priestley was an integral part of the teaching team at the first postgraduate AMT training program in Herdecke, Germany, where I first met her in 1979. There, AMT training consisted of individual and group AMT sessions, intertherapy training, and both individual and group AMT supervision. The experiences I had during my AMT training at Herdecke were deep and transformative. I have devoted my life to teaching AMT in academic settings and practicing as a clinician in various contexts: psychiatry (Scheiby, 1999, 2005), medicine (Scheiby, 2002a, 2013), palliative care (Scheiby, 2005; Stewart et al., 2005), with children (Scheiby, 1988), with people who have been through traumas (Scheiby, 2002b, 2010), and in education and supervision (Scheiby, 1998, 2001). In 1982, Inge N. Pedersen and I integrated AMT-inspired training elements as the basis for mandatory experiential training for all students in the 5-year full-time music therapy program at Aalborg University in Denmark. The program provides individual, group, and intertherapy music therapy education and supervision at the bachelor's and master's levels.

Theoretical Tenets

AMT is a synthesis of psychoanalytic theory and music therapy, drawing upon the theories of Sigmund Freud, Melanie Klein, Carl Jung, and in later work, from the psychoanalytic body psychotherapist Alexander Lowen. As AMT has developed in different ways, depending on the psychoanalytic training of the therapist, there are some variations in the theoretical tenets of AMT across practitioners. AMT involves the use of musical and verbal processing and expression of the client's work on issues, themes, resources, and challenges. Musical improvisation is the primary avenue for gaining insight from the unconscious and conscious layers of the psyche.

Hadley (2002) discussed influences on Priestley's work in three areas.[1] In the first area, *intrapersonal* concepts, Priestley's understanding of the self is shaped by the Freudian structural model that includes the *moral* superego, the *thinking* ego, and

---

[1] The material presented here about Priestley's reliance on concepts of Freud, Klein, and Jung is based on Hadley's (2002) analysis and summary of Priestley's original work (Priestley, 1975, 1994).

the *instinctual* id. The person is healthy and able to function well when these aspects of the personality are well balanced, but pathology, when present, suggests a lack of balance. Priestley believed that unconscious material could have detrimental effects and thus should be brought into consciousness, giving the person freedom in responding to situations. Improvised music was seen as the way into the unconscious. Priestley also understood from Klein that people have fragile egos that must be protected, and that one of the ways of protecting the ego is by splitting it into the good and bad parts of the mother. To be fully healthy, people must be aware of these projections and integrate them into the self. Priestley also came to believe in Jung's concept of the *shadow*, the part of the psyche that contains lost memories, impulses, and ideas that are not acceptable and therefore are repressed. She believed that the shadow must be acknowledged and accepted in order for the person to reach his or her fullest potential. The common point of these theories is that to function at the highest level, people must become aware of the unconscious aspects of themselves, deal with them, and integrate them into their awareness.

The second area of Priestley's work, *interpersonal* concepts, relates to the previous one in that unconscious aspects of a person are seen as influencing his or her functioning. Priestley believes that many problems in adult relationships stem from projections of unintegrated aspects of oneself onto other people. Therapy, then, involves breaking patterned responses to situations through corrective emotional experiences that are provided through AMT.

The third area, which Priestley calls the *ineffable* but Hadley (2002) says could be considered *transpersonal*, are moments "where our sense of time is altered and we stand still and wonder" (Hadley, p. 37). Priestley believes that these moments are products of the improvisation, but are not necessary for the therapy to take place.

AMT is also based on the work of psychoanalytic body psychotherapist Lowen. Priestley (1994, Essay 3) used Lowen's emotional spectrum as a way of mapping emotional function. The author and Pedersen (1989) drew upon Lowen's work in developing psychodynamic movement work, used as a basic training method to help sensitize music therapy students to their bodies' signals so that they can use personal body sensations and somatic awareness as pathways to understanding orientation, directions, forms, intensity, and transference–countertransference in the therapist–client relationship. Psychodynamic movement work helps people to connect to feelings and expressions and to recognize them through body sensations.

Music Therapy Applications

AMT Musical Techniques

A fundamental function of the music therapist is that of a highly skilled listener. The two basic guidelines are to (1) listen from a nonjudgmental stance and (2) pay attention to everything observable. Every aspect has meaning: the client's voice, the content of the narrative, body language, and the music. One listens beyond what is being played, sung, and spoken. The meanings that arise guide the choice of therapy techniques. In this context, a technique is defined as an intervention or action initiated by the music therapist. A technique is chosen to elicit a certain musical, bodily, or verbal/vocal response from the client or to shape the client's spontaneous musical experience. It can stand alone as an intervention strategy and can also be combined with other techniques. Whether or not to accompany the client musically is left to the music therapist's judgment, guided by what serves the client best. When not playing, the music therapist serves as an active listener. Priestley classified her techniques as individual techniques, techniques for dyads, and group techniques. Within each category four methodological objectives guide the technique: (1) exploration of conscious material, (2) accessing unconscious material, (3) strengthening the ego, and (4) accessing somatically internalized material.

Individual Techniques in the Exploration of Conscious Material

The techniques described in the following material are important components of individual AMT work:

- *Holding.* The music therapist holds or contains the client emotionally, providing a musical matrix that helps the client feel held, comparable to the image of a baby being held by a parent. This holding offers the client a safe, structured environment. Any musical parameter or musical form can be used as a holding structure: a rhythm, a repeated harmonic progression, a melodic motif, a pulse, a certain timbre, or a tonality. This technique also includes silences as part of the intervention and the music.

- *Splitting.* Based on Klein's (1932) concept of the infant's experience of the mother as having good and bad parts, this technique is used when the client seems to have many experiences that involve polarities and conflicts between opposing parts. It is particularly helpful when the client projects split parts of the self onto other persons. The goal is to resolve conflicts and opposing forces within the client and facilitate integration. For example, a client might often experience the victim role, as one abused by the mean abuser or attacker. With the help of the music therapist, the client can take turns in the music, experiencing both roles. With guidelines from the client, the music therapist plays the opposite role. Another client may often become trapped in a child–parent dynamic. To become aware of this pattern, the client can experience the different roles of being the child or the parent in music while the music therapist takes on the opposite role. Yet another client might sense imbalance in the way that his or her masculine and feminine sides manifest themselves psychologically. Through splitting, the client can experience either gender in the music, working toward integration of the masculine and feminine aspects in life.

- *Free association.* This technique is useful when the client is not yet able to verbalize his or her issues clearly. Repressed material in the form of images or emotions will often surface during improvisation. The music therapist's role is to musically accompany or reinforce what is heard. Encouraging a client to vocalize this uncensored material often opens up the ability to speak about that which was previously unspeakable.

- *Programmed or spontaneous regression.* The client is instructed to use the music to return, or perhaps spontaneously returns, to an earlier age in life when unresolved conflicts, traumas, or problematic events took place. The client now has an opportunity to relive challenges in music, together with the music therapist as a witness, and resolve them in a safe, creative context. The music therapist helps to establish the musical stage and provides the musical support for the client's emotional expression in the improvisation. Priestley speaks about the importance of connecting to the inner child. This technique is often used to help a client connect to the healthy part of that inner child.

- *Entering into somatic communication.* This technique is used when the client's emotions and conflicts are manifested in somatic symptoms. In this case, the client can improvise an experience of being the symptom, while the music therapist musically expresses the client's bypassed emotion.

Techniques for Dyads

Dyadic techniques can be used with couples, in work with two siblings, or with parent and child. Depending upon the couple's issues, the role of the music therapist is to invent improvisation themes and rules that help clients to work on and process the challenges that they experience. Priestley (1975) writes that the general aim and outcome of a joint session is "to preserve a partnership while the feelings about it are being explored and expressed, in such a way that growth and development can take place and another, more creative, relationship interaction may emerge" (p. 154). The needs of both parties should be identified at the beginning of the therapy. Often the challenge for couples is that one is not listening to what the other is saying or is misinterpreting what is being said or done. In this case, the music therapist can suggest musical dialogues in which the couple communicates through music, with the music therapist as a third ear and a witness. Sometimes improvisations between the couple and the music therapist can open up themes that have been previously unspoken. In the music, the music therapist might act as model for self-expression and show the couple how to verbally express how one feels in relation to the other. The music therapist might focus on the relational rhythms in the relationship. Is there a rhythm? A style of articulation? A tempo? Is it staccato? Is it too fast or too slow for the individuals? Have they forgotten to play and be creative together? Improvisations can take the form of a solo, a duet between partners, a duet between one partner and the music therapist, or a trio.

Group Techniques

Priestley (1994) defines the general work areas for group members as becoming aware of their feelings, expressing these feelings, identifying and establishing an identity, developing the ability to defend their identity in a group, and building skills in interpersonal relating. Techniques for individuals can be also used in a group setting. It is important to identify the goal of the group, as it will guide the music therapy interventions.

Generally, the leader introduces the members to the group's purpose, then each member articulates what he or she would personally like to work on. After this, group members start out improvising together, using the music to identify the themes for the session. Verbal processing follows the music, and it is up to the group members to decide how to move forward with the material that surfaces. The group leader facilitates identifying an improvisation title, image, or rule that addresses either the needs of the members or the need of one member.

At an intermediate stage of the group, the leader may need to facilitate group cohesion. For example, the music therapist might suggest that the whole group improvise about a certain image, such as the archetypal image of rain falling into a brook that turns into a river and eventually feeds into the sea, or he or she might suggest that the whole group start together in music and try to find a common rhythm or pulse. After the rhythm or pulse has been established, the music therapist invites pairs to play together in duos while the rest of the group listens. The improvisation concludes with everyone playing together.

Music therapists can also apply procedures and techniques in music that are drawn from verbal analytical group psychotherapies. Note, however, that the processing medium is improvised music rather than verbalization. For example, when one group member is sharing a dream, it can be processed musically. That group member may assign different roles or symbols in the dream to other group members to be expressed in music. The dream is processed chronologically in music. Although the dreamer is the solo player, some group members accompany the dreamer. Afterward the whole group processes the experience verbally. Groups can also be excellent media for family reenactments, using improvised music to work through projected family patterns and roles.

In sum, the group leader takes an analytical stance, waiting and letting the group members take charge and decide for themselves what is important to work on and letting them figure out, on their own, how the improvisation should be structured, how long or short it should be, and who takes which roles. The music therapist is trained to pick up key words or symbols/metaphors from the clients' verbalizations, and facilitate creative titles and ways to motivate the group members to start an improvisation. Sometimes there is no need for an agreed theme/issue/title. The group members may already begin to improvise and it will be up to the music therapist's clinical judgment to know if there is a need or no need for an agreed theme/issue/title. The title serves as a beginning structure/anchor/focus for the clients to start out with so they feel more secure when that is needed. For clients who have a tendency to intellectualize and be heady it might not be helpful to have a title to start out with as it encourages the clients to stay in their heads rather than listen more deeply to emotions and bodily sensations. The leader functions as a kind of translator, facilitating interpersonal and intrapersonal communication in the music.

Techniques for Accessing Unconscious Material in Individual Sessions, Dyads, and Groups

Access to unconscious material through music can be assisted by a focus on symbols, guided imagery, dream work, myths, and/or images that the client sees through the inner eye during playing and meditation. Insights from these types of interventions are then related to the material on which the client is working. Often, when improvising without a title, images come up to which clients cannot connect. These images can be material for further improvisations, to explore their connection and meaning. In work with clients who cannot or will not process verbally, visual art using drawing or clay (to indicate symbols emerging from the music) or bodily expression (e.g., psy-

chodynamic movement) can be used to process what is experienced in music.

Techniques for Strengthening the Ego in Individual Sessions, Dyads, and Groups

Many clients present with poor ego strength. The next techniques are intended to help the client develop greater ego control.

- *Reality rehearsal.* The client musically takes a step that is needed in his or her life (e.g., going to a job interview, moving away from parents, showing up for the first day of school). During the improvisation the client focuses on inner obstacles, fears, anxieties, ambivalences, or destructive urges that stand in the way.
- *Exploring relationships.* The client musically explores feelings related to significant persons in life, the music therapist, his or her partner, or other group members.
- *Affirmations and celebrations.* To prevent the client's dependency on approval, the music therapist rarely gives verbal affirmations. However, it is important to support the client in celebrating positive occurrences in life.
- *Subverbal communication.* The client and the music therapist improvise together without guidelines and do not engage in verbal processing before or after the music. This technique can be very useful when a client is verbally defensive, when words seem meaningless, or when there might be relationship challenges between the client and the music therapist.
- *Patterns of significance.* The client improvises on feelings in relation to significant events in his or her life such as a death, a birth, a marriage, or losses. The music therapist accompanies the client using the holding technique.
- *Programmed regression.* This technique helps the client access unexpressed feelings from the past, using the music to go back to a certain age in life. Insight might surface that explains certain behaviors, fears, and/or traumas.

Gathering Information and Setting Goals

I discourage my AMT trainees from examining the client's chart too intently before actually working with him or her, so that the clinical judgment of other team members does not taint their music therapy assessment. At the same time that Priestley (1975) suggests that music therapists should have general goals, she also states that there should be no goal at all.

> Any setting of an external aim for the client imposes a limitation on the therapy. In trying to achieve such an aim, valuable developments outside it will be passed by. . . . Even to have as an aim the removal of symptoms can be threatening to a client. . . . So from saying that there is one overriding aim to stating that there should be no aim at all, I will veer to the direction of believing that the client and therapist between them produce a mutual aim, with the therapist dominating the direction of the central work and the client that of the periphery. (pp. 194–195)

For persons with severe cognitive deficits (e.g., developmental disabilities, aphasia, traumatic brain injury, autism, coma), the working goal is derived from the client's musical/vocal and bodily communication, combined with team- or caretaker-defined goals set for the client.

Procedural Phases

Generally, each single AMT session can be understood as a cycle, as illustrated in Figure 17.1.

There is a good deal of flexibility in how the cyclic model is used. It can be repeated within the same session. There may be sessions where no words are exchanged and there is only music, or the opposite may occur. The entire session may be regarded as one long improvisation where what is needed in the moment takes priority over rules. A client might avoid playing or singing. This often occurs when the client has a tendency to intellectualize or might not want or be able to verbalize what just happened in the music. A description of the

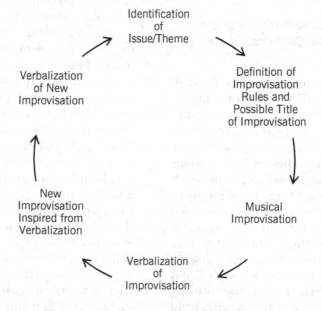

FIGURE 17.1. Procedural phases in AMT.

recommended methodological steps in a session follows.

Identification of Issue, Challenge, or Theme

The therapeutic focus can be a problem, concern, challenge, or an internal or external conflict with which the client is struggling. It can be a troubling emotion, a nightly dream, a fantasy, or a hallucination—anything intrapersonal or interpersonal on which the client wants to work. It can be about searching for resources. If something to work on does not readily come to mind, the music therapist and client can improvise together, with no title for a while, and receive help from the music. In the music, issues or themes often surface quickly and can be identified and used as work material.

Another way to access work material for the improvisations is to observe the client's body language. When working with nonverbal clients, body language or sounds are often the main cues for improvising. Which rhythms are present in the body? What is the tempo of the breathing? What emotional expression is in the face or eyes? Is the body tense, heavy, shaking, or seemingly lifeless? The client's postures and/or gestures can also provide cues.

After identifying an issue or theme, the client and music therapist agree upon an improvisation title that captures the essence of the client's issue or work focus. Developing a title that is suggestive enough to stimulate improvisation—but not so limiting or so fixed that it stops the process of bringing forth the client's feelings, associations, or insights—is an important aspect of the process. In work with high-functioning clients, it is important to let the client develop the title. The idea is to get the client to take responsibility rather than the therapist rescuing or taking over. Within the first 10 minutes of the session, what needs to be worked on has already presented itself, consciously or unconsciously and verbally or nonverbally.

Definition of Roles during Improvisation

In this step the client defines his or her own role and that of the music therapist, which helps the client take responsibility outside of the session for important decisions and choices that must be made in life. When roles are not clarified in the session it can cause confusion and make the client feel unsafe, both in the music and in the verbal processing. The music therapist asks direct questions about his or her role in the improvisations. For example: "Shall I play with you or be an active listener?" "Shall I reinforce your sounds or just play what comes to my mind?" If parts of a dream are being musically dramatized and reexperienced, certain symbols might be delegated to the music therapist or to the client. At times, defined roles are not needed in an improvisation processing a dream. That may be when the client is expressing the need to free associate and see what comes up. It may also be when a client has the need to work with the ability to deal with the unknown and with uncertainties in life.

Improvising the Title

In this phase the client improvises according to the title or theme and the agreed-upon role, with or without the music therapist. Here it is important to pay attention to which instruments are selected: percussion, wind, string, vocal; the instruments' sizes; and/or their material of metal or wood. Where and how are they arranged: close to or distant from the client? Can the client make eye contact with the music therapist? Is the client hiding behind the instruments? Does the client use the instruments the music therapist selected? How does the client use the instruments and/or the voice? Does the client use the same instruments in each session or pick different ones from session to session? Does the client move while playing or singing?

These observations are part of a music therapy assessment and are based on listening to the qualities of the musical elements. These elements can be categorized as affective, relational, developmental, cognitive, kinesthetic, creative, energetic, aesthetic, spiritual, and imaginative. The first step is to identify and describe the use of parameters: rhythm, melody, harmony, tempo, phrasing, themes or motifs, dynamics, choice and use of instruments and voice, musical idioms, range, articulation, and timbre. This musical information is combined with other sources such as verbal information and the client's diagnosis, history, cultural context, processed themes or issues, the place of the session in the treatment cycle, and client-expressed treatment goals. All these areas can provide information for an accurate assessment on which to base goals and objectives. This articulation of goals represents a departure from Priestley's writings. Yet in actual practice she incorporated some goal-oriented thinking. The client's own verbal and nonverbal comments related to the music take priority in the assessment process. During playing or singing, the music therapist automatically does some analysis of the improvised music, at an internal level. I discussed additional issues surrounding AMT assessment in a previous work (Scheiby, 2002b).

Verbalization Phase (Translating Music into Words)

The AMT philosophy is that verbalization is useful because it helps integrate the nonverbal musical and bodily experiences with cognition. If feeling states remain out of consciousness, behavior may remain impulsive and disconnected from the self. Verbalization can facilitate the building of a bridge between intrapersonal and interpersonal experiences gained during the playing, vocalization, or movement. Verbalization can enhance congruence between inner and outer realities and help clients identify emotions and understand the deep roots of those emotions. Verbal identification of musical patterns can help clients

gain insight into life or behavioral patterns that they are interested in changing.

Training

I developed a 4-year postgraduate AMT training program based upon the advanced training that I received from Mary Priestley. The first year provides individual AMT therapy to the trainees so they can work with their challenges, resources, images, dreams, needs, ambitions, and emotions. An account on the personal experience and professional impact of this first phase of training, from the perspective of an AMT trainee, has been documented by Abrams (2013). The second year is devoted to inter-therapy training, renamed *inter music therapy* (IMT). The third year is devoted to individual AMT supervision, and the fourth year to group AMT supervision. The individual and group AMT supervision training components are based on the trainees' work with clients. Supervision is provided through musical or verbal processing and is based on the material that trainees bring to supervision. The theoretical part of the training consists of log writing and readings that relate to the trainees' work with their current clients. A list of AMT literature is given to the trainees to ensure their familiarity with this literature base. They are encouraged to publish articles and give presentations to help them become comfortable communicating about their work method. Once they have finished the training, they are expected to continue to receive music therapy supervision on a weekly basis from an experienced analytical music therapist.

Examples from AMT Practitioners

AMT is currently practiced in Europe, the United States, Canada, Israel, and Japan with the following populations and contexts: adult, adolescent, and child psychiatry; medical hospitals and rehabilitation facilities; special education for children; mentally challenged adults; hospice and palliative care; adults, adolescents, children and couples in private practice; forensic populations; adolescents in psychiatric day treatment programs; wellness, growth, and prevention; community music therapy; and music therapy students and supervisees. The examples that follow are drawn from personal communications with two practicing AMT music therapists, one from individual supervision and the other from work in a psychiatric hospital.

AMT Individual Supervision

In AMT supervision, any theme or issue is processed musically or through visual art or bodily expression. Suzannah Scott-Moncrieff, an AMT supervisee and self-employed music therapist, shares her experience using live improvised music in AMT supervision (S. Scott-Moncrieff, personal communication, June 30, 2012). She says that the musical interventions during supervision may not always be "holding or reflecting" but can also be "bold and confronting." When we play together, the music often helps her imagine a braver version of herself as a clinician. In music therapy with her clients, she easily utilizes the well-developed, supportive musical interventions she has experienced in supervision. It is sometimes challenging when the music of her supervisor is different from her own, but that reminds her that she can allow herself to be that way with her clients, too. Using live, improvised music in supervision can release playfulness and spontaneity. She has taken this lightness into her own clinical work by allowing her playfulness to shine with her clients. The music created in supervision sessions allows her to be in her "clients' shoes," as well as deeper in her "own shoes as a music therapist." It continues to be a vital way of keeping her clinical work "fresh and music-centered."

AMT Group Music Therapy in Psychiatry

Audrey Morse (personal communication, January 29, 2013) conducts five types of AMT music therapy groups at a psychiatric hospital: a drum circle group, a musical relaxation group involving improvisation and body awareness, a songwriting group, and two listening groups. She explains: "AMT aspects of my work are apparent in the connections I help patients achieve between music and other aspects of their lives, and in symbolic musical communication with patients who have impaired verbal communication (e.g., due to psychosis or mood disorders)." Tolerance of individual expression in AMT group therapy is a necessity. An analytically informed group goal is the achievement of the ability to tolerate and accept "musical disorganization," as these two qualities help clients tolerate and accept living with the symptoms of psychiatric illness. The groups are a mix of patients with high and low cognitive functioning. At the beginning of Audrey Morse's groups, each patient chooses an instrument from a selection in the middle of the room. The initial musical selection functions as an assessment tool, particularly with regard to the patient's rhythmic organization and interpersonal relational abilities. Throughout the session group members are encouraged to communicate feelings through instruments or vocalization. Emphasizing musical communication creates a setting wherein patients can learn to manage themselves in a nonverbal way. In drum circle groups the music assessment is kept brief so the group can focus on giving each member a turn being the musical leader. "The leadership experience allows for the experience of empowerment, of being in control of the situation, and crucially of being heard, so members feel that what they communicate has importance."

Research

In addition to a variety of reconstructive case studies describing AMT individual and group music therapy interventions and significant outcomes (e.g., see also Kowski, 2003; Pedersen, 2002, 2003), a number of qualitative research studies and one quantitative research study have been conducted, and two mixed methods studies are in process.

Qualitative research includes Auf der Heyde's (2012) study of interpersonal rhythms in the AMT treatment of a client with a history of cumulative trauma, exploring whether and how rhythmic interactions within musical improvisations could facilitate the repair of ruptures in such rhythms. Her close rhythmic analysis of improvised interactions can help music therapists assess clients' level of trauma and tailor interventions to move them out of the repetitious rhythms of hyper- and hypoarousal.

Cooper (2011) used archival material from Priestley's work, housed at Temple University (*www.temple.edu/musictherapy/home/dbs/amt_priestley.htm*), to examine how Priestley musically implemented AMT techniques for exploring conscious material, accessing unconscious material, and strengthening the ego. The results of the study present clinical considerations necessary for applying each AMT technique and the clinical/musical goals of the analytical music therapist.

Pedersen (2007) conducted a phenomenological study on countertransference used as a clinical concept by interviewing four music therapists working with musical improvisation in adult psychiatry. Among several findings, she reported that (1) countertransference experiences emerge as a moment of surprise; (2) the therapist–patient relationship is a main tool in working with severe mentally ill patients; (3) music therapists are very present in countertransference experiences; and (4) the act of simultaneously playing music helps music therapists remain present.

Eyre (2007) used Bruscia's (1987) Improvisation Assessment Profiles in a reconstructive case study in which she analyzed improvisations during the course of five individual sessions that Priestley had held with a patient with schizophrenia. Eyre sought to document whether significant changes occurred and how these changes were manifested in the client's images, life events, and music improvisations.

Through a multimodal phenomenological inquiry Hadley (2001) showed that AMT is linked to and reflects many of Priestley's actual *lived* biographical contexts and experiences. Hadley's work emphasizes that Priestley's unique approach to music therapy developed out of her personal context.

Kim (2013), in a case study, examined group music therapy work with six older Korean immigrant women residing in New York City. The women received weekly group music therapy sessions for a 6-month period. The method was strongly influenced by AMT, as Kim is trained in that method. With each client belonging to four major subculture groups (Korean, immigrant, older adult, and female), attention was directed to the impact of these subcultures on group dynamics and the therapeutic process. The study addressed the assessment, treatment, and evaluation of the group music therapy process. Data were analyzed using a variety of qualitative methods. Based on the findings of the study, the author suggested that music therapists should take into account cultural considerations and the gender roles of their clients to better serve them.

Langenberg and her colleagues (Langenberg, Frommer, & Tress, 1993) conducted many studies on AMT; for example, they employed a qualitative hermeneutic research approach to investigate and describe how the phenomenon of the *resonator function* can operate to create meaning in clinical improvisations in an AMT-informed music therapy context. They found that the resonator function occurs in a number of contexts, providing evidence that the therapist can resonate with the music of the client/improviser. In additional studies, Mahns (1998) studied the meaning of improvisation in music therapy with school children in a study of symbol development in AMT with children; and Marom (2004) conducted a qualitative inquiry into the spiritual experiences of music therapists, including an AMT-trained music therapist conducting hospice care.

One quantitative study, a randomized controlled trial (RCT; Scheiby et al., 1999), focused on how group music therapy with patients with early- or middle-stage dementia can affect levels of depression, anxiety, agitation, and quality of life. I practiced the AMT group music therapy method in the study. The outcome demonstrated a significant decrease in levels of depression, anxiety, and agitation and a significant improvement in quality of life for the group music therapy participants.

I am currently conducting a small mixed methods study examining the effect of AMT group music therapy interventions on levels of anxiety and motivation with patients recovering from medical traumas. My hypothesis is that during music psychotherapy treatment, neural networks that will eventually help in recovery from medical and psychological trauma are built and reinforced. A portable brain scanner is under development for the purpose of collecting quantitative data in relation to self-directed neuroplasticity during and after AMT treatment. Figure 17.2 shows a client in AMT with a headset that collects data, and Figure 17.3 shows incoming data from the headset. The therapeutic environment and instrument selection are consistent, and the same room is used for every session. An appropriate selection of acoustic and musical instrument digital interface (MIDI)-based instruments for AMT is available, including Sound Beam (an interactive MIDI hardware and software system) and an iPad 2. Another mixed methods research study I am conducting is examining the effect of AMT supervision, making use of the same quantitative measurement instrument as well as qualitative measures.

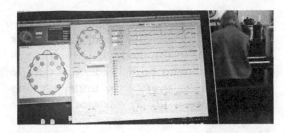

FIGURE 17.3. Incoming data from the headset.

Conclusions

AMT is a form of psychodynamic music therapy in which the primary agent of change is the improvised music in combination with verbal processing, if the client is able to verbalize. AMT is founded on the belief that improvised music making in the context of the therapeutic relationship between client and music therapist can release what is stored in the unconscious and facilitate change. Searching for meaning is essential, and the primary goal is the facilitation of integration between unconscious and conscious; among body, mind, and spirit; between past and present; as well as integrating what is expressed and experienced emotionally in music with the cognitive and spiritual levels of awareness. The AMT approach can be applied to a variety of clients and in a variety of contexts.

Training in AMT occurs at an advanced academic level and involves individual and group music therapy self-analysis as well as direct and indirect individual and group supervision, where processing in music is essential. Developing psychotherapeutic skills; improvisatory skills, using a multitude of idioms in both tonal and atonal expressive resources; and self-experiential

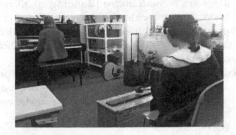

FIGURE 17.2. A client in AMT with a headset that collects data.

training with an AMT-trained MT are mandatory. Audio- or videotaping the sessions is important to the method, as the recordings can be used both inside and outside the sessions to deepen the understanding of the process. Often, the work includes body movement and/or expression through visual art in conjunction with the music.

The road to the unconscious is through improvised music. An AMT therapist understands that the client's unconscious has an impact on the music therapist's unconscious. Therefore, both musical and extramusical transference and countertransference phenomena are sources of information and navigation tools for the music therapist. Numerous instruments are needed so the client can choose an instrument that has the sound and material that appeals to him or her in the moment. Both the instruments and the improvised music are often used as transitional objects or projection tools.

ACKNOWLEDGMENT

I wish to thank Katie Colton for assistance in editing.

REFERENCES

Abrams, B. (2013). A perspective on the role of personal therapy in analytical music therapy training. In K. E. Bruscia (Ed.), *Self-experiences in music therapy education, training, and supervision* (pp. 304–314). Gilsum, NH: Barcelona.

Auf der Heyde, T. M. C. (2012). *Interpersonal rhythms disrupted by a history of trauma: An in-depth case study of analytical music therapy* (Doctoral dissertation, City University of New York). ProQuest, UMI Dissertations Publishing, 3499217.

Bruscia, K. E. (1987). *Improvisational models of music therapy*. Springfield, IL: Charles C Thomas.

Cooper, M. L. (2011). *A musical analysis of how Mary Priestley implemented the techniques she developed for analytical music therapy* (Doctoral dissertation, Temple University, Philadelphia). ProQuest, UMI Dissertations Publishing, 3509047.

Eyre, L. (2007). Changes in images, life events and music in analytical music therapy: A reconstruc-

tion of Mary Priestley's case study of "Curtis." *Qualitative Inquiries in Music Therapy, 3*, 1–31.

Hadley, S. (1998). Exploring relationships between life and work in music therapy: The stories of Mary Priestley and Clive Robbins (Doctoral dissertation, Temple University, Philadelphia). *Dissertation Abstracts International, 59*(10), 3690A.

Hadley, S. (2001). Exploring relationships between Mary Priestley's life and work. *Nordic Journal of Music Therapy, 10*(2), 116–131.

Hadley, S. (2002). Theoretical bases of analytical music therapy. In J. T. Eschen (Ed.), *Analytical music therapy* (pp. 34–48). London: Jessica Kingsley.

Kim, S. A. (2013). Re-discovering voice: Korean immigrant women in group music therapy. *Arts in Psychotherapy, 40*, 428–435.

Klein, M. (1932). *The psycho-analysis of children.* London: Hogarth Press.

Kowski, J. (2003). Growing up alone: AMT therapy with children of parents treated within a drug and substance abuse program. In S. Hadley (Ed.), *Psychodynamic music therapy: Case studies* (pp. 87–104). Gilsum, NH: Barcelona.

Langenberg, M., Frommer, J., & Tress, W. (1993). A qualitative research approach to analytical music therapy. *Music Therapy, 12*(1), 59–84.

Mahns, W. (1998). *Symbolbildungen in der analytischen Kindermusiktherapie: Eine qualitative Studie über die Bedeutung der musikalischen Improvisation in der Musiktherapie mit Schulkindern* [Symbol development in analytical music therapy with children: A qualitative study of the meaning of improvisation in music therapy with school children]. Unpublished doctoral dissertation, Aalborg University, Aalborg, Denmark.

Marom, M. K. (2004). Spiritual moments in music therapy: A qualitative study of the music therapist's experience. *Qualitative Inquiries in Music Therapy, 1*, 37–76.

Pedersen, I. N. (2002). *Opbygning af alliance. Musikterapi med en teenagepige fra børnepsykiatrien med diagnosen infantile autism* [Building up alliance: Music therapy with a teenage girl from child psychiatry with diagnosis of infantile autism]. *Musikterapi I Psykiatrien. Årsskrift 3.* Aalborg: Musikterapiklinikken 7–21.

Pedersen, I. N. (2003). The revival of the frozen sea urchin: Music therapy with a psychiatric patient. In S. Hadley (Ed.), *Psychodynamic music therapy: Case studies* (pp. 375–388). Gilsum, NH: Barcelona.

Pedersen, I. N. (2007). *Countertransference in music therapy: A phenomenological study on countertransference used as a clinical concept by music therapists working with musical improvisation in adult psychiatry* (Doctoral dissertation, Aalborg University, Aalborg, Denmark). Retrieved from *www.mt-phd. aau.dk/phd-theses/Alfabetical+list+of+PhD+theses.*

Priestley, M. (1975). *Music therapy in action.* London: Constable.

Priestley, M. (1980). *The Herdecke analytical music therapy lectures* [Analytische Musiktherapie] (B. Stein, Trans.). Stuttgart, Germany: Klett-Cotta.

Priestley, M. (1994). *Essays on analytical music therapy.* Gilsum, NH: Barcelona.

Scheiby, B. B. (1988). *Musikterapi: psykoterapi som kunstnerisk erkendelsesmetode og akademisk disciplin* [Music therapy: Psychotherapy as artistic method of insight and academic discipline]. *Matrix, Journal for Psychotherapy, 5*(3), 37–84.

Scheiby, B. B. (1998). The role of musical countertransference in analytical music therapy. In K. E. Bruscia (Ed.), *The dynamics of music psychotherapy* (pp. 213–247). Gilsum, NH: Barcelona.

Scheiby, B. B. (1999). Music as symbolic expression: Analytical music therapy. In D. J. Wiener (Ed.), *Beyond talk therapy* (pp. 263–285). Washington, DC: American Psychological Association.

Scheiby, B. B. (2001). Forming an identity as a music psychotherapist through analytical music therapy supervision. In M. Forinash (Ed.), *Music therapy supervision* (pp. 299–335). Gilsum, NH: Barcelona.

Scheiby, B. B. (2002a). Improvisation as a musical healing tool and life approach: Theoretical and clinical applications of analytical music therapy improvisation in a short- and long-term rehabilitation facility. In J. T. Eschen (Ed.), *Analytical music therapy* (pp. 115–153). London: Jessica Kingsley.

Scheiby, B. B. (2002b). Caring for the caregiver: Trauma training in music and transfer of terror into meaning through community music therapy training. In J. V. Loewy & A. F. Hara (Eds.), *Caring for the caregiver: The use of music and music therapy in grief and trauma* (pp. 92–105). Silver Spring, MD: American Music Therapy Association.

Scheiby, B. B. (2005). An intersubjective approach to music therapy: Identification and processing of musical countertransference in music psychotherapeutic context. *Music Therapy Perspectives, 23,* 8–17. Audio excerpts to accompany the article available at *www.wmich.edu/musictherapy/ mtp.html.*

Scheiby, B. B. (2010). Analytical music therapy and integrative medicine: The impact of medical trauma on the psyche. In K. Stewart (Ed.), *Music therapy and trauma: Bridging theory and clinical practice* (pp. 74–87). New York: Satchnote Press.

Scheiby, B. B. (2013). Analytical music therapy for pain management and reinforcement of self-directed neuroplasticity in patients recovering from medical trauma. In J. Mondanaro & G. Sara (Eds.), *Music and medicine: Integrative models in pain medicine* (pp. 149–179). New York: Satchnote Press.

Scheiby, B. B., & Pedersen, I. N. (1989). *Psychodynamische Bewegung innerhalb eines musiktherapeutischen Konzepts* [Psychodynamic movement in a music therapeutic context]. In H.-H. Decker-Voigt (Ed.), *Diplom-Aufbaustudium Musiktherapie, 3* (pp. 70–74). Lilienthal/Bremen, Germany: Eres.

Scheiby, B. B., Tomaino, C., Ramsey, D., Asmussen, S. M., Shah, V., & Goldstein, A. (1999). *The effects of a music therapy intervention on the levels of depression, anxiety/agitation, and quality of life experienced by individuals diagnosed with early and middle stage dementias: A controlled study.* Unpublished document, Institute for Music and Neurologic Function, Beth Abraham Health Services, Bronx, NY.

Stewart, K., Silberman, R. J., Loewy, J., Schneider, S., Scheiby, B. B., Scott-Moncrieff, S., et al. (2005). The role of music therapy in care for the caregivers of the terminally ill. In C. Dileo & J. V. Loewy (Eds.), *Music therapy at the end of life* (pp. 239–250). Cherry Hill, NJ: Jeffrey Books.

CHAPTER 18

Neurologic Music Therapy

Corene P. Hurt-Thaut
Sarah B. Johnson

Music has always been recognized for the powerful and therapeutic effects that it can have on human behavior across cultures. In 1950 the profession of music therapy was established to formalize the use of music as a therapeutic tool. Although many years of clinical outcome research have demonstrated the therapeutic effects of music on various populations, insufficient understanding of basic mechanisms involved in the perception and performance of musical tasks has often made it difficult to reproduce functional, goal-oriented, therapeutic applications of music with consistent results. At a training session in 1999 Michael Thaut introduced Neurologic Music Therapy (NMT) as a research-based system of standardized clinical techniques, based on diagnostics and functional goals of individual patients, which use music for sensorimotor, speech and language, and cognitive training. Because the clinical applications in NMT are based on current basic science and clinical research, NMT techniques result in consistent and functional results.

Thaut believed that in order to rationally translate musical experiences into therapeutic experiences, the following question needed to be answered first: What are the mechanisms through which music psychologically and physiologically influences human behavior in a therapeutically meaningful and predictable way? Music therapists have often tried to answer this complex question by conducting clinical outcome research studies to validate and quantify the effects of music in therapy. Unfortunately, outcome research does not tell a therapist how to translate music into therapy, which is the prerequisite for good music therapy research and clinical practice. Thaut (2000) suggested that growth of the scientific and medical acceptance of music therapy would depend on the development of a model that (1) explains the therapeutic effect of music on behavior, based on scientific evidence; (2) provides the framework to systematically and creatively transform a musical response into a therapeutic response; and (3) leads to the development of a systematic clinical methodology to select applications and predict the therapeutic outcome and benefits of music in therapy. The research conducted by Thaut and the research team of the Center for Biomedical Research in Music in Fort Collins, CO, combined with research done by neuroscientists and therapists around the world, has helped to clarify the answers to his questions. This scientific groundwork, in conjunction with collaborative work between music therapists and other therapeutic professionals in the clinical setting, has led to what is today known as NMT, with current information available at *www.nmtacademy.co.*

History

In 1968 Gaston identified an important concept that forms the foundation of music in therapy. He spoke of "the unique potential of rhythm to energize and bring order" (p. 17). In 1991 Thaut and his research team at Colorado State University published the first in a series of research papers that would become the foundation for investigating just how important rhythm is for movement of both the upper and lower extremities in normal and neurologically impaired individuals. Thaut, Schleiffers, and Davis (1991) investigated auditory rhythm as a timekeeper to modify the onset, duration, and variability of electromyographic (EMG) patterns in the biceps and triceps during the performance of a gross motor task. The results revealed a decreased variability in muscle activity during a motor task, with auditory rhythm indicating a more efficient use of the muscles, which could lead to a patient's ability to perform a task with more accuracy and for a longer period of time.

A similar study by Thaut, McIntosh, Prassas, and Rice (1992) investigated the effect of auditory rhythm on temporal parameters of the stride cycle and EMG activity in normal gait. In the rhythmic condition, subjects improved stride rhythmicity between the right and left lower extremities,

showed delayed onset and shorter duration of gastrocnemius muscle activity, and increased integrated amplitude ratios for the gastrocnemius muscle. These results provided evidence that more focused and consistent muscle activity occurs during push-off when a rhythmic auditory cue is present, due to a priming effect that results in a more efficient recruitment of motor units in the spinal cord. The conclusions of this study led to the further exploration of the effect of rhythmic auditory cuing on temporal stride parameters and EMG patterns in patients with hemiparetic gait due to a stroke, which also demonstrated similar results (Thaut, Rice, McIntosh, & Prassas, 1993).

Basic science and clinical research supporting the use of music in the rehabilitation of movement of both the upper and lower extremities with many different types of neurologic disorders have continued to grow over the last 20 years. Recent studies investigating the effects of rhythmic auditory stimulation on gait with Parkinson's disease (de Dreu, van der Wilk, Poppe, Kwakkel, & van Wegen, 2012; Kadivar, Corcos, Foto, & Hondzinski, 2011), traumatic brain injury (Hurt, Rice, McIntosh, & Thaut, 1998), multiple sclerosis (Baram & Miller, 2007; Conklyn et al., 2010), spinal cord injuries (de l'Etoile, 2008), and spastic diplegic cerebral palsy (Baram & Lenger, 2012; Kim et al., 2011) continue to show the significant impact of rhythm on gait kinematics through better posture, more appropriate step rates (step cadence) and stride length, and more efficient and symmetric muscle activation patterns in the lower extremities during walking. A Cochrane review of music therapy for acquired brain injury (Bradt, Magee, Dileo, Wheeler, & McGilloway, 2010) suggested that rhythmic auditory stimulation may be beneficial for improving gait parameters in patients with stroke, including gait velocity, cadence, stride length, and gait symmetry, with these conclusions based on studies of rhythmic auditory stimulation, an NMT technique.

Theoretical Tenets

The *rational scientific mediating model* (R-SMM) explores the premise that the scientific basis of music therapy is found in the neurological, physiological, and psychological foundations of music perception and music production and the influence of music on functional changes in nonmusical brain and behavior function (Thaut, 2000). The R-SMM was designed to promote understanding of how brain systems perceive, respond, and relate to music in order to build a meaningful connection between musical and nonmusical behaviors. Only when this connection is made can music be translated into consistent therapeutic applications. The R-SMM is comprised of four steps that are necessary to develop a valid model of music in therapy that will consistently modify behaviors in the cognitive, affective, and sensorimotor domains:

- Step 1, *musical response models*, requires basic science research, which can help us understand music as an aesthetic object in which psychological and physiological responses are elicited through the perception and performance of musical stimuli. Berlyne (1971) identified the central nervous system as an arousal-seeking system that seeks aesthetic input to satisfy the senses. Since music is an aesthetic object, it can be used as a mediator in the therapeutic process as a supplementary response that simulates a desired response in areas of cognition, affect, and motor performance. Psychological, collative, and ecological properties of music stimuli provide a structure that can help focus attention, increase motivation, and excite the senses, thereby meeting arousal needs.

Example: Thaut, Rice, and McIntosh (1997) reported that when moving to a rhythmic auditory cue, an individual's time stability is enhanced by rhythmic synchronization throughout the whole duration and trajectory of the movement, not just at the end points of the movement coincidental with the rhythmic beat. Therefore, when we move to music, we do not move *on* the beat, but we scale our movement *between* the beats.

- Step 2, *nonmusical parallel models*, involves identifying processes in nonmusical brain and behavior function and doing basic science research to investigate whether there are similar processes involved in musical and nonmusical perception and behaviors that are of therapeutic interest. The question that is answered in this step is whether there are parallels between affective, cognitive, and sensorimotor processes in musical and nonmusical behavior and perception.

Example: Walking is an intrinsically rhythmic movement that is based not only on the end goal for the movement but on the kinematic pattern or motion that occurs between the end points of the movement.

- Step 3, *mediating models*, involves the development of mediating models based on the similarities and parallels identified in step 2 in the affective, cognitive, and sensorimotor domains. The goal of these mediating models is to provide good theory and rationales for building future research hypotheses that would facilitate subsequent study of the therapeutically meaningful influence of music on behavior and brain function (Thaut, 2000).

Example: Thaut et al. (1992) investigated the effect of an auditory rhythmic stimulus on muscle activity and stride in normal gait and found that the rhythmic cuing (1) resulted in improved stride rhythmicity between the right and left lower extremities, (2) showed delayed onset and shorter duration of gastrocnemius muscle activity, and (3) increased integrated amplitude ratios for the gastrocnemius muscle.

- Step 4, *clinical research models*, explores whether there is research evidence that supports the use of music with clinical populations. Through good clinical research, solid clinical techniques can be developed which produce consistent outcomes when used in therapy.

Example: Research with a variety of neurologic disorders, including traumatic brain injury (Hurt et al., 1998), Parkinson's disease (McIntosh, Brown, Rice, & Thaut, 1997), stroke (Thaut et al., 1993), cerebral palsy (Thaut, Hurt, Dragan, & McIntosh, 1998), and Huntington's disease (Thaut, 2005), has provided substantial evidence for the use of rhythmic auditory stimulation as an effective tool in the rehabilitation of gait.

Over the past 20 years, basic science and clinical research have answered many of the questions in all of the steps of the R-SMM related to the use of therapeutic music applications for sensorimotor, speech and communication, cognitive, and socioemotional rehabilitation. The second step in the R-SMM has been particularly important in predicting major findings in brain research in music, related to neural systems in music processing mediating general nonmusical cognitive, motor, and language function. Today, many music therapy university programs make the R-SMM an integral part of their teaching to help students understand what is going on in the brain when it engages in musical and nonmusical tasks, and ultimately to better understand how music can be used in therapy to produce consistent results based on standards of best practice.

When reviewing the ideas of the early music therapy pioneers, many connections can be made to the R-SMM, including the music therapy course titles in the first academic music therapy programs in the United States:

- Foundations of Music in Therapy (addresses step 1)
- Psychology of Music (steps 1 and 2)
- Influence of Music on Human Behavior (step 3)
- Music in Therapy (step 4)

Music Therapy Applications

NMT is the therapeutic application of music to cognitive, sensory, and motor dysfunctions due to neurological disease of the human nervous system. When many people think of NMT, they think of typical neurological rehabilitation patients with conditions such as cerebral vascular accidents (CVAs), traumatic brain injury, and Parkinson's disease. However, NMT is not limited to these groups of clientele but encompasses neurological rehabilitation and neuropediatric, neuropsychiatric, neurogeriatric, and neurodevelopmental therapy. Therapeutic goals and interventions address rehabilitation, development, and maintenance of functional behaviors (Thaut, 2005).

NMT is a research-based system of 20 standardized clinical techniques for sensorimotor, speech and language, and cognitive training. Treatment selection is based on the diagnostics and functional goals of each individual patient. Although a therapist often addresses several functional goals during a session, each goal is addressed through a separate therapeutic music intervention based on the standardized NMT techniques (Thaut & Hoemberg, 2014).

The *transformational design model* (TDM; Thaut, 2005), is a clinical model designed to guide the thought process of the NMT clinician in order to select the best therapeutic music intervention based on the client's functional assessment needs and goals. The TDM consists of five steps:

1. Assessment: Gather diagnostic information and evaluate current functional needs.
2. Functional goals and objectives: Identify immediate and long-term changes to be addressed.
3. Nonmusical therapeutic experience or exercises: Identify an exercise outside of music that addresses the functional goal.

4. Therapeutic music experience: Translate step 3 into functional therapeutic music interventions based on:
   a. Scientific logic (current theory and/or models).
   b. Musical logic (creativity, aesthetics, good musical form).
   c. Therapeutic logic (isomorphic in structure and function).
5. Transformation: Transfer functional behavior into the client's everyday life.

All music therapists are trained to assess client needs (step 1) and develop observable, measurable goals and objectives for clients (step 2). However, step 3 requires that the therapist also think of an intervention in nonmusical terms, such as in relationship to the functional outcome behavior or an exercise that an occupational, physical, or speech therapist would employ to address the client's goals. This knowledge is essential to the appropriate selection and development of the successful therapeutic music experience (step 4). Equally important is the transformation or translation of the therapeutic experience into meaningful engagement for the client's daily life experiences (step 5).

The clinical examples in the next section of this chapter illustrate the collaborative efforts of rehabilitation therapists to move from activity-based therapy toward functional outcomes and improved therapeutic efficacy across a wide spectrum of diagnostic and age groups through the use of the TDM. All of the following examples are based on therapeutic sessions that were conducted by Sarah B. Johnson in collaboration with occupational, physical, and speech therapists, in acute adult rehabilitation, outpatient adult and pediatric rehabilitation, and community-based NMT exercise classes.

Sensorimotor Rehabilitation

In the sensorimotor domain NMT offers a variety of musical interventions and experiences to address functional motor skills such as gait and mobility, strength and endurance, coordination, balance and posture, and range of motion. These goals are addressed through three techniques: rhythmic auditory stimulation (RAS), patterned sensory enhancement (PSE), and therapeutic instrumental music performance (TIMP).

Rhythmic Auditory Stimulation (RAS)

RAS is a neurological technique used to facilitate the rehabilitation of movements that are intrinsically biologically rhythmical, most importantly gait. RAS can be used as both an immediate entrainment stimulus, providing rhythmic cues during movements, and as a facilitating stimulus for training in order to achieve more functional gait patterns (Thaut, 2005).

CLINICAL EXAMPLE: RAS for Gait Training with an Adult Who Had a Stroke

- *Step 1: Assessment.* John, a 56-year-old male who had a right middle cerebral artery ischemic stroke, presented with mild left-sided weakness and discoordination, impulsivity, and extreme distractibility. John lived alone and needed to be able to transfer, ambulate, and in general be independent with self-care.
- *Step 2: Therapeutic goal.* To be independent and safe with ambulation, using the least restrictive assistive device.
- *Step 3: Nonmusical therapeutic exercise.* Pregait and balance exercises, gait training with front-wheeled walker, with possible progression to a quad cane.
- *Step 4: Therapeutic music intervention.* RAS to facilitate pregait and advanced gait exercises, and more normalized walking parameters.
- *Step 5: Transfer.* John was discharged home with his daughter to assist with activities of daily living and to transport him to his outpatient therapy appointments.

During his regular physical therapy (PT) session, John was impulsive and unsafe and demonstrated a lack of heel strike and gait symmetry. The NMT added RAS to his PT sessions to assist with dynamic balance challenges and gait training. In addition to walking with RAS, sessions also consisted of pregait (e.g., standing weight shifts and alternately stepping forward and backward) and advanced gait exercises (e.g., walking around obstacles, frequency modulation, starting/ stopping), facilitated by rhythmic musical cues. Though John was often distractible in other situations, the musical cues served as a focal point for him during NMT interventions. His immediate rhythmic entrainment allowed him to coordinate his movements, improve his posture, sustain a stable cadence, and improve his heel strike and stride symmetry. When a familiar song was incorporated with the RAS pattern, he sang along and a greater normalizing effect to his overall kinematic gait pattern became evident.

Patterned Sensory Enhancement

PSE uses the rhythmic, melodic, harmonic, and dynamic acoustical elements of music to provide temporal, spatial, and force cues for movements that reflect functional exercises and activities of daily living (Thaut et al., 1991).

CLINICAL EXAMPLE: Exercise Group for People with Parkinson's Disease

- *Step 1: Assessment.* A group of individuals, ages 58–80, were diagnosed with Parkinson's disease or Parkinson's-like symptoms. All were ambulatory but demonstrated significant loss of trunk mobility, poor posture, and decreased strength and range of motion in upper and lower extremities.
- *Step 2: Therapeutic goal.* To increase or maintain dynamic balance as well as strength and coordination for maximal safety and independence in mobility and self-care.
- *Step 3: Nonmusical therapeutic exercise.* Upper and lower extremity exercises, emphasizing trunk mobility and core strength.
- *Step 4: Therapeutic music intervention.* PSE facilitation of exercise movements.
- *Step 5: Transfer.* Participants exhibit in-

creased stamina and greater confidence and safety in walking and daily activity.

This exercise class, co-facilitated by a PT and an NMT provides community members with Parkinson's disease the opportunity to remain mobile and independent. Traditional physical exercises, such as leg extensions, reaching forward and back, biceps curls, shoulder and wrist flexion and extension, and trunk rotations, are done while seated. Exercises are performed with hand weights, weighted dowels, weighted therapy balls, resistive exercise bands, or dowel rods. The entire session utilizes PSE, facilitated by the NMT on either the autoharp or piano, using the harmonic depth and musical flexibility of these instruments to create a dynamic musical stimulus. The PT chooses the desired exercise, and the NMT pair the movements with appropriate musical facilitation cues. Generally, in a group setting such as this, use of songs will galvanize the group members to participate and motivate them to keep working. The music is used to simulate the physical movements through temporal, spatial, and dynamic/force cues, painting an auditory picture of the desired movement and providing a musical structure to facilitate the movement goal.

Therapeutic Instrumental Music Performance

TIMP involves the playing of musical instruments to exercise and simulate functional movement patterns. Appropriate musical instruments are selected in a therapeutically meaningful way to emphasize range of motion, endurance, strength, functional hand movements, finger dexterity, and limb coordination (Thaut, 2005).

CLINICAL EXAMPLE: Facilitating Dynamic Balance for a Patient with a Traumatic Brain Injury

- *Step 1: Assessment.* Julie, a 32-year-old female, had incurred a traumatic brain injury (TBI) and resultant overall weakness from a protracted stay in the intensive care unit. She was able to ambulate with assistance and participate in self-care when she came to the rehabilitation unit, but was ataxic with her movements and significantly challenged with standing balance and gait training. Her functional balance was formally assessed by the PT, and it was determined that she had a high risk of falling, causing significant concerns for her safety at home.

- Step 2: Therapeutic goal. To improve dynamic standing balance.
- Step 3: Nonmusical therapeutic exercise. Standing and reaching outside her base of support; standing on unstable surfaces.
- Step 4: Therapeutic music intervention. TIMP to facilitate dynamic reaching and stepping.
- Step 5: Transfer. Julie wanted to be able to stand and reach safely in her kitchen so that she could begin to cook simple meals at home.

Julie's sessions were initially conducted with the help of parallel bars for safety, and she would stand and let go of one bar and then the other for short periods of time to challenge her balance. The NMT joined the PT as Julie began to regain her strength and stability. The therapists challenged her to reach for instrumental targets that were held or placed in positions that would require her to reach outside of her comfort zone. A dynamic balance challenge facilitated through TIMP, for example, might involve reaching forward for a conga drum placed on the floor while standing with her feet close together. In each session the NMT explained to Julie that the instruments provided a visual target that would deliver auditory and kinesthetic feedback to her sensory system. The strong, dynamic, and rhythmic cues of the songs provided Julie with the temporal structure to organize her movements and help her move in a more coordinated fashion. As she improved, the therapists were able to challenge her further by having her stand on different surfaces while engaged in TIMP interventions, progressing to stepping up on a 4-inch step while reaching for instrumental targets. The key element in these sessions was Julie's understanding that TIMP was not just about playing instruments in unusual ways, but rather the combination

of replicating functional movements within an organized musical experience.

Speech and Language Rehabilitation

NMT can play a large role in the development and rehabilitation of both verbal and nonverbal communication skills. Techniques in this domain are used to address speech apraxia; fluency disorders such as stuttering and cluttering; aphasia; and voice disorders that may result in abnormal pitch, loudness, timbre, breath control, or prosody of speech. Goals address issues such as functional and spontaneous speech; speech development; speech comprehension; motor control and coordination essential for articulation, respiratory function, fluency of speech, vocal production and sequencing of speech sounds; and rate and intelligibility. The goals are addressed through musical speech stimulation (MUSTIM), melodic intonation therapy (MIT), rhythmic speech cuing (RSC), vocal intonation therapy (VIT), therapeutic singing (TS), oral motor and respiratory exercises (OMREX), developmental speech and language training through music (DSLM), and symbolic communication training through music (SYCOM), all of which are based on current research in this area.

Musical Speech Stimulation

MUSTIM is the use of musical materials such as songs, rhymes, chants, and musical phrases, simulating prosodic speech gestures, to stimulate nonpropositional and eventually propositional speech (Thaut, 2005).

Melodic Intonation Therapy

MIT is a treatment technique developed for expressive aphasia rehabilitation by speech therapists. MIT utilizes a client's unimpaired ability to sing to facilitate spontaneous and voluntary speech through sung and chanted melodies, which resemble natural speech intonation patterns (Sparks, Helm, & Albert, 1974; Thaut, 2005).

CLINICAL EXAMPLE: MUSTIM, Transitioning into MIT, for Expressive Aphasia with a Patient Who Had a Stroke

- *Step 1: Assessment.* Eric, a 42-year-old male, had sustained a left-sided CVA, with severe expressive aphasia and oral apraxia. In addition to physical impairments from his stroke (right-sided hemiplegia) causing gross and fine motor deficits, he was unable to express his basic needs or communicate with his family.
- *Step 2: Therapeutic goal.* To communicate basic needs to nursing staff and family.
- *Step 3: Nonmusical therapeutic exercise.* Structured speech exercises to elicit automatic verbal responses.
- *Step 4: Therapeutic music intervention.* MUSTIM for spontaneous vocalizations
- *Step 5: Transfer.* Eric was able to verbally ask nursing staff to go to the bathroom, and he was able to say "I love you" to his wife and "How was school today?" to his two children.

Initially, all attempts at breath control and vocalizations were unsuccessful with speech therapy. When the NMT joined the speech therapist (ST) for cooperative sessions, MUSTIM was introduced using several familiar songs with well-known lyrics to access his voice through the completion of familiar musical phrases (e.g., "Country *roads*, take me *home* to the *place* . . ."). This approach became the entrance to finding Eric's voice.

Later sessions used MIT to introduce functional phrases that Eric could utilize to express himself verbally. The ST, patient, and family chose sentences that they felt were essential for his communication, for example, "My name is Eric Smith," "Bathroom, please!" and "I love you." For each phrase, the NMT created a musical replication of the normal prosody of the phrase, with an emphasis on the melodic and rhythmic components of natural speech. With the ST providing visual cues and assisting Eric in tapping the rhythm of the phrase with his left hand, the steps in the MIT protocol were followed. Eric recovered quickly from the physical impairments of his stroke and was discharged home to continue therapy as an outpatient. The ST and NMT created a DVD of these functional phrases so that he could to continue to practice at home.

Rhythmic Speech Cuing

RSC is the use of rhythmic cuing to control the initiation and rate of speech through cuing and pacing. The therapist uses the metronome to prime speech patterns or pace the rate of speech. This technique can be useful to facilitate motor planning for a patient with apraxia, to cue muscular coordination for dysarthria, or to assist in pacing with fluency disorders (Thaut, 2005).

Vocal Intonation Therapy

VIT is the use of intoned phrases simulating the prosody, inflection, and pacing of normal speech to work on inflection, pitch, breath control, timbre, and dynamics (Thaut, 2005).

Therapeutic Singing

TS is a technique that involves the unspecified use of singing activities to facilitate initiation, development, and articulation in speech and language as well as to increase functions of the respiratory apparatus (Thaut, 2005).

CLINICAL EXAMPLE: Increasing TS to Increase All Aspects of Vocal Output with a Patient with Multiple Sclerosis

- *Step 1: Assessment.* Jennifer, a 36-year-old female who was diagnosed with multiple sclerosis (MS) 7 years earlier, was hospitalized for an exacerbation of her MS, which affected her overall physical functioning. She was extremely weak, unable to support herself in an upright posture in her wheelchair, and was having difficulty speaking clearly and at an audible volume.

- *Step 2: Therapeutic goal.* To increase vital capacity and vocal/verbal output for improved communication.
- *Step 3: Nonmusical therapeutic exercise.* Posture and breathing exercises; increasing unsupported sitting time in wheelchair.
- *Step 4: Therapeutic music intervention.* TS while sitting in wheelchair.
- *Step 5: Transfer.* Increased quality of life for Jennifer to be up, in her wheelchair, able to interact and communicate with friends and family.

Jennifer was very frustrated and downhearted by the exacerbation of her MS and was not completely compliant with other therapies while working toward her functional goals. Neither VIT to address specific aspects of vocal output nor OMREX for improving speech intelligibility interested her. The NMT decided to capitalize on Jennifer's love for reggae music, working toward the goal of singing "No woman, no cry" in one breath. Because of her initial low endurance and decreased breath control, the structure required alternating singing, with Jennifer's initiating or completing phrases, and the therapist completing the remainder. Because she was motivated to sing, Jennifer was willing to get up and sit in her wheelchair for speech sessions, gradually increasing her ability to actively participate in all aspects of the sessions.

Oral Motor and Respiratory Exercises

OMREX involves the use of musical materials and exercises, mainly through sound vocalization and wind instrument playing, to enhance articulatory control and respiratory strength and function of the speech apparatus (Haas, Distenfield, & Axen, 1986).

Developmental Speech and Language Training through Music

DSLM is the specific use of developmentally appropriate musical materials and experiences to enhance speech and language development through singing, chanting, playing musical instruments, and combining music, speech, and movement (Thaut, 2005).

Symbolic Communication Training through Music

SYCOM is the use of structured instrumental or vocal improvisation to train communication behavior, language pragmatics, appropriate speech gestures, and emotional communication in nonverbal language system (Thaut 2005).

Cognitive Rehabilitation

Several NMT interventions have been developed to address cognition and learning, based on research evidence providing clinical support for the role of music to aid in memory, attention, executive function training, affect modifications, and cognitive reorientation. Cognitive training techniques in NMT include musical sensory orientation training (MSOT), musical neglect training (MNT), auditory perception training (APT), musical attention control training (MACT), musical mnemonics training (MMT), associative mood and memory training (AMMT), executive function training (MEFT), and music in psychosocial training and counseling (MPC).

Musical Sensory Orientation Training

MSOT is the use of music, presented live or recorded, to stimulate arousal and recovery of wake states and to facilitate meaningful responsiveness and orientation to time, place, and person. In more advanced recovery of developmental stages, training would involve active engagement in simple musical exercises to increase vigilance and train basic attention maintenance, with emphasis on quantity rather than quality of response (Thaut, 2005).

Musical Neglect Training

MNT involves active playing of musical instruments in performance exercises that are structured in time, tempo, and rhythm, with an appropriate spatial configuration of instruments to focus attention to neglected or unattended areas of the visual field. MNT may also involve receptive music listening to stimulate hemispheric brain arousal while engaging in exercises addressing visual neglect or inattention (Frasinetti, Pavani, & Ladavos, 2002).

CLINICAL EXAMPLE: MNT with A Patient with a Right CVA

• *Step 1: Assessment.* Nancy, a 69-year-old female, had a right-sided CVA with left hemiplegia and left inattention. Nancy gazed to the right side constantly, was unaware of her left arm and leg, and was inattentive to her left side when performing tasks of daily living. Formalized visual assessment from occupational therapy (OT) identified a visual field cut in the left visual field.
• *Step 2: Therapeutic goal.* To increase awareness of left side and promote compensatory strategies.
• *Step 3: Nonmusical therapeutic exercise.* Functional tasks oriented to the patient's left side.
• *Step 4: Therapeutic music intervention.* MNT that requires patient to engage in musical tasks on the left side of her body.
• *Step 5: Transfer.* For safety and management of daily life, Nancy needed to be able to compensate for her visual field cut in wheelchair mobility and to manage her weaker left arm to prevent injury.

Nancy was initially asked to play a paddle drum with her unaffected right hand. The drum was held in front of her, and she was to play for the entire song that the NMT was singing and playing on the Autoharp. As Nancy was able to sustain this task, the OT would gradually move the drum into different visual planes to challenge her visual tracking. The therapists then increased the challenge by placing one drum in front of Nancy and one slightly left of her midline, gradually widening the space between the two drums, requiring scanning between the left side and back to midline. Musical facilitation provided repetitive opportunities for Nancy's attention to be drawn to the left visual field in combination with the visual targets of the instruments. The auditory and kinesthetic feedback of hitting the target assisted Nancy in learning to compensate for inattentiveness to her left side.

Auditory Perception Training

APT is the use of musical exercises to discriminate and identify different components of sound, such as time, tempo, duration, pitch, timbre, rhythmic patterns, as well as speech sounds. Integration of different sensory modalities, including visual, tactile, and kinesthetic input, are used during active musical exercises such as playing from symbolic or graphic notion, using tactile sound transmission, or integrating movement to music (Gfeller, Woodworth, Robin, Witt, & Knutson, 1997).

CLINICAL EXAMPLE: A Pediatric Patient with a Cochlear Implant

• *Step 1: Diagnostic and clinical assessment information.* Samuel, age 6, recently received a cochlear implant and was working with speech therapy to develop his auditory perception of sounds in his environment.
• *Step 2: Therapeutic goal.* To increase awareness of auditory sounds in the environment.
• *Step 3: Nonmusical therapeutic exercise.* Playing a sound track of various environmental noises and having patient identify the sounds.
• *Step 4: Therapeutic music intervention.* APT by identifying instrumental sounds.
• *Step 5: Transfer.* Samuel increased his awareness and responsiveness to environmental sounds and voices, responding more consistently to his name, for example, in a group setting.

Samuel was resistant to working on auditory processing during speech therapy but enjoyed using percussion instruments while in a pediatric music group. The ST requested to work cooperatively with the NMT to engage him in APT. The NMT first assessed which instruments he was able to distinguish among and which ones appeared to be unpleasant, heard through his cochlear implant. The NMT then provided two pictures of instruments. One of those instruments was played behind him, and Samuel chose which picture he thought he had heard. Another variation involved the therapist playing or not playing an instrument that the therapists knew he was capable of hearing. The therapist would then ask him if he heard it, and he would answer "yes" or "no."

Musical Attention Control Training

MACT involves structured active or receptive musical exercises, using precomposed performance or improvisation, in which musical elements cue different musical responses as a way to practice sustained, selective, divided, and alternating attention functions (Thaut, 2005).

Musical Mnemonics Training

MMT is the use of musical exercises to address various memory encoding and decoding/recall functions. Immediate recall of sounds or sung words using musical stimuli can be used to address echoic functions. Musical stimuli can be used as a mnemonic device or memory template in a song, rhyme, or chant, or to facilitate the learning of nonmusical information by sequencing and organizing the information in temporally structured patterns or chunks (Groussard et al., 2010; Maeller, 1996).

Associative Mood and Memory Training

AMMT involves musical mood induction techniques (1) to instate a mood-congruent state to facilitate memory recall, or (2) to access associative mood and memory function through inducing a positive emotional state in the learning and recall process (Dolan, 2002; Thaut & de l'Etoile, 1993).

Musical Executive Function Training

MEFT is the use of improvisation and composition exercises in a group or individually to practice executive function skills (e.g., organization, problem solving, decision making, reasoning, comprehension) within a social context that provides important therapeutic elements such as performance products in real time, temporal structure, creative process, affective content, sensory structure, and social interaction patterns (Dolan, 2002).

Music in Psychosocial Training and Counseling

MPC is the use of musical simulations to address issues of cognitive orientation, affective expression, and appropriate social interaction to facilitate psychosocial function.

Conclusions

Over the past 20 years, the scientific, evidence-based practice of NMT has created a much-needed link between basic science and music therapy clinical practice. According to the standards of best possible practice, treatment should be selected according to (1) best available objective assessment procedures, and (2) best available objective outcome data. It only makes sense that patients deserve the best available treatment, and that is only possible if we can provide scientific evidence that explains the therapeutic effects of music on behavior and thereby establish a framework for the systematic and creative transformation of musical responses into therapeutic responses that produce consistent therapeutic outcomes and benefits.

REFERENCES

Baram, Y., & Lenger, R. (2012). Gait improvement in patients with cerebral palsy by visual and auditory feedback. *Neuromodulation, 15*(1), 48–52.

Baram, Y., & Miller, A. (2007). Auditory feedback control for improvement of gait in patients with multiple sclerosis. *Neurological Sciences, 254*, 90–94.

Berlyne, D. E. (1971). *Aesthetics and psychobiology.* New York: Appleton-Century-Crofts.

Bradt, J., Magee, W. L., Dileo, C., Wheeler, B. L., & McGilloway, E. (2010). Music therapy for acquired brain injury. *Cochrane Database of Systematic Reviews, 2010*(7), CD006787.

Conklyn, D., Stough, D., Novak, E., Paczak, S., Chemali, K., & Bethoux, F. (2010). A home-based walking program using rhythmic auditory stimulation improves gait performance in patients with multiple sclerosis: A pilot study. *Neurorehabilitation and Neural Repair, 24*(9), 835–842.

de Dreu, M. J., van der Wilk, A. S. D., Poppe, E., Kwakkel, G., & van Wegen, E. E. H. (2012). Rehabilitation, exercise therapy and music in patients with Parkinson's disease: A meta-analysis of the effects of music-based movement therapy on walking ability, balance and quality of life. *Parkinsonism and Related Disorders, 18*(Suppl. 1), S114–S119.

de l'Etoile, S. K. (2008). The effect of rhythmic auditory stimulation on the gait parameters of patients with incomplete spinal cord injury: An exploratory pilot study. *International Journal of Rehabilitation Research, 31*(2), 155–157.

Dolan, R. J. (2002). Emotion, cognition, and behavior. *Science, 298*, 1191–1194.

Frasinetti, F., Pavani, F., & Ladavos, E. (2002). Acoustical vision of neglected stimuli: Interaction among spatially convergent audio-visual inputs in neglect patients. *Journal of Cognitive Neuroscience, 14*, 62–69.

Gaston, E. T. (1968). Man and music. In E. T. Gaston (Ed.), *Music in therapy* (pp. 7–29). New York: Macmillan.

Gfeller, K., Woodworth, G., Robin, D. A., Witt, S., & Knutson, J. F. (1997). Perception of rhythmic and sequential pitch patterns by normally hearing adults and adult cochlear implant users. *Ear and Hearing, 18*, 252–260.

Groussard, M., Viader, F., Hubert, V., Landeau, B., Abbas, A., Desgranges, B., et al. (2010). Musical and verbal semantic memory: Two distinct neural networks? *NeuroImage, 49*(3), 2764–2773.

Haas, F., Distenfeld, S., & Axen, K. (1986). Effects of perceived music rhythm on respiratory patterns. *Journal of Applied Physiology, 61*, 1185–1191.

Hurt, C. P., Rice, R. R., McIntosh, G. C., & Thaut, M. H. (1998). Rhythmic auditory stimulation in gait training for patients with traumatic brain injury. *Journal of Music Therapy, 35*, 228–241.

Kadivar, Z., Corcos, D. M., Foto, J., & Hondzinski, J. M. (2011). Effect of step training and rhythmic auditory stimulation on functional performance in Parkinson patients. *Neurorehabilitation and Neural Repair, 25*(7), 626–635.

Kim, S. J., Kwak, E. E., Park, E. S., Lee, D. S., Kim, K. J., Song, J. E., et al. (2011). Changes in gait patterns with rhythmic auditory stimulation in adults with cerebral palsy. *NeuroRehabilitation, 29*(3), 233–241.

Maeller, D. H. (1996). *Rehearsal strategies and verbal working memory in multiple sclerosis* (Unpublished master's thesis). Colorado State University, Ft. Collins, CO.

McIntosh, G. C., Brown, S. H., Rice, R. R., & Thaut, M. H. (1997). Rhythmic auditory–motor facilitation of gait patterns in patients with Parkinson's disease. *Journal of Neurology, Neurosurgery, and Psychiatry, 62*, 22–26.

Neurologic Music Therapy. (n.d.). Available at *www.cbrm.colostate.edu.*

Sparks, R. W., Helm, N., & Albert, M. (1974). Aphasia rehabilitation resulting from melodic intonation therapy. *Cortex, 10*, 313–316.

Thaut, M. H. (2000). *A scientific model of music in therapy and medicine.* St. Louis, MO: MMB Music.

Thaut, M. H. (2005). *Rhythm, music and the brain.* London: Routledge.

Thaut, M. H., & de l'Etoile, S. K. (1993). The effects of music on mood state-dependent recall. *Journal of Music Therapy, 30*, 70–80.

Thaut, M. H., & Hoemberg, V. (Eds.). (2014). *The Oxford handbook of neurologic music therapy.* Oxford, UK: Oxford University Press.

Thaut, M. H., Hurt, C. P., Dragan, D., & McIntosh, G. C. (1998). Rhythmic entrainment of gait patterns in children with cerebral zpalsy. *Developmental Medicine and Child Neurology, 40*(78), 15.

Thaut, M. H., McIntosh, G. C., Prassas, S. G., & Rice, R. R. (1992). Effects of auditory rhythmic pacing on normal gait and gait in stroke, cerebellar disorder, and transverse myelitis. In M. Woollacott & F. Horak (Eds.), *Posture and gait: Control mechanisms* (Vol. 2, pp. 437–440). Eugene: University of Oregon Books.

Thaut, M. H., Rice, R. R., & McIntosh, G. C. (1997). Rhythmic facilitation of gait training in hemiparetic stroke rehabilitation. *Journal of Neurological Sciences, 151*, 207–212.

Thaut, M. H., Rice, R. R., McIntosh, G. C., & Prassas, S. G. (1993). The effect of auditory rhythmic cuing on stride and EMG patterns in hemiparetic gait of stroke patients. *Physical Therapy, 73*, 107.

Thaut, M. H., Schleiffers, S., & Davis, W. B. (1991). Analysis of EMG activity in biceps and triceps muscle in a gross motor task under the influence of auditory rhythm. *Journal of Music Therapy, 28*, 64–88.

CHAPTER 19

Community Music Therapy

Brynjulf Stige

Community Music Therapy (CoMT) practices are context-sensitive and resource-oriented, focusing on collaborative music making and attending to the voices of disadvantaged people. Practices within this orientation acknowledge that disability and disadvantage are as much a product of discrimination and marginalization as of individual impairment. CoMT is a relatively new orientation within music therapy. Only after 2000 was an international discourse established with the first books and articles that reached an international audience. As we will see, however, CoMT has many roots and a multifaceted history. In my appraisal, CoMT also has an important role to play in the development of music therapy as discipline and profession.

When the international CoMT discourse emerged at the beginning of this century, responses varied. Advocates of the orientation would receive feedback such as, "This is the future of our discipline!", or "There is nothing new here, I've been doing this for years," or even "This is professional suicide—we need to stick to the medical model." In other words, some music thera-

pists were highly enthusiastic and felt that CoMT helped them develop highly relevant ways of working. Others were very skeptical and argued that CoMT is a step in the wrong direction for the profession. What is so similar or different, dangerous or intriguing about CoMT? We discuss such questions later in the chapter, when we have a better understanding of what CoMT is or could be.

Community, music, therapy—each of these terms has multiple meanings. We could clarify by trying to define Community Music Therapy. Several scholars, myself included (Stige, 2012), have attempted to do so, but such definitions tend to end up as both difficult and disputed. There is only so much that one can do with definition when what you want to define is not an object or given phenomenon but a multifaceted and evolving social practice. Sometimes we are better served by brief portrayals of key features. One attempt of producing such a portrayal is the following: "Community music therapy encourages musical participation and social inclusion, equitable access to resources, and collaborative efforts for health

233

and wellbeing in contemporary societies" (Stige & Aarø, 2012, p. 5). If portrayals are complemented by examples, we can perhaps learn to recognize practices related to CoMT, similarly to how we are able to recognize people in a family. All members do not look the same. They are not even similar in some respects, but there is usually a complex mix of recognizable features distributed among family members. Later in the chapter I present the acronym *PREPARE*, which has been constructed to identify features (or qualities) of the *family* of CoMT.

History

Although an international discourse on CoMT only emerged in this century, there have been many precursors both in practice and in theory. I discuss some of these here, focusing on developments within the United States, United Kingdom, and Scandinavia, and with reference to a previously published investigation of the history of the orientation (Stige, 2012). A more comprehensive presentation would include a broader presentation of developments in a range of countries (Stige & Aarø, 2012).

Before we embark on a historical journey of CoMT, three caveats are worth considering. First, CoMT is an emerging movement and orientation. Discussions of relationships between music therapy and community can be traced in the literature of several decades, and the term *Community Music Therapy* has sometimes been used also, but as a specific concept, it was established internationally only this millennium. Second, the English term *community* does not translate directly to some of the languages of countries where related practices and perspectives have been developed, such as Argentina, Brazil, Germany, Japan, and Norway. This, of course, makes shared definitions even more complex to achieve. Third, a central tenet in CoMT is that practices need to be situated in local contexts—

and a local focus suggests that it is more meaningful to think in terms of several interrelated histories than of one singular development.

Consequently, we need to choose metaphors carefully when we consider the history of CoMT. The customary metaphor of historical *roots* is misleading, at least if interpreted as shared ancestry. The more specific image of *aerial roots* would be more helpful: When plants with aerial roots grow, new roots descend from the branches, push into the ground, and form new trunks. This image illuminates how the history of CoMT is manifold and still unfolds. Other relevant metaphors could be to think of CoMT as a *river* with water from several smaller streams, or—as indicated above—to think of it as a *family* of practices. The river metaphor suggests how CoMT is a blend of ideas and practices influenced by changes in the surrounding landscape, whereas the family metaphor allows for acknowledgment of the human agency involved when the relationships that shape the field are established (Stige & Aarø, 2012, pp. 49–52).

Early community-related ideas in the music therapy literature include a critique developed by the American ethnomusicologist Bruno Nettl (1956), published in the fifth *Book of Proceedings* of the National Association for Music Therapy. Nettl argued that ethnographic studies of healing rituals in traditional cultures show us something that is worth considering when developing professional music therapy. In the traditional practices to which he referred, music is integrated in social and ritual settings. Nettl contrasted this to the more limited focus on the direct effect of music on behavior that he found in modern music therapy at that time.

Although Nettl's critique was highly pertinent, community-related issues were not ignored altogether in the first decades of development of the new professional discipline. Several of the music therapy pioneers in Europe in the 1960s and 1970s, such as Juliette Alvin, Paul Nordoff and Clive

Robbins, and Mary Priestley, developed some community-oriented ideas within the gamut of notions they proposed (e.g., see Stige & Aarø, 2012, pp. 34–36). In the United States, Gaston's (1968) seminal text *Music in Therapy* had a separate section devoted to music therapy in the community. Florence Tyson was one of the American pioneers who contributed insights on relationships between community and music therapy. In the 1950s, '60s, and '70s, Tyson published several texts that focused on issues such as *outpatient music therapy*, linked to the deinstitutionalization of some music therapy services at that time (McGuire, 2004). Tyson occasionally used the term *Community Music Therapy* also, but she did not develop theoretical perspectives that inform the field today. Her focus could be described as *music therapy in the community*, whereas contemporary CoMT practices could be described as *music therapy as community* and/or *music therapy for community*.

These more contemporary notions build upon developments in music therapy theory that started to emerge in the 1980s, with scholars such as Carolyn Kenny in the United States and Canada and Even Ruud in Norway leading the way. Throughout the 1980s, Kenny (2006) developed social and systems-oriented ideas about music therapy theory that are of clear relevance for contemporary CoMT (even though she has not used this term in her writings). Kenny made a case for how music therapy practices must be understood as part of broader sociocultural systems. She also discussed the relevance of systems theory to music therapy, and she developed her theory of the Field of Play, which highlights relational and contextual aspects of music therapy processes. Similarly, Even Ruud, already in 1980, discussed implications of a more socially oriented approach to music therapy. He went beyond the scope of conventional individualized treatment objectives and suggested that music therapy has a role to play in bringing music to people who are excluded from the musical activities of a community. Further, Ruud argued that biomedical and psychological perspectives on health tend to neglect the social and cultural dimensions of human life. The problems and challenges that a person in music therapy experiences cannot be understood at an individual level only; they are linked to a range of social and cultural conditions. Ruud therefore argued that music therapy (also) must be directed towards the context of the client (see Ruud, 1998).

The 1980s witnessed efforts to articulate more specific perspectives closely related to practice. For instance, Marcia Broucek (1987) argued that music therapy historically had been an *institutionalized practice* and that there was need for *deinstitutionalization of practice* in order to meet needs of a larger proportion of the population. At about the same time, Edith Boxill (1988) developed an activist vision that she called *Music Therapists for Peace*. At the same time, in Norway, music therapists informed by participatory rights-based and sociocultural perspectives had started to explore how music therapy can contribute to the development of inclusive local communities (Kleive & Stige, 1988).

In the 1990s there was an increasing interest in the relationship between music, health, and community in the music therapy literature. The inclusion of ecological and community-oriented perspectives in influential textbooks of this decade illustrates the tendency. Leslie Bunt's (1994) *Music Therapy: An Art Beyond Words* included a chapter devoted to the discussion of music therapy as a resource for the community. Bunt also promoted the relevance of *working links* with other disciplines and professions and of a *partnership model* within research. Another influential book, the second edition of *Defining Music Therapy*, by Kenneth Bruscia (1998), specifically included a discussion of CoMT, which he related to what he described as a broader area of *ecological practices*.

Even though community-oriented practices were included in these influential publications in the 1990s, it would hardly be precise to suggest that CoMT was part of the general conception of music therapy at the beginning of the 21st century. But new publications soon started to emerge, with the Internet creating completely new conditions for discussion and debate beyond the restraints of national associations and context. *Voices: A World Forum for Music Therapy* (*www.voices.no*) was established in 2001 and became one of the vehicles for this global discourse. Soon, a new international awareness and interest evolved, with 2002 as an especially intense turning point. This year saw the publication of several articles focusing specifically on CoMT, with Ansdell's (2002) "Community Music Therapy and the Winds of Change" as probably the most influential example. Two books featuring chapters on CoMT (Kenny & Stige, 2002; Stige, 2002) were published the same year. At the 10th World Congress of Music Therapy in Oxford (UK) in 2002, CoMT was a central topic of discussion. The first edited book specifically devoted to CoMT was published only a couple of years later (Pavlicevic & Ansdell, 2004).

After this turning point, there has been a steady stream of case reports, research articles, master theses, and doctoral dissertations about CoMT, in addition to several books. This sudden yet sustained interest could hardly be understood as a response to influential publications and theoretical debates, even though some of the texts to which I have referred probably played their part. It is more plausible to think of the interest as a response to practice challenges. My claim, then, is that music therapists around the world have taken interest in the emerging CoMT literature because they have been sensitive to people's rights and changing needs in a changing society. CoMT deals with and acknowledges innovative and inclusive practices with which many practitioners were already familiar, to some degree. These music therapists have craved possibilities to discuss and develop their understanding of such practices in an informed language. This is the issue we now consider: What are the tenets that inform CoMT discourse today?

Theoretical Tenets

The rights-based and culture-centered tenets that are typical for CoMT reflect the orientation's relationship to moral and political theory, on one hand, and to developmental theory in an ecological lifespan perspective, on the other. I present these two groups of tenets and then the acronym PREPARE, which summarizes the assumptions that characterize CoMT.

Rights-Based Tenets

CoMT practices acknowledge that disability and disadvantage are as much a product of discrimination and marginalization as of individual impairment. Our capacity to act freely as individuals depends upon political freedom as well as a minimum number of conditions by which our basic needs are met. The interdisciplinary literature on human rights illuminates the relationships between freedom and well-being, which both require at least a minimal degree of equality and solidarity in society. I have previously developed an argument for CoMT as rights-based practice (Stige & Aarø, 2012, pp. 177–183) and I summarize and build on this argument here and try to clarify how needs and rights are interdependent.

The Universal Declaration of Human Rights was passed by the United Nations General Assembly in 1948, the need for it having been made all too clear by the atrocities of World War II. Even though the declaration is violated in multiple ways every day almost everywhere, its value as a worldwide consensus about the rights and responsibilities that we have as human beings could hardly be overestimated. It is common to talk of *three generations of human rights*, for which I give a brief outline of their relevance to CoMT.

The *first generation* of human rights is often labeled the *civil and political rights*. These are *freedom rights* of each individual and include the rights to citizenship and free participation in society, equality before the law, freedom of religion and self-expression, and so on. These rights require protection through legislation, and most people think of the legal profession rather than the profession of music therapy when they consider how these rights are secured in a society. It would be a mistake, however, not to consider how the music therapy profession relates to these rights. Take music therapy in prisons. Offenders ending up in the criminal justice system lose many of their human rights, especially the freedom rights but often other rights too, even though there is not always a clear rationale for why this should be the case (Connolly & Ward, 2008, pp. 81–95). Tuastad and O'Grady (2013) examine how music therapy could contribute to more humane criminal justice services that would build experiences of and pathways to freedom.

The *second generation* of human rights are *economic, social*, and *cultural rights* and include the rights to employment with a reasonable wage, housing, sufficient food, clothing, education, health care, social security, and so on. Whereas the first generation of rights focuses on individual liberty, the second focuses on welfare. These rights involve an active role for the public in provision of adequate conditions and services for everyone. South African music therapist Helen Oosthuizen has written on poverty and professional priorities, exemplifying music therapy concerns in relation to this generation of rights. She describes how her own background provides her with solid cultural understanding of affluent communities, which also are in the best position to pay for services. To prioritize working in affluent communities would clearly be easiest in practical terms. But would it be the best solution in ethical and political terms? "I need to consider that by working only in wealthy, resourced communities similar to my own community, I may be highlighting the divide between wealth and poverty. In this way, I compound our country's struggle with social inequality" (Oosthuizen, 2006).

The *third generation* of human rights includes more *collective* and *environmental* rights, such as the right to live in a peaceful society and the right to access to unpolluted air, clean water, and nature. CoMT practices related to the third generation of rights include work with conflict transformation (see Vaillancourt, 2009). Furthermore, the German music therapist Christine Simon (2013) has argued that the disregard of nature in contemporary societies cannot be disconnected from the discourse on human well-being and social justice. This view contributes to the breadth and depth of our understanding of how CoMT relates to human rights.

The idea of music therapy as rights-based practice might perhaps initially be somewhat overwhelming, given that we belong to a small profession. It could be developed into an empowering one, however, if we move beyond thinking of human rights as paragraphs in abstract treatises. Human rights do not just happen. Also, they cannot be achieved by laws and political decisions only. Rights must be actively protected and provided for in concrete situations.

Human rights imply social and ethical responsibilities; we belong to a community of rights-holders and duty-bearers (Gewirth, 1996). Building on Gewirth's philosophy, Connolly and Ward (2008) argue that human rights set minimum standards for a life of dignity rather than depicting an ideal world. Professions working in health, social care, and criminal justice should take special interest in human *agency* (the capacity to act intentionally) then, because realization of rights requires agency. Culture is a major resource for human agency, we now turn to some culture-centered tenets of CoMT.

Culture-Centered Tenets

Culture-centered tenets provide us with a framework for understanding how human agency can evolve in and through musical community. A culture-centered perspective on music therapy focuses on how our human lives evolve in social and cultural contexts and on how the individual and the environment influence each other reciprocally. A basic idea, then, is that the person develops within an ecology instead of being a product of circumstances; we are all active in co-constructing the conditions of our development (Stige, 2002). Consequently, the culture-centered tenets of Community Music Therapy imply something more substantial than adjustment of practice to the differences between cultural groups. Here I focus on the tenets that illuminate the ecology of human agency.

As humans we have an inherent capacity for action, but the form it takes and the degree to which we are able to promote change depends on our history of interacting with the environment where we develop. Action requires access to resources and therefore operates within constraints. Such constraints are not constant, however. Human agency potentially enables production of as well as redistribution of resources (Giddens, 1984). In CoMT, musical community is explored in order to create conditions for such change. For instance, Gary Ansdell (2010a) explains how experiences of musical community over time enable the development of a *community of practice*, where people are engaged in doing and learning things together.

As we have seen, to be an agent means to be able to exercise some control over the relationships of which we are part, within the constraints of an ecology. Agency evolves when individuals and communities collaborate mobilizing and distributing resources in new ways. As a multifaceted resource in our social environment, music has great potential in the service of human agency. Whether or not it operates as a positive re-

source depends on who uses it, where, and how, under which conditions.

Such a concept of agency could therefore be linked to the ecological perspective on human development advocated by Bronfenbrenner (1979) and many other socioculturally oriented psychologists. Bronfenbrenner was concerned about how human service professions focus too much on development within the isolated microsystem of the therapy room and too little on developments within other systems, including the interaction of various microsystems (*mesosystems* in Bronfenbrenner's terminology).

I now discuss the meanings within the acronym PREPARE to highlight how CoMT can contribute to the freedom and well-being of groups and individuals.

PREPARE: Synthesizing the Assumptions That Inform CoMT

The acronym of PREPARE has been developed as a mnemonic to communicate seven characteristic qualities or features of CoMT (Stige & Aarø, 2012, pp. 16–24), suggesting that CoMT is:

Participatory
Resource-oriented
Ecological
Performative
Activist
Reflective
Ethics-driven.

These qualities are related to the theoretical tenets outlined above, but they are developed from a synthesis of research on practice. Based on our (Stige & Aarø, 2012) discussion, I briefly summarize the seven qualities.

1. The *participatory* quality of CoMT refers to the valuing of democratic processes. People are encouraged to take part in ways that make a difference. This quality suggests, for example, that the expertise of par-

ticipants is valued highly. The expertise of the music therapist matters also, but CoMT is not an expert-driven practice. A participatory approach, with willingness to listen and to negotiate, characterizes CoMT.

2. The *resource-oriented* quality of CoMT includes, but goes beyond, the nurturing of personal strengths. To mobilize, create access to, and redistribute social, cultural, and material resources is part of the agenda. When relevant, a resource orientation also involves working with and relating to problems and challenges. We can think of resources as the reserves people appropriate in their daily life in order to be able to tackle problems and explore possibilities.

3. The *ecological* quality of CoMT involves working with the reciprocal relationships among individuals, groups, and networks in social contexts. The ecological quality of COMT implies exploration of systemic perspectives on practice.

4. The *performative* quality of CoMT implies that there is focus on human development through action and performance of relationships in context. This may include musical performance, but goes beyond it to include performance of self and community.

5. The *activist* quality of CoMT refers to recognition of how people's problems are related to limitations in society, such as marginalization and inequity. It also involves willingness *to act*; social change is often part of the CoMT agenda. The activist quality is perhaps more controversial than the other qualities discussed here, but logically goes together with the notion of a rights-based practice discussed above.

6. The *reflective* quality of CoMT involves collaborative attempts to understand the processes, outcomes, and broader implications of practice. Reflection often involves verbal discussion, but not exclusively. Actions, interactions, and reactions in a given situation also contribute to human understanding.

7. The *ethics-driven* quality of CoMT implies that practice, theory, and research are rights-based. Human needs and limitations are taken into consideration, but CoMT is not guided by a medical model that focuses on diagnoses and treatment plans. The values informing human rights and the intention of realizing rights in the given context guide the activity.

The qualities communicated by the PREPARE acronym relate to musical as well as *paramusical* aspects of a situation; musical processes are understood as elements of human activities in context (see Stige, Ansdell, Elefant, & Pavlicevic, 2010, pp. 298–300). A better understanding of the seven qualities could be developed by reading case examples describing CoMT practice. There are currently two anthologies with such examples. Pavlicevic and Ansdell (2004) edited an international anthology organized around headings such as "Community music therapy a challenge to the consensus model?", "But is it music therapy?", "What has culture got to do with it?", and "What has context got to do with it?" Some years later, a research-based collection of eight case studies from four different countries was published, reflecting different situations of needs and of challenged rights (Stige, Ansdell, Elefant, & Paulicevic, 2010). This research-based anthology was a central source for the articulation of the seven qualities outlined above. In addition, a textbook (Stige & Aarø, 2012) summarizes many case examples from the literature, reflecting CoMT practices across people's lifespans, and in various geographical and sociocultural contexts.

A Synthesized Example from Practice

In some detail I present a synthesized example from CoMT practice, based on my previous experience as a practicing music therapist in a Norwegian clinic for mental health. In telling a narrative about Johanna and her friends, I have synthesized elements from several case stories and also added some elements, both in order to secure anonymity and to make the synthesized example more instructive.

Visions of Johanna

"We sit here stranded, though we're all doin' our best to deny it." "What do you mean?" "Lights flicker from the opposite loft. In this room the heat pipes just cough." The music therapist was quite confused. He realized by now that Johanna was quoting the lyrics of a song, but didn't quite understand what she wanted to communicate. Johanna then decided that the music therapist might need some help: "Don't you know these lines from 'Visions of Johanna'?" "Well, eh . . ., but OK, you're into Dylan?" "No, not really, but I love Marianne Faithfull's version of this particular song. When she sings, everything is so clear and so perplexing at the same time. That's life, you know."

This sequence from Johanna's first music therapy sessions turned out to be characteristic. The music therapist sometimes found Johanna's communication enigmatic, but Johanna's motivation for participation was clear enough. She had asked for music therapy the second day after she came to the clinic. "I need to regain my voice," she said. It was not obvious to the chief psychiatrist of the mental health center what Johanna meant by that, but he agreed that music therapy could be suitable for her, even though he admitted to the music therapist that he was not sure. Johanna had just arrived in the center because of an incident of serious self-harm, and she was not diagnosed yet. "So—how do we know that there is evidence to prioritize Johanna's request for music therapy?" the doctor asked.

The music therapist did not quite know what to answer. For a few years he had tried to argue that a client's motivation should be an indication in itself and that diagnoses not always make all that much sense as an indication for music therapy. His colleagues never supported this view directly, but they had at least accepted that the music therapy services developed in the center were broad in orien-

tation, and not only linked to individualized treatment. In addition to traditional music therapy sessions, the music therapist organized open musical events in the ward, sometimes inviting people from the neighborhood as guests. He also spent considerable time trying to support clients who wanted to find out if and how they could use music as a resource in their everyday life when they left the center.

Voices of Johanna's Friends

When the fourth session of Johanna was about to begin, the music therapist was in for a surprise. Johanna did not arrive alone. "I brought a couple of friends who want to sing with me, is that OK?" Again the music therapist did not quite know what to answer. He was inspired by the CoMT literature and supportive of a broad and flexible notion of music therapy practice, but he was thinking that open ward and community events were one thing, and music therapy sessions something different. He was not convinced that blurring genres was such a brilliant idea. But would it be good to turn Johanna's request down?

From the back of his head he dug out memories of a meeting with his supervisor when they had discussed the boundaries of therapy processes. It is helpful to differentiate between boundary violations and boundary crossings, the supervisor had argued. Boundary violations are often exploitive and always harmful for the client, whereas boundary crossings only imply that therapist and client step out of the usual framework in some way. Boundary crossings are not necessarily harmful. They could, at times, even advance the therapeutic alliance and the power of the process. "Perhaps my reluctance has more to do with my own comfort zone than anything else," the music therapist reflected. He decided to give it a go and to look for opportunities to reflect on this choice together with Johanna.

The two friends that Johanna brought with her had also just recently arrived to the clinic. They had been chatting a bit the other night and decided that it would be fun to sing together. The music therapist asked them if perhaps they wanted to do some songwriting also. "Sure," Johanna responded spontaneously, but then she stopped herself. When the music therapist invited the three of them to write down ideas for the lyrics of a song, she came up with no suggestions. Her friends did, however, and after a while one of them proudly read a line she had written: "Oh, doctor, please, won't you listen to me. I don't need any beef now, I wanna be free." The three friends laughed out loud. The music therapist wondered where this would end.

In the weeks to come Johanna's music therapy sessions were converted to songwriting workshops where her friends took on a very active role. The music therapist still found Johanna's verbal communication quite enigmatic, and he observed that she did not always contribute much to the writing of song lyrics either, but she sang the songs eagerly and also expressed that they were very meaningful to her. She would say things such as "We're singer songwriters now." "Well, yes, sort of. . . . " "And we should invent a name for ourselves." After quite a bit of discussion the group ended up with the name *Free Therapy*. "You know, this is nothing like therapy, but it sure is therapeutic, so Free Therapy is a good name," Johanna argued.

After some weeks they had written a few songs with which they were pleased, and the music therapist asked Free Therapy if they wanted to share their songs and perhaps organize a little performance in the ward. They talked about it for a while, discussing if they would be ready to pull it off and also if the staff would appreciate the lyrics. They decided to give it a go.

The music therapist was pleased, but also a bit worried. Some of the songs were a bit critical, albeit in a humorous way, and sometimes the clinic and its staff seemed to be targeted in the songs. It was kind of hard to say, because the lyrics of several of the songs were not always all that easy to understand. With some hesitation he had come to the conclusion that the enigmatic quality of the lyrics perhaps contributed to their poetic quality rather than reflected a lack of clarity.

Pathways of Johanna's Journey

Johanna's music therapy journey did not evolve as a process of individual sessions only,

as the music therapist had anticipated, but ended up including a series of songwriting workshops, rehearsals, and performances. It grew into a process of reaching out, with plenty of ups and downs. Some of the Free Therapy performances went quite well. The audience listened attentively and the group's motivation for future songwriting and performances increased. Other times, things were not so clear. Perhaps the audience was just being polite? What did they really think of the songs? And why would Johanna sometimes just start singing without checking if the others were ready? These would be some of the questions to process before and after the performances of the group.

The music therapist was confused about the process more than once. Not too much of what he had learned in university about the music therapy process made sense in this context. He was not the expert who assessed the strengths and problems of a client and then offered a pertinent intervention. The process was collaborative and to some degree unpredictable. It was not arbitrary, however, he would argue to support his own sense of professional competency. Free Therapy would always evaluate the things they were doing and adjust their ways accordingly. There were plenty of predicaments to deal with, but also lots of things to celebrate.

One of the positive surprises of the process was to discover that the chief psychiatrist had become very supportive of the group. The music therapist did not know what to make of this, but the psychiatrist explained to him that he had realized that the clinic needed to focus more on recovery-oriented practice than what they had done previously. "And what would be a better example than Free Therapy of an approach focusing on people's own creative journeys toward a better and more self-directed life? It's only natural that their songs are a bit critical of the system at times." The music therapist realized that working with Free Therapy once again had put him in a situation where he did not know what to say. Had the group's performances really contributed to some change in his colleagues' understanding of their professional role, or was that too good to be true? How should he understand all this? Perhaps he needed to do some reading on personal and social recovery too.

After several weeks of workshops and performances, Johanna requested a few individual sessions with the music therapist. "I'm soon going to leave the clinic. To think of the empty life I lived before I came here scares me. I don't want to lose the connection to music that I now have developed." The individual sessions focused quite a bit on how Johanna could succeed in maintaining her connection to music when going back to a life in her own apartment, and to use it as a vehicle for establishing connections to other people too. The music therapist knew that there was a community music and theater group in the neighborhood where Johanna lived, and they decided to explore what the possibilities for participation in that group would be.

If we step back from this synthesized narrative, we can see that the process was collaborative rather than expert-driven. Both the participants' expertise and the music therapist's expertise were necessary components in the process. The music therapist struggled quite a bit with his own understanding of this experience. Challenges of professional unlearning and relearning are often involved in the development of CoMT practices (Stige, 2014), and practitioners might need a language for reflecting on processes that are collaborative, multidimensional, and open. In one attempt to develop a model of CoMT processes, we (Stige & Aarø, 2012) proposed that

> community music therapy processes can be described as movement in the direction of health, wellbeing, and social-musical change through the *interaction* of six different shifts: *Creating critical awareness* (developing information about broader contexts and challenging ideology), *Appraising affordances* (planning what is possible to do in a given context, through appraisal of problems and resources in relation to several dimensions of practice and at several levels of analysis), *Bonding and bridging* (supporting social-musical processes that connect people within homogeneous and heterogeneous communities), *Dealing with predicaments* (transforming conflicts at various level of analysis, ranging from person to group to broader communities), *Evaluating and adjusting* (examining strengths and weaknesses in all of the shifts made within the participatory process, with the aim of improving practice), and *Communicating and celebrating* (performing for broader audiences and creating and welcoming collective joy). (pp. 230–231)

Obviously, a model of CoMT processes does not help if the music therapist does not have a theoretical understanding that can support reflections on and development of the evolving relationships. The narrative above illustrates the relevance of several issues that require theoretical reflection, such as problems and possibilities linked to an expansion of contexts for music therapy practice (e.g., see Turry, 2005) and performance as an integrated element in the music therapy process (e.g., see Ansdell, 2005, 2010b). Both of these issues, in the next round, request theoretical and metatheoretical reflections on the concept of context in music therapy (Rolvsjord & Stige, 2013).

Certainly, the example we have visited also suggests that interdisciplinary theories are of relevance to CoMT. The music therapist's ponderings on boundary violations versus boundary crossings were perhaps informed by psychotherapy theory (see Gutheil & Brodsky, 2008). But more importantly (here), the example also reveals that music studies and the social sciences are highly relevant for CoMT. Music is much more than a stimulus (or personal expression, for that matter). It is often better understood as a social activity in context, what Small (1998) describes as *musicking*. As a social activity, music can build social resources through facilitating processes such as bonding within a group and bridging between groups (Putnam, 2000).

We also observed that the emerging *recovery approach* within the field of mental health (Solli, Rolvsjord, & Borg, 2013) is of relevance for the understanding of some CoMT processes, because of several shared tenets. This relevance does not suggest, however, that CoMT is limited to the recovery model. Gary Ansdell (2014), for instance, develops an ecological perspective on how music helps (in music therapy and everyday life) where he does not apply the recovery model but instead elaborates on a broad notion of human wellness and musical flourishing, focusing on musical worlds, musical experience, musical personhood, musical relationship, musical community, and musical transcendence.

Conclusions

CoMT's focus on collaborative possibilities and social responsibilities represents a contrast to more received views of what music therapy is or should be. Consider the American Music Therapy Association's (2005) definition of music therapy as "the clinical and evidence-based use of music interventions to accomplish individualized goals within a therapeutic relationship." There is a contrast between this definition and the ideas presented in this chapter: CoMT is usually not clinical by any stretch of the term. Goals may be individualized, but not necessarily, and the pursuit of them is not restricted to work within a therapeutic relationship. Processes are participatory to a degree that suggests that a term such as *intervention* should be replaced by broader terms such as *involvement* or *initiative*. And CoMT's relationship to research is more multifaceted than what is suggested by the phrase *evidence-based*.

As the synthesized example presented in this chapter reveals, there is also continuity and not only contrast. Sometimes CoMT practices evolve as extensions of more traditional approaches to music therapy. This is not always the case, however. The musical and social starting points of CoMT might request ecologically oriented practices that are very different from what we usu-

ally think of as therapy. Bruscia (1998) has made a pertinent comment when comparing traditional group therapy with ecological practices (such as CoMT):

> In traditional group therapy, the aim is to effect therapeutic change in individual members; whereas in ecological group work, the aim is to effect therapeutic change in the ecological system and the individuals that are a part of it. This means that in traditional group therapy, changes in individual members have to be generalized or applied to each member's own ecological context away from the group; in ecological work, no such generalization is necessary. In other words, the client in traditional group therapy is each individual member, rather than the group itself; the client in ecological work is both the individual and the community. (p. 230)

Perhaps the complex patterns of contrast and continuity have contributed to making CoMT controversial in some music therapy circles, but CoMT has grown into a strong movement already and many controversies are now history. One context for understanding the controversies around CoMT might suggest that some of the debates will go on, however. I am thinking of the continuous struggles within society between individualized treatment strategies, on one hand, and public health strategies on the other. Medicine's enormous advances in the 20th century clearly drove policies and professional efforts in the direction of individualized treatment. It is becoming clearer, however, that such strategies are insufficient, not least if we take equity, social justice, and the multidimensional nature of human well-being into consideration (Stige & Aarø, 2012).

The debates on how a society should prioritize individualized treatment versus public health initiatives therefore will continue to reappear in new configurations, depending on the sociocultural, material, and political realities of a society. CoMT, as a rights-based and culture-centered practice, clearly pulls music therapy in the direction of public health initiatives. Of course, ideally there should be no contradiction between individualized treatment and socialized health promotion and public health work, but the limitation of financial resources that characterizes all human societies suggests that there will be continuing political debates on the relative merit of each strategy.

Implications for the profession and discipline of music therapy are manifold. First, we need to ask how we prepare our students musically, theoretically, and ethically for the challenges of CoMT practice. Second, we need to rethink our notion of what it means to be a professional and learn how to develop a more collaborative and socially engaged role. Third, we can think of CoMT as a lasting invitation to reflect on music therapy's position in and contribution to society.

REFERENCES

American Music Therapy Association. (2005). *What is music therapy?* (American Music Therapy Association definition, 2005). Retrieved from *www.musictherapy.org.*

Ansdell, G. (2002). Community music therapy and the winds of change: A discussion paper. *Voices: A World Forum for Music Therapy, 2*(2). Retrieved from *https://normt.uib.no/index.php/voices/article/view/83/65.*

Ansdell, G. (2005). Being who you aren't; doing what you can't: Community music therapy and the paradoxes of performance. *Voices: A World Forum for Music Therapy.* Retrieved from *https://normt.uib.no/index.php/voices/article/view/229/173.*

Ansdell, G. (2010a). Belonging through musicing: Explorations of musical community. In B. Stige, G. Ansdell, C. Elefant, & M. Pavlicevic (Eds.), *Where music helps: Community music therapy in action and reflection* (pp. 41–62). Aldershot, UK: Ashgate.

Ansdell, G. (2010b). Where performing helps: Processes and affordances of performance in community music therapy. In B. Stige, G. Ansdell, C. Elefant, & M. Pavlicevic (Eds.), *Where music helps: Community music therapy in action and reflection* (pp. 161–186). Aldershot, UK: Ashgate.

Ansdell, G. (2014). *How music helps in music therapy and everyday life.* Aldershot, UK: Ashgate.

Boxill, E. H. (1988). Continuing notes: Worldwide networking for peace [Editorial]. *Music Therapy, 7*(1), 80–81.

Bronfenbrenner, U. (1979). *The ecology of human development: Experiments by nature and design.* Cambridge, MA: Harvard University Press.

Broucek, M. (1987). Beyond healing to "wholeing": A voice for the deinstitutionalization of music therapy. *Music Therapy, 6*(2), 50–58.

Bruscia, K. (1998). *Defining music therapy* (2nd ed.). Gilsum, NH: Barcelona.

Bunt, L. (1994). *Music therapy: An art beyond words.* London: Routledge.

Connolly, M., & Ward, T. (2008). *Morals, rights and practice in the human services: Effective and fair decision-making in health, social care and criminal justice.* London: Jessica Kingsley.

Gaston, E. T. (Ed.). (1968). *Music in therapy.* New York: Macmillan.

Gewirth, A. (1996). *The community of rights.* Chicago: University of Chicago Press.

Giddens, A. (1984). *The constitution of society: Outline of the theory of structuration.* Cambridge, UK: Cambridge University Press.

Gutheil, T. G., & Brodsky, A. (2008). *Preventing boundary violations in clinical practice.* New York: Guilford Press.

Kenny, C. B. (2006). *Music and life in the Field of Play.* Gilsum, NH: Barcelona.

Kenny, C. B., & Stige, B. (Eds.). (2002). *Contemporary Voices of music therapy: Communication, culture, and community.* Oslo, Norway: Unipub forlag.

Kleive, M., & Stige, B. (1988). *Med lengting, liv og song* [With longing, life, and song.] Oslo, Norway: Samlaget.

McGuire, M. G. (Ed.). (2004). *Psychiatric music therapy in the community: The legacy of Florence Tyson.* Gilsum, NH: Barcelona.

Nettl, B. (1956). Aspects of primitive and folk music relevant to music therapy. In E. T. Gaston (Ed.), *Music therapy 1955. Fifth book of proceedings of the National Association for Music Therapy* (pp. 36–39). Lawrence, KS: National Association for Music Therapy.

Oosthuizen, H. (2006). Diversity and community: Finding and forming a South African music therapy. *Voices: A World Forum for Music Therapy.* Retrieved from *https://normt.uib.no/index.php/voices/article/view/277/202.*

Pavlicevic, M., & Ansdell, G. (Eds.). (2004). *Community music therapy.* London: Jessica Kingsley.

Putnam, R. (2000). *Bowling alone: The collapse and revival of American community.* New York: Simon & Schuster.

Rolvsjord, R., & Stige, B. (2013). Concepts of context in music therapy. *Nordic Journal of Music Therapy*.

Ruud, E. (1998). *Music therapy: Improvisation, communication and culture.* Gilsum, NH: Barcelona.

Simon, C. (2013). *Community music therapy: Musik stiftet Gemeinschaft* [Community music therapy: Music creates community]. Klein Jasedow, Germany: Drachen Verlag.

Small, C. (1998). *Musicking: The meanings of performing and listening.* Hanover, NH: Wesleyan University Press.

Solli, H. P., Rolvsjord, R., & Borg, M. (2013). Toward understanding music therapy as a recovery-oriented practice within mental health care: A meta-synthesis of service users' experiences. *Journal of Music Therapy, 50*(4), 244–273.

Stige, B. (2002). *Culture-centered music therapy.* Gilsum, NH: Barcelona.

Stige, B. (2012). *Elaborations towards a notion of Community Music Therapy.* Gilsum NH: Barcelona. (Original work published 2003)

Stige, B. (2014). Community music therapy and the process of learning about and struggling for openness. *International Journal of Community Music, 7*(1), 47–56.

Stige, B., & Aarø, L. E. (2012). *Invitation to community music therapy.* New York: Routledge.

Stige, B., Ansdell, G., Elefant, C., & Pavlicevic, M. (2010). *Where music helps: Community music therapy in action and reflection.* Farnham, UK: Ashgate.

Tuastad, L., & O'Grady, L. (2013). Music therapy inside and outside prison: A freedom practice? *Nordic Journal of Music Therapy, 22*(3), 210–232.

Turry, A. (2005). Music psychotherapy and community music therapy: Questions and considerations. *Voices: A World Forum for Music Therapy.* Retrieved from *https://normt.uib.no/index.php/voices/article/view/208/152.*

Vaillancourt, G. (2009). *Mentoring apprentice music therapists for peace and social justice through community music therapy: An arts-based study.* Doctoral dissertation, Antioch University, Santa Barbara, CA. Available at *http://etd.ohiolink.edu/view.cgi?acc_num=antioch1255546013.*

CHAPTER 20

Music Therapy in Expressive Arts

Margareta Wärja

Throughout history humans have engaged in making art for the intrinsic joy, empowerment, and healing it can bring. The arts are a gateway to known and untraveled roads and bring us to ineffable worlds of human myths and history. The languages of the arts provide living fibers for making sense of life. It is where we share hopes and dreams and stories of suffering. In music, dance, paintings, poems, and theatre, we tell and show our personal stories to each other and to the community. In that telling and revealing of stories, we are changed. *Experience* is the material from which we craft these stories. Expression through the arts is, in itself, an essential and distinctive attribute of our humanity.

The different art forms and languages all intersect, like a huge, connected, and vital river system. Each mode of expression contributes unique qualities to be considered in psychotherapy and any healing endeavor. Some arts, such as music and dance, are embedded in the temporal mode. They emerge, dissolve, pass, and transform with each moment. Others, such as the visual arts and sculpting, concern themselves with shaping objects, things, and devices

in space that hold their stories and can be viewed, explored, and revisited time after time. As we engage in art activities in psychotherapy, we become open to aesthetic encounters that can improve communication and expression; increase psychological, physical, emotional, cognitive, and social functioning; and promote health and well-being. The arts provide creative and interactive processes that support change and help us find resources for living life more fully. A number of associated professions, including music, dance, art, and drama, apply the arts in therapy. The term *creative arts therapy* encompasses these separate disciplines of art therapies.

This chapter concerns the related field of *expressive arts therapy*, a multimodal approach combines the visual arts, music, dance/movement, drama, photo/filmmaking, writing, literary art, and other creative processes in psychotherapy, social services, and community work. More specifically, I describe the use of music in the larger container of expressive arts. I call this approach *music-centered expressive arts therapy*. Various psychological problems, conflicts, and traumatic experiences can be addressed through the use of imagination and creative expression. There are many ways to combine the modalities in expressive arts, many different personal styles of working, and various psychological frames upon which to draw. A common basis for the work is the interplay of experiences, emotions, behavior, and physical health that characterizes a mind–body connection (Damasio, 2010).

Over the past 25 years I have been engaged in the development and the training program of expressive arts in Sweden. Today this method is employed in mental health, psychotherapy practice, medical care and rehabilitation, geriatrics, hospice, social change endeavors, special education, clinical supervision, and organizational development. My journey in music therapy started around 30 years ago as a music therapy student at California State University, Long Beach, when I had arrived from Sweden, curious and eager to learn about the powers of music in the healing arts. The years since then have been an engaging voyage where many have guided me along the way. Some stand out for their particular perspectives and wisdom.

From early on, the theoretical and philosophical writings by Carolyn Kenny (2006) on music therapy as a whole systems approach, guided by aesthetics, influenced my thinking. The inspirational teachings and collaborations in the Bonny Method of Guided Imagery and Music with Frances Smith Goldberg, Lisa Summer, and Helen Bonny created the foundation for the way I practice and understand music therapy as a space for surrender, empowerment, beauty, and transcendence. Years of working with esteemed expressive arts colleagues Paolo Knill, Margo Fuchs, Markus Alexander, and Steve and Ellen Levine have taught me the innate powers of arts and spontaneous play. The same can be said for 20 years of teamwork with Melinda Meyer, Director of the Norwegian Institute of Expressive Arts and Communication, who has shown me the healing capacity of art making itself in

using testimony and intermodal psychodrama with survivors of torture and trauma (Meyer, 2007). My background in adult psychiatry, and lately in oncology, has included addressing a wide variety of psychological problems and existential dilemmas where the philosophical base is rooted in phenomenology, existentialism, and a body-oriented frame of reference. All of these have contributed to the practice of music-centered expressive arts therapy.

This chapter begins with an introduction to the background and theoretical foundations of expressive arts and the psychotherapeutic frame of reference in which the work is based, followed by a presentation of case vignettes demonstrating how music therapy can be applied in this field.

History

The beginning of expressive arts therapy dates back to the 1970s, when a group of pioneers in related fields of art came together at Lesley College Graduate School in Boston (now Lesley University) to exchange experiences and combine artistic disciplines in psychotherapeutic and social educational work. Eventually a therapeutic school, called *expressive arts*, was formed, where different artistic expressions and disciplines were integrated. The founders of the program were Shaun McNiff, art therapist; Paolo Knill, music therapist and performance artist; Norma Canner, dance therapist; and Elisabeth McKim, poet (McNiff, 2009). In the early days of the new discipline there was a notion of expressing outwardly what was felt and experienced inwardly as a way of *self-expression*. The foundational focus has since shifted to the power of the arts and the aesthetic experience as approached phenomenologically. The field emerged in the tradition of psychotherapy but has expanded into different domains, including organizational development, education, media and communication, social change, community integration, and peace building and conflict transformation. Educational programs are currently found at universities and private institutes in the United States, Canada, South America, Israel, and Europe.

One essential concept introduced by Knill in the 1970s is the notion of the *intermodal* aspects of expressive arts, based on our capacity for sensing (Knill, Nienhaus Barba, & Fuchs, 1995). We perceive the world through our senses: sight, taste, touch, smell, sounds, and kinesthetic. This concept of intermodality refers to the understanding that every artistic discipline is primarily based on a specific body modality (e.g., music on audition, visual art on sight), but that all stem from the body's capacity for *sensing*, a capacity in which all the senses may be involved (Levine & Levine, 2005, 2009). It is the *body* that paints, plays music, performs, and dances.

Understanding the interconnectedness of the senses in art making is essential for the practice of expressive arts therapy and informs how to proceed in a given situation. Within each art discipline, the modalities of the other arts lie in the background as potential resources. The different art forms hold innate qualities that serve the process in different ways. For example, a client in therapy may paint a picture. The client and therapist can then engage in a dialogue and relate to the picture/images in a free, nondirective, and nonreductive manner. The aesthetics of the image speak as fully as possible. A visual image will most likely also hold a sense of rhythm and maybe a tonal space, too. The image might carry a story line, a text, or a dramatic act. Maybe the images give directions for bodily movements and dance. In the course of therapy, the therapist pays attention to and follows the process closely, and, when the timing seems right, the process moves on to the use of another art form based on a different modality. How and when this so-called *intermodal transfer* takes place is a matter of context, therapeutic alliance, and issues at hand. Once again, the therapist's aesthetic

sensibility comes into play in shaping the session so that it is effective for the client.

The purpose of using art in psychotherapy is not primarily to represent or symbolize an inner experience, feeling, or relationship. Rather, it is the other way around: letting the creative process and the artwork itself provide a path of exploration that can lead to growth, affect release, and self-understanding by helping one to stay with feelings, sensations, and images while moving into the act of shaping. It is a journey that goes through liminal spaces that most likely will bring about surprises and unexpected turns along the way. The concept of *liminality* was introduced by anthropologist Arnold van Gennep (1960) and later Victor Turner (1995) to describe aspects of cultural change and rituals. This concept points to the experience of leaving the ordinary and stepping over thresholds into unknown territories to experience the *in-between* places where possible change and profound transformation can be discovered.

Theoretical Tenets

The theoretical foundation of expressive arts is grounded in the humanistic–existential orientation, where concepts intentionality, spontaneity, creativity, human potential, and responsibility are emphasized. The power of the arts themselves is at the base of the work. Playing with imagination and engaging our human capacity to shape our world is central to the practice. In developing a theoretical frame, we turn to the work of Edmund Husserl (1960) and Martin Heidegger (1953/1996) to find a philosophical base. Husserl, considered the founder of phenomenology, was active at the beginning of the last century and was critical of the prevailing psychology at the time, arguing that science had to be based on the direct/immediate experience of the world. He turned against Descartes' dualism of spirit and matter and argued that there was a great problem with this split between consciousness and nature. Husserl's (1970) phenomenology is a theory of knowledge and an approach to reality based on investigating the nature of experiencing. By paying attention to what is there, the thing will make itself known. A basic assumption is the principle of *intentionality*, which states that consciousness has a direction. Intentionality can be directed toward the world, ourselves, and itself. What do we then mean by a *phenomenon*? It is that which shows itself to us. The phenomenon is given to me immediately in the act of perception. To be able to perceive what is actually there, I put brackets around past experiences and try, as much as possible, to experience the phenomenon at hand.

Heidegger (1953/1996) formulated an existential phenomenology in which he dwelt on the question of *being (Dasein)*. His view was that we can choose to live an authentic or an inauthentic life. He argued that, in order to live authentically, we must first accept and take responsibility for our own existence. Heidegger believed that truth was potentially manifested in the arts. He used the word *poiesis* from classical Greek, which translates into *making*, and refers most often to art making but may also refer to bringing something new into the world. The phenomenon is seen as containing *multiple narratives*—that is, a phenomenon can hold many different stories and descriptions (Levine & Levine, 2005, 2009).

The expressive arts are closely related to existential phenomenology and psychotherapy. When we create, we are shaping the conditions of our existence. Existential psychotherapy is influenced by existential philosophy and concerns themes such as how we humans create meaning and how we develop a sense of coherence and trust in our lives. A set of circumstances is given at birth—a combination of heredity and environmental factors—that affects our existence and everyday lives by influencing how we decide to live. We are in a constant process of becoming; we are co-creators in shaping how our lives and personality de-

velop. As we create, we need to start with the formless and set our life experiences in motion (Levine & Levine, 2009; van Deurzen, 2010).

It is essential to be aware of the body when working with existential psychotherapy through the arts. Clients are encouraged to be aware of bodily sensations, the breath, and of grounding the body. Levine (2011) points to the neglect of the bodily experience in Heidegger's writing and turns to Merleau-Ponty and his notion of "the 'lived body,' a generalized body-awareness that underlies consciousness," that serves as a philosophical understanding of the practice (Levine, p. 40). As we consider recent research in neuropsychology, attachment, and the function of the brain, we find empirical support for this view and the necessity to work through the body in conducting psychotherapy. The body holds memories, assumptions, and stories of the past. Stern (2010) speaks of the dynamic forms of vitality in our bodies as relating to affects and feelings. There are five different dynamic events—movement, time, force, space, and intention/directionality—that give rise to the experience of vitality and to experiences of being alive. Stern points out that in the time-based arts, such as music and movement, these forms of vitalities are fundamental building blocks. The story unfolds through the body, with the accompanying feelings, and can be processed, deepened, and changed.

Neurobiological research on emotion and consciousness has brought us toward a greater understanding of these phenomena. Damasio (2010) has formulated a neuropsychological theory of the concept of mind (the self). He argues that we have preverbal minds, based solely on the affects produced in the body. At higher levels of development, autobiographical recollections and memories can be linked to thoughts and to languages. Thus we have several, parallel consciousnesses. Other researchers (Schore, 2009; Stern, 2004, 2010) have contributed to the understanding of the central nervous system and the brain. They have predicted that the future practice of psychotherapy will involve methods whereby we will be able to work directly with feelings, with expressive (arts-based) and body-oriented methodologies. Attention to verbal discursive language will diminish, and the starting point will become the immediate experience of a relationship and the feelings involved. Verbal reflection and integration can take place only after having had the experience in the *here and now*, as in intermodal expressive arts, and with other creative arts therapies. As we practice poiesis, we let images flow like dream sequences to perception through the attentive mind. The therapy room serves as space, open for images to arrive and to be shaped and explored. As we allow our stories to unfold, they transform and shape us. The spontaneous gesture, the sculpted shape, the rough painted surface, the dynamics of music and movement—all are tangible expressions of the rich imaginal tapestry in which we can meet ourselves. The way in which images and stories can help us needs to be explored with attentive presence and care.

The capacity for attachment and the creation of trust are prerequisites for growth and for reciprocal relationships. Today, the study of attachment is seen as one of the most important areas that influences the theories and practice of psychotherapy and relates to more recent research on the development of the brain in the field of neuropsychology (Shore, 2009). In psychotherapy, the development of a trusting relationship is the base. Paying attention to the ways in which communication moves in the relationship is of interest in this work. When trust is established, there is also a sense of surrender to the other. There is a readiness to give and receive experiences that enhance and deepen the mutual connection, such as communication of various affect states. Today the idea of a transitional space, or play space, as formulated by Winnicott (1971), has relevance

for psychotherapy, along with new theories of attachment and the development of intersubjectivity, which is a human relational and developmental process of sharing lived experiences. Intersubjectivity occurs in an implicit (nonverbal) relational field but can also take an explicit form as in language development. What is shared is attention, intention, and affectivity (Stern, 2004). It is a common and mutual interaction that is larger than the separate individuals. Related is the concept of mentalization, referring to the preconscious ability of mental process of understanding human behaviours and the intentions of another human being as well as one's own. These concepts of intersubjectivity, mentalization, and sharing experiences are essential in understanding how psychotherapy works as it deals with the essence of being in relationship with another person and concerns how we become human beings and how consciousness develops. A relational perspective in psychotherapy is founded on the assumption that change and transformation toward health is based on the client's capacity for intersubjectivity, mentalization, and attachment within that psychotherapeutic relationship (Stern, 2004).

Here is an example of intermodal work where movement, music, and painting are braided together in one coherent creative process. It is written in the present tense to convey the sense of here and now that characterizes an expressive arts session where the process flows between the different modalities.

CLINICAL EXAMPLE: Exploring the Potential Space of Imagination

This is an excerpt from one session with a young woman I call Maya who was referred to me from an outpatient clinic. She arrives wanting to work on issues such as loneliness and isolation, depression, dependency, and lack of self-esteem. The sudden death of her father due to an accident about 1 year earlier is the event that led her to seek help. The unspoken question is hanging in the air: Did her father in fact commit suicide? Maya speaks of aches and pains in her body and loss of feelings.

In meeting her, two images emerge in my awareness: a strong current that is deep-frozen; and a small, frightened animal pacing in the shadows. I realize that I have to begin in a slow tempo and build trust. We begin this particular session in the early phase of our work with a short dialogue in which Maya complains about her stiff body and not getting any work done at the university where she is studying to become a teacher. She goes around in circles and ends up talking of practical problems. Her narration is like a chant, where a short melody fragment is repeated over and over again. It is time for a shift, and we stand up.

I ask her to pay attention to her breathing and the sensations of her body. Can she notice if she is aware of any image? She speaks of physical sensations: heavy head, tension in her back, and legs feeling weak. I suggest that she move freely in the way her body needs to move. I mirror the dynamics of her movements. Maya stretches, kicks her legs, and yawns. I sense that she is not fully present. Then, as she lifts both arms up in the air, something happens. She stops and takes hold of her head with both hands, as in an act of protection, and mentions an image of a sturdy orange helmet. We explore the image of the helmet for a while through dialogue and then agree to continue with a short, receptive music experience (KMR–Brief Music Journeys). Maya relaxes in the reclining chair and I help her settle in. Before the music begins, I suggest that she bring the orange helmet to her attention. The short piece, "Mot den nya världen" (Towards the New World) by the Swedish composer Stefan Nilsson, fills the room. It has a gentle, soft melody that starts in the piano, is picked up by the oboe, and held in the embrace of strings. The melody moves a contained crescendo that fades away. When the music ends, I say, "Stay with whatever comes to you—any feelings, thoughts, images. . . . Then when you are ready, walk up to the art material, take the colors and brushes that attract you, and simply start to paint. Just move with the rhythm and colors. Let go of any attempt to deliberately *make* a drawing

about your experience. Stay with it, and let it just happen."

Maya stands up while painting on a fairly large piece of paper. I watch her put on transparent layers of blue and gray gouache. The shapes float, fall, and transform over the paper like fog, haze, and soft rain. I follow the birth of a strange image in a dark corner, an alien-looking creature with wings and claws. I am aware of her tension as she pounds and slaps on the colors with large brushes. The beating intensifies into a storm and stops abruptly. She bends down, sighing heavily. Silence. Waiting. I am aware of strain and pain in my body as I witness her work. Quickly she stands up and adds layers of wet paint that drip to the floor. The paper gives in, dissolves, and leaves a hole with ragged edges. She stops, looking pleased.

As we sit down to talk, Maya first speaks of her experience in the music. "I saw myself at a construction site, balancing on an iron bar high up. I must admit it was a bit strange and scary, and I felt totally lost. I noticed someone that I could not recognize, standing on another rod farther away. Suddenly this person just fell and tumbled headlong in the air. Then my head started to hurt really badly, even though I could hear that the music was so soft and friendly. Next, I came to think of a large bird that was struggling to fly."

This session represented a major shift in Maja's therapeutic journey. As we continued to work, she unraveled layers of ambivalent feelings in regard to her relationship with her father and her unsure identity as a woman. In summary, the session started with bodily movement where one image was found. This image was taken into a short music-listening experience, and further on to painting. In the last part, there was the verbal dialogue and exploration. These different steps in the intermodal approach served to open, shape, explore, and deepen the emerging material in a nonthreatening way. An experience must be lived in the moment with feelings and actions. Change happens in steps and spurts that are nonlinear and from processes and experiences of mutual sharing.

Music in Expressive Arts Therapy

We now turn to the language of music. There are many ways to use the creative arts techniques in the practice of music therapy. The focus here is a music-centered approach in expressive arts. It draws from the traditions of improvisational music therapy (Wigram, 2004), the receptive method of guided imagery and music (GIM; Bonny, 1980; Bruscia & Grocke, 2002), and the theoretical and methodological foundations of expressive arts (Levine & Levine, 2005, 2009). The core consists of the intermodal perspective, the creative process, and dialoging with images through a phenomenological and existential perspective. Warming up to the body in different ways is most often the entry to the work. In practice this approach comprises active and receptive models of music therapy.

Following the line of thought presented so far, the evolving visual images, the swirling movements of the dance, the unfolding dramatic story, and the poetic metaphors are all embedded in music. Experiencing music as a form of sensing intuitive knowledge that brings us to the body is the foundation of this kind of work. One vital function of music is to open us up to worlds of imagination and connect us with feelings that often are carried in the content of the imagery.

Important principles of music-centered expressive arts include the following:

- Using music as the main gateway for entering the play space and engaging imagination.
- Entering the work through an awareness of the body (breathing, grounding, images).
- Using active and receptive methods of music therapy:
  o Improvisations.
  o KMR–Brief Music Journeys an adaptation of GIM.
- Embracing the intermodal possibilities of music.
- Engaging in the model of decentering (described below).

- Dialoging with images through a phenomenological and existential frame.
- Using intermodal transfer to move to other art languages as ways to explore the images.
- Recognizing the implicit mutual relational field between therapist and client as the space wherein change occurs.

Decentering: Working with Change through the Arts

A model called *decentering* presents a structure for how to approach change in expressive arts (Levine & Levine, 2005). I introduce this structure here because it is relevant to the work in a music-centered approach. Decentering has its theoretical roots in systems theory and a solution-focused methodology and can be used with individuals and groups and in working with organizations and communities. To *decenter* means to leave the everyday life of habits and step into an alternative experience of the everyday world, guided by play and creativity. As we move into unpredictable terrains through the arts, we enlarge the range of play. Conflicts cannot be solved through the same kind of thinking and acting that created them. Stuck patterns and habits need to be unstuck so that new possibilities can arise. The structure of a decentering experience can be outlined in the following way:

1. *Containment:* In dialoguing about the issue of concern, the therapist stays open and reflective, asks questions and makes comments to help deepen, contain, and focus the issue. There is mutual agreement about what to focus on in the session.
2. *Warm-up:* This is a shift that most often means to stand up, warm up, and become aware of the body. Metaphorically, this is a transition where you step into another territory. It usually brings in a slightly altered state of consciousness, for example, through the use of images, guiding, grounding, and attention to the breath.

3. *Play space:* Most often the therapist invites the client to engage in some form of artistic activity. The client can be the one to initiate a creative act of some sort—for example, painting, working with clay or sculpture, dancing, improvising, or listening to music in a relaxed state. The process involves an altered state of consciousness. The problem or issue at hand is in the background but is not addressed explicitly. Instead this is a space for imagination, play, and free and spontaneous creativity.

4. *Aesthetic reflection:* When the creative part of the session has ended, there is time for an open dialogue about the aesthetic experience itself. How does it speak to you? What do the images say? What is the work bringing you now? Here the aim is to stay in the actual experience of the image. What was it like? How did it feel? How is it now? Are there any surprises?

5. *Harvest:* This is the time to come back, carefully collect the richness from being involved with the arts, and reflect on how this experience best can serve the client's needs. What was discovered? This part requires care. There is a risk of losing the poetic and multidimensional language when trying to understand and analyze. Sensitivity is needed as one moves between verbal and implicit layers of communication. In psychotherapy, there are times when silence and empathic holding are most helpful.

Playing and Shaping with Sounds, Rhythms, and Images

There are infinite ways to improvise in music: alone, in a duet, in a small ensemble, with others in a large community. Percussive instruments, gongs, xylophones, and the voice are most commonly used in this approach. For example, a client can be given one or two instruments to explore. After a period of playing and improvising, the therapist can help the client find the sounds having the greatest impact, either because of their pleasing and harmonious quality or due to their dissonance. A number of *takes* (repetitions in which different sound patterns are discovered in a sequence) can be conducted. The result may be a simple musical composition that touches the client's inner experience and brings something new. A period of reflection or *aesthetic analysis* follows, in which the process of visual and musical art making is described from a phenomenological perspective. The therapist can then bring the discussion back to the presenting problem and find resonances between the session and the material that the client initially brought to therapy. We call this a *work-oriented* approach to the arts in therapy, insofar as the emergence of a work of art that is meaningful for the client is a goal. Other examples of active and expressive ways of working in music include:

- *Sound painting:* A free associative improvisation, alone, in a duet with the therapist, or in a group where one especially explores sounds and timbre of music (the tone colors). There is a warm-up through movement, during which visual images of color are introduced to connect with feeling states of the moment. The music becomes like an expressive painting on a resonating canvas using instruments and the voice.

- *Structured improvisation:* Applying existing musical forms such as ternary form, rondo, theme and variation, or blues. A conductor may be used to structure the music.

- *Composing and songwriting:* Starting with a poem, a story, or an image that becomes the score for building the composition. Working with different takes to shape and crystallize the piece. It is conceivable to use a performance format.

- *Intermodal music psychodrama:* An adaptation of psychodrama, developed in collaboration with Meyer, wherein music is the main modality of exploring a life situation or an image. On stage, time can be moved to the past or into the future. The drama, however, is experienced in the present. This work is best done in groups and requires a clear structure, skill, and holding of a director/therapist. The aim is to assist the client in exploring the arising images; releasing and shaping them through a dramatic act involving group participants, musical instruments, and the voice; and then finally harvesting the discoveries.

The relational theoretical framework on which this work is based acknowledges the possibility of an unexpected third space opening up between therapist and client. This is the potential opening in which images come alive and in which the imagination is put into sound and motion. Thus the core of the session occurs through the engagement in music. The creative phase generally starts with warming up through attention to the body and moving to music, using active and/or receptive methods of music therapy. The images, stories, and discoveries found are then brought to a process of shaping through other art modalities. The process of intermodal transfer involves using different-size papers, gouache paints, coal, acrylic paint on canvas, clay, installation art, movement, bodily expression, musical improvisations, theatre and role play, poetry, and story writing. Staying and living with images and letting them materialize in the outer world creates a large kinesthetic image container.

When two human beings meet in a psychotherapeutic context, a particular kind of psychological meeting takes place in a sort of underlying current created by the intersubjective domain of present moments. This is what happens when we play or listen to music together; sharing happens without verbalizing. Kenny (2006) speaks to this aspect of music as direct experience in presenting a phenomenological approach to music therapy called the *Field of Play*. As two people make music together, both bring an aesthetic environment that consists of who they are and the potential they each hold. The aim of the creative process is to move toward wellness and all that it is possible to become. Kenny says that the creative process "is informed by love, the intelligence of the heart, and thus the knowledge of the self-organizing system. It assumes that given its creativity, a safe environment and appropriate resources, after trauma, a person will naturally use the creative process to facilitate reorganization and reintegration" (p. 102). The field of play has much in common with Winnicott's (1971) concept of transitional space, in which the client can explore, play, gain confidence, grow, and become increasingly more capable and independent. The act of playing is central to the development of the child: In the healthy mother–child interaction the child is mirrored and affirmed and thus develops basic trust and self-confidence. The ability of the arts to bring about direct experience is one of the founding principles of using music in expressive arts therapy. Clients seeking therapy often have difficulty in this regard. The therapist needs to initiate a playful attitude and have access to his or her own spontaneity. This stance will help clients face and make sense of large existential questions, such as the meaning of life, death, identity, belonging, dependency, love, sex, and intimacy.

Receptive Music Therapy KMR–Brief Music Journeys

Although there are no restrictions on what kind of receptive music therapy methods to use, a method called KMR–Brief Music Journeys [English translation]) has become the hallmark of the music-centered expressive arts approach at the Swedish and Norwegian institutes (Kaestele & Müller, 2013; Wärja, 2010, 2015). KMR is an adaptation of the Bonny Method of GIM and involves listening to carefully selected, short pieces of music. The purpose is to work with existential questions and various psychological difficulties. KMR grew out of my background as a GIM practitioner and has been explored in the context of expressive arts during the last 15 years. In working with

KMR, one can explore current events, dive into relationship issues, and work with problems of varying degrees. It is possible to enter into dream images, explore symptoms, address crises and traumatic events, and face concrete everyday situations (Wärja, 2013). In working with KMR, images are evoked in response to the music that is used and which is carefully selected by the therapist (Wärja & Bonde, 2014). Both small and large life events, and the emotions associated with them, come up. The music might also evoke images that serve as resources and *inner helpers*. Experiences of both conflicts and beauty assist in the integration of our lives (Wärja, 2010). The method begins with agreement as to a focus for the session, an induction involving relaxation, open listening to a short selected piece of music (mostly nonclassical), working in intermodal arts, and talking about the experience. Visual art is particularly helpful, as the art products can be considered and pondered many times. Reflecting on the music and art experiences with the therapist is done in the phenomenological manner described above. The therapist is present to hold and anchor the experience in the music.

Music is the primary *energetic mover* that is involved in the process of producing images. It provides a holding environment, a vibrational presence, movement, and vitality. There can be explicit or implicit material, symbolized images, and/or bodily sensations. There are opportunities to meet oneself fully and experience negative and positive sides to one's personality. The music lasts from 2 to 6 minutes and is chosen to be safe enough to hold and contain the person's feeling state, but also to provide some degree of dynamic movement to support exploration. The aesthetic capacity of the piece is carefully considered. The aim of KMR is to help the client surrender to the sound presence of the music and allow for spontaneous imagery to emerge.

An excerpt from the therapy process using KMR with a woman named Anna follows. We met for 15 sessions and a couple of follow-up meetings. Anna kept a journal, and we reflected on her writings together. Permission has been granted to share pieces of her texts and paintings. This was part of a pilot study in preparing for a larger randomized control study in music therapy with women treated for gynecological cancer. A cancer diagnosis usually causes a great deal of social and psychological stress. Many experience fear of recurrence and need to find strategies to handle that worry.

Gynecological cancer and its treatments are affected by social and cultural values regarding illness, death, sexuality, and femininity. Women being treated for these diseases may suffer from many different side effects, bodily changes, and problems with sexual function, health, and well-being. They must, in addition to the threat of death by the disease, also deal with the loss of female body parts, which often have strong symbolic meanings. Self-esteem is often affected, and feelings of guilt and shame are not uncommon. The experiences can be traumatic and affect the woman's self-concept and identity (Stead, Fallowfield, Selby, & Brown, 2007). Sexuality has many facets. The obvious is the sexual drive and the experience of arousal and pleasure, but there are other essential aspects of sexuality such as intimacy, physical touch, and affirmation. The prevalence of sexual dysfunction after cancer treatment is difficult to estimate. Studies suggest that between 40 and 100% of all cancer patients experience periods of sexual dysfunction (National Cancer Institute, n.d.). Sexuality and cancer are taboo areas; medical staff often hesitates to discuss problems in these sensitive areas, and patients are left to handle question and concerns themselves.

CLINICAL EXAMPLE:
Reclaiming a Sensuous Body

Anna and I met in expanded time where past, present, and future were woven together to one rich tapestry. This was a journey of descent and return. When we connect with the hidden and more unconscious side of ourselves, we are in touch with feelings such as anger, rage, hatred, envy, revenge, empowering lust, and sexual passion. What we cannot face will catch us from behind.

Coping with a diagnosis and treatment of a life-threatening illness such as cancer is a complex process. How this is done is unique to each individual and depends on many interrelating factors, such as the present life situation, past experiences, and earlier traumatic events. The kind of cancer diagnosis, treatments, and prognosis will obviously affect the person's ability to handle the stress. When the cancer is located in a place in the body associated with sexual pleasures, it may be felt as an attack to the core of one's sexuality. For Anna, it meant that she detached from her body. The hospital owned the cancer problem, and she checked out.

During our first meeting she curled up in the chair in my office, with legs tucked under like a small girl, reminding me of a fragile bird with shallow breathing. Anna told her story of being diagnosed and treated for uterine cancer, how life had completely changed, and how she had lost herself. Medical procedures had ended 1 year prior to the start of therapy and consisted of surgery, chemotherapy, and radiotherapy. Her uterus and ovaries had been removed; she experienced loss of hair, fatigue, and a minor depression. The cancer was treated in an early stage and her prognosis was good. Anna was married, had no children, and was involved in a profession that required a creative capacity. She had some previous experience of being in therapy and was familiar with reflecting about her history and the landscapes of inner worlds. There are usually many concurrent and parallel threads running through the process of psychotherapy. In this text, I focus on one major theme relating to femininity and sexuality.

Anna questioned what it meant for her to be a woman, an issue that had followed her since her teenage years. Her own mother had not been of much help here. She described her mother as absent, frail, and anxious. After cancer treatment, Anna lost faith in her body and questioned how to go on living. The capable and strong body she had developed during adulthood had betrayed her. She felt weak, sickly, and vulnerable. The relationship with her husband was strained and numb. Sex had been one vital and uniting force between them, and that was now gone. She wrote: "I think of my vagina as a tube, sewn together. Cut off from my inner space. Before, this has always been so special to me, that my vagina was an entry to my insides, my uterus. It feels like having a new body. Nothing related to the mysteries of life. My inner room is gone."

The first phase of therapy dealt with creating safety and allowing feeling layers of despair and hopelessness to surface. The approach I took was to receive, allow, and contain the fluctuating currents of fright and anguish. I invited her to sessions of KMR and spontaneous painting (an intermodal approach is inherent in KMR). Anna listened to "Songs from the Second Floor" by Benny Andersson, and in her imagination she found a safe place under a red comforter on her bed. In the music, she encountered her maternal grandmother, whom she had never met in real life. She had died of an illegal abortion when Anna's mother was a young girl. Anna connected with the fate of her grandmother, feeling the heaviness of her own destiny. Maybe she would die too. "I always knew the catastrophe would come. So when the cancer arrived, I knew; I had prepared myself. It was time to die. I even felt relieved. Maybe it is the terror of my mother and grandmother that rides my back."

For some sessions to come, we dealt with her fears and struggles of being a woman. Anna needed help to create psychological boundaries between the generations of women in her family. This was done through music listening, grounding the body, and reflecting on her experiences and journal writings. In the fourth session, we dived into a huge, desolate wasteland of losses: the loss of not having children, of her sexuality, of the relationship with her husband as it once had been, of the joyous sexual energy, of her vital life force, of her ability to create. Before mourning can begin, a time is needed for naming, sorting, and facing of what have been lost. Going into music, Anna picked a special childhood place by the sea that she had known before the divorce of her parents. The music ("Arons dröm" by Stefan Nilsson) first brought forth images of the warming sun, peace, and beauty. However, soon dark clouds, thunder, and heavy rain rolled in and stayed. There was no escape. Anna sat there in the emptiness of what was lost.

After the music she came back to her sexuality and her longing. "I feel outside life and hide in the bushes. Before cancer my husband and I had a good sex life. Now that is gone. My vagina is without blood. We live two parallel lives. I don't want that! I still have my pleasure and lust." Anna's sexual energy and passion were also connected to her creativity in general. These were the beginning stirrings of healthy anger.

We moved into the working phase—a time of descent, falling, and darkness—where hope and a new kind of strength were found. First we needed to face the overwhelming fears of cancer and how this disease intertwined with earlier painful experiences. Terror stole her will to live. She had no energy left, and no sexual desire. I brought in short pieces of Swedish folk music performed in a jazz tradition. Anna was comforted by the clear base lines, repetitive and syncopated rhythms, and pleasing simple melodies. She gasped at the realization that, in an unconscious way, she was fulfilling what had been the fate of most women of her family: to suffer, to endure, to be dependent and sickly. She had always seen herself as a radical, creative, free thinker. We worked on grounding the body, releasing tension, and taking full breaths. We listened to music that supported the sense of weight and substance of her body. She began to feel more at ease, and her body became softer. At home there were the first stumbling steps of reaching out for her husband.

In the seventh session a beautiful, graceful melody, "Innocent," by Fläskkvartetten, brought something new. "The music is sad but brings comfort," Anna commented. "It is a soft landscape with long paths. I see myself walking there. Heaven and grass. I can find hope and safety. It is just to endure this. Walk the paths and search for myself. I must explore the rooms of death and terror. I know I dare to do it." As we proceeded, Anna found both what she must do and the beauty that could help and sustain her. We dealt with two opposing forces, one wanting to die and the other wanting to live. Anna described a tough membrane between the two sides of forces

and made a drawing. The gentle, exploratory piece, "Resting Place" by Dobrogosz, took her inside the image. This music has some tension and dissonance in a persistent dialogue between two instruments, which allows for differences to coexist. Anna discovered that on both sides there are "good and bad parts and qualities." One had more anger and destructive energy, and the other had more lightness, but was also vague. The intensity of the anger frightened her at first. The other side was more familiar. At the end of one session, she asked where she could find the kinds of crayons I had in my office. I just say, "Take them with you, use them, and bring them back when you can." She looked very happy. This became the birth of Anna's art-making journey and a new integrating phase of the therapy process.

One day Anna came in carrying a whole stack of paintings and proceeded to arrange them on the floor. She moved with focused energy and knew exactly how to arrange them. The paintings had poured out of her like gushing fresh water in a spring river. They had a life of their own. The colorful images held life and expressed hope, fear, despair, and longing. They spoke of mother, father, husband, cancer, sexuality, and intimacy. A group of paintings were from the inside of her body: on the operating table, of longing to heal, protecting her organs and herself, fighting with cancer, searching for her sexuality, and facing death (see Figure 20.1). Most of the pictures had titles and short statements on the back. One difficult turn on the road was initiated by a couple of drawings that dealt with shame and sexual betrayal. This piece added depth and understanding to her sense of losing her body and her sexual identity as a consequence of cancer.

Shortly thereafter she made a large body drawing in the same size as her actual body. With the support of "Songs from a Secret Garden" by Secret Garden, she found wisdom and intelligence of more unknown female ancestors inside her body. This discovery became a turning point in our work. In the midst of profound pain was also a life that carried meaning, strength, and beauty. There was flow and openness between us. Our relationship became the stage for increased self-esteem and insight into significant rela-

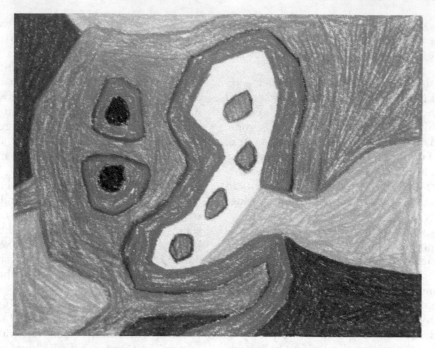

FIGURE 20.1. Anna's painting, "Death in My Uterus."

tionships. Some images became gateways into music. Images are intermodal and contain sounds, complex rhythms, vital movements, and stories. Anna took full breaths and was more present in her body. Gone was the small fragile bird. Here was a woman with flesh, bones, and feelings. She was on the way to reclaiming her sensuous body, discovering what being a woman meant to her, and embracing her sexuality in a new way.

Conclusions

This chapter has introduced the music-centered expressive arts therapy approach in which music is a gateway to the process of change and transformation in therapy. Both active and receptive music therapy methods are used in combination of all the art modalities. Music is the portal into the therapeutic process. Music speaks to the heart, connects us to feelings, and can convey meaning, beauty, and mystery. The arts have infinite possibilities and can be mixed,

fused, combined, separated, torn apart, and played with in multiple ways. Making music, painting, writing, acting, and dancing involve our senses. The capacity of music to evoke emotions is possibly the most essential function when music is applied in therapy. In this work, the concept of aesthetics—of beauty—is of uttermost importance: Aesthetic is its vital energy. Beauty speaks of flow, of grace, of soul, and of profound meaning. When we honor beauty in the therapeutic work, we also care for the whole person.

REFERENCES

Bonny, H. L. (1980). *GIM therapy: Past, present and future implications*. Salina, KS: Bonny Foundation.

Bruscia, K., & Grocke, D. (Eds.). (2002). *Guided imagery and music: The Bonny method and beyond*. Gilsum, NH: Barcelona.

Damasio, A. (2010). *Self comes to mind: Constructing the conscious brain*. New York: Pantheon Books.

Heidegger, M. (1996). *Being and time* (J. Stambaugh, Trans.). Albany: State University of New York Press. (Original work published 1953 by Max Niemeyer Verlag, Tübingen, Germany)

Husserl, E. (1960). *Cartesian meditations*. The Hague: Martinus Nijhoff.

Husserl, E. (1970). *The crisis of European sciences and transcendental phenomenology*. Evanston, IL: Northwestern University Press.

Kaestele, G., & Müller, D. (2013). *Kurze Musik-Reisen (KMR): Ein Tor Zur Innenwelt*. In I. Frohne-Hargeman (Ed.), *Guided imagery and Music Konzepte und klinische Anwendungen* (pp. 108–125). Wiesbaden, Germany: Ludwig Reichert Verlag.

Kenny, C (2006). *Music and life in the field of play: An anthology*. Gilsum, NH: Barcelona.

Knill, P., Nienhaus Barba, H., & Fuchs, M. (1995). *Minstrels of soul: Intermodal expressive therapy*. Toronto: Palmerston Press.

Levine, S. (2011). *Trauma tragedy and suffering: The arts and human suffering*. London: Jessica Kingsley.

Levine, S., & Levine, E. (Eds.). (2005). *Principles and practice of expressive arts therapy: Towards a therapeutic aesthetics*. London: Jessica Kingsley.

Levine S., & Levine E. (Eds.). (2009). *Art in action: Expressive arts therapy and social change*. London: Jessica Kingsley.

McNiff, S. (2009). *Integrating the arts in therapy: History, theory, and practice*. Springfield, IL: Charles C Thomas.

Meyer, M. (2007). *Repatriation and testimony: Expressive arts therapy*. Unpublished doctoral dissertation, European Graduate School, Saas-Fee, Switzerland.

National Cancer Institute. (n.d.). Retrieved from *www.cancer.gov/cancertopics/pdq/supportivecare/ sexuality/HealthProfessional*.

Schore, A. N. (2009). Attachment trauma and the development of the right brain: Origins of pathological dissociation. In P. F. Dell & J. A. O'Neil (Eds.), *Dissociation and the dissociative disorders: DSM-V and beyond* (pp. 107–141). New York: Routledge.

Stead, M. L., Fallowfield, L., Selby, P., & Brown, J. M. (2007). Psychosexual function and impact of gynaecological cancer. *Best Practice and Research Clinical Obstetrics and Gynaecology, 21*(2), 309–320.

Stern, D. (2004). *The present moment in psychotherapy and everyday life*. New York: Norton.

Stern, D. (2010). *Forms of vitality: Exploring dynamic expression in psychology, the arts, psychotherapy and development*. Oxford, UK: Oxford University Press.

Turner, V. (1995). *The ritual process: Structure and anti-structure*. Piscataway, NJ: Aldine.

van Deurzen, E. (2010). *Everyday mysteries: A handbook of existential psychotherapy*. London: Routledge.

van Gennep, A. (1960). *The rites of passage*. London: Routledge.

Wärja, M. (2010). *Korta musikresor (KMR): På väg mot en teori om KMR som musikterapeutisk metod* [KMR–Brief Music Journeys: Towards a theory of KMR as a music therapy method]. Stockholm: Kungl. Musikhögskolan.

Wärja, M. (2013). Konstnärlig metodik: Handledning i psykoterapi och utbildning [Arts-based methods: Supervision in psychotherapy and education]. In I. N. Pedersen (Ed.), *Kunstneriske medier i supervision af psykoterapi: Indsigt og vitalitet* [Art modalities in suprvision and psychotherapy: Insight and vitality] (pp. 85–110). Aalborg, Denmark: Aalborg Universitetsforlag.

Wärja, M. (2015). KMR–Brief Music Journeys. In D. Grocke & T. Moe (Eds.), *Guided imgaery and music spectrum: A continuum of practice*. London: Jessica Kingsley

Wärja, M., & Bonde, L. O. (2014). Music as cotherapist: Towards a taxonomy of music in therapeutic music and imagery work. *Music and Medicine, 6*(2).

Wigram, T. (2004). *Improvisation: Methods and techniques for music therapy clinicians, educators, and students*. London: Jessica Kingsley.

Winnicott, D. (1971). *Playing and reality*. London: Tavistock.

PART III

CLINICAL APPLICATIONS

INTRODUCTION

Music therapy can be applied in a variety of settings, including hospitals, schools, mental health facilities, prisons, and private settings, and with ages ranging from before birth to the oldest adults. Problems addressed include physical, emotional, medical, and learning difficulties. The chapters in this section cover some of these areas. Because this is an edited book, the chapters present a variety of views. Authors have different perspectives on, and experiences with, their topics, as well as different views of what is most important to present, so the content varies somewhat among chapters. Part III is divided into three sections focusing on children and adolescents, adults, and medical applications.

Some important areas in which music therapists work are not covered in these chapters. No chapters focus on adults with intellectual disabilities, autism, or sensory impairments, for instance. Many considerations guided decisions on what to include and what not to include, including space and the length of the book. Every area in which children may benefit from music therapy can also be applied to adults with the same disabilities, and in virtually all cases, music therapists do work with both children and adults. It is possible to apply what is written here to clients of different ages, although of course some of the issues will be different (e.g., adults are not generally part of a school system, so nobody is working on educational goals in exactly the same way as they do with younger people). Conversely, some of the areas that are presented for adults can also apply to younger people. Examples would be children with mental illness or those who have been through traumatic events.

The orientations (i.e., psychodynamic, humanistic, cognitive-behavioral) and approaches (i.e., Nordoff–Robbins Music Therapy, the Bonny Method of Guided Imagery and Music, Analytical Music Therapy, Neurologic Music Therapy, Community

Music Therapy) that were presented in Part II provide much of the basis for clinical techniques and influence music therapy clinical work in other ways, whereas most of what is done in sessions is based on the methods (receptive, composition, improvisation, re-creative) that were presented in Chapter 11. The reader will find that the knowledge of these orientations, approaches, and methods from the earlier section deepens and enriches the understanding of the clinical applications presented in this section.

These clinical applications are rich with information that readers can apply to their own work. Authors also frequently share material about people with whom they have worked (either directly from the actual work or, when the client has not provided permission to discuss his or her work, in a disguised or composite form). These case examples bring music therapy with those described in Part III to life.

SECTION A

Music Therapy for Children and Adolescents

CHAPTER 21

Music Therapy for Developmental Issues in Early Childhood

Marcia Humpal

Each time a baby is born, the family expects the infant to go through a natural progression of stages that leads to independent adulthood. Medical and scientific advances have made possible early identification of problematic conditions that may affect typical development. Unfortunately, the exact diagnoses, reasons for their occurrence, and assurance of their being easily corrected or cured may not always exist. Hopes may be dashed. Denial may set in. Families may become overwhelmed and not know where to turn for assistance.

Early intervention offers the key to helping infants and young children develop to their greatest potential. Music therapy is an effective and highly developmentally appropriate treatment modality for this population and their families.

Clientele

Definitions

Early Childhood

Early childhood is generally recognized now as a period of development with its own specific characteristics and learning styles. The National Association for the Education of Young Children (NAEYC) conducts research and publishes extensive literature on young children. Although its literature describes early childhood as a period from birth through age 8 (Copple & Bredekamp, 2009), the principles of early childhood education may be adhered to less rigorously after children reach primary grades, possibly due in part to the increasing demands in the United States for educational accountability and the testing that has resulted.

Early Intervention

Under the U.S. federal law now known as the Individuals with Disabilities Education Act (IDEA), children with disabilities are eligible for special services designed to meet their unique needs. The original Public Law 94-142, enacted in 1975, has been revised several times. Recent amendments guide services to very young through school-age children. The U.S. Department of Education's Part B of IDEA (2006) addresses services for children ages 3–21, and Part C (2011) focuses on babies and toddlers.

Early intervention services are provided through the state for infants and toddlers with disabilities who are less than 3 years of age and their families. For school-aged children and youth (ages 3–21), special education and related services are provided through the school system. These services can be instrumental in helping children and youth with disabilities develop, learn, and succeed in school and other settings (U.S. Office of Special Education, 2012).

Although music therapy is not a specifically mandated service of IDEA, it may be considered a *related service* if it is required to help a child with a disability receive an appropriate education. The website of the U.S. Department of Education includes a question-and-answer document that clarifies related services, including music therapy. This document is included and discussed in the article "Inclusion of Music Therapy in Early Intervention Programs" (Simpson, 2011).

Developmental Disability

A developmental disability is a condition that is attributable to a mental, physical, or combination of these two types of impairments that manifests prior to age 22 and is likely to continue indefinitely. IDEA lists the following 13 disability categories under which 3- through 21-year-olds may be eligible for services (U.S. Office of Special Education, 2012):

- Autism
- Deaf–blindness
- Deafness
- Developmental delay
- Emotional disturbance
- Hearing impairment
- Intellectual disability
- Multiple disabilities
- Orthopedic impairment
- Other health impairment
- Specific learning disability
- Speech or language impairment
- Traumatic brain injury
- Visual impairment (including blindness)

Developmental Delay

The term *developmental delay* applies to children from birth through age 9. It is considered one of the specific categories of developmental disability under IDEA for these ages and also is specified in Part C of IDEA as one of the criteria for early intervention services provided by states for children from birth through age 2. Part C also includes provisions for service delivery to very young children who have been diagnosed with a mental or physical condition that may put them *at risk* for developmental delay.

Under IDEA, *infants and toddlers with disabilities* are defined as individuals under 3 years of age who need early intervention services because they are experiencing developmental delays, as measured by appropriate diagnostic instruments and procedures, in one or more of the following areas: cognitive, physical, communication, social or emotional, and/or adaptive development; or have a diagnosed physical or mental condition that has a high probability of resulting in developmental delay. The term may also include, if a state chooses, children under 3 years of age who would be "at risk of experiencing a substantial developmental delay" if early intervention services were not provided.

Developmentally Appropriate Practice

Recognizing that young children learn and progress in unique ways, NAEYC set forth fundamental tenets to guide effective practices when working with very young children. This philosophy is grounded in child development theories and guided by research on how young children learn—that is, through play. NAEYC further stresses that young children progress through various stages of play, guided by caring adults who plan their environment to facilitate learning through interactive play with adults, peers, and materials that are age-appropriate. The doctrine of developmentally appropriate practice (DAP; Bredekamp, 1987) emerged from these components.

Although the initial version of DAP provided for all areas of child development and recognized that children have wide ranges of interests and abilities, many felt that it did not adequately address the needs or learning styles of young children with developmental delays or disabilities. The 2009 revision to DAP (Copple & Bredekamp, 2009) calls for the following:

- Meeting children where they are and enabling them to reach goals that are challenging yet achievable.
- Basing decisions pertaining to curriculum and learning experiences on knowledge of how children learn and develop.
- Reducing the achievement gap.
- Using a comprehensive, effective curriculum.
- Improving teaching and learning.

These guidelines acknowledge the unique needs of young children with developmental delays or disabilities. However, different accommodations or explicit strategies often need to be employed or combined with a developmental approach when working with children, depending on their specific needs (e.g., for children with autism spectrum disorder [ASD]; Humpal & Kern, 2012).

Development in Early Childhood

General Development

When we talk about normal development, we are talking about areas such as gross and fine motor, language, cognitive, and social skills. Children progress through stages in these areas that have set developmental milestones or age-specific functional skills, usually achieved within a given age range.

Babies develop from head control to control of the extremities (i.e., from top down and from the middle out). They learn to visually and auditorily track objects, people,

and then themselves in a mirror. They learn to smile, laugh, demonstrate likes and dislikes, babble, recognize their names and special people, and show affection. In the motor domain of development, they kick, reach, bat, hold, grasp, and explore objects (often by mouthing). Infants respond to touch, massage, rocking, sitting in a lap, and movement with adults, then progress to moving independently.

Toddlers are mobile. They have increasingly more functional fine motor control (e.g., thumb–finger isolation, stacking, dropping, throwing) and can follow simple directions. They use gestures, imitate, vocalize with inflections, and begin to use words. They begin to understand concepts such as up–down, in–out, loud–quiet. In addition, they demonstrate a variety of feelings (e.g., frustration, jealousy, empathy).

Preschoolers continue fine-tuning gross and fine motor skills and speech and language abilities, and they become much more social. Though they still operate concretely, they begin to experience a wider range of emotions and are better able to understand the feelings of others. During the preschool years, young children become much more independent and develop a strong sense of self. They have active imaginations, search out knowledge, love to pretend, show great curiosity and intellectual growth, and begin to reason.

All children do not attain these milestones at exactly the same point in their lives; some reach them earlier and some later but still are in the range of normal development. It is very important for music therapists to recognize the typical developmental milestones as well as the indicators or "red flags" that may signify delays or variations from the norm. Although developmental milestones are useful as guidelines for typical stages of development, it is helpful to remember that they are generalizations. Knowing the milestones helps us understand developmental progression, anticipate an approximate time to expect certain behaviors to occur, and then, if necessary, formulate a step-by-step plan for advancing or remediating this developmental process in each young child with whom we work.

Factors Affecting Typical Development

Various factors can affect a child's development and may play a part in determining whether early intervention is needed. When assessing current levels of functioning, take into consideration the following aspects of the child's history as well as his or her total environment:

- Prematurity: A child born prior to 37 weeks of gestation is considered premature and should be assessed according to his or her corrected age (gestational age at birth plus months of life) rather than actual chronological age. Children usually catch up to their chronological age between the ages of 2 and 3, although this may vary with individuals (Standley, 2003).
- Low birthweight
- Genetics
- Maternal substance abuse during pregnancy
- Parental/caregiver considerations (e.g., availability; understanding of terminology; possible cognitive, mental or physical health issues)
- Lack of stimulation
- Medical issues

When working with very young children, it is essential to include the family or caregivers in assessment and treatment. Others who work directly with the child (e.g., physical, occupational, and speech therapists; medical personnel) also can provide information and insight.

Play Skill Development

Young children learn in distinct ways that are indicative of their age and developmental level. Until the latter part of the 20th century, little attention was given to the early childhood years; they were considered simply as a downward extension of the elementary grades. Most learning theorists did refer to various stages that a child moves through as he or she progresses toward adulthood and higher-level thought processes. However, the earlier stages of learning did not become a major focus in educational circles until the doctrine of DAP gained acceptance. Based on the cognitive developmental theories set forth by Piaget (1962) and Vygotsky (1967), DAP stresses the importance of play in early childhood development and learning (Humpal & Tweedle, 2006).

Indeed, young children's play yields incredible rewards. Through play, children learn about all aspects of the world around them. Think of children playing in a sandbox. This activity is not purely recreational in nature. As the sand is poured into various containers, as water is added and the sand turns to mud, or as two children pull on the handle of the same pail, analysis, contemplation, investigation, and even negotiation are taking place. Young children learn through play.

However, some young children do not play spontaneously. Others play in rigid, repetitive ways. Some are limited by delays and disabilities that, if not addressed, will affect their ability to learn for the rest of their lives. For these children, play does not just happen. Play needs to be facilitated, and this facilitation is a big part of early intervention.

Music therapy can be a playful and highly effective treatment for young children. These little ones often need a structured and systematic play environment that will allow them to move through the developmental stages of play. Their skills may need to be bumped up from one level to the next. Recognizing the various levels of play and the different categories of play help us to design sessions and treatment plans that are developmentally realistic and thereby address the needs of each child more appropriately.

Play levels can be categorized according to their purpose or how the play is utilized. A Piagetian approach (Piaget, 1962) focuses on both areas: for what purpose the child plays and how the child plays. At a very basic level, the young child would be at the *functional* play stage (e.g., banging on drums). The *constructive* play stage (e.g., stacking drums into a tower) would be slightly more complex, as would the next *symbolic* play stage (e.g., moving to music using ribbon streamers). The most complex stage for early childhood is *games with rules* (e.g., playing a game of musical chairs), a stage that often is not totally embodied until children are well into their early elementary school years. Other theorists have analyzed play and categorize it according to the level of social interaction that it entails. From most basic, these categories of social play in early childhood generally range from *unoccupied* behavior to *solitary*, then to *onlooker* play, to *parallel, associative*, and ultimately *cooperative* play (Linder, 1990; Parten, 1932).

Having a solid understanding of the typical developmental progression of play skills can help us form a more accurate picture of each child's functioning level. Yet it is important to note that for some children (e.g., for those with ASD), the sequence and rate of development and learning may be uneven and may even be substandard in one area and highly advanced in another (Humpal & Kern, 2012; Sandall, Schwartz, & Joseph, 2001).

Musical Development

Music skills also develop along a continuum. Elements of music actually are perceived prior to birth; consistent response to auditory stimuli appears evident by 28 weeks gestational age (Whipple, 2005). Researchers tend to agree that the development of specific musical skills and abilities appear within developmental periods, which include gestational, infancy, and early childhood, and range upward through adolescence (Gooding & Standley, 2011).

From infancy, very young children typically progress through the following musical stages (Briggs, 1991):

- Reflex (0–9 months): React to changes in musical elements, use voice to play with sounds, and move body to music.
- Intention (9–18 months): Localize sound sources, recognize familiar songs, move individual body parts to music.
- Control (18–36 months): Demonstrate more accurate pitch perception, begin to sing recognizable pitches contours, remember lyrics, exhibit a large increase in rhythmic/motor control.

The manner in which young children process musical input and demonstrate musical skill seems to follow a distinct pattern. Young children begin to show an awareness of music by responding differently to various music qualities (e.g., calming to a quiet lullaby), then exhibit trust as they recognize and react to familiar melodies. They show a sense of independence by rhythmically moving to music and rhythmic stimuli and progress to having control of their musical skills by following or demonstrating melodic contours of familiar phrases, sounds, or songs (e.g., intoning the universal children's chant of *sol, mi, la, sol, mi*). Later, they are able to assume responsibility for their musical skills as they become able to maintain a steady beat (Schwartz, 2008). Furthermore, the pattern of young children's musical skill development can be divided into subsets such as responses to sound and auditory learning characteristics, responses to music, pitch/tonality ability, rhythm ability, movement ability, singing ability, instrument playing, and responses to other musical elements (e.g., dynamics) (Gooding & Standley, 2011).

Challenges

Those who work with young children with developmental issues are challenged by many factors that extend far beyond knowing that the child has a developmental delay or developmental disability. Especially challenging are the following overarching aspects.

Many Different Developmental Diagnoses

As mentioned earlier, there are 13 broad categories of developmental disabilities and five specific areas of concern for developmental delay that apply to children from birth through their early childhood years (and sometimes beyond). Each of these includes many subcategories with their own diagnostic criteria. Furthermore, assessment yields varying degrees of functioning and severity, as well as unique aspects of the individual. All of these factors affect how we develop treatment and session plans.

Variety of Treatment Options

Not only is there a wide variety of developmental issues and areas of concern, there also are countless general treatment approaches for each (e.g., applied behavior analysis [ABA]; Developmental, Individual Differences, Relationship-Based Approach [DIR®/Floortime™] for ASD [National Autism Network, 2013]). Effective treatment requires keeping abreast of the most current information and evidence-based practices both inside and outside one's particular discipline. No one size fits all; the treatment must be geared to the specific developmental issue and should be compatible with the treatment used by the family and other professionals serving the child. Furthermore, when working within a comprehensive treatment framework, music therapists should base particular music therapy interventions on solid evidence-based practice (Kern, 2011). This is achieved by considering these three components: clinical expertise, best available research evidence, and individual client factors (Sackett, Rosenberg, Gray, & Richardson, 1996).

Legal Aspects

Federal and state regulations, as well as individual insurance policies, guide how services to young children are funded. Basic education and some therapies (e.g., physical, occupational, or speech) are specifically mandated or covered. Music therapy is mentioned as a possible related service (see Simpson, 2011), but obtaining funding may be a difficult process. Although music therapy often is the therapy to which a child responds best, music therapists must be able to document that music effectively addresses the goals set up for the child, or that the child learns more effectively when music strategies are utilized. Families are diligent advocates for their children, and often their insistence provides the impetus for obtaining coverage for music therapy services.

Family Involvement

The family members or designated caregivers are an integral and required part of the young child's team and must take part in decisions regarding the child's educational plan and treatment. No one knows the child better than the family. It is not unusual for the young child to act one way at home and a totally different way in other settings. Therefore, developing a good rapport with the family is essential for continuity of educational programming and for optimum experiences that aid the child's progress.

Although family members provide essential insights about the child, they are often overwhelmed by the initial unexpected news that their child has problems. They may be in denial and unable to deal with the reality of a diagnosis. They may be afraid, angry, depressed, overbearing, or incapable of taking any action. They may be constantly on the lookout for a cure or may treat any suggestion as a threat.

Music therapists will be treating not only the child, but the family as well. Becoming aware of the family's culture and accepting the choices family members ultimately make for their children help anchor a good working partnership (Morris, 2013). We have at our disposal a magnificent tool for highlighting abilities of all levels and offering services that provide not only information and strategies, but also coping skills, healing, and food for the soul.

Clinical Work

The use of music therapy with young children with developmental issues is beneficial for many reasons. Music may be the first stimulus to which a child relates, as it occurs naturally in many settings and is a socially appropriate activity. Music therapy affords the benefit of merging extremely well with a play-based approach. Music therapists are trained to use and adapt music to all other targeted areas or methodologies by:

- Providing opportunities for participation at a child's own ability level.
- Addressing several of a child's needs in a positive and exciting medium.
- Designing pleasurable learning experiences that promote success.
- Supporting all aspects of the child's educational experiences and needs.

Settings

At the early childhood age, children with developmental issues are, first and foremost, young children. The settings in which they receive services that address their delays or disabilities are guided by established practice models for their age group. Typical service delivery is team-oriented with overlapping, shared, and supportive goals. Service is preferably delivered in settings that are considered natural (i.e., one that is typical for the majority of young children). Therefore, music therapists may provide services to young children with developmental issues in their homes, in community settings such as libraries or local recreation centers, or in schools. For some young children, specialized or more intense therapeutic approaches may prove to be more beneficial for the long-range outlook and may therefore meet the intent of being the least restrictive environment to address the child's unique needs. Families play a major role in determining appropriate and most advantageous treatment settings or approaches for young children. Let us now look at a few vignettes featuring specific types of clinical settings where music therapists often work with young children with developmental issues. Names of individuals have been changed to ensure anonymity.

The Home

Sophie was born after an uneventful pregnancy. However, shortly after birth she was diagnosed as having Down syndrome. Her mother was referred to a developmental specialist while still in the hospital. A service coordinator who was a developmental specialist met with the family in their home, arranged an assessment, and then worked with the family to determine a plan to work on Sophie's developmental issues. The team consisted of the parents, the developmental specialist, an occupational therapist, and a physical therapist.

When Sophie approached 6 months of age, her mother had recognized that she calmed to music, smiled, and would move her head as it played. The mother asked if a music therapist could accompany the occupational therapist to her next home visit. The private practice music therapist often worked as a consultant for various early intervention teams in her geographic area and arranged to make the visit. The occupational therapist shared Sophie's individualized family service plan (IFSP) with the music therapist and asked if the music therapist could provide strategies for increasing the amount of time Sophie would purposefully use her hands. The music therapist took musical instruments to the visit, taking into account Sophie's chronological and developmental ages. After assessing Sophie's fine motor skills as well as her tolerance for accepting various sensory input, the music therapist prepared a report that included suggestions for utilizing certain instruments for targeted developmental areas. She returned to the home for one more visit, where she shared and demonstrated instrument usage (e.g., a tambourine for hitting and a small maraca for later use to encourage grasping and shaking). She also shared appropriate songs for infants with the family and the occupational therapist.

Community-Based Settings

"I am so glad I found your class! My son was kicked out of library story hour before the end of our first meeting. I doubted that we would ever be able to go to any class like other children do. But now he stays with the music group and even will take turns!" This was the joyful observation one parent relayed to the music therapist after her son took part in a toddler parent–child music program held at the local YMCA.

The class was offered as a special time for young children (of all ability levels) and their caregivers to make music together. The class provided opportunities for young children between the ages of 21 and 30 months, and their families, to sing or use their voices, move, play rhythm instruments, listen, and experience music through a variety of senses. Class registration information was sent to area agencies that served infants and toddlers with developmental issues. Being in a community setting that offered a wide range of courses, the class also readily drew typically developing children.

The program utilized music to work on nonmusical skills. Using the same hello and good-bye songs at each session helped establish a routine. Repeating familiar activities plus supplementing with novel new songs each week added to the children's comfort levels and increased their attention spans. Picture cues and transition songs gave advance notice of what was to happen next and provided directions in a nonconfrontational way (e.g., "Sticks and shakers go in the box, sticks and shakers go in the box, sticks and shakers go in the box, then we'll dance with the parachute!" sung to the tune of "Skip to

My Lou"). To encourage taking turns, parents held a drum while their children struck it with a mallet as the music therapist accompanied them on the guitar. When the music therapist paused the music, the drumming also ceased. Then the dyad would exchange objects. After much practice, this intervention was expanded to back-and-forth playing: One person used both the drum and the mallet while the other waited. Throughout the class, music interventions not only addressed the unique needs of each child but also ensured that everyone was actively and successfully involved in making music.

The sessions were fun and provided great resources for families. However, they were planned in great detail, and the children's successes did not just happen. Music therapists are well suited to lead this type of class. They have unique training, skills, and expertise and can adjust and adapt music experiences to meet the needs of *all* young children. Both long-standing and recent music therapy research substantiate that young children with special needs benefit from music classes that include their typically developing peers (Humpal, 1991; Walworth, 2009). In addition, small-group music therapy experiences offer more modeling, opportunities for practice, and support for families and yield more social engagement during toy play (Hanson-Abromeit, 2011; LaGasse, 2011). Designing the class for children of various ability levels follows established early childhood practice. Recent brain research (Molenberghs, Cunnington, & Mattingley, 2009; Wan, Demaine, Zipse, Norton, & Schlaug, 2010) adds validity to this premise. Studies indicate that the mirror neuron system (MNS) in the brain is comprised of neurons that respond to actions of oneself and others. This system mirrors the behavior of others as if the observers were performing the action themselves. Music making with others (e.g., playing instruments, singing, or watching others do these things) adds a layer of multimodal activity that engages brain regions that overlap with the MNS.

Offering music therapy classes in community settings may yield other unexpected advantages for families. New friendships develop among adults, and children learn to accept differences and develop compassion. Sometimes the music therapist may catch warning signs that parents may have overlooked, such as their child's low or high muscle tone, lack of eye contact, delayed language, or extreme difficulty with transitions. The music therapist may be the first to suggest referral for further evaluation that may lead to early intervention—often the key to addressing delays before they become lifelong issues.

The above-mentioned scenario described a little boy who, later in the year, was diagnosed with ASD. His mother reported that the progress he made in his music therapy sessions and the support she received helped her accept the diagnosis and look to her son's abilities, successes, and potential rather than dwell on the negative aspects of his developmental issues.

School or Educational Settings

Children with developmental issues who are age 3 and older may be served in preschools, schools, or other educational settings. The programs in these facilities may be carried out in the regular classroom (perhaps with a special education aide), an inclusion classroom, or a special education classroom. Music therapists may take children out of their regular class setting (a *pull-out* model) or work within a classroom, seeing the children individually or in small groups. Specialized classes may receive regularly scheduled music therapy sessions or consultative services.

Music therapy service delivery may be either programmatic or based on individualized education programs (IEPs). In the programmatic model, the music therapist uses and adapts musical experiences and also engineers the musical environment to address global goals and needs of specific children while also supporting such areas as curricula or classroom themes. IEP-based music therapy addresses identified goals and objectives for specific children. In a consultative role, music therapists may work with early intervention specialists, teachers, or music teachers to adapt instructional strategies, curricula, or the environment to meet the individual needs of the children (Adamek & Darrow, 2010; Furman & Humpal, 2006).

Target Areas

The family, with recommendations from the young child's team, determines the areas to be targeted for treatment. The nature of the delay or developmental disability will, of course, guide this decision. Though different states and agencies may use different terminology, the following domains are representative of areas of focus for young children with developmental issues: physical/motor, communication, social/emotional/play, cognitive, and sensory.

Music interventions can be designed to support treatment across all these areas and may be used as a form of social routines to encourage turn taking. Young children learn through repetition, and music can offer a repetitious form of play that sets up anticipation and teaches cause and effect. Language and music both have varied accents, rhythm, and tone patterns; children respond to rhythm and intonation before words. Thus, music can be a motivator for movement as well as a precursor to speech. Participation in music can be both verbal and nonverbal, making it a wonderful vehicle for emotional expression. Music therapy research offers a variety of substantiating evidence for utilizing music across all domain areas with young children with all types of developmental issues (Swaney, 2006). Figure 21.1 offers suggestions for making music meaningful for young children with developmental issues.

- Consider children's needs when setting up the environment.
- Keep it simple—not too many choices, and not too many words.
- Utilize music for commenting and seamless transition.
- Provide opportunities for **response.**
- Ask: "More?"—encourage *any type* of communication to continue.
- Repeat, repeat, repeat, and repeat! Young children learn through repetition.
- Capture their attention and build anticipation.
- Vary the tone of your voice—**be expressive**.
- Slow down.
- Get up close and at the child's level.
- Adjust the pace and use musical *pregnant pauses* . . . **wait!** Give enough time for the child to respond.
- Use age and developmentally appropriate instruments and materials:
  - Commercially available smaller versions (e.g., maracas);
  - Mallets with two heads;
  - Rhythm sticks that are cut in half (easier to hold and less likely to accidentally hit a neighbor);
  - Conventional objects used in **unconventional** ways (e.g., a vibrating pen with the tip removed makes an adapted mallet that encourages a grasp and gives extra sensory input; placing rubber shelf liner on a desk or a wheelchair tray helps anchor a tambourine or a drum in place so that it can be more easily played).
- Have enough of the same instruments and props so that parallel play can peacefully exist.
- Have some instruments that can be played by sharing (e.g., xylophones with extra mallets; large drums that can accommodate several children at a time).
- Provide adaptations and modifications to songs, instruments, or props if needed.
- Employ technology to encourage communication, capture and increase attention, improve fine motor skills, and anchor concepts (numerous free or low-cost music apps are available online).
- Use live, unaccompanied, or simple accompaniment (it is less confusing for relaying information).
- Play recorded instrumental music to enhance movement exploration.
- Use repetitive words and sound effects.
- Utilize contrasts (e.g., play–stop, loud–soft, fast–slow).
- Include multicultural examples.
- Share wiggles, tickles, bounces, and nursery rhymes with infants and toddlers (and their families).
- Keep your expectations at a realistic level. Don't give a triangle and beater if the child can't isolate a finger and a thumb; instead, **adapt** or **modify** (e.g., you hold the triangle, the child holds beater).
- Present concrete experiences that can be *bumped up* to a higher level of play.
- Enjoy yourself while sharing the joy and benefits of music with little ones. Their enthusiasm will reward your efforts!

FIGURE 21.1. Tips for making music meaningful for young children with developmental issues.

Applications to Other Disciplines

Young children who have, or are at risk for, developmental issues can be found across all walks of life. Because music is so much a part of early childhood, its therapeutic efficacy can extend across an entire gamut of settings. Music therapists who possess a solid understanding of early childhood development, musical development, and various types and characteristics of developmental issues can work in conjunction with families and professionals in a variety of settings and disciplines (Humpal, Kaplan, & Furman, 2013).

Music therapy can be at the heart of programs that address the needs of at-risk families who are helped to more appropriately and effectively parent young children (Abad & Williams, 2007). Music therapists can work in tandem with specialists such as audiologists or speech–language pathologists to enable preschool recipients of cochlear implants to perceive and understand the musical input that is part of a young child's world (Gfeller, Driscoll, Kenworthy, & Van Voorst, 2011). Forthcoming chapters introduce the reader to even more settings in which young children with developmental issues may reap the benefits of the clinical application of music therapy.

Conclusions

Early childhood is a unique time. Never again in our lives will we change and learn so quickly. The developmental process goes through numerous stages, each with its particular characteristics and underpinnings for progression to more advanced skill acquisition. Young children learn in a variety of ways, seeking to understand the world around them. Being aware of developmental milestones as well as a wide range of strategies and interactions helps those of us who live or work with young children be more effective in supporting all kinds of learning.

Young children with developmental issues face obstacles that may be daunting to themselves and to their families. Fortunately, early intervention offers many of these children an avenue of support that can rectify problems or lessen the effects of a disability. Music therapy can provide an especially appropriate type of early intervention.[1]

Development and learning advance when children are challenged to achieve at a level just beyond their current mastery, and when they have many opportunities to practice newly acquired skills. Musical interventions can be extremely motivating, and can be enjoyed at various developmental levels and stages of play, and within many different environments. Music can be used throughout the child's day and in many ways. Music therapy can be the therapy that supports and enhances the goals of all other therapies and treatments. The strategies and therapeutic benefits of music that are developed and facilitated can thereby enhance the whole child, as well as those who share in his or her world.

[1]Readers can learn more about various aspects of music therapy for young children by accessing *imagine*, the online early childhood music therapy magazine, at *http://imagine.musictherapy.biz/Imagine/home.html*.

REFERENCES

Abad, V., & Williams, K. (2007). Early intervention music therapy: Reporting on a 3-year project to address needs with at-risk families. *Music Therapy Perspectives, 25*(1), 52–58.

Adamek, M., & Darrow, A.-A. (2010). *Music in special education* (2nd ed.) Silver Spring, MD: American Music Therapy Association.

Bredekamp, S. (1987). *Developmentally appropriate practice in early childhood programs serving children from birth through age 8*. Washington, DC: National Association for the Education of Young Children.

Briggs, C. (1991). A model for understanding musical development. *Music Therapy, 10*(1), 1–21.

Copple, C., & Bredekamp, S. (2009). *Developmentally appropriate practice in early childhood programs serving children from birth through age 8* (3rd ed.). Washington, DC: National Association for the Education of Young Children.

Furman, A., & Humpal, M. (2006). Goals and treatment objectives, setting, and service delivery models in early childhood and early interventions settings. In M. Humpal & C. Colwell (Eds.), *Effective clinical practice in music therapy: Early childhood and school age educational settings* (pp. 82–96). Silver Spring, MD: American Music Therapy Association.

Gfeller, K., Driscoll, V., Kenworthy, M., & Van Voorst, T. (2011). Music therapy for preschool cochlear implant recipients. *Music Therapy Perspectives, 29*(1), 39–49.

Gooding, L., & Standley, J. (2011). Musical development and learning characteristics of students: A compilation of key points from the research literature organized by age. *Update: Applications of Research in Music Education, 30*(1), 32–45.

Hanson-Abromeit, D. (2011). Early music therapy intervention for language development with at-risk infants. *imagine, 2.* Retrieved from *http://imagine.musictherapy.biz/Imagine/archive_files/imagine%202%281%29%202011.pdf*.

Humpal, M. (1991). The effects of an integrated

early childhood music program on social interaction among children with handicaps and their typical peers. *Journal of Music Therapy, 28*(3), 161–177.

Humpal, M., Kaplan, R., & Furman, A. (2013). *E course: Music therapy in early childhood: Meaningful music from infancy to kindergarten.* Silver Spring, MD: American Music Therapy Association. Available at *www.musictherapy.org.*

Humpal, M., & Kern, P. (2012). Strategies and techniques: Making it happen for young children with autism spectrum disorders. In P. Kern & M. Humpal (Eds.), *Early childhood music therapy and autism spectrum disorders* (pp. 162–180). Philadelphia: Jessica Kingsley.

Humpal, M., & Tweedle, R. (2006). Learning through play: A method for reaching young children. In M. Humpal & C. Colwell (Eds.), *Effective clinical practice in music therapy: Early childhood and school age educational settings* (pp. 152–173). Silver Spring, MD: American Music Therapy Association.

Kern, P. (2011). Evidence-based practice in early childhood music therapy: A decision-making process. *Music Therapy Perspectives, 29*(1), 91–98.

LaGasse, B. (2011). Research snapshots 2011: Music and early childhood development. *imagine, 2.* Retrieved from *http://imagine.musictherapy.biz/Imagine/archive_files/imagine%202%281%29%202011.pdf.*

Linder, T. (1990). *Transdisciplinary play-based assessment: A functional approach for working with young children.* Baltimore: Brookes.

Molenberghs, P., Cunnington, R., & Mattingley, J. B. (2009). Is the mirror neuron system involved in imitation?: A short review and meta-analysis. *Neuroscience and Biobehavioral Reviews, 33*, 975–980.

Morris, I. (2013). Culture matters: Latin American cultural attitudes toward disability and their implications for music therapists working with young children. *imagine, 4.* Retrieved from *http://imagine.musictherapy.biz/Imagine/home.html.*

National Autism Network. (2013). *Treatment specific resources.* Retrieved from *http://nationalautismnetwork.com/index.html.*

Parten, M. (1932). Social play among preschool children. *Journal of Abnormal and Social Psychology, 27*, 243–269.

Piaget, J. (1962). *Play, dreams, and imitation in childhood.* New York: Norton.

Sackett, D. L., Rosenberg, W. M. C., Gray, J. A. M., & Richardson, W. S. (1996). Evidence based medicine: What it is and what it isn't. *British Medical Journal, 312*, 71–72.

Sandall, S., Schwartz, I., & Joseph, G. (2001). A building blocks model for effective instruction in inclusive early childhood settings. *Young Exceptional Children, 4*(3), 3–9.

Schwartz, E. (2008). *Music, therapy, and early childhood: A developmental approach.* Gilsum, NH: Barcelona.

Simpson, J. (2011). Inclusion of music therapy in early intervention programs. *imagine, 2.* Retrieved from *http://issuu.com/ecmt_imagine/docs/imagine-2-1-2011/15.*

Standley, J. (2003). *Music therapy with premature infants: Research and developmental interventions.* Silver Spring, MD: American Music Therapy Association.

Swaney, B. (2006). Articles published in music therapy journals through 2005 categorized by special education topics. In M. Humpal & C. Colwell (Eds.), *Effective clinical practice in music therapy: Early childhood and school age educational settings* (pp. 207–215). Silver Spring, MD: American Music Therapy Association.

U.S. Department of Education. (2006, August 14). Rules and regulations. *Federal Register, 71*(156). Retrieved from *http://idea.ed.gov/download/finalregulations.pdf.*

U.S. Department of Education. (2011, September 28). Early intervention programs for infants and toddlers with disabilities. *Federal Register, 76*(60139). Retrieved from *www.federalregister.gov/articles/2011/09/28/2011-22783/early-intervention-program-for-infants-and-toddlers-with-disabilities.*

U.S. Office of Special Education. (2012). Categories of disability under IDEA. Retrieved from *www.parentcenterhub.org/repository/categories/#dd.*

Vygotsky, L. (1967). Play and its role in the mental development of the child. *Soviet Developmental Psychology, 12*, 62–76.

Walworth, D. (2009). Effects of developmental music groups for parents and premature or typical infants under two years on parent responsiveness and infant social development. *Journal of Music Therapy, 46*(1), 32–52.

Wan, C. Y., Demaine, K., Zipse, L., Norton, A., & Schlaug, G. (2010). From music making to speaking: Engaging the mirror neuron system in autism. *Brain Research Bulletin, 82*, 161–168.

Whipple, J. (2005). Music and multimodal stimulation as developmental intervention to neonatal intensive care. *Music Therapy Perspectives, 23*, 100–105.

CHAPTER 22

Music Therapy for Children with Intellectual Disabilities

Beth McLaughlin
Ruthlee Figlure Adler

Music has long been valued as an important therapeutic and educational tool in the treatment of individuals with intellectual disabilities (ID). It has been reported that people of school age who were institutionalized in the late 19th century participated in music experiences as part of their educational training (Farnan, 2002). Edouard Seguin, a well-known educator at that time, "advocated the use of music to teach listening skills, speech and to develop gross and fine motor skills" (Davis & Farnan, 2008, p. 81). In the 1940s, music therapy was used primarily to teach social skills and to provide an environment in which group members could actively participate and build social relationships through the music experience. Today, people with ID are contributing members of our society but face many challenges due to limitations in communication, social skills, and adaptive behaviors. In this chapter we explore how deficits in these areas impact growth and development and how music therapy can play an integral role in contributing to foundational skills that promote learning and independence

Clientele

Definition

Prior to 2010, a person with an ID was commonly referred to as having a developmental disability or mental retardation. In October of 2010, President Barack Obama signed legislation that replaced the term *mental retardation* with *intellectual disability*. Known as Rosa's Law, the mandate assured that all federal health and education policy would follow a statewide trend to remove any reference to mental retardation in favor of more positive terminology. Publicity generated by discussions of the implications of this change in terminology increased awareness among some of the general public of the effects of labeling and of the feelings of those being labeled.

The American Association of Intellectual and Developmental Disabilities (AAIDD;

2010) states that an intellectual disability originates before age 18 and is "characterized by significant limitations both in intellectual functioning and adaptive behavior as expressed in conceptual, social, and practical skills." A person with an ID has an intelligence quotient (IQ) of 70–75 or below and exhibits limitations in the following adaptive behaviors:

- Conceptual skills: communication including understanding and responding appropriately to language, concept development (numbers, money, time), literacy, self-direction;
- Social skills: interpersonal relationships with family and peers, social responsibility, self-esteem, following rules, avoiding victimization and making choices;
- Practical skills: activities of daily living, including eating, dressing, toileting, mobility, preparing meals, taking medication, using transportation, maintaining a safe environment, occupational skills. (Farnan, 2007, p. 81)

Because of these limitations, the rate of development and ability to learn for children with an ID is slowed or delayed as compared to their typical peers. They have difficulty acquiring new skills or generalizing information to new environments or situations. Important milestones such as sitting up, crawling, walking, or talking occur later than for those of the typically developing child. For instance, at 9 months, typically developing children start showing a preference for favorite toys, begin to babble, point to objects of interest, and play peek-a-boo. They are able to use both hands together, sit without support, and crawl. Children with ID at this age may have difficulty standing without support, have poor reciprocity when interacting with a caregiver, and may not respond to their own name. If a child has not developed imitation skills by the age of 3, has difficulty following directions, or does not make eye contact, there is a strong possibility of a developmental delay that could be related to an ID. The rate at which a person with ID will develop academic, social and vocational skills, and the supports needed for his or her success depends upon the extent of the impairment.

Although IQ scores measure only part of a person's cognitive ability, certain ranges of IQ scores are typically associated with general levels of functioning and can help to further identify the challenges of those identified with ID. An IQ score under 35 is one indicator of a severe or profound ID. Although individuals in this range may develop strong relationships with family, teachers, and other people of significance to them, they will have very limited communication and will require support for meeting personal needs and accessing the community. Those with an IQ score between 35 and 50 may be considered to have a moderate ID, and they will always need some level of support but are able to learn functional communication, make personal choices, participate in community and family events, and develop some independent living skills. People with mild ID have an IQ between 50 and 70 and the potential to read and write, learn vocational skills, live independently, and contribute to the community (Davis & Farnan, 2008).

Causes

Although there are many different causes of ID, the four most common factors include genetic conditions, problems during pregnancy, difficulties during labor and delivery, and health issues. Genetic conditions may include Down syndrome, fragile X syndrome, autism, Angelman syndrome, or Williams syndrome, to name a few. Problems that occur during pregnancy may be a result of poor nutrition or excessive alcohol consumption, infections such as rubella, or abnormal fetal development such as spina bifida. Problems occurring during labor and delivery may be a result of oxygen deprivation, premature or multiple births, or infections such as meningitis or encephalitis. Finally, health problems that can contribute to an ID include poor nutrition, certain childhood diseases such as whooping cough or measles, exposure to poisons such as lead or mercury, and accidents such as near drowning or those that cause severe head injuries (Harris, 2010).

With improvements in prenatal care and continued advances in assessment procedures for determining risk factors in newborn babies, the cases of children with ID have decreased in recent years (Harris, 2010). In addition, early intervention programs have played a significant role in providing support to families and early educational opportunities for young children. These services can maximize resources for dealing with potential developmental challenges and decrease the need for special education services later, during the school-age years.

Challenges

According to a 2010 report of the U.S. Department of Education, more than 545,000 children between the ages of 6 and 21 with ID are receiving special education services. These services are individualized to meet the specific needs of each child, regardless of the disability, and address the challenges that affect the ability to learn the necessary skills to function with optimum independence in the most integrated setting. Although there is great diversity among this population, the primary emphasis in their education is on developing communication and conceptual skills, the acquisition of social skills, and learning to complete activities of daily living. The long-range goal of an educational program that focuses on these adaptive skills is to enable individuals with ID to become independent and productive adults who are contributing members of their community. Given the many needs of this population, an effective program requires a collaborative environment that provides proactive behavioral supports and teaching strategies rooted in best practice (Farnan, 2007).

Goals and Areas of Need

Communication and Conceptual Skill Development

Because of the overall delay in cognitive development in this population, language is slow to develop and requires early and intensive intervention. The acquisition of language and the ability to communicate effectively to meet one's needs is critical for functioning successfully in today's world. The extent of the language delay depends on the severity of the disability. Without an effective system of communication, children will often develop a repertoire of inappropriate behaviors to meet or express their needs. These behaviors may include aggression, tantrums, self-stimulation, or destruction of property. When children are given the tools that allow them to communicate, they become empowered to meet their needs, manage their behaviors, and interact with others in meaningful and socially appropriate ways. An important aspect of establishing communication skills is to provide opportunities for generalization. The more pervasive and profound a disability, the greater the challenge in establishing a successful and functional communication system that works across environments.

Social Skills

Learning appropriate and adaptive social skills is critical for anyone's success but can be particularly challenging for the individual with an ID. Understanding shared rules and expectations for conversations, greetings, physical contact, dress, and eye contact requires skills that enable people to function and interact with others in school, at work, and in the community. The absence of these skills can isolate people with ID from their peers and limit their options for a meaningful and productive life. Because of the delays occurring in the early childhood years, these children may not have had the opportunities to learn from peers through play; they may not have had opportunities to develop friendships or had the benefit of observing appropriate social behaviors in natural environments. Indeed, many young people with ID have experienced rejection or bullying from others who have limited understanding of their challenges, resulting in their withdrawal from social situations and low self-esteem.

Activities of Daily Living and Other Practical Skills

Activities of daily living (ADLs) include, but are not limited to, personal grooming, brushing teeth, toileting, caring for personal belongings, preparing simple meals, and eating with appropriate utensils. Other important practical skills include using public transportation to access the community, developing vocational skills, and maintaining a safe living environment. Being able to independently participate in these activities not only enhances the quality of life for individuals with ID but also increases their eligibility for community and employment services in the most integrated setting upon reaching adulthood. Individuals with ID are challenged by a number of factors that inhibit their ability to perform these tasks at the highest level of independence. For example, they may have difficulty understanding the sequence involved in completing the task or in processing the request; they may lack conceptual skills, such as one-to-one correspondence needed to set a table or the inhibition to respond appropriately to strangers in the community; they may have difficulty with the motor planning and coordination required to put on their shoes or brush their teeth.

Clinical Work

The Role of the Music Therapist

Music therapists who serve the needs of children and adolescents with ID in a school-based setting are an integral part of a team comprised of parents, professionals, and paraprofessionals who share responsibility for developing and implementing program goals and interventions that support the student across environments (Adler et. al., 2006). There are many opportunities for music therapy to support the acquisition of the functional skills described above. However, in order to structure an intervention to target the appropriate behavior or skill sequence, planning must be done in collaboration with the teacher, social worker, occupational and/or physical therapist, speech and language pathologist, and family members who know, work, and live with the child. Together they help identify the challenges to learning that will be the shared focus of the educational or treatment team. Beyond the classroom, the music therapist often assumes a role of working with the family to develop music interventions targeting specific areas for use in the home. These areas might include increasing independence, developing coping skills to deal with anxiety around transitions, or helping the child to be included in cultural celebrations practiced at home and in the community.

Music Therapy for Communication and Conceptual Skill Development

When an individual is able to successfully interact with the world through meaningful and relevant experiences, language and cognition develop in natural and reciprocal ways. Music is a natural part of our world. Singing and moving with music are activities in which people of all ages can engage spontaneously, providing a means of expression, exploration, and self-discovery. Music invites participation through the joy of shared listening, dancing, or music making. If language is learned through meaningful interaction with people, things, and events, then music is a natural environment in which learning can take place. A music therapist is trained to structure the environment in ways that actively involve children by engaging their faculties and stimulating channels of learning. By facilitating children's movement, singing, playing of instruments, and listening, music therapists are able to reinforce a range of communication skills that includes initiating communication, listening, sequencing, developing concepts, acquiring vocabulary, and vocalizing (Adler, 1988).

Using visuals to depict different feelings, such as smiling, frowning, surprised, or laughing faces, while singing a song helps children with ID visually, receptively, and aurally express themselves. The following example illustrates how a multisensory approach to teaching feeling awareness can help students better understand and communicate their feelings across environments.

CLINICAL EXAMPLE from Ruthlee Figlure Adler

Katie was a 10-year-old with intellectual disabilities whose limited expressive language inhibited her ability to communicate her thoughts and feelings to and about others. In our music therapy sessions, we included several different sets of visuals depicting feelings, including happy, sad, afraid, sleepy, and angry faces, as well as those found in the Mayer–Johnson Boardmaker® (Mayer-Johnson, 2004) program. We sang songs about feelings, including "If You're Happy and You Know It," and original songs. We also played musical instruments to express our emotions. Once Katie could match sets of visuals, we began writing original story songs about her feelings. We also created a set of "feelings" cards for her to carry with her and encouraged her teachers, therapists, and family to help her use them to express how she felt in various settings and situations outside of music therapy and in the community.

Singing encourages expressive and receptive language, strengthens self-image, develops body awareness, and provides emotional release. It also reinforces the ability to follow directions and can teach self-help skills through embedding a task sequence in a song. It helps develop vocalization, verbalization, and inflection while building vocabulary. Moreover, targeted song intervention can help to remediate specific speech impairments by helping the child to slow the rate of speech, practice repeated speech sounds, develop breathing awareness, and generally increase vocal production in a nonthreatening, fun activity. The therapist's voice, as well as the voices of peers, provides encouragement and support. Vocal improvisation, imitation, open-ended chants, lyric completion, and/or question-and-answer songs encourage spontaneous use of the voice. It is important to select music with a strong rhythmic beat, relevant vocabulary, and accessible vocal range. Incorporating visual aids provides additional reinforcement. When students are able to fully explore their voices with contrasting sounds of high–low, fast–slow, loud–quiet, happy–sad sounds, they are internalizing these concepts for further comprehension. Body movement can be added to reinforce vocal directions. Kazoos or harmonicas can be used for those who do not sing as a way to stimulate blowing, vocalization, and humming. Working with a speech therapist to develop these experiences is important to maximize the learning and developmental impact for each individual.

Movement and instrumental activities provide a natural and motivating means of teaching and reinforcing dynamic concepts (e.g., loud–quiet, fast–slow), positional concepts (e.g., up–down, in–out, left–right) and language concepts (e.g., attributes such as colors, size, length, shape). A music therapist will design activities to incorporate these basic concepts while actively engaging students in the movements that help to internalize the information being taught. For example, songs about the weather can support language and cognition by adding simple movements that mimic the gross motor skills associated with recreational activities such as skiing, swimming, or hiking. Removable pictures of seasonal activities can be presented on a picture board or programmed into an iPad or an alternative augmentative communication device such as a DynaVox. The American Sign Language signs that depict these activities provide a visual focus that further reinforces vocabulary. A rain stick and a repeated glissando on a xylophone can help to orchestrate a song about a rainstorm that starts with a quiet sprinkle, then crescendos to the sound of a gong, ending with the quiet shake of a thunder tube.

The music therapy literature contains many examples of music used to facilitate the development of speech and language. LaGasse (2011) used Neurologic Music Therapy (NMT) techniques to improve speech intelligibility and functional communication with a 6-year-old boy with Down syndrome. Music therapy helped him to learn functional phrases and to generalize them to his environment, thereby improving the intelligibility of his speech, increasing his use of alternate means of communication, and decreasing the frustration he felt whenever his speech was not understood.

Wheeler (2013) suggests that using songs that require a vocal response by leaving a space in the music can assist these children in acquiring many skills and achieving many goals, including initiating communication, increasing the frequency and variety of spontaneous vocalizations, and repeating simple words or sounds on cue.

Perry (2003) studied the use of improvisational music therapy on the development of intentional communication in children with ID. Through a qualitative research study with 10 school-age children who did not use any form of symbolic communication consistently, she was able "to describe the patterns in the communication of children with varying levels of preintentional and early intentional communication and

how the consequences of disability affected children's communication" (p. 231). As a result of her study, she was able to present the children's communication levels and describe them as they related to their interactions within the music therapy environment. These findings are important because they provide a greater understanding of children with rudimentary levels of communication while placing "musical interaction within the scheme of general communication development" (p. 242).

Music Therapy for Social Skills

Music therapy plays an important role in providing an environment that supports the teaching and generalizing of social skills. Through structured group music therapy sessions, participants develop prosocial behaviors by learning to acknowledge their peers, take turns, and work cooperatively through shared music making. They learn "not only to act, but to act together" (Gaston, 1968, p. 19). They also learn important management skills, such as waiting for musical cues to play instruments and modulating their movements or vocal responses to match the tempo or dynamics of the music. Moreover, a trained music therapist has the skills to adapt the interventions to facilitate the successful inclusion of each member in the music therapy experience.

Transitions to new environments can be disorganizing for many students with ID, causing anxiety and provoking negative behaviors (see McLaughlin example in Adler et al., 2006, pp. 192–193). Starting and ending music sessions with quiet music and dim lights is a proactive way to help students relax and prepare for a new direction or move to the next class. A good-bye song that includes information about what is coming next eases the transition and provides a predictable outcome to the routine.

Singing songs that include the names of group members in their lyrics is a meaningful way of acknowledging individuals while helping students to develop awareness of themselves and their peers. Additional reinforcement can be offered for younger children by lightly touching the student's shoulder while his or her name is being sung, or using a mirror so that the students can see themselves at the appropriate time. Prompting children to point to themselves when their name is sung or to another child when they hear that name extends the interaction and promotes social reciprocity.

Including students as helpers for passing out instruments provides a functional means of teaching students how to recognize their peers and acknowledge them by name (e.g., "Here you go, Susie," or "Your turn, Joe"). Opportunities for teaching reciprocal social exchanges (e.g., "Thank you" and "You're welcome") occur naturally as each individual gives and receives an instrument. Finally, because the helper is getting his or her instrument last, he or she is learning to delay gratification and develop the ability to wait.

Playing instruments within a group structure has the potential for teaching a range of social skills, including maintaining eye contact by attending to the therapist or a peer model maintaining impulse control by playing, resting, or adjusting tempo according to musical cues; and peer awareness by performing with the group. Incorporating the musical structure of chorus-verse-chorus inherent in many songs provides a predictable form that can be adapted to teach these important skills.

Boxill (1985) utilizes an opening song in which members are acknowledged by name and involved in various ways. She describes "Our Contact Song" as "the first reciprocal musical expression, the first two-way musical communication, the first overt musical indication initiated by the client of an awareness of the existence of another" (p. 80). Bitcon (2000) suggests a number of Orff–Schulwerk techniques that focus on psychosocial dynamics. She emphasizes the importance of accepting participants' contributions without requiring verbal explana-

tions. Bitcon further illustrates the diverse possibilities for using the Orff–Schulwerk approach by presenting suggestions for its use in getting acquainted, expressing feelings, forming identity, sharing news, dealing with rules, and increasing spirituality and trust.

Robbins and Robbins (1991) describe their work with a girl with a moderate ID, brain injury, and emotional instability. The therapists used a number of instrumental songs and techniques to develop her sense of self and the ability to communicate with the world and included her in a production of The Children's Christmas Play (Nordoff & Robbins, 1970). Through her involvement in music therapy, she developed self-confidence, a sense of pride, and improved social skills, which generalized to both school and home.

CLINICAL EXAMPLE from Ruthlee Figlure Adler

Ben, diagnosed with central nervous system (CNS) dysfunction, multiple cerebral disabilities, and low social and expressive language skills, began individual music therapy sessions with me while in high school. Initially, he played piano by ear but did not verbally or socially interact with others before or after the song ended. In our 50-minute individual music therapy sessions he learned to read notated music and began answering simple questions about the pieces or selections. However, if he played an incorrect note, he would immediately stop playing and repeat the music starting once again at the beginning. (This form of perseveration also occurred in his written work at school, where he would retrace individual letters or words until he made a hole in the paper and had trouble "moving on" with the assignment.) Through music therapy, Ben learned to continue playing a piece until the end without mentioning the "wrong note." He also learned to follow directions, accept constructive criticism and honest praise, and make decisions regarding the tempo, notation, dynamics, etc., of a piece. He was able to verbally share simple information about his favorite pieces and composers with others as well as me. These new skills and improved self-esteem carried over to the classroom and later into the workplace where Ben now successfully completes assignments and projects and is a contributing member to our society.

Music Therapy for ADLs and Other Practical Skills

A music therapist can support the acquisition of daily living skills by providing activities that motivate the child to become actively engaged with the learning environment. Dance activities that involve moving hands and feet in isolation help teach self-awareness and differentiation of body parts needed for dressing. Playing mallet instruments helps to develop the bilateral skills needed for hand washing. Singing a song that provides the steps in a learning sequence can motivate a child to sustain his or her attention to a specific task.

Keith (2013) suggests using action listening songs to cue specific behaviors, such as gross or fine motor movements, verbal responses, or ADLs. Goals can include improving receptive and expressive language skills, improving self-care, and following directions.

Functional motor skills are needed to perform basic tasks such as reaching to put groceries away, bending to pick up an item, or twisting at the trunk to perform hygiene tasks after using the toilet. Bilateral coordination is needed for paper-and-pencil tasks, using the telephone, or opening a jar. Having the ability to plan and carry out motor actions (motor planning) and maintaining balance are necessary to assess and navigate the environment in order to follow multistep directions such as standing up, going to the sink, and rinsing a bowl (Case-Smith et al., 2010). A collaborative focus on functional motor development is an effective approach to meeting the needs of individuals who face profound challenges in acquiring and generalizing some of the most basic motor skills. In 2000, a transdisciplinary group of professionals, including those from physical therapy (PT), occupational therapy (OT), and adapted physical education (APE) from Wildwood School, where Beth McLaughlin works, identified five students from the adolescent program who were making little to no progress acquiring the most basic motor skills. These students were unable to sustain motor activity or to generalize motor skills to their daily activities, had poor endurance and attention, and required highly structured and repetitive functional tasks. A daily, 30-minute integrated program was designed for these students with a focus on facilitating development of the following motor skills: pushing and pulling; maintaining a grasp and carrying; bending, stooping, and reaching; initiating and sustaining motor tasks; improving body awareness; increasing endurance; improving motor planning; and participating in recreational games and movement.

To support this program, the music therapist designed interventions with input from the PT, OT, and APE to provide an environment for further generalization of these skills through music. The targeted functional motor skills and supporting music therapy interventions are explained in Table 22.1.

Embedding a task sequence in a familiar melody can be an effective means of teaching a simple skill (Kern, Wakeford, & Aldridge, 2007). Using the melody to the children's song "Here We Go Round the Mulberry Bush," lyrics can be substituted for putting on shoes or brushing teeth. Following this format, young children with ID can be taught to master these daily living skills in a step-by-step progression. Incorporating a familiar melody allows for other members of the team, as well as family members, to remember the lyrics and melody, while sequencing the steps necessary for achieving these important daily living skills.

TABLE 22.1. Functional Motor Skills and Supporting Music Therapy Interventions

Functional motor skills	Supporting music therapy interventions
Pushing and pulling	• Maintain grasp on prop or instrument while performing push–pull movements
Maintaining grasp and carrying	• Maintain grasp on prop or instrument while performing push–pull movements • Maintain grasp on prop (stretchy band or parachute) while walking or moving in or out of circle
Bending, stooping, reaching	• Perform movement sequence with/without instruments involving stooping and reaching • Play instruments or perform movements with full arm extension
Initiating and sustaining motor tasks	• Sustain shaking movement with parachute while music is played
Improving body awareness	• Move body forward/backward and side to side with musical cues • Maintain orientation of body in space during movement activity (facing center of circle, facing partner, walking in line) • Walk in intended direction while playing an instrument • Play instruments on different body parts • Play instruments in different body positions (kneeling, side sitting, standing, long sitting, cross-legged)
Increasing endurance	• Sustain shaking movement with parachute while music is played • Perform two-step movement sequence for three repetitions of a song phrase
Improving motor planning	• Perform movements or instrumental accompaniment with appropriate movement gradation • Change body orientation in dance activity • Hold instrument in one hand while playing with opposite hand
Recreational games and movement	• All of the above

Polen (2013) suggests using precomposed songs from the clinical repertoire to support the development of targeted adaptive behaviors. She recommends songs from Nordoff and Robbins's *Children's Play Songs* that address specific goals and outcomes for clients. The "Shoe-Tying Song" provides a teaching sequence for learning to tie shoes. The "Penny-Nickel-Dime-Quarter-Dollar Song" teaches money values. Fill-in-the-blank songs such as "A Rainy Day" provide opportunities for the client to complete lyric phrases by choosing appropriate clothing or activities, depending on the weather.

CLINICAL EXAMPLE from Beth McLaughlin

Kyle was an 8-year-old boy who had been attending Wildwood School since age 5. He had an ID with limited verbal communication. His language was primarily echolalic, with poor comprehension. Kyle was taking medication that required monitoring of his blood pressure several times throughout the school day. He was terrified of the blood pressure cuff and resisted having it put on his arm.

In spite of his lack of verbal communication, Kyle was very engaged by song lyrics that were sung as an accompaniment to stories read in class. His teacher approached me with the challenge of developing a song intervention that would help Kyle tolerate having his blood pressure taken. Together with the school nurse, we task-analyzed the sequence they would use, and I developed a song that was sung to one of his preferred melodies, "Turkey in the Straw." I recorded it on a cassette tape and gave it to his teacher. She played it for him once while taking her own blood pressure, then had him complete the sequence himself with the music providing the steps for him to follow. He showed no resistance and from that point on, went independently to the nurse's office at the appointed times with the tape recorder in tow.

Applications to Other Disciplines

As noted in the preceding examples, music therapists who work with individuals with ID integrate their work with many other disciplines to benefit the clients they serve. The American Music Therapy Association clearly states in its professional documents "an expectation of professional practices that fosters collaboration with other service providers and team members" (Allgood, 2006, p. 111). The Baltimore County Public School District has identified collaborative opportunities shared by professionals providing educational services to students with ID, including teachers, music therapists, and art therapists. These opportunities include ideas for structuring the classroom, managing behaviors, sharing resources, and supporting teaching strategies across environments (Ritter-Cantesanu & Kauffman, 2012). Collaborating with teachers, social workers, OTs, PTs, and speech and language pathologists is essential when developing music therapy interventions that support the acquisition of specific skills. Task analyses that have been developed through best practice in other professional fields are needed resources that inform and assure the integrity of music therapy practice.

The following example illustrates how families are also an important resource for the music therapist working with individuals with ID.

CLINICAL EXAMPLE from Beth McLaughlin

Tina was a young girl at Wildwood with agenesis of the corpus callosum, a neurological birth defect that had a significant impact on her overall development. She presented with a seizure disorder, poor impulse control, delayed language, and difficulty performing certain motor tasks. At 5 years of age, Tina was still in diapers, and her parents' attempts at toilet training were met with little success. Tina loved books and was particularly engaged by songs written and sung by her music therapist that accompanied familiar stories. She would sit for extended periods and attend to the songs in her music therapy group and to the recordings provided her family for use at home. Since this was the only time that Tina would sit, her mother suggested that I write a song to help them with her toilet training program. They provided me with specific language being used, the steps they were following, and where the process was breaking down. Tina could sit on the toilet but would not stay there. She enjoyed social reinforcement as well as primary rewards. The song intervention was designed not only to sequence the steps being taught, but also to increase the duration of her sitting as well as inform her of the reinforcement she could expect at predictable intervals. After 2 weeks, Tina's family reported that she was completely toilet trained.

The success of this intervention was due to the collaboration between the therapist and the family. Although this skill was not taught following specific steps provided by a task analysis, the song was developed in partnership with the parent and individualized to include behavioral expectations and language that was relevant to the child. The music sustained her attention, motivated her to follow the steps in the sequence, and assured her success

Music therapists are frequently called upon by teachers, families, and other related service providers to provide original or recorded music to promote relaxation, aid in transitions, accompany social stories, and reinforce basic concepts taught in the classroom. They often provide consultation to music educators to provide support and develop strategies so that students with ID can be successfully included with typical students in the music classrooms. Social workers working with family support organizations collaborate with music therapists to provide assessments that help families access community music therapy services for their child in the home.

Conclusions

The elements of music—melody, rhythm, form, harmony, and timbre—can be used to create an environment that motivates people with intellectual and developmental challenges to grow and engage with their world. A melody can comfort a child in distress. Rhythm provides a pulse that can unify a group. Form has a temporal structure that creates a predictable and secure environment. Harmony creates mood in music through tension and resolution. Timbre is the unique quality of tone particular to each voice or musical instrument. A music therapist is trained to use these elements as tools to create movement, singing, and instrumental experiences that promote cognitive development, social interaction, and skill acquisition. Through movement a child develops self-awareness, movement control, and self-confidence. Singing activities teach listening, language concepts, sequencing, and communication skills. Playing instruments provides opportunities for taking turns, following directions, improving eye–hand coordination, and practicing

behavioral control. The fundamental skills that develop through these experiences can help individuals with ID become capable adults with the skills and adaptive behaviors they need to live in today's world.

Farnan (2007) states that "services for individuals with intellectual and developmental disabilities need to be person centered, provide positive behavior supports, produce evidence based practice and provide for self determination, social inclusion, full participation, self sufficiency, [and] personal responsibility" (p. 85). The music therapist plays an important role in providing services and supports that enhance quality of life and promote integration through meaningful music experiences. As we have discussed, music therapy provides an environment that is inherently inclusive, structured for success, and individualized to maximize each person's active participation. As students with ID experience success and satisfaction in any endeavor, they are developing a positive sense of self.

In her book Esteem Builders, Borba (1989) outlines five essential components found in individuals with high self-esteem: security, selfhood, affiliation, mission (purpose), and competence. Music therapy has the potential to contribute to each of these building blocks in positive and meaningful ways. When designed prescriptively, music therapy provides a secure structure that is consistent, with clear expectations and experiences adapted to assure success. Students feel safe and nurtured while given the freedom to express themselves within the defined limits of the musical experience. As they continue to engage successfully and expand their repertoire of activities and skills, they develop self-awareness and grow in their ability to contribute positively to the group process. When students contribute to songwriting activities or perform with a group, they develop a sense of affiliation as their contributions are acknowledged and appreciated by adults and peers. Their willingness to try new things and take new musical risks increases as they gain a sense of purpose and commitment to the music and to the group. As their ideas are embraced and incorporated into the group process, they gain a sense of ownership and competence, giving them the confidence to develop new skills and build new relationships. When students experience success, they feel more competent to make appropriate behavioral choices, accept challenges, and contribute to their school, home, and community.

REFERENCES

Adler, R. F. (1988). *Target on music: Activities to enhance learning through music.* Rockville, MD: Ivymount School.

Adler, R. F. (2006). Goals and treatment objectives, settings, and service delivery models for the school age years. In M. Humpal & C. Colwell (Eds.), *Effective clinical practice in music therapy: Early childhood and school age educational settings* (pp. 68–81). Silver Spring, MD: American Music Therapy Association.

Adler, R. F., Allgood, N., Furman, A., Humpal, M., Kaplan, R., McLaughlin, B., et al. (2006). Noteworthy examples. In M. Humpal & C. Colwell (Eds.), *Effective clinical practice in music therapy: Early childhood and school age educational settings* (pp. 192–206). Silver Spring, MD: American Music Therapy Association.

Allgood, N. (2006). Collaboration: Being a team player. In M. Humpal & C. Colwell (Eds.), *Effective clinical practice in music therapy: Early childhood and school age educational settings* (pp. 110–119). Silver Spring, MD: American Music Therapy Association.

American Association of Intellectual and Developmental Disabilities. (2010). *Intellectual disability: Definitions, classifications and systems of support* (11th ed.). Washington, DC: Author.

Bitcon, C. H. (2000). *Alike and different* (2nd ed.). Gilsum, NH: Barcelona.

Borba, M. (1989). *Esteem builders: A K–8 self-esteem curriculum for improving student achievement, behavior and school climate.* Fawnskin, CA: Jalmar Press.

Boxill, E. H. (1985). *Music therapy for the developmentally disabled.* Rockville, MD: Aspen Systems.

Case-Smith, J., & O'Brien, J. C. (2010). *Occupational therapy for children* (6th ed.). St. Louis, MO: Mosby.

Davis, W. B., & Farnan, L. A. (2008). Music therapy with children and adults with intellectual disabling conditions. In W. B. Davis, K. E. Gfeller, & M. H. Thaut (Eds.), *An introduction to music therapy: Theory and practice* (3rd ed., pp. 79–115). Silver Spring, MD: American Music Therapy Association.

Farnan, L. A. (2002). Music therapy for learners with profound disabilities in a residential setting. In B. Wilson (Ed.), *Models of music therapy interventions in school settings* (2nd ed., p. 165). Silver Spring, MD: American Music Therapy Association.

Farnan, L. A. (2007). Music therapy and developmental disabilities: A glance back and a look forward. *Music Therapy Perspectives, 25*(2), 80–85.

Gaston, E. T. (1968). Man and music. In E. T. Gaston (Ed.), *Music in therapy* (pp. 7–29). New York: Macmillan.

Harris, J. (2010). *Intellectual disability: A guide for families and professionals.* New York: Oxford University Press.

Keith, D. R. (2013). Mild–moderate intellectual disability. In M. Hintz (Ed.), *Guidelines for music therapy practice: Developmental health* (pp. 305–334). Gilsum, NH: Barcelona.

Kern, P., Wakeford, L., & Aldridge, D. (2007). Improving the performance of a young child with autism during self-care tasks using embedded song interventions: A case study. *Music Therapy Perspectives, 25*(1), 43–51.

LaGasse, A. B. (2011). Developing speech with music: A neurodevelopmental approach. In A. Meadows (Ed.), *Developments in music therapy practice: Case study perspectives* (pp. 166–181). Gilsum, NH: Barcelona.

Mayer–Johnson, Inc. (2004). *The picture communication symbols* (PCS). Solana Beach, CA: Author.

Nordoff, P., & Robbins, C. (1970). *The children's Christmas play.* Bryn Mawr, PA: Theodore Presser.

Perry, M. R. (2003). Relating improvisational music therapy with severely and multiply disabled children to communication development. *Journal of Music Therapy, 40*(3), 227–246.

Polen, D. W. (2013). Severe to profound intellectual and developmental disabilities. In M. Hintz (Ed.), *Guidelines for music therapy practice: Developmental health* (pp. 335–370). Gilsum, NH: Barcelona.

Ritter-Cantesanu, G., & Kauffman, B. (2012). *El-*

ementary CALS best practices: Related service collaborative opportunities, music and art therapy. Unpublished document.

Robbins, C. M., & Robbins, C. (1991). Self-communications in creative music therapy. In K. E. Bruscia (Ed.), Case studies in music therapy (pp. 55–72). Gilsum, NH: Barcelona.

U.S. Department of Education. (2010). 29th annual report to Congress on the implementation of the Individuals with Disabilities Education Act, 2007 (Vol. 2). Washington, DC: Author. Available at www2. ed.gov/about/reports/annual/osep/index.html.

Wheeler, B. L. (2013). Individuals with severe and multiple disabilities. In M. Hintz (Ed.), Guidelines for music therapy practice: Developmental health (pp. 399–440). Gilsum, NH: Barcelona.

CHAPTER 23

Music Therapy for Children with Autism Spectrum Disorder

John A. Carpente
A. Blythe LaGasse

Leo Kanner first used the term *autism* in 1943 when describing a small group of children who exhibited unusual behaviors and social skills. The word *autism* was selected due to its Greek origins, meaning *self*; it was previously utilized to describe adults with mental health disorders who demonstrated introverted behaviors. One year later, in 1944, Hans Asperger also used the term *autism* to describe children (Asperger, 1944/1991); however, his observations were of children with large vocabularies. Although the first mention of these autism disorders occurred in the 1940s, it wasn't until the 1980s that the diagnosis of *infantile autism* was included in the third edition of the *Diagnostic and Statistical Manual of Mental Disorders* (DSM-III; see Volkmar, Reichow, & McPartland, 2012). Since this first inclusion, the diagnosis has continued to evolve within DSM, leading to the current diagnosis of *autism spectrum disorder* (ASD).

The incidence of ASD has risen drastically in the past two decades, with a current prevalence of 1 in 88 children (Centers for Disease Control and Prevention [CDC], 2013). The cause of rising rates is unclear, and researchers suggest that there could be several contributing factors, including increased public awareness, broader diagnostic criteria, and diagnosis substitution (Lord & Bishop, 2010). The rising incidence may also be due to environmental factors, genetics, autoimmunity, and/or the interaction of these factors. The rapidly increasing incidence of autism has impacted policy and led to a heightened need for treatments that are evidence-based (Lord & Bishop, 2010). In this chapter we review the common characteristics of ASD and the impact that music therapy can have in the treatment of children with ASD.

Clientele

Characteristics

Although its causes remain unknown, ASD is generally accepted as a neurological disorder present at birth (American Psychiatric Association, 2013). The clinical guide used to define ASD is the fifth edition of the *Diagnostic and Statistical Manual of Mental Disorders* (DSM-5; American Psychiatric Association, 2013). Individuals with ASD generally exhibit challenges in the ability to relate and communicate with others, such as difficulties in responding contextually and initiating conversations, misreading of nonverbal cues and interactions, and/or challenges in developing and establishing age-appropriate relationships. In addition, individuals with ASD are generally highly sensitive to changes in the environment and may be overly dependent on routines and repetition. It is important to note that symptoms of ASD fall along a continuum from mild to severe.

ASD is a puzzling and heterogeneous disorder that manifests in various ways depending on the developmental level and chronological age of the individual. The diagnostic criteria for ASD contain two core features (American Psychiatric Association, 2013): (1) social communication and interaction impairments and (2) restricted interests/repetitive behaviors. The category of restricted interests/repetitive behaviors includes reactivity level (hyper- or hypo-) to sensory input (American Psychiatric Association; Wing, Gould, & Gillberg, 2011).

Impairments in Social Communication and Social Interaction

According to DSM-5 (American Psychiatric Association, 2013) social communication and social interaction impairments are defined based on deficits in three main areas: (1) social–emotional reciprocity, including awkwardly approaching social situations, and/or difficulty exhibiting typical back-and-forth conversations, and/or challenges in the ability to share interests and emotions (e.g., empathy, sympathy), and/or initiate or respond to a social interaction; (2) nonverbal communication, including difficulties in (or lack of) communicating, and/or understanding and/or integrating verbal and nonverbal cues, such as facial expressions, eye contact, and body gestures; and (3) establishing relationships, involving difficulty in the abilities to initiate, and/or develop, and/or maintain, and/or understand relationships.

Repetitive and Restricted Behaviors

DSM-5 (American Psychiatric Association, 2013) defines restricted and repetitive behaviors within four areas: (1) stereotyped or repetitive motor movements, including engaging in the same act over and over again, repeatedly vocalizing the same phrase, insisting on the same routine, and/or obsessing on a familiar topic; in addition, repetitive motor movements such as hand flapping, toe walking, rocking, swaying, and pacing are also indicated in this area; (2) insistence on sameness, involving the dependence on routines, rituals, and/or ritualized patterns of verbal and/or nonverbal behavior (interrupting routines, rituals, and/or self-stimulatory behaviors) may result in the individual having a *meltdown* (e.g., tantrumming, hitting, biting); (3) fixated interests, including a preoccupation with objects, interest of intense or abnormal focus, and/or preservative interests (i.e., repeating verbal or nonverbal behaviors); and (4) hyper- or hyporeactivity to sensory input, involving an over- or underresponsive reaction to climate, sounds, textures, touch, smell, or visual input.

Etiology

Autism is commonly understood to be a neurodevelopmental disorder that involves a complex interaction of genetic and environmental factors (Thurm & Swedo, 2012). Neurological studies indicate that there are observable brain-based differences in structure and neurological function that affect behaviors (Thurm & Swedo). Although the cause is not understood, researchers are investigating the role of genes, hormones, autoimmunity, and environment in the disorder. Complicating researchers' ability to identify a cause is the nature of a spectrum disorder, whereby children involved in studies represent a heterogeneous population affected by different factors (Thurm & Swedo). Given the rising rates of ASD, Lord and Bishop (2010) suggest that research of sound methodology is required to better understand this complex disorder. Furthermore, regardless of the cause of the disorder, there is a clear need for effective treatment methods that can help increase success and independence.

Clinical Work

The purpose of music therapy for individuals with ASD is to provide these clients with clinically intended musical experiences, such as improvisation, receptive music, precomposed music, and/or songwriting that target core features of autism: relating, communicating, socializing, sensory integration, motor functioning, and cognitive functioning. This section of the chapter presents several music therapy methods and techniques used to treat individuals with ASD.

Music therapy practice has a long history of treating children with autism (Alvin & Warwick, 1991; Hintz, 2013; Kaplan & Steele, 2005; Kern, Wolery, & Aldridge, 2007; Kim, Wigram, & Gold, 2008, 2009; Nordoff & Robbins, 2007), and the literature is replete with clinical writings and research studies on the topic. The clinical writings demonstrate how various approaches to music therapy—such as developmental (Schwartz, 2008); Developmental, Individual Differences, Relationship-Based Approach (DIR®/Floortime™; Carpente, 2012; Greenspan & Weider, 2006); interactive (Oldfield, 2006); Creative Music Therapy (Nordoff & Robbins, 2007); family-centered (Thompson, 2012); applied behavior analysis (Martin, 2012); improvisational (Kim, Wigram, & Gold, 2008, 2009; Robarts, 1996); and psychoanalytic (Lecourt, 1991)—have been used with in-

dividuals with ASD to foster nonverbal expression and communication, socialization, behavior management, self-awareness, sensory integration, and musical and interpersonal relatedness.

In addition, empirical studies have shown that individuals with ASD may exhibit special musical abilities, particularly in pitch perception (Heaton, 2004; Thaut, 1988), as well as an affinity for music. Furthermore, empirical efficacy studies have shown that music therapy is effective in increasing socialization and communication (Finnigan & Starr, 2010; Kern et al., 2007) and decreasing perseverative behaviors (Brownell, 2002).

The therapeutic process and clinical direction, in terms of goals and interventions, vary considerably depending on the therapist's training and working approach. Some music therapists may formulate nonmusical goals in the areas of communication, cognition, speech, and so forth. Others, however, implement music-centered goals, such as musical relatedness, musical interrelatedness, and so forth, within the context of the relationship.

This section introduces music therapy interventions and techniques that are based on our clinical experiences and are derived from two perspectives: (1) relationship-based clinical work and (2) Neurologic Music Therapy (NMT).

Relationship-Based Music Therapy Framework

Here we discuss music therapy methods, techniques, and interventions within a relationship-based framework that focused on fostering the child's musical–social–emotional skills in the areas of musical relatedness, communication, and thinking. Thus, the areas of assessment and intervention are grounded in the child's ability to musically attend to, engage with, adapt to, and interrelate with musical play and musical interrelatedness (Carpente, 2012, 2013).

In a relationship-based framework the therapist works directly with the core features of ASD (relating and communicating). The therapist and the child work together in musical play though improvisation, composition, and re-creative experiences (Bruscia, 1998). The therapy process, including assessment and intervention, takes place within the coactive musical experiences (musical play) between the child and therapist, with roles, relationships, and dynamics guiding the therapy process.

Improvisatory Experiences

Music improvisation experiences, also known as clinical improvisation, have been an effective method in the treatment of children with ASD, targeting goals of relatedness, communication, joint attention, and social–emotional skills (Carpente, 2009; Kim et al., 2008; Nordoff & Robbins, 2007). In the improvisational approaches, therapists usually employ a nondirective approach working on a variety of instruments and using movement with music to address areas involving self-expression, communication, body awareness, anxiety and aggression, sensory integration, socialization, and communication (Carpente, 2013; Nordoff & Robbins, 2007).

When working within improvisational experiences, the therapist generally follows the child's musical lead by spontaneously creating music to engage the child's musical and nonmusical responses. The therapist incorporates every response the child offers within a musical framework, enabling the child and therapist to interact and develop their own unique therapist–child relationship (Carpente, 2013). During this musical–clinical process, the therapist gains insight into the child's musical–emotional strengths and challenges that pertain to relating, communicating, and thinking, while also considering and supporting the child's individual skill differences that impede his or her engagement in higher levels of musical interaction (Carpente, 2012, 2013).

CLINICAL EXAMPLE

Mary is an 8-year-old girl diagnosed with ASD. She presents with difficulties in her ability to self-regulate, process sensory information, and plan movement (i.e., motor plan). These biological factors appear to impede her capacity to engage in musical play in a related and communicative manner. In addition, she presents with both an under- and overreactive sensory system (mixed reactivity) and generally withdraws from interactions by becoming self-absorbed (underreactive) or by engaging in constant motion, seeking sensory stimulation, and screaming (overreactive). Improvisational experiences centered on following Mary's musical and emotional lead while providing her with the sensory support needed to foster reciprocal and intentional musical play.

Mary walks into the treatment room to start her ninth session. The therapist, playing the guitar and singing, improvises music based on Mary's emotional "being" as well the tempo of her walking movement. The music consists of a simple melody based in F mixolydian, harmonically moving between Eb and F major. Mary walks slowly to the snare drum, seeming unaware of the therapist's music, as the music reflects her movement. Mary stops walking for no obvious reason; the therapist, reflecting her pause, vamps on an A diminished chord, repeating the triad using finger picking while vocally sustaining an Eb note, waiting for Mary to respond or react in some fashion. Mary socially references the therapist and offers a smile. The therapist responds by smiling back and continuing the music, resolving the melody and harmony to F. Mary looks away, and again the music follows her lead, this time pausing, waiting for her response. Does Mary realize that she is controlling the music? Does she realize that the therapist and music are there to engage her in play? Does she realize that the therapist is following her lead?

Mary recognizes the musical alteration, looks and smiles in the therapist's direction, once again closing a circle of communication (Greenspan & Weider, 2006) as the musical theme continues and moves into a B section. This momentary interaction is followed by Mary's initiating play on the snare drum, as she picks up both mallets and begins to beat the basic beat of the original theme. Does she realize that she came into the basic beat on her own? Does she realize that she is engaged in a related musical experience? The therapist quickly picks up on Mary's beating and clinically decides to introduce an emotionally charged and rhythmic type of improvisation, modulating to a D minor progression that includes D minor, G minor/B♭, B minor 7♭5, E minor 7♭5/B♭, and A7, played in a detached manner while altering the timbre of his voice. Singing nonverbally, the therapist improvises a motif around Mary's beating, mirroring her beats with a melody note.

After three to four measures, Mary withdraws from the interaction. The therapist, continuing vocally with the melodic theme, places the guitar down and moves in front of the drum to provide Mary with visual support through modeling and gestures while singing. Mary appears responsive as she picks up the mallets and begins playing again. The therapist, while singing, also begins to play on the same drum using different mallets, providing Mary with emotionally charged musical experiences along with modeling as a means to foster her engagement and relatedness in musical play.

After eight to ten measures, it appears that Mary is getting overstimulated, as evidenced by her unorganized beating and loud, unrelated vocalizations. The therapist begins to decrease the tempo and dynamic range of the improvisation, while altering his singing to a falsetto range, and limiting the visual input of his drumming. Mary continues to display difficulty regaining self-regulation and shared attention. Thus, the therapist, while singing, provides her with sensory input such as deep pressure in her forearms. The singing melody accompanies the sensory input. This combination appears to help Mary self-regulate and regain musical attention. She slowly turns to face the therapist and joins his singing by vocalizing a variation of the original theme. Her vocalizations appear to capture the emotional qualities of the improvisation in regard to pitch, tempo, dynamics, and affect. After approximately 25 measures, the therapist initiates a decrease in tempo, letting Mary know that the musical experience may be coming to a conclusion. Mary follows the changes, slow-

ing down the tempo and dynamic range of her singing, and finally initiating the last note of the improvisation by singing the tonic (D).

Re-Creative Experiences

Re-creative music experiences involve the child's learning, performing, and/or reproducing a form of music, whether vocally and/or instrumentally (Bruscia, 1998). It provides the child with musical structure, predictability, and a defined musical role within the experience. Re-creative experiences may include precomposed and orchestrated pieces, as well as composed music designed for a specific client. The choice of music is based on the client's challenges, strengths, individual differences, and developmental capacities. Clinical goals may encompass the areas of self-regulation, shared attention, musical perception, problem solving, communication, and sharing ideas.

CLINICAL EXAMPLE

Eric is a 9-year-old boy with ASD who has participated in music therapy for four sessions. During musical play, Eric displays the capacity to self-regulate and engage; however, his interactions are fragmented and intermittent. During moments of musical engagement, Eric exhibits difficulty with grading his force of movement and depth perception, resulting in his constantly playing the drum and cymbal very loudly. Although Eric displays a propensity for rhythm, his playing appears to be mostly reflexive, and he exhibits challenges in the areas of intentionality and relatedness.

The precomposed song "Fun for Four Drums" (Nordoff & Robbins, 1968) helps facilitate Eric's ability to (1) focus and engage for a sustained period of time, (2) engage in a continuous flow of relational music experiences, and (3) explore and integrate a range of tempos and dynamics. The main idea of this music activity is that each of the four drums is cued to a distinct piano accompaniment. In order for Eric to play the correct drum, rhythm, tempo, and dynamics, he must listen to and discriminate each of the four piano accompaniments. Although this song has been presented to Eric in three prior consecutive sessions, each time it is presented, the therapist alters and varies the drum parts and piano accompaniment as a means of maintaining Eric's alertness, shared attention, music perception, and overall responsiveness to the changes. Thus, although the musical structure and form of the song are familiar to Eric, the therapist improvises within the predictable structure by altering the dynamics and tempo range, as well as the order in which the drums are presented musically. After eight sessions of working with this song, Eric showed improvement in his ability to engage and relate in a continuous flowing manner, and he increased his range of tempos and dynamics when playing the drum.

Composition Experiences

Composition or songwriting experiences involve the therapist and child in the process of writing songs, lyrics, and/or instrumental pieces (Bruscia, 1998). Generally, the therapist facilitates the songwriting experience/process based on the child's interaction, participation, relational dynamics, and developmental capacities.

Children diagnosed with ASD who possess expressive language skills as well as the ability to engage conversationally may display challenges in their ability to think abstractly, for example, about feelings, empathy, and theory of mind. The basis for their interactions may be based on concrete topics and memory-based thinking. Songwriting experience can offer the child an opportunity to develop the ability for symbolic and abstract thinking and can also foster shared problem-solving and collaborative experiences, as well as the capacity to explore life's themes and inner world experiences (Bruscia, 1998).

Generally, for children with ASD to engage in songwriting experiences, they should display some capacity to express words and ideas, as well as to engage in some form of conversation.

CLINICAL EXAMPLE

Derek is a 12-year-old boy who displays the ability to engage in musical play in a related manner. He also exhibits the capacity to engage in conversation and to share ideas. However, the focus of Derek's conversations tends toward concrete and familiar topics, such as movies, television programs, and current events. He has difficulty initiating ideas that pertain to feelings and emotions, and he exhibits a limited capacity to respond to unexpected events that occur during sessions. In addition, Derek's ability to bridge ideas with the therapist's during sessions is limited. When confronted with abstract and unfamiliar topics, Derek tends to withdraw from the interaction by scripting stanzas from familiar movies or songs, or by becoming angry and tangential in his behavior.

Songwriting was introduced to Derek as a means for him to organize and bridge his ideas with those of the therapist, while providing him with creative opportunities to facilitate abstract and symbolic thinking. The song outlined below illustrates how this type of music experience helped facilitate self-expression, while also providing the therapist a window into the child's thoughts, ideas, feelings, and insight.

During session 35, Derek appears to be preoccupied and anxious. The therapist asks if something is bothering him, to which Derek replies, "No! Well, yes, I think so. No! Forget about it." He then asks if they can play music, and the therapist replies, "Sure we can. What would you like to do or play?" Derek, still seeming anxious, has difficulty responding to the therapist's open-ended question. Recognizing that Derek is having a difficult time engaging and responding, the therapist asks him if he would like to write a song. Derek replies, "OK. What should we write about?" The therapist then engages him in dialogue while providing him with musical choices for the song (e.g., harmony, dynamics, tempo, style). The dialogue begins to take form and a theme emerges that deals with Derek's feelings of loneliness and abandonment, as he begins to discuss how upset he is about his friend from school moving out of state. The therapist, empathizing and reflecting his feelings, helps Derek articulate his ideas in song form. This is followed by Derek's expressing his thoughts in a continuous, flowing manner, soon becoming lyrics for an emerging song:

Verse 1
I stayed up late last night all alone missing you
It's been so long since we spoke ya' know?
and you know you're so far away
Preoccupied in the everyday things
and simply forget the small things that become
   large.

Pre-chorus
It's been deep in my thoughts like a pain in
   wild.

Chorus
Time passes by and I'm still not shaken,
but just frustrated
and can't stop thinking
of how it used to be.

Verse 2
I ran into a cathedral
a message of a new chapter comes to me
I stumble outside and feeling is no different.

Pre-chorus
It's been deep in my thoughts like a pain in
   wild.

Chorus
Time passes by and I'm still not shaken,
but just frustrated
and can't stop thinking
of how it used to be.

Neurologic Music Therapy

The second framework is the NMT model. NMT is defined as the systematic application of music stimuli to facilitate functional changes in cognitive, communicative, or sensorimotor skills (Thaut, 2005). NMT is an evidence-based approach to music therapy, where the current research literature is considered when making treatment decisions. This includes research evidence from basic music neuroscience studies (music perception and production) to clinical models in music therapy and related fields. A clinician in this methodology utilizes the transformational design model (TDM) to develop functional and generalizable music therapy interventions that address core needs of the individual. The TDM begins with completion of an assessment and the formalization of client goals. The therapist then considers functional nonmusical exercises that could be utilized to reach the goals. This is followed by an isomorphic translation of the nonmusical exercise into an exercise where music directly facilitates the identified need. The final step is generalization from the music experience to the normal environment. Thus, the TDM leads the music therapist through thoughtful consideration of the child's needs and the development of music stimuli that will directly address those identified needs. Although clinicians practicing NMT will often develop treatment protocols to address common needs, high-quality music-making experiences are a cornerstone of this method. For the purpose of this chapter, three NMT techniques and their functional applications are illustrated.

Auditory Perception Training

In NMT sensory regulation is addressed using the technique of auditory perception training. This technique serves two purposes: (1) It helps children achieve optimal auditory sensory functioning within their environment, and (2) it helps decrease children's sensitivity to environmental stimuli. Researchers have demonstrated that children with ASD react differently to environmental stimuli, whether via perseveration, sensory seeking behaviors, avoidance behaviors, or poor attention (Liss, Saulnier, Fein, & Kinsbourne, 2006). These reactions may be due to differences in their neurophysiological processing of stimuli, including poor habituation to sound and atypical responses to new stimuli (Guiraud et al., 2011). These studies serve as the basis for utilizing music stimuli as a way to decrease sensitivity, increase regulation, and decrease auditory hypersensitivity. These improvements are achieved through various experiences in which the child has the opportunity to receive multisensory stimulation that is anticipatory (rhythmic deep pressure) or practice attending to relevant stimuli in the presence of nonrelevant stimuli. As the child demonstrates decreased hypersensitivity in the controlled environment, novel environments are utilized for generalization with replacement behaviors.

CLINICAL EXAMPLE

Patrick was a 9-year-old boy diagnosed with ASD and sensory processing disorder. He regularly wore sound-reducing headphones, though when in environments with "noise," would cover his ears and scream. Within a familiar environment, if he heard unfamiliar stimuli he would discontinue the task at hand and repeatedly scream, "I'm scared." This behavior was observed when air conditioning would turn on, cars would pass by, and people would enter the room (who couldn't be seen). Auditory hypersensitivity led to the family's inability to take their child to even typical environments to complete activities such as shopping; this sensitivity also disrupted the classroom at school.

The music therapy experience initially involved exposing the child to predictable music stimuli. Within 2 weeks, Patrick was able to remove his ear coverings in the music therapy session. As often seen in children with auditory hypersensitivity, when he was in control of the sounds, they could be extremely loud without causing any distress. Patrick was then engaged in experiences that required him to focus his attention on musical stimuli (such as the music therapist playing a guitar) while moving around a familiar and quiet environment. Once he mastered this skill, his vision was removed though covering eyes with a hoodie or wearing a blindfold (with an assistant as a safety guard). The child again practiced following the selected sound source (such as the guitar) through the clinic with no competing stimuli. This was then practiced with competing stimuli, such as a piano or another instrument being played, so that the child had to focus attention on the selected stimuli while ignoring the competing stimuli. Once the child mastered this skill, the exercise was repeated in novel environments

including the hallway of the clinic building, outside, and in a music practice hallway. The child was challenged to focus on the relevant stimuli and ignore all nonrelevant stimuli. Patrick would be asked to stop what he was doing for that moment, focus on the environmental stimuli, and identify it—at which point the blindfold/hoodie would be removed and he would visually pair what he heard with what he saw. Eventually this exercise was completed without the blindfold and a replacement for the musical sound source was gradually introduced (rhythmic tapping on his leg), which allowed for this practice to occur in other novel environments where the music therapist would not be present. This process decreased Patrick's dependence on ear covering, allowed him to walk through noisy environments without behavioral outbursts, and helped him to maintain focus on a selected stimulus.

Developmental Speech and Language Training

Developmental speech and language training through music (DSLM) is the use of age-appropriate musical experiences that target speech and language skills. This technique involves the creation of musical experiences that directly facilitate the targeted speech needs, including prelinguistic, receptive, and expressive language skills. Once the area of need is identified, the nonmusical or functional skill is considered. For example, with expressive communication, the functional *real-world* skill could be asking for wants or needs. The music therapist would take this real-world exchange and create a musical experience that would target the functional skill, initiating communication for wants/needs. The musical structure then provides the opportunity for the child to practice this skill, using music as an anticipatory cue for response and a medium to increase engagement in the communication experience.

The DSLM technique is based in principles of child engagement, language learning, and research demonstrating that children with ASD process music better then speech (Lai, Pantazatos, Schneider, & Hirsch, 2012); however, there is also initial clinical efficacy. Lim (2010) demonstrated that children with ASD who had more severe communication deficits made greater improvements in communication with the DSLM technique. Wan et al. (2011) demonstrated that rhythm and melody, along with playing pitched drums, improved speech production in nonverbal children with ASD. This initial evidence supports the use of musical materials for communication in children with ASD.

CLINICAL EXAMPLE

Keith is a 6-year-old boy who is on the autism spectrum and who has limited speech production and no other form of communication. During the assessment, Keith's preferred musical items included the cabasa, drums, and shakers. In order to promote the use of speech communication, a musical exercise is crafted that focuses on the target response of expressive speech communication of wants. A song structure is created that creates an opportunity for Keith to be engaged in a rewarding musical experience that also provides opportunities to communicate. Since Keith showed a preference for some instruments, those instruments are included in the experience, along with novel instruments to promote further musical exploration.

In this experience, the song structure was created in ABA (where the musical material in the A sections is the same and changes in the B section) form, where the A section would provide the opportunity for Keith to play an instrument while the music therapist played the piano or guitar and sang an age-appropriate song germane to the experience. The A section of the song would conclude with Keith being instructed (through the music) to put down the instrument. The B section would then provide an opportunity for Keith to choose a new instrument. The music in this section would provide cues for the clear anticipation of a response, and rhythm would be utilized through the response period to support the speech production. Although a

functional sentence might be uttered (e.g., "I want that one"), any sentence that is initiated and clearly communicates choice would be acceptable—the goal isn't to teach a phrase, but rather to promote appropriate communication for the task at hand. Upon Keith responding that he wants to play the cabasa, the A section is repeated and he has the opportunity to play the selected instrument. Communication-based exercises would be repeated with different stimuli and manipulatives. Eventually, the music support during the response would be decreased, and Keith would have opportunities to practice the same skill in the nonmusical environment.

Social Competence Training

Another area of need in children with ASD is that of reading and responding to social cues. Social competence training provides opportunities for children to practice social skills that are necessary for functioning, including turn taking, on-topic responses, joint attention skills, and reading body language/expressions. Several studies have demonstrated that music therapy experiences can be beneficial to social skill acquisition (Finnigan & Starr, 2010; Kern & Aldridge, 2006; Kern et al., 2007). The individual's primary needs and situations where these social skills could be practiced are considered first. A musical experience is then created to add motivation, anticipation, and repetition to practicing the social experience. The social experience may be completely musical in nature (e.g., joint attention through shared playing of an instrument) or may lead to the practice of the skill (e.g., music to cue the following of eye gaze). Once the skill is demonstrated within musical tasks, the music is faded, and the skill is practiced in the nonmusical context.

CLINICAL EXAMPLE

Marigold is a 10-year-old girl diagnosed with ASD. During the assessment, social competence, including joint attention skills, was identified as primary. In order to work on triadic joint attention (i.e., two people attending to an object after one initial reference, via gaze, to the object), the experience as it occurs in the typical environment is considered and a music experience that emphasizes this skill is created. For Marigold, this music experience involves successive steps from playing an instrument with the therapist, to looking at the therapist's eyes to determine what they will play next, to looking into a peer's eyes to determine what he or she will play next. The actual act of looking at an object and relaying meaning from that gaze, then jointly participating in an activity using that object, is completed throughout the music experience. The music begins with lyrical directions, but moves into using structure within the music to signify different components of the skill. Eventually, this skill would be practiced in a nonmusical context where joint attention can be used for nonverbal social communication.

Applications to Other Disciplines

Working collaboratively with other disciplines provides clinical–musical opportunities to support other professionals (e.g., occupational therapists, speech and language pathologists) in their work with children with ASD. Working within a relationship-based framework, the music therapist can provide improvisational music experiences that enhance the interaction between the child and other professional by creating music that is built around their interactions (Carpente, 2012). Another collaborative technique includes coaching the other professional on how to work in music with clinical intent and purpose within their scope of practice (Carpente). This may involve guiding the other professional to shape or alter the music experience based on the child's affect, responsiveness, reaction, movement, and/or vocalization.

Collaborations with other disciplines are encouraged within the methodology of NMT. Treatment collaborations allow for the consideration of different perspectives, expertise, and research knowledge with the ultimate goal of providing the client with the best treatment to reach the desired outcomes. When working with children with ASD, the NMT clinician can collaborate with members of the child's treatment team, inclusive of other therapists and teachers. Once the treatment team determines the areas of needs, the music therapist can utilize the TDM to create music therapy experiences that facilitate the meeting of the nonmusical skill or need.

In addition to providing live/interactive music therapy applications on the treatment team, the music therapist can also develop materials and accommodations that can be utilized by the entire treatment team in the music therapist's absence. For example, if a child is demonstrating difficulty initiating of speech, rhythmic exercises can first be implemented in the music therapy session to practice speech initiation. The use of rhythm can be faded to rhythmic tapping on the client's leg or another rhythmic body movement while attempting speech production. This is a simple accommodation that could be utilized across therapy sessions and in the school setting to help the client communicate more independently.

Another example of materials that can be utilized across disciplines is the use of simple songs to help with routines, transitions, or behavioral/social compliance. This can be a song helping a child to remember the steps that are appropriate to follow when blowing his or her nose and discarding the tissue. The music therapist can create a transition song that the treatment team utilizes to help the child shift from one activity to another. These accommodations can be developed with the comfort of the treatment team in mind, as some members may not want to or feel comfortable singing. For example, the accommodation could incorporate melody and rhythm, a rhythmic chant, or a recording of the composed song.

Conclusions

With the incidence of ASD increasing in recent years, there is a continued need for evidence-based treatment methodologies to address the core needs of children affected by the disorder (Lord & Bishop, 2010). Researchers have demonstrated that children with ASD often have a unique attraction to music or enhanced musical abilities (Heaton, 2004; Thaut, 1988). Furthermore, research has revealed that children with ASD show increased cortical activation when exposed to music over speech stimuli (Lai et al., 2012), indicating atypical processing that may be favorable to musical stimuli. These factors may make music engagement a particularly effective method for addressing core features of ASD. Researchers in the field of music therapy have demonstrated initial efficacy of music therapy as an intervention to facilitate the acquisition of social and communicative skills. Although there are different approaches within the field of music therapy, therapists practicing in each methodology and approach are focused on using or working in music to help children with ASD reach their full developmental potential. These music therapy interventions allow children with ASD to experience the world in a different way, with the intention of improving their functional skills and everyday lives.

REFERENCES

Alvin, J., & Warwick, A. (1991). *Music therapy for the autistic child* (2nd ed.). Oxford, UK: Oxford University Press.

American Psychiatric Association. (2013). *Diagnostic and statistical manual of mental disorders* (5th ed.). Arlington, VA: Author.

Asperger, H. (1991). "Autistic psychopathy" in childhood. In U. Frith (Ed.), *Autism and Asperger syndrome* (pp. 37–92). Cambridge, UK: Cambridge University Press. (Original work published 1944)

Brownell, M. D. (2002). Musically adapted social stories to modify behaviors in students with autism: Four case studies. *Journal of Music Therapy, 39*(2), 117–144.

Bruscia, K. E. (1998). *Defining music therapy* (2nd ed.). Gilsum, NH: Barcelona.

Carpente, J. (2009). *Contributions of Nordoff-Robbins music therapy within the developmental, individual-differences, relationship (DIR)-based model in the treatment of children with autism: Four case studies* (Unpublished doctoral dissertation). Temple University, Philadelphia, PA. Available from ProQuest Dissertations and Theses database (UMI No. AAT 3359621).

Carpente, J. (2012). DIR®/Floortime™ model: Introduction and considerations for improvisational music therapy. In P. Kern & M. Humpal (Eds.), *Early childhood music therapy and autism spectrum disorders: Developing potential in young children and their families* (pp. 145–161). Philadelphia: Jessica Kingsley.

Carpente, J. (2013). *The Individual Music-Centered Assessment Profile for Neurodevelopmental Disorders (IMCAP-ND): A clinical manual.* Baldwin, NY: Regina.

Centers for Disease Control and Prevention. (2013). Data and statistics. In *Autism spectrum disorders.* Retrieved from *www.cdc.gov/ncbddd/autism/data.html.*

Finnigan, D., & Starr, E. (2010). Increasing social responsiveness in a child with autism: A comparison of music and nonmusic interventions. *Autism, 14*(4), 321–348.

Greenspan, S. I., & Weider, S. (2006). *Infant and early childhood mental health: A comprehensive developmental approach to assessment and intervention.* Washington, DC: American Psychiatric Association.

Guiraud, J. A., Kushnerenko, E., Tomalski, P., Davies, K., Ribeiro, H., & Johnson, M. H. (2011). Differential habituation to repeated sounds in infants at high risk for autism. *NeuroReport, 22*(16), 845–849.

Heaton, P. (2004). Interval and contour processing in autism. *Journal of Autism and Developmental Disorders, 35*(6), 787–793.

Hintz, M. (2013). Autism. In M. Hintz (Ed.), *Guidelines for music therapy practice in developmental health* (pp. 50–86). University Park, IL: Barcelona.

Kanner, L. (1943). Autistic disturbances of affective contact. *Nervous Child, 2,* 217–250.

Kaplan, R., & Steele, A. L. (2005). An analysis of music therapy program goals and outcomes for clients with diagnoses on the autism spectrum. *Journal of Music Therapy, 42*(1), 2–19.

Kern, P., & Aldridge, D. (2006). Using embedded

music therapy interventions to support outdoor play of young children with autism in an inclusive community-based child care program. *Journal of Music Therapy, 43*(4), 270–294.

Kern, P., Wolery, M., & Aldridge, D. (2007). Use of songs to promote independence in morning greeting routines for young children with autism. *Journal of Autism and Developmental Disorders, 37*, 1264–1271.

Kim, J., Wigram, T., & Gold, C. (2008). The effects of improvisational music therapy on joint attention behaviors in autistic children: A randomized controlled study. *Journal of Autism and Developmental Disorders, 38*, 1758–1766.

Kim, J., Wigram, T., & Gold, C. (2009). Emotional, motivational, and interpersonal responsiveness of children with autism in improvisational music therapy. *Autism, 13*(4), 389–409.

Lai, G., Pantazatos, S. P., Schneider, H., & Hirsch, J. (2012). Neural systems for speech and song in autism. *Brain, 135*(Pt. 3), 961–975.

Lecourt, E. (1991). Off-beat music therapy: A psychoanalytic approach to autism. In K. E. Bruscia (Ed.), *Case studies in music therapy* (pp. 73–98). Gilsum, NH: Barcelona.

Lim, H. A. (2010). Effect of "developmental speech and language training through music" on speech production in children with autism spectrum disorders. *Journal of Music Therapy, 47*(1), 2–26.

Liss, M., Saulnier, C., Fein, D., & Kinsbourne, M. (2006). Sensory and attention abnormalities in autistic spectrum disorders. *Autism, 10*(2), 155–172.

Lord, C., & Bishop, S. L. (2010). Autism spectrum disorders: Diagnosis, prevalence, and services for children and families. *Social Policy Report, 24*(2), 1–27.

Martin, L. (2012). Applied behavior analysis: Introduction and practical application in music therapy for young children with autism spectrum disorders. In P. Kern & M. Humpal (Eds.), *Early childhood music therapy and autism spectrum disorders: Developing potential in young children and their families* (pp. 101–116). Philadelphia: Jessica Kingsley.

Nordoff, P., & Robbins, C. (1968). *Fun for four drums: A rhythmic game for children with four drums, piano and a song*. Bryn Mawr, PA: Theodore Presser.

Nordoff, P., & Robbins, C. (2007). *Creative music therapy: A guide to fostering clinical musicianship* (2nd ed). Gilsum, NH: Barcelona.

Oldfield, A. (2006). *Interactive music therapy in child and family psychiatry: Clinical practice, research and teaching*. London: Jessica Kingsley.

Robarts, J. (1996). Music therapy for children with autism. In C. Trevarthen, K. Aitken, D. Papoudi, & J. Robarts (Eds.), *Children with autism: Diagnosis and intervention to meet their needs* (pp. 134–160). London: Jessica Kingsley.

Schwartz, E. (2008). *Music, therapy, and early childhood: A developmental approach*. Gilsum, NH: Barcelona.

Thaut, M. H. (1988). Measuring musical responsiveness in autistic children: A comparative analysis of improvised musical tone sequences of autistic, normal, and mentally retarded individuals. *Journal of Autism and Developmental Disorders, 18*(4), 561–571.

Thaut, M. H. (2005). *Rhythm, music and the brain*. London: Routledge.

Thompson, G. (2012). Family-centered music therapy in the home environment: Promoting interpersonal engagement between children with autism spectrum disorder and their parents. *Music Therapy Perspectives, 30*(2), 109–116.

Thurm, A., & Swedo, S. E. (2012). The importance of autism research. *Dialogues in Clinical Neuroscience, 14*(3), 219–222.

Volkmar, F. R., Reichow, B., & McPartland, J. (2012). Classification of autism and related conditions: Progress, challenges, and opportunities. *Dialogues in Clinical Neuroscience, 14*(3), 229–237.

Wan, C. Y., Bazen, L., Baars, R., Libenson, A., Zipse, L., Zuk, J., et al. (2011). Auditory–motor mapping training as an intervention to facilitate speech output in non-verbal children with autism: A proof of concept study. *PLoS One, 6*(9), e25505.

Wing, L., Gould, J., & Gillberg, C. (2011). Autism spectrum disorders in the DSM-V: Better or worse than the DSM-IV? *Research in Developmental Disabilities, 32*, 768–773.

CHAPTER 24

Music Therapy for Children with Speech and Language Disorders

Kathleen M. Howland

The development of speech and language skills in children is an astounding feat of both nature and nurture. It is highly complex and yet appears to evolve with the greatest of ease—that is, until something disrupts it.

In the past, researchers thought of an infant as *tabula rasa*—a blank slate upon which language and culture would be written. We now know that a baby is capable of many skills, music and speech perception chief among them. For example, a fetus in the final trimester in the womb differentially responds to previously heard music and stories when compared to novel songs and stories (DeCasper & Spence, 1986; James, Spencer, & Stepsis, 2002). An infant that is only 6 weeks old is able to distinguish all of the sounds of the world's languages (Dehaene-Lambertz & Dehaene, 1994), changes in musical meter of the culture's music, and the musical meter of other cultures (Hannon & Trehub, 2005; Soley & Hannon, 2010).

In a recent article on music and early language acquisition, Brandt, Gebrian, and Slevc (2012) propose that in the newborn brain, music is fundamental to learning language. They postulate that infants use musical aspects of language—namely rhythm, timbre contrasts, and melodic contour—as a platform for the later development of syntax (grammar) and semantics (meanings of words).

Because of the shared characteristics between singing and speaking, neuroscientists have begun to research the use of singing as a way to treat speech abnormalities (Wan, Ruber, Hohmann, & Schlaug, 2010). Much work has begun in this area, primarily with adults who have neurogenic disorders (e.g., strokes, Parkinson's disease) and more recently, children with autism. The objective of this chapter is to provide music therapists and other interested therapists with the most up-to-date approaches to treating developmental speech and language disorders using music as a clinical intervention. Music provides therapists with a motivating, nonthreatening, and enjoyable medium that is quite natural to children. Music therapy is based on the innate capabilities of nearly every child to perceive and produce elements of music—rhythm and pitch. The versatility of music affords therapists numerous ways to address the same task, especially tasks that require numerous repetitions in order to master.

The terms *speech* and *language* often occur together, as in the title *speech–language pathologist* (SLP). Speech and language are, however, two distinct skills that need to be defined separately, for they present very different profiles and require different treatment approaches. This chapter begins by addressing speech disorders and then moves on to language disorders.

The literature for pediatric speech–language disorders to date is limited. In part this limitation could be due to controversy regarding diagnostic criteria (Morgan & Vogel, 2008a) and the various etiologies that can cause a disorder. For example, dysarthria (poor speech intelligibility) can be caused by congenital conditions (e.g., cerebral palsy, Down syndrome), as well as acquired injuries (e.g., traumatic brain injury) in children. To complicate the grouping of subjects for research, there are different types of dysarthria (e.g., hypokinetic, hyperkinetic, ataxic). Thus the heterogeneity of the disorder can confound research efforts. Lastly, the numbers of children needed for formal research studies can be very difficult to recruit in any one area.

The American Speech–Language–Hearing Association has a National Center for Evidence-Based Systematic Reviews (*www.asha.org/members/ebp/EBSRs*). Reviews are conducted to inform evidence-based practice guidelines. There are limited reviews for the diagnostic categories addressed in this chapter, and the disorders that have reviews (apraxia, dysarthria, and pragmatics) report a lack of studies on which to base efficacious practices, a lack of definition for diagnostic classifications, poorly controlled studies, and limited numbers of subjects (Gerber, Brice, Capone, Fujiki, & Timler, 2012; Morgan & Vogel, 2008a, 2008b).

Much of the literature for treating speech and language disorders using music comes from work with adults who have acquired neurogenic disorders such as Parkinson's disease, strokes, and brain injuries. Music therapists working with children should be well read in the research published for both adults and children in music therapy as well as speech–language pathology. They should understand the presenting characteristics of the diagnosis, the neurological foundations of the diagnosis, and promising clinical approaches based on the rational scientific mediating model (Thaut, 2005). Clinicians would then have an informed basis from which to replicate promising practices, make adaptations to enhance the efficacy of a practice for children, and create novel approaches based on what has been attempted before.

Clientele

Children from birth through adolescence may present with a variety of speech and language disorders that can be congenital or acquired in origin. They may be genetic or an anomaly; they may present as mild, moderate, or severe; they may interfere with communication severely or mildly. A speech–language pathologist (credentials CCC-SLP) should do an assessment to identify the diagnosis and provide descriptions of how the condition impacts communication. The identification of treatment goals by the SLP is of key importance to the music therapist.

Clinical Work

Speech

Speech is a motor act involving the coordination of respiration (breath), phonation (voicing), and articulation. Disorders at any one level, or at more than one level, can negatively impact the intelligibility of speech and the success of communication.

Speech intelligibility is calculated as a percentage of an utterance that can be understood. For example, an unfamiliar listener may judge a child's speech to be less than 50% intelligible. Essentially, that listener is discerning an occasional intelligible word from which he or she is trying to guess the child's intent. In terms of speech intelligibility, a good rule of thumb is to know that a 3-year-old child should be intelligible to nonfamiliar (nonfamilial) listeners.

Speech–language pathologists generally consider four levels of motor function in identifying root causes, and thus treatment targets, for motor speech disorders:

1. *Disorders of respiration.* Poor breath support compromises the efficient vibration of the vocal folds, which reduces the quality and quantity (volume) of sound produced. A listener would hear a breathy or quiet voice that makes speech difficult to understand. Frequent breaths might be observed during speech and/or singing.
2. *Disorders of phonation.* Poor closure of the vocal cords can result in a breathy or *creaky* sounding voice. This may be due to poor respiratory control driving the vocal cords in motion, or it could be related to pathologies of the vocal folds. SLPs must refer a client with a voice disorder to an otolaryngologist (ear, nose, and throat specialist) for an evaluation to rule out cancer or other disease processes as the basis of the disorder. Music therapists should also make such a referral prior to initiating treatment.
3. *Disorders of articulation.* Poorly coordinated or weak muscles will create indistinct and poorly intelligible speech sounds. For example, if the lips are not pressed together properly, a /p/ will not have the popping quality that it should.
4. *Disorders of resonance.* The connection of the soft palate to the nasal cavity occurs only for the English sounds of /m/ as in music, /n/ as in none, and /ŋ/ as in sing. When the muscles of the soft pal-

ate are weak or the junction of the soft palate and nasal cavity is poorly coordinated, the voice will sound hypernasal or stuffy, as if the person has a cold.

The major disorders of speech include the following diagnostic categories: dysarthria, articulation and phonological disorders, apraxia, and stuttering. Each is described below with a reference for presenting characteristics and recommended treatments and activities in music.

Dysarthria

Presenting characteristics of dysarthria include poor vocal quality (hoarse or breathy) and poor articulatory precision (slurred or mumbled sounding speech). It is a motor speech disorder caused by damage or poor functioning at the level of the central nervous system (the brain and spinal cord) or the peripheral nervous system (spinal or cranial nerves). The overall result is poor speech intelligibility.

There are several types of dysarthria: flaccid (associated with Down syndrome), spastic, dyskinetic, and ataxic. Children with Down syndrome typically present with *flaccid dysarthria* due to their enlarged tongues plus the hypotonicity of the muscles of the tongue, lips, and soft palate. Their vocal quality can be described as *stuffy* sounding (hypernasal), and their articulatory efforts are imprecise and sluggish. *Spastic dysarthria* is characterized by a harsh, strained, or strangled vocal quality. *Dyskinetic dysarthria* can be hyper- or hypokinetic (too much or too little movement that results in undershooting or overshooting targets). *Ataxic speech* may also have a harsh vocal quality and is notable for being slurred and indistinct. Poor motor control and organization are aspects of this subtype. A knowledgeable SLP can identify which subtype the child presents.

In recent years, the treatment of adults with dysarthria, especially those who have Parkinson's disease, has focused on improving respiration and phonation. This protocol is called the *Lee Silverman voice treatment* (*www.lsvtglobal.com*) program, also known as *think loud*. In Neurologic Music Therapy (NMT), the protocol is known as vocal intonation therapy (VIT; Thaut, 2005). In both approaches, the primary focus is on loud productions (as measured by sound level meters) and sustained phonations (on vowels and certain consonants that provide resistance, such as /s/). The sustained phonations are timed with a stopwatch. Research studies describe improved consonant production (Dromey, Ramig, & Johnson, 1995), tongue strength and motility (Ward, Theodoros, Murdoch, & Silburn, 2000), and rate of speech (Ramig, Countryman, Thompson, & Horii, 1995) just by working on respiration and phonation. This approach contrasts with traditional articulation therapy for dysarthria that addresses speech sounds in a hierarchical fashion: first in isolation; then in syllables, phrases, sentences; and finally in conversational speech. This conventional approach is tedious, with generally limited success. It is most impressive that focusing treatment on respiration can improve articulation. It reinforces the underlying etiology that this is a motor speech disorder and not a phonological disorder.

Singing is a positive context in which to practice sustained phonations and loudness. Precomposed or original songs give the music therapist a variety of materials with which to maintain a child's interest. Recordings of these songs allow children to practice at home with their families, which is key to realizing positive outcomes.

Traditionally oral motor exercises (OMEs) have been used to strengthen the muscles of the speech system, primarily the tongue, lips, and cheeks. An evidence-based systematic review of non-speech-related OMEs on speech by McCauley, Strand, Lof, Schooling, and Frymark (2009) reported insufficient evidence to support or refute the use of OMEs for speech enhancement. If a music therapist is collaborating with a speech therapist who feels that OMEs would be helpful, the music therapist can indeed incorporate these drills in a musical context that could be compelling and motivating. Thaut (2005), in his description of oral motor and respiratory exercises (OMREX), recommends the use of wind instruments (flutes, kazoos, recorders, and slide and tin whistles) as musical ways to build respiratory control and muscle strength of the lips and cheeks. Tonguing the instruments in call-and-response patterns can facilitate rapid movement of the tongue tip, which is important in speech articulation. There are whistles that are graduated to provide more resistance as a child develops strength (see Web Resource list at end of chapter).

Music therapy is an ideal clinical intervention for dysarthria because it can infuse repetitive tasks with meaning and enjoyment. It also contextualizes the sustained phonations and loudness productions into something purposeful.

A metronome can be used to slow a song down for improved success. As a child's articulation improves, the metronome can be increased by 5%, a change that is barely noticeable to the ear but creates a greater and assumable demand on the motor system. Another strategy to employ is elongation of syllables. This can give a poorly coordinated motor system more time to organize itself when the demand for syllable productions is decreased. Word or sound targets can be written with a pause, sung with an elongated syllable preceding them (*I feel\^\^\^fine*), or sung with a longer vowel (*muuuusic*) to support motor organization of the /z/ sound in "music". In subsequent trials, the pauses and elongations can be decreased and then eliminated as the motor system performs better.

Good breath control can be taught and reinforced by increasing phrase lengths in songs. All of these techniques can be used naturally in music activities and should be communicated to the speech therapist and family to generalize to speech conditions.

Articulation and Phonological Disorders

Children make naturally occurring speech errors as they develop speech skills. For example, a 2-year-old child might say *pay* for the word *play* because articulating two consonants together is so demanding. A 5-year-old, in contrast, should not be making those reductions on a regular basis. A naturally occurring error becomes a disorder when it persists too long.

Motor systems typically lag behind the development of cognitive–linguistic systems (knowledge of the word play and desire to use it conversationally). There are developmental scales that define the ages at which speech sounds should be occurring (see Web Resources section for references). A music therapist who treats childhood disorders should be thoroughly familiar with these scales to facilitate the development of age norms and sequences in speech and language.

When children have difficulties articulating age-appropriate speech sounds, or when developmentally appropriate speech errors persist, they should be referred to, and evaluated by, an SLP. The number of errors may be minimal and may or may not impact overall intelligibility. If the patterns of errors are systematic and numerous, thus significantly reducing intelligibility, the child may be diagnosed with a phonological disorder. A child with this disorder classification may make a variety of errors. For example, a child may collapse the syllable structure of a word to make it easier to say. He or she might say *heter* for *helicopter* or *amblance* for *ambulance*. A more serious pattern of errors is the deletion of final consonants. For example, a child who says *be* could mean *beat, beach, beef, beak, beam, bean*, and so forth. Another phonological disorder may be indicated by the omission of whole classes of sounds, such as deleting or substituting fricatives (i.e., consonants made by constricting airflow to create a hissing sound) such as /s/ in *sat*, /ʃ/ as in *she*, or /z/ as in *zoo*. A child may say *tat* for

sat, tee for *she*, and *do* for *zoo*. These last two error classes significantly and negatively impact speech intelligibility. They are too far from the intended target to be well understood by a listener, especially one not familiar with the child. The evaluating speech therapist will have a detailed treatment plan targeting one or more of these phonological processes in specified sequences. Much thought goes into these treatment plans and it is important for the music therapist to rely on the expertise of the SLP in order to optimally support the client's progress with musical interventions.

Speech therapists work on targeted speech sounds in various positions in words. If a child was working on the sound /p/, for example, drills of /p/ in the initial position would include *pat, Pete*, and *pick*. Drills in the medial position would include *apple, supper*, and *tapping*. In the final position, words such as *tap, stop*, and *cap* would be practiced. It is important for the music therapist to know on which speech sounds to focus by closely collaborating with the speech therapist. It is recommended that the music therapist adopt the same type of cuing that the SLP is using. Kinesthetic cues can be very helpful for articulatory placement. For example, in order to say the sound /ʃ/ as in *hush*, the lips must be rounded. The kinesthetic prompt would be to circle your lips with your finger as the child observes.

Once the targets have been identified by the SLP, the music therapist can create songs and activities that include the sounds in words that are both true words and protowords (i.e., made-up syllables, e.g., *scat* singing). The lyrics can include other words that have not been practiced to see if the ability to produce the targeted sounds has generalized to nonrehearsed words. Producing these sounds in nonrehearsed contexts would indicate notable progress. Some songs that are commercially available work nicely for articulation therapy. One example is "Sunshine on My Shoulders," by John Denver. It is a good song for practicing fricatives such as /s/ as in _sun_ and /ʃ/ as in _shine_. The accompanying book is also very engaging.

Instruments that make sounds similar to a speech sound can be used to work on the sound in isolation. For the sound /ʃ/, the ocean drum is wonderful. The opposing drum head can be used with a hand or beater to tap out plosives (i.e., an oral stop; a consonant that is made by blocking a part of the mouth so that no air can pass through) _pa ta ka, pa pa pa_, and _pa ta pa_. The afuche cabasa can help the child sustain the /ʃ/ sound, as in _sshhhh_, and short bursts of the affricate (i.e., consonants that begin as stops, such as [t] or [d], but release as a fricative, such as [s] or [z])] /t ʃ/ as in _cha cha cha_. Note that some sounds can be sustained and some cannot. Knowledge of phonetics is important in knowing how to structure activities for practice.

Composed songs are a key asset for creating varied, compelling, and customized opportunities for practice. The focus of the songs can be single words, phrases, or whole sentences, depending on the level of speech competencies and treatment needs. Call-and-response singing is a useful technique for many developmental speech disorders. With a very young child, it may be helpful to involve the parent so the child can have a model for turn taking; this is especially so with children diagnosed on the autism spectrum.

Apraxia

Effortful, groping, or unsuccessful speech attempts are presenting characteristics of apraxia. The word _apraxia_ comes from the Greek _praxis_, which refers to _action_. Apraxia is a disruption in the action of speech at the level of the brain. It is a movement disorder that is not caused by weakness, paralysis, sensory loss, or poor comprehension. The brain is unable to send properly programmed and sequenced commands to the speech mechanism. Speech becomes worse with increasingly complex phonetic combi-

nations and with repetitions (in this case, practice does not make perfect).

The key differences between apraxia and dysarthria rest on the effortful articulatory attempts for the former and the sluggish, imprecise productions of the latter. Videos are available online (e.g., YouTube) to help advance one's clinical skills in identifying key features of these disorders. It is highly recommended that a clinician use these for professional development.

Strand (1995) reports the following principles as most often suggested in the treatment of developmental apraxia:

1. Use of intensive, paired auditory and visual stimuli (e.g., songbooks such as _Sunshine on My Shoulders_ [Denver & Canyon, 2003]) are very supportive.
2. Production of sound combinations versus training phonemes in isolation.
3. Focus on movement performance drill (repetitions are easily programmed in music activities).
4. Use of repetitive productions in systematic drills (call-and-response is a good way to engage a child in lots of trials).
5. Well-planned hierarchies of stimuli (identified by the SLP).
6. Use of decreased rate with proprioceptive monitoring (metronomes are helpful to begin productions slowly and increase speed).
7. Use of carrier phrases (e.g., "I see a_____," "I want a_____," "I have a_____"); carrier phrases fit nicely into repetitive music such as the blues.
8. Use of paired movement sequences with suprasegmental facilitators such as stress, intonation, and rhythm (these elements are shared in speech and music and can be varied endlessly; for example, "I want TWO cookies" vs. "I want two COOKIES").
9. Establishment of core vocabulary that is meaningful and functional for the child (excellent opportunities for songwriting).

Melodic intonation therapy (MIT), first developed for adults with aphasia, is a promising protocol for children who are verbally apraxic. I use the word *promising* because the application of this protocol to children is not yet documented, but it still meets many of the guidelines set out by Strand (1995), noted above. In a systematic review of studies of young children with apraxia by Roper (2003), the efficacy of MIT was defined as "meager at best" (p. 4). This is due to a small number of studies, subjects, and individual modifications to the protocols, confounding a review of the method. A music therapist considering using MIT with apraxia should review this article to better understand these confounding variables.

It stands to reason that the application of MIT has a good theoretical basis for a treatment modality and should be explored for the efficacious application to individual clients. The following are key elements to consider:

1. The employment of rhythm provides anticipatory cues for articulatory productions. Rhythm serves as an effective external organizer to control the rate of movement, particularly when internally generated impulses are inadequate. The example of the word *music* at a slower rhythm (*muuuusic*) gives the brain and articulators an extra partial second to maximize precision of the second syllable.

2. The protocol can help train the auditory–motor system by providing models for clients to listen to and watch, thereby allowing for internal rehearsals without the effort of articulation or auditory processing of their effort. They can focus on perception without the burden of production.

3. It provides face-to-face contact, which engages the *mirror neuron system* (i.e., the system that helps us learn to do something by watching another perform it).

4. It uses high-frequency, contextually relevant phrases that facilitate successful communication in everyday situations. For example, a learning phrase might be "My name is _____" or "I'm hungry now." This approach contrasts with the bottom-up work of traditional articulation therapy at the sound and word level.

5. The production of syllables typically happens more slowly in music than in speech, which gives a poorly organized motor system more time to maximize function.

6. The intonation patterns engage the right hemisphere, which may support articulation that is typically programmed from the left hemisphere.

7. The continuous voicing in music increases the connection between syllables and words.

8. MIT use two pitches, with the higher of the two pitches emphasizing the stressed syllable of words. A child might benefit from elongating the duration of the difficult syllable or speech sound to provide more time for the motor system to organize itself. In the example given above, the word *ambulance* may be challenging because it is composed of three syllables. The first syllable could be elongated as *ammm* in addition to stressing *BU*, with the higher of the two pitches or with a slight increase in loudness.

9. The left hand is used to tap the rhythm of the phrase. Thaut (2005) describes the employment of rhythm as a way to drive the optimization of motor control.

10. There are hierarchical levels that increase the length of the unit and diminish dependency on the clinician's prompts and models. The clinician drops out and the client continues independently.

Zipse, Norton, Marchina, and Schlaug (2012) published the case study of an adolescent who had experienced an extensive left-hemispheric stroke. This child received 80 intensive (5 days/week) sessions of MIT training. Neuroimaging showed increased volume of the arcuate fasciculus (AF) in the right hemisphere following treatment. Located between the temporal and frontal lobes, the AF is an important structure that has a primary responsibility in auditory–motor mapping. It connects the language area in the temporal lobe to the speech area in the frontal lobe. Other evidence for neural changes in the AF can be found in research with singers. Halwani, Loui, Ruber, and Schlaug (2011) report that highly trained singers (professionals and those in conservatory programs) have increased volume of the AF compared to instrumentalists and to nonsingers. In adults, damage to the AF results in reduced verbal output (Johnson & Holcomb Jacobson, 1998). The number of fibers and volume of the AF significantly increased after intensive MIT training in adults who have Broca's (nonfluent) aphasia following a stroke (Schlaug, Marchinga, & Norton, 2009).

The correlation of damage to the AF in developmental apraxia is not known, so the following is a treatment hypothesis based on the neuroscientific studies cited above and my clinical success with MIT. If MIT and singing have independently been shown to be productive in increasing the size of the AF, and the AF may be damaged in people with developmental apraxia, then a clinician may want to include both MIT and the NMT protocol of therapeutic singing (TS; Thaut, 2005) in treatment. This protocol works with the child's strength—his or her ability to sing and the natural desire to participate in musical activities. The ease of singing is important when speaking is challenging and frustrating. Both protocols (MIT and TS) have the potential to improve auditory–motor coupling that could generalize to speech. Given the restrictions of clinical visits posed by insurance companies and family budgets, it would be important to include both treatment activities, rather than just one or the other, to improve successful outcomes in potentially less clinical time. TS can easily be employed in the home for more practice. Recordings of treatment songs for the child to sing, with and without the therapist's voice, can be made, ideally with family members singing along as well. An article by Norton, Zipse, Marchina, and Schlaug (2009) can be very helpful in learning further about the rationale and procedures for MIT.

Stuttering

Presenting characteristics for stuttering are repetitions (*w-w-w-what are you doing?*), prolongations (*sssssso what?*), blocks (no speech sounds), or circumlocutions (substituting a word for one that cannot be articulated).

Stuttering affects the fluency of speech by disrupting the flow of speech and creating communication breakdowns. There is also a strong psychological component to the experience of being a stutterer. The development of the child's self-esteem can be negatively impacted, particularly if he or she is socially ostracized or teased for the disorder.

When a child is young, generally less than 7 years of age, the speech therapist will work with the family to support the child, encouraging family members to yield to the child's efforts to communicate. A fast-paced family system can sometimes exacerbate developmental stuttering. The family is encouraged to slow the pace of communications down to give the child a chance to contribute. After the age of 7, stuttering treatment with the child can focus on fluent stuttering, relaxation techniques, and increasing overall fluency. Fluent stuttering is a term that relates to easing into a word that the speaker knows will be stuttered. This is a different approach than trying to eliminate stuttering all together. The therapist is instructing the child to work with versus against the stutter.

Easy onset of voicing is an important approach to achieving fluent stuttering. Voice onset can be abrupt and harsh in stutterers.

Good airflow is key to producing an easy onset. Children need to learn to inhale deeply and exhale slowly while keeping a relaxed, open-mouth posture. After several repetitions of easy breaths, they add an open /a/, as in _father_, while maintaining the relaxed oral posture. The phonation should begin softly to encourage a gentle onset of the vocal cords. When children are competent at that level, they begin to phonate at louder levels and graduate to syllables, words, phrases, and conversational speech. These early steps can all be contextualized in singing warm-up exercises similar to traditional choir exercises (once again employing TS). Young children will benefit from using drawings to follow changes in loudness and pitch. I have drawings that look like crescendo and decrescendo symbols, as well as wavy lines that represent pitch and/or loudness. Children like to use their fingers or toy cars to follow the lines. They enjoy making their own lines on paper or using a toy with a screen that erases marks with a sliding lever. Through music exercises, they can learn to gain more control over their motor system.

Reducing anxiety and inducing relaxation may be very helpful with children who stutter. The therapist can lead the child in a music and progressive relaxation experience, guiding him or her with images of progressively more stressful speaking situations (these situations would have been identified prior to this exercise). It is important that the imagery prompt the child to monitor the level of relaxation while imagining him- or herself remaining fluent. Note that stuttering is primarily a motor speech disorder and not a psychological one. Use relaxation as adjunctive to the primary treatment.

As noted above, TS (Thaut, 2005) may be useful in enhancing both the anatomy and physiology of the brain for fluent speech productions. It also emphasizes children's strengths in being able to sing when speaking is difficult and less successful.

Language

Language is the use of symbols (speech sounds, letters, signs, icons) in a rule-governed system to convey and receive meaning. The domain of language includes both expressive and receptive forms and includes both verbal and written communication. The components of language (i.e., vocabulary and grammar) allow us the magnificent human skill of generating novel and unique utterances each time we talk. This is known as _propositional speech_.

Receptive vocabulary makes possible the comprehension of another's communication. The listener decodes the words that another says to understand what he or she means. Receptive language skills include following directions and understanding figurative and literal statements. Comprehension can be difficult to assess if a child is not able to express what he or she understands. When working with a child who appears to have receptive language problems, it is of the utmost importance to refer him or her for a hearing evaluation prior to initiating treatment. It is also important to consider the possibility of intellectual deficits; referrals to a neuropsychologist would be necessary in this latter condition.

Speech–language pathologists describe five different domains or skill sets in language: syntax, semantics, morphology, phonology, and semantics. These domains are described below.

Syntax refers to the rule-governed system that we typically think of as grammar. It is the classification of nouns, pronouns, verbs, adjectives, adverbs, etc., and the rules that dictate their usage and placement in relation to each other. For example, English syntax dictates that we say _three white mice_ instead of _white three mice_. During typical language acquisition, the rules for the sequencing of adjectives are learned along with many other aspects of grammar. Generally, disorders of syntax are indicated by a lack of complexity in utterances. Children with autism often present with syntactic errors. They typically do not use pronouns or adjectives and adverbs. Children with intellectual deficits have appropriate but not elaborate syntax.

Semantics refers to the meaning of words. It is the ability to learn that a four-legged animal in a pasture is not a dog (the four-legged creature with which he or she is familiar), but, in this case, a goat. It is learning that the word *dogs* means more than one. The language development of people with autism is characterized by the slow acquisition and restricted use of word classes (Schopler & Mesibov, 2010). For example, the word *dog* may mean only the child's dog or the dog with which he or she is familiar at home. The child does not generalize the word *dog* to all dogs. A disorder of semantics can involve a lack of generalization, as noted in the last example and in vocabulary restrictions. For example, synonyms for *sad* can include *glum, melancholy, depressed, down, blue, despondent, forlorn, heartbroken*, and so forth. Extensive language allows us to communicate the nuances of our thoughts, desires, opinions, and feelings. A person with a semantics disorder might have access only to the word sad.

Morphology refers to the smallest unit of language that expresses meaning. These grammatical units are called morphemes. Morphemes include the plural -*s*, the prefix *a*- (which means *not*, as in <u>a</u>*typical*), and the suffix -*ed* on a verb to denote past tense (e.g., *play<u>ed</u>*). Speech therapists record language samples of a child telling a story and then count the morphemes. For example, the sentence, *The boys are fishing*, would receive 6 points for each of the four words plus the plural -*s* and present progressive -*ing*.

Phonology is the sound system of language. Each language has its own particular sound system. For example, English contains the phonemes *l* and *r*, as in *lice* and *rice*, whereas Asian languages do not use these *phonemes*, and thus speakers of these languages have a difficult time distinguishing them when they learn English. Speech–language therapists use the International Phonetic Alphabet (IPA) to describe speech sounds. This system is different from the orthographic representation (letters of the alphabet) we use in writing. For example, the word *ought* is recorded phonetically as /ɔt/. It is made up of two sounds, although it is written with five letters. The letter *w* is recorded as /dʌbəlju/, which describes the sequence of phonemes (sounds) that represent that written letter. Phonetic transcriptions allow a therapist to record what the child said versus what he or she intended. The example given above for *ambulance* would be transcribed as /æmblæns/. This represents the two syllable production and not the intended three syllable reference. The IPA is a key skill for music therapists to develop because they are then able to record what the child said—for example, /pe/, instead of what was intended, /ple/, in voicing the word *play*. This is especially helpful in recording nonverbal vocalizations.

Pragmatics is the social use of language; it includes many elements beyond language per se, such as social appropriateness, body language, eye contact, initiation, turn taking, and termination of topics in a conversation. Examples of *social inappropriateness* would be speaking to an elder or teacher in the casual way one would talk to a peer. *Body language* refers to the proximity of one to another and the use of gestures and facial expression. People on the autism spectrum are generally considered to have pragmatic disorders due to their lack of eye contact and inability to engage in conversational turn taking.

Songwriting is a very powerful intervention for children with language disorders because it provides them with a very motivating activity to use language meaningfully. It is a versatile intervention that allows children to use language that is both literal and figurative and to build new vocabulary. The best of all circumstances is to broaden songwriting into a theatrical setting that includes sets, costumes, makeup, and interacting with others. Working in a theatrical setting allows for more than one child to be engaged, interacting with others, using language, and experiencing the social norms of language use. While sacrifices of grammar and word choices are conventions used in songwriting, they should not be exercised in songwriting activities with children who have language disorders. Proper grammar and appropriate word choices should be the objective. Redundancy in lyrics can reinforce comprehension of a targeted aspect of language, whether it is morphological or semantic.

Songs in general can contribute to language learning in several ways. Schon et al. (2007) state that the emotional aspects of songs may arouse attention and interest. The melody may enhance phonological discrimination, as pitch changes often correlate with syllable structure. The changes in the auditory signals for music are slower than those for speech, which may give a poorly developed language comprehension system more time to correctly perceive and decode the signal. Lastly, Schon et al. note that the consistent mapping of musical and linguistic structure may optimize learning mechanisms. The songs of *Schoolhouse Rock!* (Yohe & Newall, 1996) are an ideal model in the application of these elements. They are catchy, well-written tunes that reinforce academic concepts through repetition.

Applications to Other Disciplines

The use of music in the treatment of all childhood disorders is a significant plus for any therapist. It allows one to quickly build a strong working relationship, which is important in overcoming resistance, anxiety, and dread. While I have made many recommendations for music therapists to reach out to colleagues in speech therapy, I strongly believe that we are entering into an era where other therapists will be seek-

ing out the expertise of music therapists more frequently. Books and films about the power of music are very popular in our culture and in the media. Physicians and therapists who work with children are naturally going to want to enhance their practices with these resources. The research revealing the power of music in rehabilitation can now be consulted for habilitative work with children.

I recommend that colleagues such as physicians, speech–language pathologists, occupational therapists, child life specialists, and neuropsychologists establish a collaborative network with music therapists in their area for consultation and co-treatment opportunities. A consultancy arrangement would provide colleagues with general or specific musical approaches and resources for their clients' specific needs. Co-treatment sessions would provide client-specific interactions as well as an opportunity for a colleague to observe and learn about the use of music as a clinical intervention. Please refer to the Web Resources listed below to find a music therapist in your area. Note that there are specializations among music therapists (e.g., Neurologic Music Therapy, Nordoff–Robbins), and one should be clear about the expertise that is sought.

Conclusions

Speech and language development is a tour de force in the life of a child. It typically unfolds with little effort on the part of the child. When that natural trajectory is disrupted, however, the child and family members have to make a substantial effort to help the child develop age-appropriate skills. The music therapist is uniquely trained to facilitate this process with creative, meaningful, engaging activities that allow for repetition, variation, and growth. Ideally this treatment process is conducted with the speech therapist and the music therapist working in close collaboration, as treatment goals can be complex and change fairly frequently as the child makes progress.

Although a diagnosis should guide the work, it should not cloud our assessment and treatment skills or tools. For instance, if a child presents with the initiation difficulties associated with apraxia, the easy-onset exercises described under stuttering might be useful. Call-and-response singing is listed under articulation and phonological disorders, but it is quite useful with a variety of conditions. The music therapist should build a toolbox that is versatile and has defined applications for varied skills in speech and language. The following recommendations for music therapists who treat speech and language disorders are meant to facilitate their professional development in this area.

- Know typical speech and language development. I believe it is important for music therapists to have experiences working or playing with neurotypical children at some point in their career as a way to build skills in working with children who have disorders.
- Develop good working relationships with SLPs in your area who treat pediatric disorders. Create a process for referrals and nurture positive working relationships. Attend SLP conferences to learn alongside your colleagues.
- Study the language of speech–language pathology. Become competent in the terms that are specific to SLPs (e.g., *semantics, phonology*). See resources below.
- Read case studies and research publications in music therapy and speech therapy to identify best practices in the field.
- Take a class in human growth and development and/or speech–language development specifically.
- Co-present with speech therapists at both speech therapy and music therapy conferences.
- Publish case studies, noting theoretical foundations for employed protocols.

- Consider the opportunity to investigate clinical protocols with formal research methods.
- Publish songs and activities that have proven effective in your work.
- Learn the IPA to take accurate phonetic transcriptions of children's utterances. For example, *gonna go* would not be transcribed as *going to go*. You would use phonetic symbols to transcribe /gʌnə go/.
- In clinical work, focus on meaningful, contextually valid speech productions so clients can be empowered to express their wants, needs, opinions, and feelings in their home and school environments.
- Use technology to provide home-based activities. Recordings of songs are a key and important tool for carryover.

REFERENCES

Brandt, A., Gebrian, M., & Slevc, L. R. (2012). Music and early language acquisition. *Frontiers in Psychology, 3,* 327.

DeCasper, A. J., & Spence, M. J. (1986). Prenatal maternal speech influences newborns' perception of speech sounds. *Infant Behavior and Development, 9,* 133–150.

Dehaene-Lambertz, G., & Dehaene, S. (1994). Speed and cerebral correlates of syllable discrimination in infants. *Nature, 370,* 292–295.

Denver, J., & Canyon, C. (2003). *Sunshine on my shoulders.* Nevada City, CA: Dawn.

Dromey, C., Ramig, L., & Johnson, A. B. (1995). Phonatory and articulatory changes associated with increased vocal intensity in Parkinson disease: A case study. *Journal of Speech and Hearing Research, 38,* 751–764.

Gerber, S., Brice, A., Capone, N., Fujiki, M., & Timler, G. (2012). Language use in social interactions of school-age children with language impairments: An evidence-based systematic review of treatment. *Language, Speech and Hearing Services in Schools, 43*(2), 235–249.

Halwani, G. F., Loui, P., Ruber, T., & Schlaug, G. (2011). Effects of practice and experience on the arcuate fasciculus: Comparing singers, instrumentalists, and non-musicians. *Frontiers in Psychology, 2,* 156.

Hannon, E. E., & Trehub, S. E. (2005). Tuning in to musical rhythms: Infants learn more readily than adults. *Proceedings of the National Academy of Sciences, 102,* 12639–12643.

James, D. K., Spencer, C. J., & Stepsis, B. W. (2002). Fetal learning: A prospective randomized controlled study. *Ultrasound in Obstetrics and Gynecology, 20*(5), 431–438.

Johnson, A. F., & Holcomb Jacobson, B. (1998). *Medical speech–language pathology.* London: Thieme.

McCauley, R. J., Strand, E., Lof, G. L., Schooling, T., & Frymark, T. (2009). Evidence-based systematic review: Effects of nonspeech motor exercises on speech. *American Journal of Speech–Language Pathology, 18,* 343–360.

Morgan, A. T., & Vogel, A. P. (2008a). Intervention for childhood apraxia of speech. *Cochrane Database of Systematic Reviews, 2008*(3), CD006278.

Morgan, A. T., & Vogel, A. P. (2008b). Intervention for dysarthria associated with acquired brain injury in children and adolescents. *Cochrane Database of Systematic Reviews, 2008*(3), CD006279.

Norton, A., Zipse, L., Marchina, S., & Schlaug, G. (2009). Melodic intonation therapy: Shared insights on how it is done and why it might help. *Annals of the New York Academy of Science, 169,* 431–436.

Ramig, L. O., Countryman, S., Thompson, L. L., & Horii, Y. (1995). Comparison of two forms of intensive speech treatment for Parkinson disease. *Journal of Speech and Hearing Research, 38*(6), 1232–1251.

Roper, N. (2003). Melodic intonation therapy with young children with apraxia. *Bridges: Practice-Based Research Synthesis, 1*(3), 1–7.

Schlaug, G., Marchinga, S., & Norton, A. (2009). Evidence for plasticity in white-matter tracts of patients with chronic Broca's aphasia undergoing intense intonation-based speech therapy. *Annals of the New York Academy of Sciences, 1169,* 385–394.

Schon, D., Boyer, M., Moreno, S., Besson, M., Peretz, I., & Kolinsky, R. (2007). Songs as an aid for language acquisition. *Cognition, 106,* 975–983.

Schopler, E., & Mesibov, G. B. (2010). *Communication problems in autism.* New York: Plenum Press.

Soley, G., & Hannon, E. E. (2010). Infants prefer the musical meter of their own culture: A cross-cultural comparison. *Developmental Psychology, 46,* 286–292.

Strand, E. (1995). Treatment of motor speech disorders in children. *Seminars in Speech and Language, 16*(2), 126–139.

Thaut, M. (2005). *Rhythm, music and the brain.* New York: Routledge.

Wan, C., Ruber, T., Hohmann, A., & Schlaug, G. (2010). The therapeutic effects of singing in neurological disorders. *Music Perception, 27*(4), 287–295.

Ward, E. C., Theodoros, D. G., Murdoch, B. E., & Silburn, P. (2000). Changes in maximum capacity tongue function following the Lee Silverman voice treatment program. *Journal of Medical Speech Language Pathology, 8*(4), 331–335.

Yohe, T., & Newall, G. (1996). *Schoolhouse Rock!: The official guide.* New York: Hyperion Books.

Zipse, L., Norton, A., Marchina, S., & Schlaug, G. (2012). When right is all that is left: Plasticity of right-hemisphere tracts in a young aphasic patient. *Annals of the New York Academy of Sciences, 1252,* 237–245.

WEB RESOURCES

American Speech–Language–Hearing Association: *www.asha.org.*

Apraxia information: *www.apraxia-kids.org.*

Center for Biomedical Research in Music: *http://colostate.edu/depts/cbrm.*

International Phonetic Alphabet: *www.langsci.ucl.ac.uk/ipa.*

Kinesthetic cuing for articulation: *www.promptinstitute.com.*

Music and Neuroimaging Laboratory at Beth Israel Hospital: *www.musicianbrain.com.*

National Institute on Deafness and Other Communication Disorders: *www.nidcd.nih.gov/Pages/default.aspx.*

Whistles: *www.therapro.com.*

CHAPTER 25

Music Therapy for Children with Sensory Deficits

Greta E. Gillmeister
Paige A. Robbins Elwafi

When a child has impaired or absent functioning in one or more of the senses, it is considered a sensory deficit. This chapter addresses children who have sensory deficits in the form of hearing or visual impairments as well as those who may experience a dual diagnosis of both impairments. The music therapist working with children with hearing or visual impairments has a responsibility to learn about the impairment of each child and how it affects his or her life. Music therapy treatment should be designed around those needs.

Hearing and vision play a fundamental role in our development. From birth, children use their senses to observe and learn from the environment around them. The child with a hearing or visual impairment lives in a world where hearing is different from listening, and looking is different from seeing. It isn't a quiet, dark, or lonely world, but one where much can be learned and synthesized through other senses. The music therapist should strive to respect this different way of learning and be willing to enter that world without judgment or fear.

We are continually surprised by the diversity of needs and abilities among children with sensory deficits. The facilities in which we work employ several staff with sensory deficits. This professional experience has shaped our attitudes toward the children with whom we work in music therapy. Daily, we see and hear about the joys, challenges, and uniqueness of sensory impairments. Our respect for the disabilities and for those affected by them has grown due to the relationships we have developed with coworkers. It has also helped us to see the essential reasons for addressing the needs of the whole child.

Children Who Are Deaf or Hard-of-Hearing

Over the years, I (Greta E. Gillmeister) have experienced a number of moments during my music therapy practice of working with children who are deaf or hard-of-hearing that were significant in the child's development of hearing. One of those first moments occurred during my initial year working with pre-schoolers who were deaf or hard-of-hearing. I was working with a 4-year-old girl who was deaf but also had a severe intellectual deficit. In the classroom, it was difficult to gain and focus her attention. Her affect was generally flat, and her participation was minimal unless the teacher or classroom assistant prompted her. However, within a music therapy session, the student was easily engaged in tasks, and her face lit up with smiles. The student was typically seen in a group setting, but on this particular day, she was the only one present in her class, so I worked with her individually. She had recently undergone surgery for her cochlear implant and during the first map-ping session, which is also known as the acti-vation session, the audiologist had difficulty setting the levels of sound comfort. The stu-dent had not shown any indication that she was "hearing" anything. When she came to music therapy, she participated as usual, but when we played the large floor drum and she struck it hard with a mallet, she put her hand over her ear and began to cry. At the time, I was not aware of the outcome of the initial mapping session, and I felt terrible for "making a student cry." The teacher, though, was excited. She immediately comforted the student by telling her it was OK, signed/said "How exciting! You heard the drum!", and immediately took her to audiology. This was the first time the student had indicated that she was hearing anything and that the levels were set too high.

That day impacted me in several ways. Not only did I get to witness the first time a stu-dent showed awareness of hearing, but I also got to be a part of a team that was working together to meet the needs of the child. The teacher returned later and thanked me for bringing a unique and valuable service to the school.

As a music therapist working with chil-dren who are deaf or hard-of-hearing (D/HH), it is beneficial to have a basic under-standing of the impairment, its causes, the culture of individuals with hearing loss, current technology, treating the child as a whole, and how to deliver a therapeutic ses-sion in a meaningful manner. Children do not need to have normal hearing to enjoy music and singing. All children are born with some music aptitude (Barton, 2006). The role of the music therapist is to nurture that enjoyment and reinforce the benefits of music engagement with children who are D/HH. When children are learning, it is important for them to listen, look, and feel—not just to hear, see, and touch (Es-tabrooks & Birkenshaw-Fleming, 2006). Music is a multidimensional tool for engag-ing all the senses and enhancing children's learning and communication skills.

Clientele

Hearing loss, or *deafness,* is a partial or total inability to hear and can be present at birth (congenital) or become evident later in life (acquired). The distinction between congenital and acquired deafness specifies only the time that the deafness appears. It does not specify whether the cause of the deafness is genetic (inherited). Acquired deafness may or may not be genetic in origin. For example, it may be a delayed-onset form of genetic deafness, or it may be caused by damage to the ear from noise, ill-ness, or diseases. Similarly, congenital deaf-ness may be caused by a genetic disease or may be due to prematurity, postnatal infec-tions, or ototoxic drugs, which are nonge-netic. Additional causes include infections to which the mother was exposed during pregnancy (American Speech–Language–Hearing Association, 2014).

Hearing impairment is not a unitary dis-order; hearing loss varies in type and sever-ity from one person to another (Barton, 2010; Estabrooks & Birkenshaw-Fleming, 2006). There are four different types of hearing loss: conductive, sensorineural, mixed, and central. The Centers for Dis-ease Control and Prevention (2011) de-scribes each type. *Conductive* hearing losses are caused by disease or obstructions in the outer or middle ear, usually affect all fre-quencies of hearing, and do not result in severe losses. *Sensorineural* hearing losses result from damage to the delicate sensory hair cells of the inner ear or a problem with the auditory nerve. These hearing losses can range from mild to profound deafness. They often affect certain frequencies more than others. *Mixed* hearing losses are those in which there is a problem in the outer or middle ear and the inner ear. *Central* hearing losses result from damage or impairment to the nerves or nuclei of the central nervous system, either in the pathway to the brain or in the brain itself.

After a child is diagnosed with a hearing loss, one of the first issues is whether or not the child will use *assistive hearing devices* and, secondly, whether the child will be raised using manual communication or as an *oral child* (Darrow & Grohe, 2002). For those who choose to use assistive hearing devices, there are various types and in turn varying levels of perception of hearing. The type and degree of loss will help to determine which type of assistive hearing device will be most effective for an individual. One type of device is the *hearing aid*. A conventional hearing aid is worn externally and is used to amplify and modulate sound for the wearer. A bone-anchored hearing aid is based on conduction of sound to the inner ear through the bones of the skull and places a conductor close to the auditory bones to amplify the sound. Individuals with conductive hearing losses or unilateral hearing losses, and those with mixed hearing losses who cannot otherwise wear *in the ear* or *behind the ear* hearing aids, will benefit from this type of assistive device. Finally, a *cochlear implant* (CI) may be used. CIs, which are surgically placed, are designed for persons with severe to profound losses (typically bilateral), who receive marginal to no benefit from conventional hearing aids. A CI uses a hearing processor to send digital approximations of sound directly to the auditory nerve and is used for an individual whose inner ear is damaged or not intact.

Persons who are deaf or hard-of-hearing use a variety of methods and systems for communication. The communication types are a result of different philosophies, methodologies, and cultural beliefs within the population of individuals who are deaf or hard-of-hearing. The types of communication methods include (1) American Sign Language, (2) fingerspelling, (3) manual communication, (4) oral communication, (5) cued speech, (6) simultaneous communication, and (7) total communication (Gfeller & Darrow, 2008). *American Sign Language* (ASL) is a natural language with its own grammar and syntax and is widely used in the United States. In a *fingerspelling* conversation, one person manually spells out each word, letter by letter, to another using the hand shapes that form the manual alphabet. A combination of sign language and fingerspelling for both expressive and receptive communication is considered *manual communication. There are four major systems of manual communication: Seeing Essential English (SEE), Signing Exact English (SEE II), Linguistics of Visual English (LOVE), and Signed English. Oral communication* denotes the use of speech and speech reading as the primary means for the transmission of thoughts and ideas with D/HH persons. Educators who believe in oral communication emphasize the teaching of speech and speech reading together with amplification. *Simultaneous communication* denotes the combined use of speech, signs, and fingerspelling simultaneously. *Total communication* is a philosophy of communication that implies acceptance, understanding, and use of all methods of communication to assist a child who is D/HH in acquiring language.

Upon discovering that their child has a hearing impairment, many (hearing) parents are disappointed by the thought that their child will never enjoy music. It is often a misconception that individuals with hearing losses cannot or do not enjoy music; children with hearing loss are fully capable of learning, enjoying, and playing music (Barton, 2006; Chen et al., 2010). Children's responses and preferences will depend upon the severity and type of their hearing loss as well as the type of their assistive hearing device (if they have one) (Gfeller & Darrow, 2008). Hearing aids amplify sound and provide a much more natural signal with regard to music than cochlear implants. However, the electrical circuitry of a hearing aid may be set to emphasize certain frequencies important for speech, which consequentially may not make music sounds as pleasant or natural. CIs often transmit only portions of the total sound wave, which can alter the perception of the music. Chen et al. (2010) found that the duration of musical training correlated with music perception in prelingually deafened children with cochlear implants. Children with implants who had a longer duration of musical training received higher scores for the performance of pitch perception, suggesting that, in addition to the severity, type of hearing loss, and assistive hearing device, the amount of exposure to music can affect music preferences and success. It has been my experience (Greta E. Gillmeister), as a music therapist working with D/HH children, that each child is very complex, as are his or her responses to and preferences for music. Learning about the child plays a key role in developing effective treatment plans and applications for therapeutic sessions.

Clinical Work

Music therapists working in school programs for students who are deaf or hard-of-hearing must be flexible and sensitive to the overall goals and objectives of the program (Darrow & Grohe, 2002). The therapeutic goals and objectives will depend greatly upon the school's philosophy of deaf education. Music therapists must also recognize and understand their students' position regarding Deaf culture so that they can design an approach that meets the needs of the program and the students. Recognition begins with understanding the difference between *Deaf* and *deaf*. Deaf, with an uppercase *D*, refers to a culture. Individuals who identify themselves as Deaf are part of

a community that is held together with the common language of ASL. They share their own history, social beliefs, traditions, and values. Deaf, with a lowercase *d*, refers to medical deafness. It is defined by the pathology of hearing loss rather than a culture of individuals.

Within the educational setting, I create goals and objectives by combining information gained from a child's individualized education plan (IEP), observation, and consultation with the classroom teachers and other related professionals who work with the child. The use of active and receptive music engagement provides opportunities to see a child's responses to music and preferences. Often, the emphasis of music therapy interventions with children who are D/HH is on the linguistic objectives; however, other therapeutic goals are supported by participation in music applications. These goals include behavioral, academic, and motor skills, as well as social interaction and self-concept, but can also be designed to indirectly address listening, hearing, and communication skills.

Music therapy goals for children with impaired hearing often center around linguistic and communication needs, including language, auditory training, and speech. When it comes to auditory development, hearing and listening are not the same (Berkowitz, 2012). *Hearing* is simply the act of perceiving sound. *Listening*, however, requires concentration and the conscious effort to process meaning from the words and sentences being heard. Young children are exposed to much language passively. As an infant, their mothers may sing lullabies to soothe them; they listen to their parents and siblings, the television, a radio playing in the background, or even strangers as they pass by in public. This listening leads to learning. This language input and learning are often neglected in young children who are born D/HH.

Listening skills need to develop from the simplest to the most complex. Auditory skill tasks are based upon a hierarchy of auditory skill development and begin with detection: that is, identifying the absence or presence of sound (Berkowitz, 2012; Darrow & Grohe, 2002). It then proceeds to discrimination, or differentiation among sounds. This leads to identification, the recognition of a sound, and culminates in comprehension, the most complex skill set, which attaches meaning to a sound.

Language input precedes language output (Darrow & Grohe, 2002); music can be used as a tool to benefit children's oral communication and linguistic goals. They learn attentive listening, a skill that fosters their phonological awareness, phonemic awareness, and overall fluency (Hachmeister, 2010). Using songs coupled with a book nurtures auditory and visual discrimination, eye–motor coordination, visual sequential memory, language reception, and, most importantly, promotes comprehension and dialogue (Wiggins, 2007). Berkowitz (2012) discusses the importance of creating opportunities for naturally occurring listening situations and interactions for children who are D/HH. Music engagement facilitates opportunities to practice the give-and-take in communication skills by providing an environment in which children need to focus their auditory attention and take turns with interactions. Participation in music interventions encourages the use of both receptive and expressive communication skills.

Music interventions create a motivating way to engage children while addressing the skill areas of voice inflection, articulation, rate of speech, and fluency. Singing helps with voice inflection, while rhythm activities can assist with reinforcing prosody of speech. It has long been recognized that faulty speech produced with a normal rhythm is far more intelligible than imperfectly articulated speech with an abnormal rhythm (Estabrooks & Birkenshaw-Fleming, 2006). Motor development is beneficial for all young children; for children who are D/HH, movement activities can also be used as to promote communication goals through listening, speech, and language. Movement activities can require careful listening to the musical cues with or without verbal in-

structions (Gfeller, Driscoll, Kenworthy, & Van Vorst, 2011). In addition to linguistic objectives, music therapy interventions can also enhance the overall development of children with impaired hearing.

Children with hearing impairments learn age-appropriate academic skills. Songs that include repetition can help to reinforce academic concepts, and the use of music can assist in directing attention to task. Group music therapy can also provide an outlet for the students to explore instruments and sounds and develop their personal preferences. Creating music provides opportunities to develop self-concept within a nurturing environment. A structured music activity can offer an opportunity to practice even the most basic social needs. Music is often a cooperative group event that facilitates social interactions such as turn taking, communication, and expressing wants and needs within the session.

Within the educational setting, it is important to consider the behavioral needs of the child. Consistent expectations similar to those of their classroom will help with transitioning and predictability within the music therapy session. A number of children in my facility have secondary diagnoses, and in some cases a syndrome causes their hearing impairments and may also affect behavior. Some of these diagnoses include autism, Down syndrome, Smith–Magenis syndrome, and neonatal abstinence syndrome. To build consistency within the therapeutic group setting, it is suggested to address those areas of need specific to each child's diagnosis. Often, the music therapist will need to follow a behavioral plan designed by a specialist. The music therapy environment should help to reinforce age-appropriate behaviors of the child too. These skills include turn taking, following directions, engaging in on-task behavior, sharing, complying, and developing motivation for learning.

It is graduation day for the kindergartners at the deaf oral school, and I watch my class of 5- to 6-year-olds perform the last song of the year for their families. The song is "What a Wonderful World." They are all singing, smiling, and attending to me as I accompany them on the guitar. Some are singing while others are using a combination of singing and Signing Exact English, but they are all together. Earlier in the day, the students paraded outside wearing tissue paper wings with pipe cleaner antennae, and each student released a butterfly as part of a school tradition. The butterfly is a symbol of transformation. From caterpillar to butterfly, it grows, develops, and spreads its wings to head out into the world, much like the journey of these new graduates. Throughout their attendance at the school, the students have not only learned academic and social skills, but also how to listen and communicate. The goal of group music therapy is to develop and reinforce those skills through a musical environment. The final student presentation of their song demonstrates the combination of all those skills. At the end of the graduation, I listened to the president of the parents' association talk about her son's progress over the 3 years he attended the school. Her speech began with the statement, "Thank you for giving my son a voice to sing."

Children with Blindness or Visual Impairment[1]

Brady screamed and cried throughout our first several music therapy sessions. Certain sounds in the environment and specific instruments would turn him into an emotional roller coaster. Brady had very limited use of his hands. He initially refused to touch any instruments presented to him and required physical prompts to play. Brady has cortical visual impairment and cerebral palsy. His visual impairment was fairly severe in that he presented as having little to no vision at all. His parents had been told that Brady was blind and would never be able to see. As the

[1]A variety of language can be used to describe children who are blind or have visual impairments. Professionals use different approaches to the use of language, and the language chosen is based largely upon one's comfort level or professional experiences.

vision professionals at the agency I (Paige Robbins Elwafi) work for got to know Brady, they found that the opposite was true. Brady did have some vision, and his vision might actually improve with proper stimulation. Since Brady was unfortunately not receiving vision services at school, I tried my best to provide time during our individual sessions to work on vision goals, such as using the light box to reach and touch an instrument. I still remember the joy that his mother and I felt the first time we observed him using his vision to look at a chime tree while illuminated on the light box. Brady was happy too! Over time Brady was slowly able to become more comfortable with touching and strumming the strings on the guitar. After 2 years of working on this goal, Brady was able to participate in a community recital where he strummed the guitar while I sang his favorite song. He stole the show!

Clientele

Children who have blindness or visual impairment face many obstacles and challenges that they, along with their caregivers, must work to overcome. The reality is that they are children first, with the same basic needs and hopes of typically developing children. Given the wide range of visual impairments and causes of blindness, the abilities among these children are diverse. The music therapist should focus on the child instead of his or her disability or visual impairment. This approach gives the whole child the greatest opportunity for developing independence.

The Visual System and Visual Impairment

A basic understanding of normal functioning vision is beneficial for the music therapist working with individuals who have visual impairment or blindness. The visual system consists of the eyes, the optic nerves, and the brain (Clark, 2012). Vision begins with the eyes, which take in light and images and send that information to the brain via the retina and optic nerves. Additional protective structures such as the orbit, eyelids, and tears fulfill important functions that help protect the eye from injury (Codding, 1984). Clark explains that vision is processed in different parts of the brain, but the eyes, optic nerves, and brain work together to bring in and process complex sensory input through the visual system.

Individuals who have a visual impairment are rarely totally blind or unable to see anything with either eye (American Foundation for the Blind [AFB], 2008). Many children have some usable vision or *functional vision*. *Vision loss* refers to having trouble seeing, even when wearing contact lenses or glasses (Elwafi, 2013). *Legal blindness* is defined as a "central visual acuity of 20/200 or less in the better eye with the best possible correction, and/or a visual field of 20 degrees or less" (AFB). A person with low vision will likely have an acuity from 20/70 to 20/200 in the better eye with the best possible correction (Clark, 2012).

Visual impairment occurs when problems arise in the eyes, the optic nerves, or the brain. Problems can arise in one, two, or all three parts of the visual system (Clark, 2012). Visual impairment can be categorized as due to (1) acuity loss, (2) field loss, and/or (3) processing difficulties. The effects of visual impairment vary greatly because the problems can occur in different parts of the visual system.

Acuity loss, also called *ocular problems*, affects the sharpness and clarity of images and can usually be corrected by the proper refraction with prescription glasses or contact lenses (Clark, 2012). *Field loss* can occur in any part of the visual field and may include central, partial, or total field loss, as well as loss of light perception. A third category of visual impairment is *visual processing problems*. Roman-Lantzy (2007) explains that cortical visual impairment results in damage to the visual processing centers and pathways in the brain. This type of damage can occur before, during, or after birth and ranges in severity.

Visual impairment is as diverse and dynamic as the visual system. It can range from problems that can be corrected to some extent with glasses to complex neurological issues requiring higher levels of intervention. Different types of visual impairment can occur at the same time as well. Some types of visual impairment can change over time, either improving or worsening.

Three common visual impairments of the optic nerve include optic nerve hypoplasia (ONH), septo-optic dysplasia (SOD), and optic atrophy (Clark, 2012). ONH can occur in one or both eyes and the effects on vision can vary, accompanied by acuity and/or visual field deficits (Simmons & Stout, 1993). Both ONH and SOD result from underdeveloped optic nerves; however, SOD is accompanied by complex medical issues and midline brain abnormalities (Simmons & Stout). Individuals with ONH or SOD are known to display behaviors resembling autism spectrum disorder. Some of these behaviors include sensory sensitivity, echolalia, difficulty relating to others, and language delay.

Cortical (or cerebral) *visual impairment* (CVI) is the primary visual impairment involving the brain. CVI is complex and often accompanied by additional neurological and physical problems, such as sensory sensitivities, cerebral palsy, seizure disorder, and cognitive impairment (Roman-Lantzy, 2007). Some documented causes of CVI include structural abnormalities, cerebral vascular accident, and head injury (Roman-Lantzy).

Individuals with CVI have strong basic color preferences, enjoy light gazing, find visual complexity difficult, and may experience field loss as well as preferred fields (Roman-Lantzy, 2007). Looking and touching an object at the same time, or visually guided reach, is a complex task for a child with CVI. The auditory sense will likely be much easier to access for the child with CVI than his or her vision. This is important to note for the music therapist, because the music therapy setting can be monitored to minimize auditory stimulation for a child with CVI (Elwafi, 2013). Music therapists can use silence and space creatively in the music to give the child with CVI opportunities to work on vision goals, such as visually guided reach and looking at instruments.

We live in a visual world. Approximately 85% of what we learn occurs through the use of our eyes or through *incidental learning* (Robb, 2003). The development of a child who has a visual impairment can be very similar to that of a typically developing child, but Codding (1984) explains that a child's sight or lack of sight has a direct impact on his or her development.

For the child who has blindness or visual impairment, the outside world can be more difficult to access and explore than for a sighted child (Elwafi, 2013). Blindness and visual impairment are widely misunderstood and can be accompanied by many stereotypes. Darrow and Johnson (1994) explain that the parents, family members, and teachers of the child who has a visual impairment are one of his or her most important influences. Codding (1984) stresses the importance of providing the child with opportunities to practice independence and encourage feelings of self-worth. These opportunities can also be given to caregivers to encourage confidence in the child's natural development.

Although visual impairment is a low-incidence disability (LaVenture & Allman, 2007), the variety of needs that results from the impairment is quite diverse. Factors affecting the child's future independence should be considered. Darrow and Johnson (1994) found in a survey of 699 junior and senior high school students that, out of 10 disabilities and medical conditions, blindness was ranked as the least accepted. The high unemployment rate among individuals who have visual impairment or blindness is also important. Education, sensory awareness, social development, and mobility skills are essential to navigating these challenges.

Education

The education of a child who has a visual impairment should be designed to meet the whole child's needs. LaVenture and Allman (2007) explain that this can be a challenge for the child, caregivers, and education team because the child must learn how to obtain information through other senses. This can be accomplished by the child learning to read and write Braille, how to use screen reader software and magnification devices, and how to travel safely. Learning these essential life skills requires input from a variety of professionals that may include a teacher of the visually impaired (TVI), an orientation and mobility instructor, an assistive technology specialist, and an ophthalmologist (LaVenture & Allman).

A *functional vision assessment* is an important tool that can be developed in the educational setting or in a medical setting (LaVenture & Allman, 2007) and is conducted by trained professionals to assess a child's remaining and useable vision and how the child uses that vision. For example, the functional vision assessment can identify if there is a field preference, if magnification is effective, if ideal lighting is beneficial, and some techniques for helping improve the child's functional vision (if possible). The music therapist working with a child who has a visual impairment can obtain information from a functional vision assessment to adapt the music therapy environment (Elwafi, 2013).

Sensory Awareness

Developing a child's auditory and tactile skills is important in preparing him or her for the future, but it should be done in a thoughtful and careful way. It is common to see increased sensory sensitivities, especially to touch and exploring the environment. The music therapist can provide a rich yet nonthreatening tactile environment to motivate the young child who has a visual impairment to explore and learn. This can be done with a variety of instruments, preferred textures, and stimulating music experiences.

The auditory environment can become quite overstimulating, creating too much information to be processed for an individual with blindness or visual impairment. The ability to process auditory information can be dramatically impaired with accompanying multiple disabilities. A simplified auditory environment with minimal background noise can be ideal for a child who has a visual impairment or blindness, especially in the music therapy session. The use of silence and space in the music can also be helpful to aid in auditory processing.

Social Development

Children who have visual impairment or blindness often struggle with social skills. We learn social skills by watching others—that is, through incidental learning. Children who have a visual impairment or blindness miss these visual learning opportunities, so instead they must be taught how to interact and play with others. Gourgey (1998) warns that visual impairment may cause problems in early attachment and later when peers may avoid a child who does not respond to visual cues. Overall, these social challenges affecting individuals who have a visual impairment may cause them to appear developmentally delayed.

Codding (1984) recommends that structured social learning opportunities be provided to children who have visual impairment or blindness to avoid a significant delay in development. Gourgey (1998) suggests using music therapy experiences such as musical storytelling and songs that practice greetings in a group setting to teach social awareness. Sound localization and auditory discrimination can also be addressed in a group setting by directing the children to come forward when they hear the sound of a specific instrument (Gourgey).

Some children who have a visual impairment may display odd behaviors or mannerisms. These behaviors can be self-stimulatory or functional, depending upon the child and the function of the behavior. Visual behaviors such as close viewing, head posturing, and nystagmus can provide neurological input or assist the child in

gaining access to functional vision (Jan & Groenveld, 1995). Light gazing, eye pressing, and finger flicking are some behaviors that can provide neurological input, but can also cause unneeded social attention or be harmful (Jan & Groenveld). Lack of eye contact and rocking are some behaviors that a child who has a visual impairment may engage in that may look similar to, and be mistaken for, characteristics of autism spectrum disorder. Individuals who have blindness and visual impairment may sway, rock excessively, and flap hands when needing movement (Jan & Groenveld).

Differentiating the function of these behaviors is important, especially for the child or adult who has a visual impairment. When making the decision to change these behaviors, Hughes and Fazzi (1993) recommend substituting behaviors with more appropriate sensory stimulation if the individual's ability to learn is being hindered. Codding (2000) documented the use of music to reduce self-stimulatory behaviors in individuals who have a visual impairment. Gourgey (1998) suggests modifying rocking movements with improvised music and song phrase completion to modify echolalia. In addition, understanding and using social nuances, gestures, and nonverbal language can be difficult. These skills must be taught and practiced.

Mobility Skills

One of the most helpful experiences that I have had in my work with individuals who have visual impairment or blindness occurred when I was blindfolded and asked to walk to the end of the hallway on my own. The short trip down the hall, which took much longer without the use of my vision, gave me a sense of the importance of orientation and mobility. Martinez and Moss (1998) define *orientation* as knowing where one's body is in space and the direction that one would like to go. *Mobility* is defined as carrying out the plan to move.

Professionals who specialize in direct instruction, contributing to the IEP team and educating the public, are *orientation and mobility* (O&M) instructors (Elwafi, 2013). O&M instructors focus on developing safe and independent travel abilities in individuals with visual impairment or blindness. Some O&M goals might include cane skills, spatial concepts, sensory awareness, and traveling independently via the use of public transportation (Martinez & Moss, 1998). The music therapist can coordinate treatment with the O&M instructor when addressing O&M concerns with clients. The O&M instructor can be a good source for the music therapist in learning about vision and the effects of visual impairment (Elwafi, 2013).

I was conducting a small-group music therapy session for children who have multiple disabilities and visual impairment. My cotherapist and I asked the parents, who participate in the group as well, to provide some suggestions on what we should offer their children. One parent made the point that when her child hears music, he cannot see what is making the music. She asked if we could provide some music experiences that would give her child the opportunity to learn about musical instruments in a way that was meaningful to him. I was taken aback by her request and realized just how much I take my own eyesight for granted. Following that session, we designed music experiences for each group session in which the children got to "meet the instrument." In those sessions we explored a new instrument by listening to recorded and live performances, as well as allowing the children to touch and experience the instrument with their hands. The children got to learn about a variety of instruments, such as the trombone, the cello, the violin, the flute, and a string bass. The hands-on experiences provided these children with an opportunity to learn in the most meaningful way to them.

Clinical Work

Music therapists who work with children who have visual impairment or blindness will find it most helpful to their clinical practice to learn about vision, the basic types of visual impairments, and most importantly, how those impairments affect the lives of their clients. It is important to determine what role music therapy can play in the child's development and learning.

A comprehensive music therapy assessment should examine the child's cognitive, social, behavioral, visual, mobility, and sensory development. I recommend gathering medical and educational information, as well as musical responses in the assessment (Elwafi, 2013). It is important to keep in mind that the development of most children who have visual impairment or blindness will likely be delayed due to the role of incidental and visual learning.

Following a comprehensive assessment, the music therapist will determine the needs of the child and the specific ways in which music therapy could address those needs. A variety of goals and objectives can be further developed and treatment planned for the child. Some common goals in clinical work with those who have a visual impairment include improving communication, developing tactile skills, and encouraging independence. Codding (1984) also suggests goal domains such as cognition, sensory–perceptual skills, and movement. The music therapist can address musical skills and development through adaptive music instruction and by introducing Braille music (Elwafi, 2013). Music therapy experiences designed to meet the goals and objectives for each child's specific needs should encompass a multisensory approach. Some recommended music therapy experiences include songwriting, structured musical play, and improvisation (Elwafi, 2013); detailed music therapy experiences and accompanying procedures that can address a variety of needs are provided in my previous book chapter (Elwafi) created for children who have blindness and visual impairment.

Young children's development can be supplemented with the involvement of early intervention and vision professionals through community agencies. These vision professionals can provide suggestions for developing the child's vision or working with his or her functional vision. The music therapist will benefit from consulting with vision professionals to learn about appropriate adaptations for their clients. In the following section I discuss common visual and auditory suggestions that can be used in the music therapy setting.

The visual environment, which typically includes lighting and the arrangement of objects in the music therapy room, should be considered and possibly adapted to meet the visual needs of the child who has low vision. Some children who have visual impairment will benefit from a well-lit room and additional task lighting. Others will respond better visually and sensorially in a room with low lighting. Children with CVI tend to do better in rooms with low lighting, whereas children with retinitis pigmentosa may have difficulty seeing in low lighting. It is best to ask the child or caregivers what the child's preference is or to consult the functional vision report. An important consideration for mobility is to ensure that the environment is uncluttered and easy to navigate. When offering visual material such as books, pictures, or sheet music, the therapist should avoid materials that are visually cluttered or that use complex shapes and colors. The therapist should consider whether enlarging printed material or providing large print could benefit the client.

The auditory environment offers an opportunity for the music therapist to learn about the effects of low vision or no vision on auditory processing. Extraneous sound and background music in the music therapy setting could be disorienting or distracting for the individual who has visual impairment or blindness (Elwafi, 2013). The music therapy setting should be monitored for extraneous noise or talking, especially when engaging in lyric discussion.

Another important auditory tool for the music therapist is narration. *Narration*, in this context, occurs when a sighted person who is present with an individual who has visual impairment describes the visual environment, providing details such as who or what is in the room, what action is occurring, or other relevant visual information (Elwafi, 2013). It is especially important to use narration when working with a child with very low vision or no vision, especially before touching the child, giving him or her an instrument, or taking something from the child. Narration is suggested for use with all ages of children who have visual impairment or blindness, even infants. Narration provides a learning opportunity, refines listening skills, and informs the child of his or her surroundings (Elwafi, 2013).

Applications to Other Disciplines

When accommodating a child with a sensory deficit, some special considerations will need attention. For children who are deaf or hard-of-hearing, it is important to maintain an acoustically appropriate learning environment (Berkowitz, 2012). Providing rooms with acoustic treatments such as carpet, drapes, and other soft wall treatments can help minimize reverberation. Closing doors and eliminating fans can limit background and ambient noise. It is recommended that classroom noise levels should not exceed 30–35 decibels (Cochlear Americas, 2004).

Children with hearing loss and their siblings need to share experiences and commonalities with others (Paticoff, 2012). Organizing, facilitating, and maintaining an appropriate and meaningful support group for children with hearing loss and their siblings ensure the success of a complete family support group, providing invaluable rewards to all involved. Likewise, the emotional support of the child who has visual impairment is key to his or her development. As documented by Darrow and Johnson (1994), the impact of isolation can be overwhelming for the child and the family. The chance to meet and make friends with others who have sensory deficits that affect their family is very meaningful. Healthy and balanced support for the family and child contributes to a strong sense of identity and acceptance of the child with a sensory deficit.

The child who has a visual impairment requires support on a variety of levels to be successful in the classroom setting. First, it is essential that the child's visual impairment be documented by an eye doctor and noted on the IEP or its equivalent. A trained professional, typically an O&M instructor or a teacher of the visually impaired, should evaluate the child for vision services to be designed and implemented. State schools for the blind are residential facilities, but can be of help in assessing the child for appropriate services. Parents and guardians must act as advocates for their children, and they too may need support in that role.

In the process of advocacy and coordination with a school, it is important to keep in mind that this endeavor should be a joint effort. Communication between home, school, and other providers is essential to creating well-balanced and coordinated services for the child with a sensory deficit. For children with sensory deficits who are being mainstreamed, preparation should start before they enter the classroom. The classroom teacher may not have had a child with a sensory impairment and may feel unprepared. Communicating questions early and often will help address those concerns. Also, it is important to involve classmates in the preparation. The teacher can talk about differences and special needs of the child with a sensory impairment. Asking a professional who specializes in that sensory deficit to visit or having a "cool" adult with the sensory deficit talk to the class can educate and familiarize the teacher and classmates. Finally, helping the child with the sensory deficit talk about his or her assistive technology can help address peer questions and curiosity.

Conclusions

When a child is identified with a sensory deficit, his or her life changes. Suddenly he or she is bombarded with appointments with specialists, therapists, and doctors. I (Greta E. Gillmeister) have listened to mothers talk about their past experiences of feeling guilty for having to decline a playdate because it was the same time as her child's speech therapy, or occupational therapy, or physical therapy, or audiology appointment, or any other number of specialist visits. The time it takes to address the needs of a child with a sensory deficit can reduce the time that child has for other developmental opportunities. The sensory deficit itself may also contribute to some delays. Often during the journey, the focus may seem to be directed toward the deficit and not the child. In music therapy children can engage in meaningful opportunities that incorporate their needs and practice their skills, but that are delivered in a motivating and enjoyable setting where they are free to be creative. Their progress can be measured through goals and objectives; however, seeing their smiles, watching them "steal the show," or receiving the thanks of a parent for "giving my child a voice to sing" is immeasurable.

REFERENCES

American Foundation for the Blind. (2008). *Key definitions of statistical terms*. Retrieved from *www.afb.org/section.aspx?SectionID=15&DocumentID=1280*.

American Speech–Language–Hearing Association. (2014). *Causes of hearing loss*. Retrieved from *www.asha.org/public/hearing/Causes-of-Hearing-Loss*.

Barton, C. A. (2006). Bringing music to their bionic ears: Nurturing music development in children with cochlear implants. *Loud and Clear, 1*. Valencia, CA: Advanced Bionics.

Barton, C. A. (2010). *Music, spoken language, and children with hearing loss: Definitions and development*. Retrieved from *www.speechpathology.com*.

Berkowitz, L. (2012). Auditory learning in preschoolers: Tips for professionals. *Volta Voices, 19*(3), 36–39.

Centers for Disease Control and Prevention. (2011). *Types of hearing loss.* Retrieved from *www.cdc.gov/ncbddd/hearingloss/types.html.*

Chen, J. K., Chuang, A. Y., McMahon, C., Hsieh, J. C., Tung, T. H., & Li, L. P. (2010). Music training improves pitch perception in prelingually deafened children with cochlear implants. *Pediatrics, 125*(4), e793–e800.

Clark, K. (2012, June). *"Fingering" it out!: Emergent literacy for infants and toddlers, including those who are blind or visually impaired.* Cincinnati, OH: Bureau of Early Intervention Services Training.

Cochlear Americas. (2004). *Cochlear implant resource guide: Meeting children's needs at school.* Englewood, CO: Cochlear Americas.

Codding, P. (1984). Music therapy for visually impaired children. In W. B. Lathom & C. T. Eagle (Eds.), *Music therapy for handicapped children: Vol. I. For the hearing impaired, visually impaired, deaf–blind* (pp. 43–96). Washington, DC: National Association for Music Therapy.

Codding, P. (2000). Music therapy literature and clinical applications for blind and severely visually impaired persons: 1940–2000. In C. Furman (Ed.), *Effectiveness of music therapy procedures: Documentation of research and clinical practice* (pp. 159–198). Silver Spring, MD: American Music Therapy Association.

Darrow, A., & Grohe, H. S. (2002). Music therapy for learners who are deaf or hard-of-hearing. In B. L. Wilson (Ed.), *Models of music therapy interventions in school settings* (2nd ed., pp. 291–317). Silver Spring, MD: American Music Therapy Association.

Darrow, A., & Johnson, C. (1994). Junior and senior high school music students' attitudes toward individuals with a disability. *Journal of Music Therapy, 31*(4), 266–279.

Elwafi, P. (2013). Visually impaired school children. In M. Hintz (Ed.), *Guidelines for music therapy practice in developmental health* (Vol. 3, pp. 270–304). University Park, IL: Barcelona.

Estabrooks, W. E., & Birkenshaw-Fleming, L. (2006). *Hear and listen! Talk and sing!: Songs for young children who are deaf or hard of hearing and others who need help learning to talk.* Washington, DC: Alexander Graham Bell Association for the Deaf and Hard of Hearing.

Gfeller, K. E., & Darrow, A. (2008). Music therapy in the treatment of sensory disorders. In W. B. Davis, K. E. Gfeller, & M. H. Thaut (Eds.), *An introduction to music therapy and practice* (3rd ed., pp. 365–404). Silver Spring, MD: American Music Therapy Association.

Gfeller, K. E., Driscoll, V., Kenworthy, M., & Van Vorst, T. (2011). Music therapy for preschool cochlear implant recipients. *Music Therapy Perspectives, 29*(1), 39–49.

Gourgey, C. (1998). Music therapy in the treatment of social isolation in visually impaired children. *ReView, 29*(4), 157–162.

Hachmeister, J. C. (2010). Learning through singing: How music helps children with hearing loss. *Volta Voices, 17*(4), 20–23.

Hughes, M., & Fazzi, D. (1993). Chapter five: Behavior management. In *First steps: A handbook for teaching young children who are visually impaired* (pp. 57–68). Los Angeles: Blind Children's Center.

Jan, J., & Groenveld, M. (1995). Visual behaviors and adaptations associated with cortical and ocular impairment in children. *National Newspatch*, 2–9.

LaVenture, S., & Allman, C. (2007). Special education services: What parents need to know. In S. LaVenture (Ed.), *A parents' guide to special education for children with visual impairments* (pp. 3–35). New York: AFB Press.

Martinez, C., & Moss, K. (1998). Orientation and mobility training: The way to go. *See/Hear, 3*(4). Retrieved from *www.tsbvi.edu/seehear/fall98/waytogo.htm.*

Paticoff, M. (2012). Creating a successful support group program for children. *Volta Voices, 19*(3), 24–27.

Robb, S. (2003). Music interventions and group participation skills of preschoolers with visual impairments: Raising questions about music, arousal, and attention. *Journal of Music Therapy, 40*(4), 266–282.

Roman-Lantzy, C. (2007). *Cortical visual impairment: An approach to assessment and intervention.* New York: AFB Press.

Simmons, S., & Stout, A. (1993). Chapter three: The eye. In *First steps: A handbook for teaching young children who are visually impaired* (pp. 23–34). Los Angeles: Blind Children's Center.

Wiggins, D. G. (2007). PreK music and the emergent reader: Promoting literacy in a music enhanced environment. *Early Child Childhood, 35*(1), 55–61.

CHAPTER 26

Music Therapy in the Schools

Katrina Skewes McFerran

The ability of music therapists to discern the needs of individuals and groups and design tailored musical programs that match those identified needs means that music therapists are positioned to make a unique contribution in schools. The use of music therapy in schools is traditionally documented with goals and objectives and supported by session notes and some form of regular evaluation of the program. This classic, treatment model approach (Gfeller & Davis, 2008) is well suited to schools that have historically adopted a behavioral orientation. However, "the times, they are a changin'" (Dylan, 1964).

Clientele: Students in Mainstream Schools

Educational pedagogy is increasingly focused on the value of individualized learning, which embraces the recognition that each child learns in context (Karpov, 2003) and that drawing on students' unique interests to shape learning experiences is more effective than teaching a set curriculum. This recognition has been driven by many

forces, including the information age, wherein all people have access to information via the Internet and teachers are no longer the vestibules of knowledge, which they impart through teaching. British pundits such as Sir Ken Robinson (Robinson & Aronica, 2008) are calling for a *learning revolution* in this context, with a greater emphasis on creativity and passion and a lesser emphasis on rote learning and regurgitation. American educational philosopher Maxine Greene (1995) has long emphasized the importance of creativity in learning, and she argues forcefully for the need for social change that begins in educational contexts, so that information is not simply accepted, but is critically considered.

These strong currents in educational discourse are juxtaposed with government requirements for objective, competitive comparisons between schools, learners, and teachers, resulting in considerable tension. In the United States, this need for objective comparison was actualized by President George W. Bush's policy initiatives (No Child Left Behind; U.S. Government, 2001), with a focus on evidence-based services as a basis for educational reform, in an attempt to redeem poor academic achievement across the country. This, and similar policies across the globe, led to an unequal focus on *core* subjects and *agreed-upon* curriculum—a focus that contrasts sharply with other policy initiatives driven by an emphasis on learning rather than teaching and that acknowledge that learning happens best when there is an atmosphere of well-being. Health, safety, happiness, achievement, and contribution are central and explicit values driving the new wave in British educational policy, as seen in policy documents from England and Wales (UK Government, 2005) and Scotland (Scottish Government, 2006). A similarly dichotomous situation exists in Australia, with policy initiatives of both types—on the one hand, emphasizing individual learning, whereas on the other, pressuring to excel on standardized tests of knowledge acquisition. This dichotomized environment is the context into which music therapists enter a school.

Theoretical Tenets

The situation within music therapy is no less complex than the larger policy situation (Rickson & McFerran, 2014). Conflicting theoretical perspectives also exist inside music therapy, although these are rarely discussed in the literature. Instead, there is a tendency to focus on *how* to do music therapy with particular groups of people, without including a more theoretically grounded discussion of *why* it might be done that way. Overtly acknowledging the different theoretical influences on my work has been helpful for understanding why I intuitively respond in one way with a particular person and quite differently with another. This approach involves being "guided by what best suits the adolescent in the moment" (McFerran, 2010a, p. 57) and is endorsed by research that shows that flexibility in offering different approaches is more effective than being loyal to one model when working with young people

who have some kind of psychopathology (Gold, Wigram, & Voracek, 2007).

Four of the most common theoretical influences informing why music therapists make different decisions in their school-based practices are humanistic, psychodynamic, developmental, and ecological theories (McFerran, 2010a). Each theoretical framework presupposes different beliefs about how music can benefit well-being and (theoretically) leads to different intentions and positions on the part of the therapist. Figure 26.1 illustrates the logical consequences of adopting each particular theoretical position, which are subsequently described in more detail.

Humanistic Approach

Music therapists who are informed by humanistic theories focus on encouraging young people in schools to express themselves musically and provide positive feedback on their participation by creating music with them. Many music therapists address humanistic aims to explain their practice in schools, but it is surprisingly rare for authors to overtly label their work as humanistic. Derrington (2012) says that "being able to use and connect through music is always my primary aim" (p. 209), and then describes how other goals emerge from this fundamental achievement, including improvements in social and emotional dimensions of learning. The nature of my own work with groups in schools is similarly driven by the young people's musical interests, whether they have learning disabilities (McFerran, 2009) or are working with grief and loss (McFerran & Teggelove, 2011). Nöcker-Ribaupierre and Wölfl (2010) also foster positive experiences of shared music making to provide opportunities for strengthening connections between diverse groups of classmates and preventing the expression of anger against migrant children. In each case, the therapist adopts a position of engagement and offers acceptance of any expression of the young person's mu-

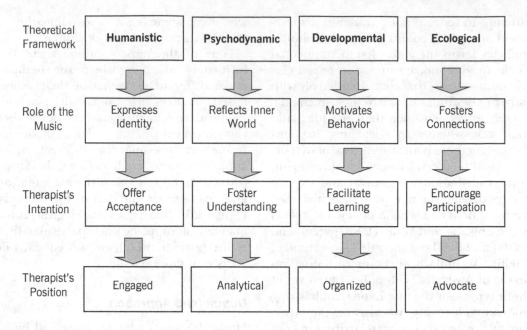

FIGURE 26.1. Four different theoretical approaches to music therapy in schools. Adapted from McFerran (2010a, p. 55) with permission of Jessica Kingsley Publisher.

sical identity, which is why these examples can be aligned with the theoretical premises of humanistic theory.

Psychodynamic Approach

A psychodynamic orientation requires the music therapist to adopt an analytical position, in which meaning is made from the ways that young people engage in music, and a greater understanding of that meaning is fostered. Although it is less common for music therapists to describe their work in schools as analytical, many music therapists interpret the musical behaviors of young people in sessions in an attempt to understand the meaning of the experience. Mahns (2003) explores the reasons for a boy's selective mutism within music therapy sessions in a school in Germany, encouraging the boy to explore issues of anger and familial conflict that ultimately lead to the return of his vocal expression. In my own work with bereaved teenagers, I have often adopted a psychodynamic lens to encour-

age the exploration of emotions and changing identity in response to grief and loss (McFerran, 2010b). Bosco (2002), utilizing aspects of a psychodynamic approach in response to 9/11, used story songs in mainstream schools to foster understanding and coping. The emphasis on deepening understanding of the inner world through musical expression is critical to approaches that incorporate psychodynamic theory, and this practice is often included in subtle ways in music therapy practice in schools.

Developmental Approach

Music therapists adopting a developmental orientation tend to be goal driven, organizing the structure of the session to facilitate the acquisition of particular skills and relying on music to provide a motivational framework as well as positive rewards for achievements. Authors may describe this work as *educational* music therapy or *behavioral* music therapy depending on the cultural context. For example, Register's research (Register, Darrow, Standley, & Swedberg, 2007) has shown how effective music can be in improving literacy outcomes for students with learning difficulties. Similarly, Kennedy and Scott (2005) were able to show a significant improvement in the story retelling and speaking skills of middle school students with English as a second language after 12 weeks of music therapy sessions. Baker and Jones (2005) worked in a school for refugees and used music to support the stabilization of their behavior in this radically new cultural context. All of these authors describe highly structured and consistent music therapy interventions that are well matched to quantitative research designs that can determine whether learning goals have been achieved. The achievement of externally observable and measurable goals is a fundamental premise of behaviorally oriented developmental approaches.

Ecological Approach

The term *ecological approach* refers to practices that demonstrate a consciousness of the wider contexts in which young people exist and the importance of engaging with these. This approach is becoming more commonly reported in the literature, with music therapists frequently describing a focus on participation in music making beyond the walls of the therapy room. The theoretical underpinning for this approach have been most clearly described in community music therapy discourse and illustrated through case studies such as Elefant's (2010) descriptions of a group program that introduced children with special needs into a mainstream school context. Her emphasis on advocacy of the students' right to participate in mixed-ability groups signifies a shift in approach within music therapy. Oosthuizen (2006) also describes an innovative approach to school-based work in South Africa that emerged from her own questions about inequity and human rights and her determination to discover a music therapy

practice that has value beyond an affluent, Western context. Rickson (2009) describes a consultancy with a bilingual school in Thailand where she empowered teachers to use music in planned ways to facilitate student learning, with positive outcomes. It would be wrong to think that ecological approaches are only suitable for faraway places, however; there are also countless local examples of an increasing expanded understanding of why music therapists might focus their intentions beyond the individual in front of them and include family members and teachers in the musical experience (Jacobsen & Wigram, 2007; Kern, Wolery, & Aldridge, 2007).

A Contemporary Eclectic Approach

The eclectic approach (McFerran, 2013) described in this chapter transcends the distinctions between these different theoretical approaches and integrates them into a contemporary approach to working as a music therapist in schools. This type of integration requires a consciousness of why particular musical opportunities could be suggested to the various players in the school. It equally ensures an ability to explain the rationale behind what happens in music therapy sessions to school staff from an informed position, rather than relying on assumptions about how effective a particular *activity* has been proven to be in achieving x, y, and z in another school with an entirely different type of young person. In reality, most music therapists working in schools do blend their theoretical approaches, depending on what needs young people present with on a given day and what interests they might have in music therapy. However, adopting an overtly eclectic approach ensures that the music therapist does not imply that he or she is working in a treatment model focused on skill acquisition, even while actively implementing humanistic or psychodynamically informed methods in the session. It is a useful framework when the music therapist is inclined to change his or her plan if it does not capture the interest of the young person, if a better idea is suggested, or if a person's needs on that day suggest something different than the original assessment. This flexibility contrasts with the rigidity involved in holding to the structure that was planned for the session, or requiring that the young person participate in songs that are known to the therapist rather than playing an instrument that has engaged the young person's interest. Instead of focusing on what to do as predetermined by a treatment plan and externally derived evidence, a contemporary eclectic approach emphasizes constant reflection on how we might best harness music for a particular client in this present context and often leads to a spontaneous experience that is led by the young person(s).

Moving away from an expert-directed treatment model also expands the goals of music therapy beyond what the music therapist might think is most helpful for the young person. Instead, the eclectic approach demands a mutual and collaborative negotiation about *musicking* together, referring to the full range of possibilities for musical participation described by Small (1998), who uses *music* as a verb, rather than a noun. In this form of therapeutic relationship, the young person's musical interests and abilities are taken as the basis for the encounter, as in the resource-oriented music therapy approach described by Rolvsjord (2010) for working in inpatient mental health. If the young person(s) is passionate about hip-hop, for example, then that preference provides a starting point for negotiating a focus. Equally, the music therapist must contribute his or her knowledge about how those interests might be utilized by fostering understanding, offering acceptance, achieving nonmusical outcomes, and/or encouraging participation. This emphasis on process and the collaboration rather than on treatment and cure is in keeping with the changing philosophy of education, which focuses on *individualized*

learning rather than *teaching*. It is worth noting that this eclecticism does not forgo our expertise as therapists, however, and it is critical for music therapists to remain conscious of the ways in which young people may use music both to promote and to hinder their mental health (McFerran & Saarikallio, 2013).

Clinical Work

Establishing a program in a mainstream school is not the same as establishing one at a special school, a hospital, or a community mental health program. A school is not designed to provide services for people with problems and pathologies. All children are required to attend school and to participate in learning so that they are able to grow up with the capacity to contribute to society. Although "well-being services" do exist in most schools, these are usually oriented toward promoting resilience and removing the obstacles that are impeding learning. A music therapy program should be aligned with this orientation in order to flourish and to allow the music therapist to make a valued contribution to the school. Focusing on the most problematic and vulnerable young people would be very limiting (see Rickson & McFerran, 2014, for more commentary).

Since pathology and problems are not the focus in this approach, the first stage of developing a music therapy program involves an assessment of the system—the school itself—and what needs could be addressed through musicking experiences. This kind of assessment requires observation and listening, as does a traditional assessment process. But instead of observing individuals, the music therapist focuses on the culture of the school by listening to the issues identified by school leaders and other well-being staff. It might be that there are bullying issues in the school, a high level of poverty in the local community leading to health and hygiene problems, a large group of students affected by bereavement, or a lack of satisfaction within the teaching team.

CLINICAL EXAMPLE: Assessing the School System

It is always somewhat intimidating to present at staff meetings in a new school. I like to include active music making because it is the easiest way for people to experience what I can do in the school, but this inclusion of music brings up resistances in staff who have a lot to do and may also have reservations about their own musical abilities. As I begin to chant the song I had composed for a call-and-response activity, I feel nervous—will they sing back to me, or just sit there in silence? In reality, they always join in, and today is no exception. I ask them to begin tapping the 1, 2, 3 rhythm on their legs, then call out the first line of the "Army Rap."

> I don't know but I've been told (you say it back)
> Staff in schools have hearts of gold (you say it back)
> I don't know but it's been said
> Teachers have a lot of cred
> I don't know but it's for sure
> We should all be paid much more
> Most important job there is
> To help Australia move ahead
> 1, 2
> 1, 2, 3, 4
> 1, 2, 3, 4!

By the time the humorous ditty is complete, they are laughing at a blooper I have made, and at their own pleasure in participating. They see and feel how overcoming their self-consciousness has led to a sense of achievement and engagement. I begin to explain how we might turn that experience into an opportunity for learning or for addressing a need in the school if we were in the classroom.

In addition to listening to key players among the school staff, it is important to develop a sense of the capacity for musicking within the community. This involves providing lunchtime workshops so that students can come and see what a music therapist might have to offer. Another strategy is to attend classes taught by willing teachers and make suggestions about how music could be used to increase engagement in the activity, showing them how it would work, and then gradually encouraging them to lead the activities.

CLINICAL EXAMPLE: Identifying Musical Capacity in the School

"What are you here for then?" asks the confused 15-year-old student, Maria. She has now attended two hip-hop workshops and still cannot grasp why I am not "teaching" them anything. I am thrilled with the question, since she is a powerful influence in the group, and her ambivalence is impacting the level of overall engagement. "I'm here to help you create a hip-hop song," I say. "I'm not here to do it for you or teach you about it. I know you love this kind of music, and I want to give you a space where you can discover and express that. I think you'll be amazed at what you're already capable of achieving." The group members nod, and Maria seems satisfied.

As the months go by, Maria becomes the leader of a small hip-hop dance troupe within the school. She describes how she wants to create a culture of hip-hop in the school where everyone knows that it is not just for "losers," and students become more interested in the genre. It is hard work, and she has to learn many leadership skills about how to break down her dance moves to teach others, how to cope with the fact that students often don't turn up to lunchtime workshops, and how eventually, the group doesn't even perform. I maintain a regular dialogue with her, being transparent about what she needs to do to engage the group, and, although it does not come naturally to her, she comes prepared to many groups with music and moves to share.

In the meantime, Maria begins attending school more regularly, and a number of staff comments that she seems to have reengaged with the school community after being on the verge of dropping out of school. She is also excited about the opportunity to connect with a hip-hop choir that provides some workshops in the school later in the year, although she doesn't take advantage of the opportunity very often. My sense is that she is still surprised to have been taken so seriously and doesn't quite believe in herself yet, but that this experience has impacted her sense of identity and may influence decisions she makes in the coming years. In an interview with Maria, she describes how it has been hard, but that my encouragement helped her learn to lead and be patient, because she'd never done anything like that before and she wanted to share it with other students within the school, not just outside school. She appreciated the opportunity for the students to be independent in the program, saying, "It makes us better leaders."

Once the various players within the school community gain an experiential understanding about how a music therapist works, it is possible to focus on why that understanding might be helpful. As noted above, music therapists contribute a unique ability for designing programs that harness the musical capacity in the school toward greater well-being and connectedness. Combining the issues that have been identified by staff and students with tailored musicking programs that can be evaluated and developed can lead to powerful change within the school.

CLINICAL EXAMPLE: Tailoring the Program to Meet the Needs of the School

Some of the teachers within the school were unhappy about the distinctions that were made between older and younger students. They felt that their younger students were not taken seriously within the school community and not given the opportunity to truly participate in many of the regular school activities. I observed that one of the teachers of the younger students was very musical, and that her classes were filled with songs. Separately, I knew that a group of older students were learning a range of body percussion activities that involved sequences of tapping, clapping, and stomping. I suggested that the older students come and lead activities in the younger class, fostering connections between different age groups in the school through shared, cre-

ative activity. This activity had the additional benefit of addressing some cultural distinctions in the school, where many students seemed to separate themselves into groups by ethnic background.

The program was a success, and the young students were thrilled by the musical games the older students led them through. As music therapist, I spoke with the older students before each session and helped them to think about how they might structure the activities. In the early sessions, I led a number of the games, but as the weeks went by, I did less and less. When a performance opportunity arose, we asked if the youngest students could open the show, and they impressed the entire school with their body percussion sequences. The older students were quite embarrassed to be on stage on this first occasion, but when the next opportunity arose to perform some months later, they were more confident and also performed their own, more complex sequence, which led to rapturous applause from their peers in the school community.

The level of interaction in the schoolyard increased between the younger and the older students across the duration of the program. Sometimes this involved greeting one another by name, but more often there would be a call-and-response of quick percussion movements. In addition, the teachers felt that the younger classes had been publicly witnessed and included within the school events. In fact, it had become clear that the lack of inhibition shown by the younger students sometimes made them better performers, and a new sense of respect for their contribution existed as a result—they no longer provided just the "cute" factor. The older students had developed leadership skills and confidence in their ability to participate musically, and teachers commented that one of the older boys seemed to have better control over his temper, which had previously been causing challenges in the schoolyard. In all these ways, musicking had allowed other people in the community to discover unexpected potentials in their peers and to admire their abilities, both musically and as players in the school.

Some young people in the school may benefit from the more specialist skills that music therapists have to offer as qualified therapists. Having the ability to understand mental illness and bereavement is a significant resource that a school may wish to utilize. Grief and loss are common experiences for students; indeed, bereavements that have occurred many years ago may still be impacting a young person's ability to participate fully in school. Similarly, early intervention with young people who are showing signs of anxiety and depression can be very helpful. If particularly vulnerable groups of young people are identified for service within a school cohort, then a different emphasis is required in the theoretical orientation adopted within the school context.

CLINICAL EXAMPLE: Providing Therapy Services

The well-being coordinator in the school mentions that there are a number of students who seem to be struggling with bereavement in the school that year. Together, we plan a bereavement support group to co-facilitate, with the aim of supporting the young people who choose to participate and also refreshing the well-being coordinator's toolbox with some new ideas for using music. The students all bring a song to the first session that is meaningful and related in some way to the person who has died. After a warm-up game, each young person plays his or her song (either from the phone or the computer), while the rest of us sit around and listen. At times, I gently remind group members how important it is to actually listen, including the well-being coordinator and the students, and after a couple of songs, we had grown comfortable enough to sit together silently for the duration of the song. After each song, I ask the young person to describe why he or she had shared that song and the personal meaning. The answers are powerful, and there are tears—which makes some of the students and the well-being coordinator uncomfortable, since the students need to return to the classroom after the group and don't want to be conspicuous in their vulnerability. We are careful to let them know that sharing is important, and that so is coping. When they

are reticent about coming each week and crying, we reinforce the point that our focus is on coping strategies, but that it is important to hear their story and their situation. Their trust in the well-being coordinator helps them to accept this, and the support they feel from being with people who understand gives them the courage to keep coming.

The following week, we again begin with a warm-up facilitated by my colleague, who emphasizes how deeply she cares about them and how she really wants them to know that things are going to be OK. I then lead a song-writing process, where we choose a song that the whole group finds relevant to grieving and then begin the process of changing the words to tell our own story. The group chooses an old R 'n' B song called "I'll Be Missing You" (Puff Daddy, 1997), and the well-being coordinator is surprised to find that the song sounds familiar and the riff that is used in it from an old song by the Police ("Every Breath You Take," 1983). One of the group members independently downloads a karaoke version of the song from YouTube on to her phone, and we begin to brainstorm ideas immediately, with the music running off her phone in the background.

We continue to work on the song for the next two sessions, and I also introduce group instrumental improvisation as a way to express and get relief from feelings. We improvise separate improvisations on happy, angry, sad, and then happy again during the next session, and although there are no more tears, the group members engage seriously in the activity, and we talk about the importance of sharing and expressing emotions in a way that doesn't hurt others. The well-being coordinator also leads discussions about issues that she feels are relevant to the group, and by the final session we have shared songs, improvisations, completed the lyric substitution, and recorded the group singing and rapping the song, after which we give them a copy of it on CD as a closing gesture. We evaluate the group by comparing scores on a depression measure before and after the process and are happy to find that two of the group members who were struggling the most have moved from being at risk to a less vulnerable score by the conclusion. All group members experience a sense of connectedness to one another that has been facilitated by sharing their stories, expressing their emotions authentically, and making music together.

Applications to Other Disciplines

Another important role that music therapists play in a school context is to facilitate learning outcomes. The age of the students is an important influence on the different kinds of musicking experiences that may be suitable to motivate learning, and the vast range of skills that a music therapist has developed through his or her training means that a range of genres can be considered. Songwriting and singing are often the most comfortable activities for teachers, since most people are familiar with some styles of songs—either from their own adolescence or sometimes through their students. Various technologies that are widely available also mean that teachers are easily able to look up songs on YouTube themselves and often need only encouragement to feel empowered enough to do so. Whether the topic is literacy or health and well-being, having the class work as a group on a songwriting project can take many forms. It may simply be a lyric substitution, or it can expand to a full video project including performers, production crew, and postproduction of the clip. The combination of the teacher's knowledge of learning outcomes and the music therapist's ability to show how steps toward achieving outcomes can be transformed into engaging activities through music can be very successful.

CLINICAL EXAMPLE: Sharing Songwriting Skills

After the teachers had experienced my musicking in the staff meetings and watched me run programs in the school grounds, as well as with the well-being coordinator, a number expressed curiosity about how music could be used in their classroom. One English literature teacher took advantage of an opportunity when I was returning a student to class and she was teaching about how to write sonnets. She pulled me in to the classroom and asked if I knew about sonnets. I honestly replied that I didn't, and she began to explain them to me and to the class. Sonnets are highly rhythmical in nature, and it was obvious that they would form the basis for a rap song. I explained this to the teacher and the class, and some of the students expressed immediate relief that they weren't going to be made to sing. I agreed to return to the class next week, and that we would work on it together.

When I return, a number of discussions have already taken place, and the teacher has encouraged three of the students to play guitar as part of the sonnet. It becomes more of a chant than a rap, and different groups take responsibility for speaking the various verses out loud before passing to the next small group. I am only needed in the classroom for 15 minutes, since the teacher has already generated the lyrics with the students, and so I spend some additional time with the beginner musicians, helping them to choose a chord progression that all can play and trying to encourage someone to take responsibility for keeping the pace so that it doesn't become a dirge.

I visit the classroom three more times, mostly for rehearsals. There are a lot of dynamics between different groups of students, with a number of new students of Asian background who don't speak much English and another large group of students from local Arab families sharing loud jokes and laughter, as well as a range of people from other cultures, including white Australian. Eventually, the players decide not to perform the piece in a public venue, since many people are shy, and the musicians have had a lot of fun but do not respond well to the kind of pressure they would be under to create a reasonable performance. The teacher reports in interview that she is very satisfied with the experience as it was, since they extended their interest in sonnets and also worked together as a cohesive team during some parts of the musicking. She is confident that she would be able to use music again in her teaching the following year, and I am equally confident in her abilities.

Conclusions

Depending on the different needs and interests of players in the school, the way I approach each program is different, as seen in the case examples. When a psychodynamic orientation was suitable, I oriented myself appropriately and provided a safe and containing space in which analysis was used. When connectedness and participation were the focus, I ensured that my role was less centralized and that the players took responsibility, both for identifying the specific needs and for leading the musicking experiences by drawing on their own musical resources. I also contributed to ensuring that opportunities for developing musical resources were manifested by applying for funding to bring musicians into the school to run percussion workshops, and later by connecting the school with a hip-hop youth choir that operated locally. When personal development and expression of identity seemed important, I focused on positive experiences that engaged the young people in ways in which they were able to discover their musical potential. And when learning objectives were prioritized, I shared my expertise about using age-appropriate musical genres and helped the teachers and well-being coordinator to feel confident that they would be able to use music as well.

Making a contribution to a mainstream school requires a different orientation than the traditional treatment model, where the music therapist is regarded as the expert who will fix a young person with problems. Schools are oriented toward goals of growth and development, and they are increasingly required to provide individually tailored learning opportunities that do more than promote rote learning and obedience. Music therapists have the option of adopting a blended and eclectically informed theoretical approach to developing programs in mainstream schools (McFerran, 2012). By drawing on our capacity to conceptualize musicking opportunities that meet the needs expressed by players

in the school, as well as critically observed using our analytic skills, we can make a unique contribution. Schools are in need of opportunities to build connections among diverse groups of students and teachers. Leadership is torn by competing demands from government. Students are often more focused on their personal worlds than their academic outcomes. Music therapists can potentially make a sustainable difference within mainstream schools by building musical cultures that encourage meaningful engagement and authentic self-expression. Actualizing these goals requires openness to collaboration, a capacity to leave our own egos at the door while we foster musical leadership in others, and a desire to make a difference.

REFERENCES

Baker, F., & Jones, C. (2005). Holding a steady beat: The effects of a music therapy program on stabilising behaviours of newly arrived refugee students. *British Journal of Music Therapy, 19*(2), 67–74.

Bosco, J. (2002). From chaos to creative expression: The New York City Music Therapy Relief Project (in response to 9-11). *Early Childhood Connections: Journal of Music- and Movement-Based Learning, 8,* 7–18.

Derrington, P. (2012). "Yeah, I'll do music!": Working with secondary-aged students who have complex emotional and behavioural difficulties. In J. Tomlinson, P. Derrington, & A. Oldfield (Eds.), *Music therapy in schools: Working with children of all ages in mainstream and special education* (pp. 195–211). London: Jessica Kingsley.

Dylan, B. (1964). *The times, they are a-changin'.* New York: Columbia.

Elefant, C. (2010). Whose voice is heard?: Performances and voices of the Renanim Choir in Israel. In B. Stige, G. Ansdell, C. Elefant, & M. Pavlicevic (Eds.), *Where music helps: Community music therapy in action and reflection* (pp. 189–218). Farnham, UK: Ashgate.

Gfeller, K. E., & Davis, W. B. (2008). The music therapy treatment process. In W. B. Davis, K. E. Gfeller, & M. H. Thaut (Eds.), *An introduction to music therapy: Theory and practice* (3rd ed., pp. 429–486). Silver Spring, MD: American Music Therapy Association.

Gold, C., Wigram, T., & Voracek, M. (2007). Effectiveness of music therapy for children and adolescents with psychopathology: A quasi-experimental study. *Psychotherapy Research, 17*(3), 292–300.

Greene, M. (1995). *Releasing the imagination: Essays on education, the arts and social change.* San Francisco: Wiley.

Jacobsen, S. L., & Wigram, T. (2007). Music therapy for the assessment of parental competences for children in need of care. *Nordic Journal of Music Therapy, 16*(2), 129–143.

Karpov, Y. V. (2003). Development through the lifespan: A neo-Vygotskian approach. In A. Kozulin, B. Gindis, V. S. Ageyev, & S. M. Miller (Eds.), *Vygotsky's educational theory in cultural context* (pp. 138–157). Cambridge, UK: Cambridge University Press.

Kennedy, R., & Scott, A. (2005). A pilot study: The effects of music therapy interventions on middle school students' ESL skills. *Journal of Music Therapy, 42*(2), 244–261.

Kern, P., Wolery, M., & Aldridge, D. (2007). Use of songs to promote independence in morning greeting routines for young children with autism. *Journal of Autism and Developmental Disorders, 37*, 1264–1271.

Mahns, W. (2003). Speaking without talking: Fifty analytical music therapy sessions with a boy with selective mutism. In S. Hadley (Ed.), *Psychodynamic music therapy* (pp. 53–72). Gilsum, NH: Barcelona.

McFerran, K. S. (2009). Quenching a desire for power: The role of music therapy for adolescents with behavioural disorders. *Australasian Journal of Special Education, 33*(1), 72–83.

McFerran, K. S. (2010a). *Adolescents, music and music therapy: Methods and techniques for clinicians, educators and students.* London: Jessica Kingsley.

McFerran, K. S. (2010b). Tipping the scales: A substantive theory on the value of group music therapy for supporting grieving teenagers. *Qualitative Inquiries in Music Therapy, 5*, 2–49.

McFerran, K. S. (2012). Commentary: Music therapy in schools: An expansion of traditional practice. In G. McPherson & G. Welch (Eds.), *The Oxford handbook of music education* (pp. 667–670). New York: Oxford University Press.

McFerran, K. S. (2013). Adolescents and substance use disorders. In L. Eyre (Ed.), *Guidelines for music therapy practice in mental health* (pp. 167–189). University Park, IL: Barcelona.

McFerran, K. S., & Saarikallio, S. (2013). Depending on music to feel better: Being conscious of responsibility when appropriating the power of music. *Arts in Psychotherapy, 41*(1), 89–97.

McFerran, K. S., & Teggelove, K. (2011). Music therapy with young people in schools: After the Black Saturday fires. *Voices: A World Forum For Music Therapy, 11*(1). Retrieved from *https://normt.uib.no/index.php/voices/article/view/285/442.*

Nöcker-Ribaupierre, M., & Wölfl, A. (2010). Music to counter violence: A preventative approach for working with adolescents in schools. *Nordic Journal of Music Therapy, 19*(2), 151–161.

Oosthuizen, H. (2006). Diversity and community: Finding and forming South African music therapy. *Voices: A World Forum for Music Therapy, 6*(3). Retrieved from *https://normt.uib.no/index.php/voices/article/view/277/202.*

Register, D., Darrow, A., Standley, J., & Swedberg., O. (2007). The use of music to enhance reading skills of second grade students and students with reading disabilities. *Journal of Music Therapy, 44*(1), 23–37.

Rickson, D. (2009). The use of music to facilitate learning and development in a school in Thailand: An exploratory case study. *New Zealand Journal of Music Therapy, 7*, 61–85.

Rickson, D., & McFerran, K. (2014). *Creating music cultures in the schools: A perspective from Community Music Therapy.* Gilsum, NH: Barcelona.

Robinson, K., & Aronica, L. (2008). *The element: How finding your passion changes everything.* New York: Penguin.

Rolvsjord, R. (2010). *Resource-oriented music therapy in mental health care.* Gilsum, NH: Barcelona.

Scottish Government, Education Department. (2006). *Getting it right for every child.* Retrieved from *www.scotland.gov.uk/Resource/Doc/161343/0043786.pdf.*

Small, C. (1998). *Musicking: The meanings of performing and listening.* Hanover, NH: Wesleyan University Press.

UK Government, Department of Education. (2005). *Every child matters: Youth matters.* Retrieved from *www.education.gov.uk/consultations/downloadableDocs/EveryChildMattersSummary.pdf.*

U.S. Government, Department of Education. (2001). *No child left behind: A desktop reference.* Retrieved from *www.ed.gov/admins/lead/account/nclbreference/reference.pdf.*

SECTION B

Music Therapy for Adults

CHAPTER 27

Music Therapy for Adults with Mental Illness

Gillian Stephens Langdon

**CLINICAL EXAMPLE: "I'll Be Good to You":
A Journey to the Outside through Music
Therapy**

I'll never know what pain may have caused Edgar to exit planet Earth and morph into Jordo #1, but I was privileged to witness the little moments of his return.

He tolerates me calling him Edgar with my earthly therapist insistence, which I tell myself I do to help him. But I think deep down I am afraid of the capacity of the mind to go so far away, and that stops me from ever using his alien name. For me, however, there is a poignancy in the smile that began to dawn on his face. But let me start at the beginning.

When I first met Edgar, it was on the long-term unit with David, the music therapist and leader of the hospital band. "He plays Jimmy Hendrix," David announced, handing Edgar a guitar. His fingers flew over the frets but never touched down, as he kind of fluttered his hands over the strings. The result was the look of a guitar player but the sound was chaotic and blurred. Later, when he begins attending one of my music therapy groups, I remember to bring an extra guitar and he plays in this same "as if" style. He plays this way while I play my chords and other songs. It is sort of irritating, but I don't want to discour-

age him. If this "idea" of playing helps him to come to group, I figure it's OK.

I notice after a few weeks that his fingers are beginning to actually touch down on the strings and a little coherent sound is emerging. Because of this, one day I say "Edgar, I'm going to play the opening song now. Can you follow me and then play your song after? It's in A." "A?" he asks and proceeds to follow my chords for a few seconds. Then he drifts off as if playing a solo. Over the weeks his fingers begin pressing hard enough to make a sound we all can share. His own music starts to have more form, and he is singing but so softly it is impossible to make it out. "What's the name of that?" a group member asks. "'I'll Be Good to You' Brothers Johnson," he answers.

Now David starts including him in the hospital band, and he even plays a couple of shows in the hospital. He stands up, his tall, awkward frame holding the electric guitar playing a little lead. Sometimes David leans over and reminds him "BflatGminor . . ." Sometimes he is playing in his own world.

I guess other people are beginning to see the change in him because one day he comes into the music therapy group and says "Had dinner downstairs." "Where was that?" "Downstairs . . . and you can smoke!" he adds with a boyish grin. "Oh, the transitional residence." "Yeah. That's it." The social worker is transitioning him to the residence that was created by locking the doors of the bottom in-patient wards and adding a ramp to the outside.

I am happy when I hear this plan because Edgar has been institutionalized for so long that it would probably be scary for him to feel like he was totally out. This way he can feel like he's on a ward while he gets used to the door being open. "You leaving?" other group members ask. They are impressed. Hardly anyone leaves this long-term ward. "Yep. Leaving soon."

I call the social worker to let her know how well Edgar is doing, the changes I have seen in his music, and how he speaks of the residence. "Really?" she says, sounding surprised, "I thought he didn't like it!" "No, he talks about it in every group!" I say. "Well, then I'll try again. You know the interview didn't go so well. The lady with the harsh voice—you know her—she yelled at him in front of everyone. 'You can't come in here like that! You need to shower—and with real soap!' He said he never wanted to go back." I protest, "But he says all the time, 'It's nice downstairs. Good food and you can smoke.'" "Well, I'll have to try again," and she does. She helps him organize his clothes and shower before the next interview, and this time he is accepted.

Now the social worker tells us she is referring Edgar to the outpatient clinic in the community for day programming because that is where we have the band rehearsals on Fridays. "That's his life! It's the only thing that he is interested in," she says. But next week, in the music therapy group inside the hospital, instead of an empty chair, Edgar is sitting there holding the guitar as always, as if nothing had changed. When I ask him about his week, he acts like everything is normal, so I don't pry and none of the members of the group do either, but I can feel the tension in the room.

At the door, when all the other group members have left, I say in more like a statement than a question, "Rough week." He stands there, his tall frame in the doorway. His arms are limp at his sides and his head is cast down, "I'm not strong as I used to be. . . . It's tough . . . tough out there. I'm not so strong." And then he shuffles out to line up with the others at the door. I find out later that when

he was at the clinic, the doctor spoke to him, and Edgar told him he was hearing voices telling him to kill himself, so they brought him back right away. I'm sure they'll never let him out again. I feel my heart sink.

Yet a few weeks later I get a call from the social worker. "We're going to try again with Edgar. I'm going to go with him in the van to the clinic in the community. The band is everything to him."

Soon Edgar is traveling by himself every day in the van to the outpatient clinic and living in the residence downstairs. He is a regular member of the outpatient music therapy group as well as attending the band rehearsals on Fridays. He often plays "I'll Be Good to You." The band has a great arrangement of that song now. In one concert the band plays for the hospital, and we've really got it down! Edgar starts it off with the guitar alone playing the first two melody lines—clear as a bell. Then as he hits the last two beats on the dominant seventh chord we all come in—percussion, bass, piano, and guitar—and the lead singer belts out "I wanna know . . ." and the song takes off with Edgar playing a solo in the middle. It's a little weaker musically lately, because Edgar wants to sing the vocals now, but what a thrill when you can hear a snatch of vocal here and there, and he's holding it all down!

But it's a long journey. We see him exploring his world. I see him at the subway station once. He is standing on the landing as I come down the stairs from the train one evening. He is just standing there. I am surprised and delighted so I run up to him and say, "Hey, Edgar, how are you doing?" He looks uncomfortable, shifting his tall body around. He says, "All right." I chat about the band rehearsal tomorrow and then say good-bye. But next week, when we have someone interviewing the band members for a presentation, he describes me as "She's OK. But she's nosey—like a woman." I realize how far away he probably was at the train station and how foolish for me to barge into his world unexpectedly. The next time I see him, I pretend I don't see him. Better perhaps for me to appear in context—the music therapist or the keyboard player in the band.

One time I see him at the clinic throwing bits of paper with deliberation into each corner sewer opening. And I know not to let him know that I notice. Maybe I *am* nosey! At other times I see him outside the clinic smoking, and I say, "There's rehearsal. You coming?" He says "Oh. It's now? I'm coming," and he hurries to get ready.

But let me go back to that smile I see today. He is playing "I'll Be Good to You" for the outpatient music therapy group. They love seeing him play! A new member, a woman about his age, comes into the group. She sits opposite him while he is playing. She is so happy. She smiles at him like he is her brother. Now she starts singing, "weather, whether good or bad, happy or sad." He looks up as he sings and smiles at her. At the end of the group, I ask if he heard her singing with him. He says, "Yes. It was nice! Nice!" He emphasizes the *s* sound. "Different song, though—but that's OK," he adds with a chuckle.

On Thanksgiving in the music therapy group we make up a song about what group members are grateful for. When it's Edgar's turn, he says, "Soap. I'm grateful for soap."

It's the journeys of the very long-term clients like Edgar that are so remarkable. When the music therapy work, along with the treatment team, creates a path to empowerment and freedom, it is truly a celebration.

It is an exciting time for music therapists working with this population. For years, music therapists have witnessed the enlivening effects of music making and have spoken of working with the healthy self. Yet often other professionals passing by a music therapy session, although startled at times at the energy and laughter in the sessions, simply pass these effects off with remarks like, "Yes, they all like music," or witness the hard work of the music therapists as "patients having fun."

With the technology available to do brain scans, we can now see these enlivening effects as music being processed throughout the brain (Levitin, 2006), involving physical, emotional, and perceptual centers. In addition, there is research on

> the idea that the brain can change its own structure and function through thought and activity. . . . The neuroplastic revolution has implications for, among other things, our understanding of how love, sex, grief, relationships, learning, addictions, culture, technology, and psychotherapy change our brains. (Doidge, 2007, pp. xix–xx)

In the future we may find that the work of music therapy, besides having psychological benefits, may be shown to have lasting effects on the brain itself.

Clientele

Music therapy in adult psychiatry spans a great range of functioning, and the music therapy work depends on where the person is along this continuum. In my position in an urban, long-term state psychiatric center, I have often worked with people who have been in the psychiatric hospital system for years, with the primary diagnoses being schizophrenia and schizoaffective disorder, as well as some patients with depression and some with bipolar disorder. Information on these and many other psychiatric diagnoses is found in the fifth edition of the *Diagnostic and Statistical Manual of Mental Disorders* (DSM-5; American Psychiatric Association, 2013). The first two of these diagnoses, schizophrenia with *schizoaffective disorder*, are characterized by "delusions, hallucinations, disorganized speech (e.g., frequent derailment or incoherence), grossly disorganized or catatonic behavior, negative symptoms (i.e., diminished emotional expressions or avolition" (American Psychiatric Association, p. 99) and schizoaffective disorder, also characterized by "an uninterrupted period of illness during which there is a major mood episode (major depression or mania) concurrent with . . . schizophrenia" (American Psychiatric Association, p. 105). There are several types of *depressive disorders*, with the common feature being "the presence of sad, empty, or irritable mood, accompanied by somatic and cognitive changes that significantly affect the individual's capacity to function" (American Psychiatric Association, p. 155). *Bipolar and related disorders* include what has traditionally been known as manic–depressive disorder (bipolar I disorder) as well as other disorders that include some type of cyclic disorders, wherein people experience both manic and depressive episodes at some point (American Psychiatric Association, pp. 123–154).

The people with whom I work are often from economically disadvantaged situations or from disrupted homes, having spent their childhood years in foster care. Some are children of immigrants sent from rural settings into the complex urban scene. Many have turned to drugs and alcohol to self-medicate and, in the process, have had run-ins with the legal system. Many have spent time in jail. Many, due to the above factors, have had little education, although many are also highly intelligent. Some have a college education, supportive families, and are not poor, yet hounded and incapacitated by their symptoms. Some people are silent, others are angry and agitated. Some are unpredictable and apparently unreachable.

Preferences in music have a huge range, often depending on age and culture. The music therapist has to meet all clients where they are and with what music makes them comfortable, whether it be salsa, R&B, reggae, rock, rap, classical, or the latest musical trend. The work may be done through improvisation, fill-in songs, familiar songs, songwriting, and various combinations of music and words. The needs of these patients may also be addressed with what is called *Community Music Therapy* (Ansdell, 2002; Stige & Aarø, 2012), through therapeutic performance (Jampel, 2006) or vocal work (Austin, 2008), or through any of a number of other interventions (see Crowe & Colwell, 2007; Eyre, 2013; Wheeler, Shultis, & Polen, 2005). The setting may be an inpatient psychiatric hospital, an outpatient clinic, a shelter, or private practice.

Clinical Work

I would like to bring the reader into the world of the music therapist through three vignettes from my work in an urban psychiatric hospital. Although there are many types of work, these provide a glimpse into what the work looks like. The first, from the beginning of the chapter, is of a client who has been hospitalized for years with a diagnosis of schizophrenia, undifferentiated type, discovering his musician's identity and moving from an inpatient to outpatient setting. The second is music therapy with a young adult survivor of severe, prolonged childhood trauma with a diagnosis of schizoaffective disorder. The third is a man diagnosed with schizophrenia, paranoid type in an acute state, filled with rage and fear, on the admissions unit.

In the vignette at the beginning, of Edgar, we can see the beneficial aspects of music therapy such as grounding, enlivening, community building, and community reintegration. The work of grounding occurred at the beginning, as we see his fingers unable to touch down on the frets of the guitar. Edgar is so lost in his mental world that he is unable to communicate much of his music, not to mention words, to others. As he receives acceptance from the therapist and the group, he begins to trust. The therapist pushes him gently to follow her and then play his song, helping him differentiate his inner world from the outer world of the therapist. Now the group can focus on listening to his music. As his music becomes clearer, he becomes grounded in a reality we all can share. As he grows in this way, he is able to become more confident and self-assured as he develops his identity as a member of the band. The band becomes his community and his point of reference as he transitions to living outside the hospital.

In the vignette of Edgar we see an example of two aspects of music therapy with adults with mental illness. The first aspect occurs in the initial encounter, when Edgar is involved in a music therapy group incorporating musicians and nonmusicians and focusing on goals of socialization, impulse control, and self-expression. The primary techniques used by the music therapist are improvisation, fill-in songs, song creation, and the use of precomposed songs. Improvisation deserves some reflection here to see exactly what is meant in this context. Bruscia (1987) describes improvising as

> inventive, spontaneous, extemporaneous, resourceful, and it involves creating and playing simultaneously. It is not always "art" however, and does not always result in "music" per se. Sometimes it is a "process" which results in very simple "sound forms." Music therapists strive to improvise music of the highest artistic quality and beauty, however, they always accept the client's improvising at whatever level is offered, whether consisting of musical or sound forms, and regardless of its artisitic or aesthetic merit. (pp. 5–6)

Adults diagnosed with mental illness have often lost their sense of self, and their relationship to others and to society has become disturbed. Improvisation is a way to assist them because it allows the client to

> experience him or herself in relation to others on two levels, the actual and the symbolic: the actual, in a very real interaction of his or her sounds with those of others; the symbolic, in that the music contains expression of emotions, thoughts, and memories. (Stephens, 1983, p. 29)

The second aspect of music therapy is illustrated with Edgar's entrance into the hospital band as a performing musician. In this aspect, the work is to support Edgar in his rediscovery of his identity as a musician, working toward a product (the songs) and supporting a developing awareness of, and being with, others (the members of the band). This is typical of what occurs in Community Music Therapy. "The aim is to help clients access a variety of musical situations, and to accompany them as they move

between 'therapy' and wider social contexts of musicing" (Ansdell, 2002, n. p.).

But not all music therapy work with the mentally ill involves musicians. Many people are not musicians and many are survivors of severe, prolonged trauma. Research points to the high prevalence of trauma in the psychiatric population (Muenzenmaier et al., 2005; Muenzenmaier, Schneeberger, Castille, Battaglia, Seixas, & Link, 2014). In fact, there is a growing movement away from the diagnosis of schizophrenia, looking instead into trauma as the origin of symptoms that have traditionally been seen as symptoms of schizophrenia, such as hearing voices (Romme, Escher, Dillon, Corsteins, & Morris, 2009; Longden, 2013).

Working within a trauma-informed perspective, it is important to understand that brain research has been able to show that

> reminders of traumatic experiences activate brain regions that support intense emotions, and decrease activation in the central nervous system (CNS) regions involved in (a) the integration of sensory input and motor output, (b) the modulation of physiological arousal, and (c) the capacity to communicate experience in words. (van der Kolk, 2006, p. 277).

In other words, the survival mechanisms of trauma often shut down the ability to speak, process, and heal, and the ability to self-regulate is impaired.

The author, with other members of the trauma committee, developed a model for working with trauma symptoms such as dissociation, difficulties in affect regulation, and flashbacks or nightmares while providing a forum for discussing tools for coping with daily challenges (Borczon, Jampel, & Langdon, 2010). In the next vignette we can see how the combination of music and words in a music–verbal therapy trauma group addresses some of the needs of a survivor of severe, prolonged childhood trauma.

CLINICAL EXAMPLE: "Don't Want No More Suffering"

I have known Beth for many years now. When I first met her, she was 20 years old and had just been transferred from a hospital upstate. The frightening news of her arrival traveled around the hospital like wildfire. We had all heard the tales of the staff injuries—the scenes of four people trying to hold her down as her lithe body moved fast, slipping through their hands, and the hitting and flailing starting all over again.

The treatment team asks me for a music therapy consultation, and I feel fearful. But I am pleased to be asked, even though I know it is probably just a ploy to get me to work with her.

The consult is planned thoughtfully. It is scheduled during a time the whole ward will be at a program, so the setting will be less stimulating to her. And a staff member will sit in with me.

I have carefully selected the instruments. The conga drum could help to ground her. If she chooses to play, it could contain a hard slap and perhaps channel her aggression, with support from the guitar or piano, into a structured beat of a musical line. I also choose the tambourine for its easy handling and for being light enough to not be too injurious if thrown. The xylimba (a six-note wooden instrument) is next because of its beauty and ease of playing, with its five-note pentatonic scale, making it virtually impossible to make a mistake. She won't feel compelled to find the "right" notes. I also bring my guitar to create an intimate sound and an accompaniment for an improvisation or a song. And the room in which we are to meet, fortunately, has a piano. I bring songbooks, especially the ones with popular songs.

I walk in. Beth is sitting calmly on a small couch, looking a little shy beside the therapy aide. I try to hide my fear with a smile. As I set the xylimba and mallets on a chair, I tell her we can play the instruments and maybe also sing some songs. Right away she takes the mallets and starts playing the xylimba. I quickly unpack the guitar to offer her some support through playing harmonies to match her melody. She begins to smile and laugh, her rhythmic melodies combining with the guitar to weave a beautiful creation.

She sees the books I have brought. "Maybe we can play a song?" She picks one out and I play it on the piano. Beth sits next to me on the piano bench and sings in a loud, unmusical way, but she is playful and creative, and I realize that I am no longer afraid. The therapy aide is laughing also.

Clearly, Beth finds in music a safe space—a place for play and delight, a place where she is in control and competent, a place where she can be heard and where she may be able to build community. Music becomes the foundation of our relationship over the years that follow, through her struggles, progress, and regressions.

She also loves to dance, and I notice how she moves her body, gyrating down close to the ground, rhythmically and beautifully but almost too open, as if her body is in complete abandon with no boundaries—and no protection—and then she laughs and suddenly stops dancing.

Beth habitually leans back in her chair, somewhat precariously. But when we begin to play music, she focuses intently, leaning forward with the chair and her feet firmly on the floor. She often chooses the conga drum. It allows her to ground herself. The conga connects directly to the floor and it can be played gently or loudly, providing her with a range of expression that she so desperately needs.

She often asks to sing for the annual holiday show, where she always wants to sing "Lean on Me" in a kind of monotone—out of tune, but sincerely. She is shy in singing in front of an audience, often wanting me to sing with her, and in the middle she stops singing. But she has the audience with her. That is the thing: as terrifying as she can be, she has won the hearts of most people. Everyone wants her to succeed.

Beth later joins the music–verbal therapy trauma group, which uses words and music to integrate the different needs of the trauma survivors. Here Beth is able to express in music what is impossible for her to say in words, while at the same time providing a place where she can begin to look and speak of specific events, finding tools to help with trauma symptoms and sharing the challenges in her daily life. In this group she finds community, connecting with peers who have also experienced severe traumatic events throughout their lives. Beth always insists that we do the opening song (a "check-in" song) exactly the same as when we began years ago. I see how music is her point of contact in difficult times when she becomes speechless but also how, even when her words are organized and her outer look is happy, the music expresses a deeper troubled side to her. Music provides grounding and a balance for her emotions. And I see that she is able to express joy through music in the smile that spreads across her face and her laughter after playing music.

Over time, Beth becomes a role model for younger clients as they join the group. She reassures a young woman not to feel guilty about reporting her uncle's abuse. "It's good you told. Someone has to help you. You did the right thing." Another time she says, "You need to stop hurting yourself. It doesn't do any good. I used to cut myself and all that, but it doesn't do any good, so I stopped." If only she could follow her own advice.

In one group, Laura, another group member, has been eloquently sharing techniques she learned in another hospital to help with symptoms of trauma. We have been talking a lot in this group, and I feel it is time to play music to try and integrate any feelings that may accompany these thoughts. As soon as I mention music, Beth slams her hand against the drum. Laura immediately slams her hand on a drum near her. I quickly grab chords on the piano to match their intensity. I want them to feel validated, that their rage or strong feelings are heard and honored. I attempt to create a structure to contain the sound, supporting a basic beat. Then I begin to create musical phrases supported by harmonies on the piano. They hear me and, I think, feel how the music is holding them. This sense of holding allows them to play with these emotions, expressing the unspeakable, harnessed into a musical form that is manageable. It is clear that there is a split between their intellectual understanding of trauma and their underlying rage and feeling out of control. With the music, we are trying to integrate these different aspects.

Now Beth is on the upswing and staying in a residence outside of the hospital. She is returning once a week to the music–verbal therapy trauma group. After several weeks she returns to the group in complete silence, locked inside herself. This withdrawal goes on for several weeks. She travels back from her residence, only to be silent for the whole group. On the third week I escort her from downstairs, again in silence. She sits near the piano and before we formally open the group, Beth reaches over and plays a note on the piano. Without a word, I play a note back. She plays another note, and we go back and forth playing random notes. Soon she bursts out laughing, and so do I. The music has helped her break out of her silent prison and return to us.

As the group progresses she opens up verbally about what is happening in her life—the challenges and the anger she is feeling. She describes her hopelessness at being able to change destructive patterns. As she describes a challenging situation, the group helps her to see that she actually said "no" to her potential abusers. After this intense discussion, she is eager to play a musical improvisation that I initiate and that appears to provide release for the whole group, given members' eagerness to join in.

Today, Beth is feeling well and eager. I suddenly notice, as she tries out a song for the holiday show, that she is singing on key. Her range has opened—the notes can travel into her chest and up in her throat. I have been so used to her voice that I thought she couldn't match the notes, so I hadn't thought about it much. But here she is singing "The Greatest Love of All." "I found the greatest love of all inside of me"—all the words memorized and the melody right there—not perfect, but there—a sign of a deeper healing. Something is changing.

In one session, we are singing the "Don't Want No More" song that I put together based on a traditional spiritual using A-minor, D-minor, and E-major. The minor key creates a feeling of openness, and the rather lilting melody can convey a sort of contained sadness—or, if played with more drive, can convey a stronger feeling, even anger. It can be sung fairly slowly but has a rhythm that carries it along. Beth sings, "Don't want no more suffering . . . suffering . . . suffering." The group joins her, "Don't want no more suffering," as she resolves it as, "I want to be happy instead." And then Beth begins another lyric with a different tone of voice, "Don't want no more tears . . . tears . . . tears." We follow, expanding this feeling, and Beth resolves it into, "I want Jesus to be happy." My mind conjures up the image of the *Pieta* with Jesus in Mary's arms after the crucifixion. But simultaneously, I imagine images of the baby Jesus in the manger. In Beth's world, even the "Great Comforter" has to be taken care of.

Soon it's time to end the group. I ask the members what song they would like to end the group with. One of the quieter members of the group mumbles something. "What is it?" "La Bamba," she answers. I decide to go with this suggestion. The upbeat rhythm of this song and its familiarity make it perfect for moving us from inner reflection to creating boundaries. The familiar verses and the predictable chorus create safety. The laughter connects us together and prepares everyone to leave the group and join the rest of the community. "*Para bailar la bamba.* . . . In order to dance *la bamba* you need a little grace, a little grace for me, for you and onward, onward *arriba, arriba!*"

Over the years, we have been able to witness how music can assist trauma survivors in their healing process. In reviewing this vignette, we can see many of the symptoms of trauma and how the needs of these survivors of severe, prolonged trauma can be addressed through music.

The first encounter with the music therapist is a consultation. Here the music therapist is able to assess the strengths and needs of the client and to begin to form a relationship. In an assessment, the music therapist is able to

> observe and interpret the ways in which the client uses the musical media available to him or her and consequently identify treatment goals from within the musical media themselves. Second, it allows the therapist to make some determination about the actual music therapy experiences that will be most beneficial for the client. (Meadows, Wheeler, Shultis, & Polen, 2005, p. 29)

"The central task of the first stage [of recovery] is the establishment of safety" (Herman, 1992, p. 155). In the first music therapy meeting with Beth, safety is created in the staffing, the choice of instruments, and the containment that occurs in supporting her music, and with the therapist's use of chords and predictable rhythmic patterns on the guitar. Safety then continues to be conveyed in the group through (1) the establishment of routines such as the check-in song; (2) the presence of two coleaders (one of whom can assist if a client is experiencing difficulties); (3) not speaking of the specifics of the trauma, but rather leaving that to individual therapy when he or she is ready; (4) creating a closing song; and (5) validating affect through musical improvisation supported by the therapist. Herman (1992) also emphasizes the role of relationship in the healing process:

> Recovery can take place only within the context of relationships; it cannot occur in isolation. In her renewed connections with other people, the survivor re-creates the psychological faculties that were damaged or deformed by the traumatic experience. These faculties include the basic capacities for trust, autonomy, initiative, competence, identity, and intimacy (Erikson). Just as these capabilities are originally formed in relationship with other people, they must be reformed in such relationships. (p. 133)

In the music therapy consultation, we can see the beginnings of establishing a healthy relationship, evident in the playfulness of the musical interaction. Beth is able to sing and play to create connection instead of making contact and feeling heard by lashing out uncontrollably and needing to be bodily restrained. Within the music–verbal therapy group the client can continue this work in the company of other trauma survivors, through music and words. The predictable rhythms, phrases, and forms (e.g., verse and refrain) of music, in addition to a feeling of safety, help survivors modulate their emotions during hyperaroused states.

The physicality of playing an instrument or singing helps with grounding and, with the support of the music therapist, assists the client in returning to the present from a dissociated state, often helping to decrease numbing and flashbacks. Words are used to share specifics of the trauma survivors' current life experiences, to recognize destructive patterns, and to articulate strategies for change. Words of encouragement from peers help to instill feelings of hope for the future.

When Beth continues to return to the hospital after discharge, we see an example of what seems to be dissociation and how music therapy is able to use musical *play* to recreate a connection and help Beth return to the present to tell her story. She moves from hopelessness to empowerment through the integration of words and music in the music–verbal therapy trauma group, first making contact through the playful music, then being able to verbally share the details of her struggle to negotiate the challenges of functioning in the community and her feelings of hopelessness. Her peers and the group leaders then reframe her story and, finally, her emotions and those of the group are integrated through a musical improvisation, without having to shut down.

We can see how Beth is able to work on healing the split between her words and feelings in her improvisations with one of the group members who is verbally proficient but affectively disconnected. Sutton (2002) explains this process:

> Feeling grounded in one's own body while processing and assimilating the emotional impact of traumatic experience is accessible when one is musically engaged with a therapist. . . . Music offers experiences of ourselves as embodied in sound and in silence. . . . In this way, access to the medium of music in a spontaneous yet boundaried environment can be of use to those traumatized. (p. 35)

This grounding is also evident in the change in Beth's singing voice. In this re-gard, Austin (2008) notes: "Recovering one's true voice requires re-inhabiting the body. . . . Cutting off the breath by constricting the throat, chest or abdomen can sever the connection to feelings and dramatically affect the quality of the speaking and singing voice" (pp. 24–25). And: "The process of finding one's voice, one's own sound, is a metaphor for finding one's self" (p. 21).

In Beth's work in the music–verbal therapy trauma group we can see how the combination of words and music is used. Nolan (2005) articulates the value of the musical–verbal component: "Verbal processing may contribute toward client awareness of internal sensations, feelings and thoughts related to external events and relationships, as well as . . . therapist understanding of the affective, cognitive and relational material which surfaces during musical experiences in music therapy" (p. 8).

In the final segment of the "Don't Want No More Suffering" song, we see that in music, when we sing words, we can move beyond the shell of the word itself into the expression within it. We go to the essence of the word without needing to describe, explain, or justify its meaning. As group members join in this expression, they have room to bring themselves into the word and also experience the release, as seen in Beth's example. And most importantly, music can give voice to the unspeakable.

> [Music] frequently offers the only bridge from . . . inner world to outer reality. It may provide the only means to give expression, in a safe way, to inner feelings. . . . The therapist is not so much concerned with the forms or refinements of the medium, as with its use as a vehicle by which inner reality can come to the surface, and be heard and experienced and examined in the light of day. (Tyson, 2004, p. 250)

Finally, we see the need for closure following Beth's singing of "Don't Want No More Suffering." In Borczon's (1997) words, "The conclusion of any session . . . must not be too abrupt, since the clients may have been experiencing many different levels of emotion, and with these experiences there must be a sense of closure before the sessions ends" (p. 27).

CLINICAL EXAMPLE:
Critical Improvisation:
Connecting with a Client in an Acute State

I am gathering the patients for my music therapy group on the admissions programming area. As I walk down the hall, I hear a man screaming. He has come to the unit agitated and is now sitting alone in an empty, tile-floor room, making his shouts echo all over the unit. "No! No! No! Can't! Can't! Can't! Trapped! Trapped! Angry! Angry! Angry!"

The sound of his voice causes a shiver to run down my spine, and I quickly pass the door, trying to be invisible. I close the music therapy door as quickly as I can. The group members are already seated around the table with the usual instruments—tambourines, maracas, cabasa, xylimbas, and small drums. The congas are also there. I take my guitar and face the group. The piano is behind me. I begin the check-in song, singing hello and asking how each one is, with the group reflecting it back.

At this point Omar, who has been a regular client member in the men's music–verbal therapy trauma group, arrives at the door with this man shouting behind him, "No! No! No! Angry! Angry! Angry!" Omar announces, "This man needs music therapy!" I try to calm myself by taking a few deep breaths and go to the door, hoping I can dissuade him. "I don't think he's ready for group," I say. Omar insists, "You need to help him. He needs music therapy." I am thinking, "This is wonderful—such a validation!—if only I were not so afraid!" I negotiate, "OK, Omar, I'll try to work with him—but only of you stay in the group to help me." Omar is built like a football player. He is stunned and a little chagrined. He obviously was not planning to attend music therapy today. But he agrees, "OK." He guides Robert into the room. Robert is still shouting, but I forge ahead, trying to get a word in as Robert stops shouting momentarily. "In this group sometimes we sing a song." I was thinking of

"Here Comes the Sun" or "I Can See Clearly Now," I say, strumming chords on the guitar. I am trying to shift his focus with the sound and rhythm of the guitar. At the same time, I am trying to find a song to engage him—something contemporary from his youth and with a clear beat that might move him from his agitated loop. I decide to go in this direction rather than to try and mirror his agitation in the music, which I am feeling might add to his distress at this time.

He starts screaming again but manages "can see clearly," so I try and play it, while he continues shouting. Then he bangs the drum with all his might. I wonder if he is going to break the drum or pick it up and throw it. He hits the drum hard again. Finally I say, "Don't break the drum." Omar puts his arm over the drum, and Robert, unseeing, hits Omar's arm once and then appears to realize what he has done and stops. Looking at me, Omar says, "It's all right." Robert quiets down for a moment, then says, "They're after me! It's not safe! I'm in trouble with the law. I'm in trouble!" I say, "We try to make this room safe. It's safe here in this room." Robert says, "How can it be safe? It's not safe!" I say, "It's safe because we have rules—three rules: no throwing instruments, no hitting anyone, and respect everyone." Robert looks a little relieved. He has stopped shouting. Pedro, another client, leans over to him and says, "You know, today is the first day of the rest of your life." I focus on other clients now. "Is there anything you would like to do in music?" Pedro answers, "Can you play the song from 'Lady Sings the Blues'?" I play it, and soon it is time to end. I thank everyone for their generosity. And truly I am impressed by how much they have come together to help this desperate man.

In later sessions when Robert, continuing to be agitated, tries to pound the xylimba with his fists, the group members help me to offer him the mallets, while I hurriedly grab my guitar to try and entrain this agitated sound into music. As he hears the pounding of the mallets becoming musical notes, supported by the guitar or piano and the instruments of other group members, he appears to be captivated by the sound, is able to create a musical improvisation, and ends by smiling. He begins to recognize music therapy as a place to calm down and express himself both verbally and musically. One day he looks straight at me and says "You have empathy!" Another client replies, "She is *not* your enemy!"

In an acute setting, where one often finds clients like Robert, it is essential that the therapist be willing to communicate more with music than with words. Often the sound of the music can change the mood or short-circuit a loop or transform an angry interaction, giving the therapist a chance to support a common group rhythm or to set some rules. For this client in the acute state, I would like to return to the essential relationship in music therapy with this population. As stated by Stewart (2002), the aims are:

- To provide an experience of consistency, reliability, structure and boundary
- To provide opportunities for primarily non-verbal communication, play and relating
- To provide an experience of transformed self and self–other relationships through shared musical play
- To help develop an experience of trust, cohesion and belonging
- To provide an experience of being listened and responded to and thought about. (p. 32)

Robert is able to feel heard and to begin to listen to others and recognize, through the structured musical work, that he is an accepted and respected part of the group.

It is gratifying to see the dramatic changes that can take place in the moment, allowing a severely distressed person to get relief and to be able to feel safe.

Applications to Other Disciplines

The most important point in conducting music therapy is recognizing the value of collaboration. In Edgar's case, the social worker and I communicated closely from our different perspectives about his reactions and feelings in regard to discharge.

A discharge plan was created that was in harmony with his emotional, creative, and empowerment needs. The discharge of this person who was institutionalized so long became a success.

In the music–verbal therapy trauma group, we see an ongoing collaboration of the two coleaders (music therapist and psychologist), weaving an effective dance of words and music, creating a safe space and sharing techniques. This collaboration can extend beyond a single coleader to a team, allowing for a variety of modalities, including other creative arts therapies, to help individuals find expression for difficult emotions, and providing possibilities for the group members to heal from deep trauma (Muenzenmaier, Margolis, et al., in press).

In Robert's story, the referral comes in an unusual way—from another client—who recognizes the power of music from his own experience in a music–verbal therapy trauma group. He collaborates, or rather insists, that I take on this case, which ultimately brings Robert, through music, to a place of order that helps calm his inner storm.

I am reminded by my cotherapist in the music–verbal trauma group, psychologist Faye Margolis, of the story of the blind men and the elephant. Each touches a different part of the elephant, and each thinks they know the elephant. As both verbal and nonverbal clinicians are able to integrate our knowledge and techniques, we are more fully able to understand and meet the real needs of people with a diagnosis of mental illness (Faye Margolis, personal communication, November 15, 2012).

Conclusions

These three clinical examples are just a sampling of the ways in which music therapy attempts to reach adults with mental illness. As can be seen, music is used in many ways. With Edgar, the emphasis is on using his love for the guitar as a channel to connect him to the physical world and eventually to others around him, and his playing in a band and performing for an audience giving him a feeling of self-esteem and purpose. With Beth, we see how the latest understanding of trauma work helps to understand and inform her treatment through music, creating safety, and helping her to regulate her emotions through steady, predictable rhythms and phrases, and the opportunity to express in music what she is unable to express in words alone. With Robert, we see the faster-paced work of meeting in music a person who is in an acutely troubled state—where there may only be a few sessions of treatment, where the music therapist has to be more directive and set more limits, and where music is used to engage more extreme forms of behavior. We see how the sound of the music can sometimes cut through an agitated state and create a pattern that can carry someone along.

In my years of working as a music therapist, although I am often a witness to great pain and hopelessness, still I am able to experience the healing power of music, not just in the people I work with but within myself as well. Since the work of music therapy requires the therapist to enter into the music, I experience the healing myself in every session. "[Music] has a unique power to express inner states and feelings. . . . And there is, finally, a deep mysterious paradox here, for while music makes one experience pain and grief more intensely, it brings solace and consolation at the same time" (Sacks, 2007, pp. 300–301).

REFERENCES

American Psychiatric Association. (2013). *Diagnostic and statistical manual of mental disorders* (5th ed.). Arlington, VA: Author.

Ansdell, G. (2002). Community music therapy and the winds of change. *Voices: A World Forum for Music Therapy, 2*(2). Retrieved from *https://normt.uib.no/index.php/voices/article/view/83/65.*

Austin, D. (2008). *The theory and practice of of vocal psychotherapy: Songs of self.* London: Jessica Kingsley.

Borczon, R. M. (1997). *Music therapy: Group vignettes.* Gilsum, NH: Barcelona.

Borczon, R., Jampel, P., & Langdon, G. (2010). Music therapy with adult survivors of trauma. In K. Stewart (Ed.), *Music therapy and trauma: Bridging theory and clinical practice* (pp. 101–127). New York: Satchnote Press.

Bruscia, K. (1987). *Improvisational models of music therapy.* Springfield, IL: Charles C Thomas.

Crowe, B. J., & Colwell, C. (2007). *Music therapy for children, adolescents, and adults with mental disorders.* Silver Spring, MD: American Music Therapy Association.

Doidge, N. (2007). *The brain that changes itself.* New York: Penguin Books.

Eyre, L. (Ed.). (2013). *Guidelines for music therapy practice: Mental health of adolescents and adults.* Gilsum, NH: Barcelona.

Herman, J. (1992). *Trauma and recovery.* New York: Basic Books.

Jampel, P. (2006). *Performance in music therapy with mentally ill adults* (Doctoral dissertation). Available from ProQuest Dissertations and Theses database (UMI No. 3235696).

Levitin, D. J. (2006). *This is your brain on music.* New York: Penguin Books.

Longden, E. (2013). Listening to voices. *Scientific American Mind, 24*(4), 34–39.

Meadows, T., Wheeler, B. L., Shultis, C. L., & Polen, D. W. (2005). Client assessment. In B. L. Wheeler, C. L. Shultis, & D. W. Polen (Eds.), *Clinical training guide for the student music therapist* (pp. 27–56). Gilsum, NH: Barcelona.

Muenzenmaier, K., Castille, D. M., Shelley, A.-M., Jamison, A., Battaglia, J., Opler, L. A., et al. (2005). Comorbid posttraumatic stress disorder and schizophrenia. *Psychiatric Annals, 35*(1), 51–56.

Muenzenmaier, K., Margolis, F., Langdon, G. S., Kóbayashi, T., Rhodes, D., & Rifkin, L. (in press). Transcending bias in diagnosis and treatment for women with serious mental illness. *Women and Therapy.*

Muenzenmaier, K., Schneeberger, A., Castille, D., Battaglia, J., Seixas, A., & Link, B. (2014). Stressful childhood experiences and clinical outcomes in people with serious mental illness: A gender comparison in a clinical psychiatric sample. *Journal of Family Violence, 29,* 419–429.

Nolan, P. (2005). Verbal processing within the music therapy relationship. *Music Therapy Perspectives, 23*(1), 18–28.

Romme, M., Escher, S., Dillon, J., Corstens, D., & Morris, M. (2009). *Living with voices: 50 stories of recovery.* Herefordshire, UK: PCCS Books.

Sacks, O. (2007). *Musicophilia.* New York: Knopf.

Stephens, G. (1983). The use of improvisation for developing relatedness in the adult client. *Music Therapy, 3*(1), 29–42.

Stewart, D. (2002). Sound company: Psychodynamic group music therapy as facilitating environment, transformational object and therapeutic playground. In A. Davies & E. Richards (Eds.), *Music therapy and group work: Sound company* (pp. 27–42). London: Jessica Kingsley.

Stige, B., & Aarø, L. E. (2012). *Invitation to community music therapy.* New York: Routledge.

Sutton, J. P. (2002). Trauma: Trauma in context. In J. P. Sutton (Ed.), *Music, music therapy and trauma* (pp. 21–39). London: Jessica Kingsley.

Tyson, F. (2004). Guidelines toward the organization of clinical music therapy programs in the community. In M. McGuire (Ed.), *Psychiatric music therapy in the community: The legacy of Florence Tyson* (pp. 243–252). Gilsum, NH: Barcelona.

van der Kolk, B. A. (2006). Clinical implications of neuroscience research in PTSD. *Annals of the New York Academy of Sciences, 1071*, 277–293.

Wheeler, B. L., Shultis, C. L., & Polen, D. W. (2005). *Clinical training guide for the student music therapist.* Gilsum, NH: Barcelona.

CHAPTER 28

Music Therapy in Addictions Treatment

Kathleen M. Murphy

Addiction is defined as a chronic, relapsing brain disease characterized by compulsive drug seeking and use, despite harmful consequences" (National Institute on Drug Abuse, 2012, p. 5). Persistent drug and/or alcohol use has been found to change the structure and functioning of the brain. These changes, which disrupt the way critical brain structures interact to control and inhibit behaviors, can be long-lasting and are thought to lead to the persistent, repetitive, and often self-destructive behaviors associated with addiction (National Institute on Drug Abuse, 2012).

A diagnosis of *substance-related disorder* is given when individuals have an intense need to use alcohol or drugs that gradually takes over their life (American Psychiatric Association, 2013). Most recent estimates indicate that 22.2 million Americans, age 12 or older, are classified with substance dependence or abuse disorders (Substance Abuse and Mental Health Services Administration, 2012). Ten classes of substances are included in this group of disorders, which is divided into two categories: substance use disorders and substance induced disorders (American Psychiatric Association, 2013). A diagnosis of substance use disorder is used to describe a state of chronic relapse and compulsive drug taking (American Psychiatric Association, 2013). Substance use disorders range from mild to severe. Substance induced disorders include "intoxication, withdrawal, and other substance/medication-induced mental disorders" (American Psychiatric Association, 2013, p. 227). A complete list of substance-related disorders is found in Table 28.1.

Clientele

Individuals who enter substance abuse treatment are often broken—physically, mentally, emotionally, and spiritually. Every aspect of their life has been affected—family, school, work, and community—often leading to unemployment, homelessness, and a life of crime. At some point, those who abuse sub-

TABLE 28.1. DSM-5 Substance-Related Disorders

- Alcohol-related disorders
- Caffeine-related disorders
- Cannabis-related disorders
- Cocaine-related disorders
- Hallucinogen-related disorders
- Inhalant-related disorders
- Opioid-related disorders
- Sedative-, hypnotic-, or anxiolytic-related disorders
- Stimulant-related disorders
- Tobacco-related disorders

stances may *hit bottom*, becoming *sick and tired of being sick and tired* (a commonly stated reason by those in treatment) and voluntarily enter treatment. More often than not, though, those who abuse substances do not enter treatment voluntarily; they are usually pushed into treatment as a result of an intervention by family, employers, friends, or the legal system (Straussner, 2004). Relapse, picking up the drug of choice after a period of abstinence, may also motivate individuals to enter treatment.

Substance abuse treatment occurs across a continuum of settings with the focus of treatment changing in each phase, beginning with detoxification. *Detoxification* is defined as "a set of interventions aimed at managing acute intoxication and withdrawal" (Center for Substance Abuse Treatment, 2006, p. 4). In this phase of recovery, individuals may experience uncomfortable withdrawal symptoms such as severe depression, increased agitation and restlessness, nausea, sweating, anxiety, and/or agitation. These symptoms are caused by the brain's reaction to the cessation or drastic reduction of the abused substance (National Institute on Drug Abuse, 2012). In addition to these physical symptoms, unpleasant feelings, many of which have been suppressed by the substance of choice, may surface or worsen.

From detoxification, individuals will move into *rehabilitation*, which takes place in an inpatient and/or outpatient treatment setting. This phase of treatment focuses on (1) education about addiction and the disease process; (2) the development of healthy coping skills; (3) the importance of Alcoholics Anonymous (AA), Narcotics Anonymous (NA), or other self-help groups; and (4) personal care. The last phase of treatment is *relapse prevention*, which helps the client move from a structured treatment environment to an unstructured outpatient environment. The focus on treatment in this phase is applying the principles and techniques for sober living that were presented in treatment, including increased awareness of and response to relapse warning signs, managing cravings and triggers, and identifying and using supportive resources (Gray & Gibson, 2004).

Clinical Work

Goals

Because of the widespread effects of addiction, treatment needs to be multifaceted, focusing on (1) the addictive process; (2) development of a social support network; (3) physical, cognitive, mental, and spiritual issues related to recovery; (4) the physiological effects of addiction; and (5) the healing of the body and mind (Borling, 2011). Music therapists need to consider these areas when working in substance abuse treatment settings. Borling recommends a treatment approach that addresses the biophysical, psychoemotional, and psychospiritual issues related to recovery. It should be noted that, although each of these areas is discussed in a linear fashion here, treatment does not progress in that manner. When planning music therapy experiences, the music therapist should always ask: "What does the client need from the music today?" It may be the case that a client in the late stages of recovery needs to focus on relaxation and ways to address physical tension. Conversely, a client in early recovery may need to work on spiritual issues.

Biophysical

Physical recovery is the first hurdle in addictions treatment. The brain and the body need to heal from prolonged substance abuse. Withdrawal from substances is usually accompanied by uncomfortable physical and emotional symptoms (see Table 28.2). These symptoms, which usually are the opposite of those observed when the client is under the influence, often lead to cravings and, in some cases, relapse (American Psychiatric Association, 2013). Most acute withdrawal symptoms resolve within 14 days; however, many individuals experience protracted withdrawal, also known as postacute withdrawal. Protracted withdrawal includes the continued presence of withdrawal symptoms as well as "*non*-substance-specific signs and symptoms that persist, evolve, or appear well past the expected timeframe for acute withdrawal" (Center for Substance Abuse Treatment, 2010, p. 2; see Table 28.3).

Typical music therapy goals for physical recovery include strategies for managing withdrawal symptoms, relaxation and

TABLE 28.2. Physical and Emotional Withdrawal Symptoms

Physical symptoms

- Sweating
- Racing heart
- Palpitation
- Muscle tension
- Tightness in the chest
- Difficulty breathing
- Tremor
- Nausea, vomiting, diarrhea

Emotional symptoms

- Anxiety
- Restlessness
- Irritability
- Insomnia
- Headaches
- Poor concentration
- Depression
- Social isolation

TABLE 28.3. Possible Symptoms of Protracted Withdrawal

- Anxiety
- Sleep difficulties
- Problems with short-term memory
- Alcohol or drug cravings
- Impaired executive control
- Anhedonia
- Difficulty focusing on tasks
- Irritability
- Unexplained physical complaints
- Unexplained physical complaints
- Reduced interest in sex

Note. From Center for Substance Abuse Treatment (2010, p. 4).

stress management techniques, and education about the importance of incorporating these techniques into daily life (Borling, 2011). Increased pain perception and insomnia are also common withdrawal symptoms, regardless of the substance used. Education on nonpharmacological methods to manage pain and sleep difficulties, and techniques to improve sleep hygiene, are additional goals to be addressed (Murphy, 2010).

Psychoemotional

Once detoxification is complete, emotional issues that were suppressed by substances may begin to surface. These symptoms, including depression, anxiety, anger, and other problems in living, may also be indicative of an underlying mental illness (Center for Substance Abuse Treatment, 2010). Cognitive strategies that were used to maintain a distance from the addiction, such as denial, rationalizing, and minimizing, may also be exposed as individuals move through the recovery process (Borling, 2011). Goals for this level of recovery include becoming aware of and starting to change faulty thinking, working through denial, increasing self-esteem, making choices and behavioral changes, acceptance of unmanageability and powerlessness, decreased isolation, increased emotional exploration and expression, ability to use a support system, and increased authenticity and honesty (Borling, 2011, 2012).

Psychospiritual

Addiction is a disease of the mind, body, and spirit; however, central to sustained recovery is *spiritual healing* and adoption of spiritual principles (Alcoholics Anonymous World Services, 2001). In addiction treatment, spirituality is related to the search for meaning. Jung believed that addiction resulted when a habit replaced the spiritual center and that spirituality might be the best solution for individuals who are addicted to drugs and/or alcohol (Sandoz, 2001).

Spirituality is the cornerstone of 12-step recovery programs. In Alcoholics Anonymous, spiritual awakenings are considered to be the mechanism of change (Alcoholics Anonymous World Services, 2001). Recovery involves transformation. Working through the steps facilitates movement through this transformative process as individuals in recovery strive to (1) turn their lives over to a higher power of their understanding, (2) ask for removal of character defects, and (3) seek to know and carry out the will of their higher power through prayer and meditation. It is important to remember that one's higher power does not have to be the "God of the Churches" (Borling, 2011, p. 345), though it can be. AA reminds those in recovery that they do not have to "consider another's conception of God" (Alcoholics Anonymous World Services, 2001, p. 46). The emphasis is on one's willingness to believe in something greater than the self, in whatever form that may take. Music therapists need to be open and accepting, encouraging clients to explore their spiritual beliefs in order to define their higher power. Additional psychospiritual goals addressed in music therapy include making meaning of one's life, forgiveness, self-acceptance, and understanding true freedom.

Summary

These goal areas have been delineated as a means of describing the aims of music therapy in substance abuse treatment and not as a means of prescribing a treatment process that will lead to sobriety. Music can affect the body, mind, and spirit simultaneously; clients may have a *spiritual awakening* or experience a decrease in anxiety during a drumming experience that was chosen as a means to reduce physical tension or build community. Music therapists should be open to work with *whatever the music experience brings up*, in whatever goal area seems to be primary. It is also important for music therapists to be familiar with AA/NA principles and steps so they can engage clients in music experiences that will facilitate a deeper awareness and understanding of true recovery.

Music Therapy Methods

Re-Creational Methods

The performance of precomposed music is the earliest use of music therapy reported in the literature. These early reports describe the benefits of performance groups for those in substance abuse treatment (e.g., Miller, 1970). Re-creative methods (Bruscia, 1998a) (the use of precomposed songs or instrumental music) are used to address biophysical (i.e., using musical performance as a way to channel and release physical tension) and psychoemotional (i.e., promoting sober fun, improving mood, socialization) goals. Therapeutic sing-alongs—those that are goal-directed or focused on a theme related to recovery—are often used in early recovery to develop group cohesion and tolerance of others. In later stages, they can be used as a means to identify and communicate feelings (Murphy, 2013).

CLINICAL EXAMPLE

"Singing for the Soul" is a therapeutic vocal re-creation group that I've conducted in a short-term residential treatment program. The goals were to (1) provide clients with an opportunity to engage in a creative experience within a supportive environment, (2) increase tolerance for the music preferences of others, (3) improve mood and attitude, and (4) experience the benefits of group singing. Participants took turns choosing songs with a positive or uplifting theme for the group to perform. Clients who were musicians, or I, provided live musical accompaniment. All group members were encouraged to participate in whatever way felt comfortable. Levels of participation included listening, playing handheld percussion instruments, singing, and/or dancing. The group ended with participants sharing their experiences and describing any physical, mental, emotional, and spiritual effects related to the music experience. This was followed by a brief psychoeducational discussion on the benefits of singing in recovery.

Receptive Methods

Receptive methods are those in which the client listens and responds (verbally, nonverbally, or through another medium) to live or prerecorded music verbally (Bruscia, 1998a). These methods are used to address biophysical, psychoemotional, and psychospiritual goals across all stages of substance abuse treatment. The receptive methods most commonly used in substance abuse treatment are described in the following material.

MUSIC-ASSISTED RELAXATION

Music-assisted relaxation (MAR), with or without imagery, is used for stress reduction, anxiety management, meditation, and spiritual development. MAR (i.e., music listening combined with progressive muscle relaxation or stretching) is commonly used to address biophysical goals related to recovery, which include decreasing physical

tension and stress. The music used should be 3–7 minutes in length, have a lyrical melody, predictable harmony, minimal dynamic changes, and tempo between 58 beats per minute (bpm) and 78 bpm. Music considered New Age or environmental generally works best for clients in detoxification or the early stages of recovery.

MOVEMENT

Movement, both structured and improvisational, is used to address biophysical goals related to recovery, including releasing physical tension and connecting to one's physical body (Borling, 2012; Gardstrom, Carlini, Josefczyk, & Love, 2013). Structured movement (e.g., line dances, therapist-created movement sequences) may add some levity and light-heartedness to treatment as clients attempt to perform the movement sequences (Gardstrom et al.). Psychoemotional goals such as physically feeling the weight of negative emotions and letting go of unwanted feelings can also be addressed through movement experiences (Gardstrom et al.). In early recovery, clients may be reluctant to move, due to decreased energy levels, increased fatigue, and muscle aches. Music therapists should take this possibility into consideration and use movement experiences that match the energy and ability levels of the clients.

DISCUSSIONS

Song discussions are used to address psychoemotional and psychospiritual goals. As noted by Bruscia (1998b), songs "express who we are and how we feel . . . they articulate our beliefs and values" (p. 9). Songs are useful in recovery because they describe life experiences cognitively (lyrics) and emotionally (music). Songs can unfreeze emotions, at times bringing the most stoic client to tears. The emotional response may be related to the personal meaning a client ascribes to the lyrics, to an emotional state, or to a memory. Verbal processing after a song can help clients reconnect with and learn from their emotions. Using open-ended questions that focus on the feelings and the body, as opposed to thoughts, can help to draw a client deeper into the experience, giving access to his or her emotional world.

In early recovery, songs can be used to develop a therapeutic relationship between client and therapist or among group members. Listening to music in a group puts few demands on participants yet opens the door for relationship building. Song discussions often provide opportunities for group members to share their stories and come to the realization that they are not alone in their recoveries.

In all stages of recovery, songs can be used to explore and/or gain new perspectives on concepts related to the 12 steps (see Table 28.4), such as powerlessness, unmanageability, and surrender. Issues related to recovery, such as denial, change, empowerment, self-esteem, shame, and guilt, can also be addressed through song discussion. The most powerful songs are those in which the music matches the emotional tone of the lyrics. As an example, the song "Addicted" (sung by Kelly Clarkson) may be considered a musical and lyrical portrait of the unmanageability and powerlessness that is the hallmark of active addiction. Each stanza of the song focuses on a different aspect of these two concepts. Clients experiencing intense cravings often choose the lyrics that describe the incessant intruding thoughts that are then attributed to their experiences of powerlessness. Other clients choose lyrics from the bridge as representative of the false promises they make to themselves or others about entering treatment or ending their substance misuse.

Finally, clients are often reminded of the lies and false promises they make to themselves and others about entering treatment or ending their substance misuse after listening to "Addicted:"

Recovery requires a transition from a destructive lifestyle to one that is healthy and fulfilling. Songs can be used to help

TABLE 28.4. The 12 Steps of Alcoholics Anonymous

1. We admitted we were powerless over alcohol—that our lives had become unmanageable.
2. Came to believe that a Power greater than ourselves could restore us to sanity.
3. Made a decision to turn our will and our lives over to the care of God *as we understood Him.*
4. Made a searching and fearless moral inventory of ourselves.
5. Admitted to God, to ourselves, and to another human being the exact nature of our wrongs.
6. Were entirely ready to have God remove all these defects of character.
7. Humbly asked Him to remove our shortcomings.
8. Made a list of all persons we had harmed, and became willing to make amends to them all.
9. Made direct amends to such people wherever possible, except when to do so would injure them or others.
10. Continued to take personal inventory and when we were wrong promptly admitted it.
11. Sought through prayer and meditation to improve our conscious contact with God, *as we understood Him*, praying only for knowledge of His will for us and the power to carry that out.
12. Having had a spiritual awakening as the result of these Steps, we tried to carry this message to alcoholics, and to practice these principles in all our affairs.

Note. From *www.aa.org/en_pdfs/smf-121_en.pdf.* Copyright by AA World Services, Inc. Reprinted by permission.

clients move from contemplating change to actually making a change. "In the Journey" (Martin Sexton) is a musical recounting of all that can be lost, and the accompanying sense of regret and despair that will be experienced if one does not change. "I Choose" (Indie Arie), on the other hand, is an uplifting and motivating song whose lyrics describe the decision to make a positive change. Used in tandem, these songs can serve as a decisional balance tree, helping clients to understand the outcomes of choices that are made on both a cognitive and emotional level.

Song dedications are used to bring closure to treatment, especially in longer-term

(90+ day) programs, where relationships between clients have begun to form. Clients are asked to bring in songs that convey a sense of hope and encouragement for a group member who is about to be discharged. The verbal discussion following the music listening gives all group members opportunities to authentically share their hopes and fears for the client who will be leaving. Additionally, group members are able to offer their gratitude for the support and encouragement that they received.

Songs are also used to help clients explore their relationship with their higher power. An example would be the lyrics from the song "Crossroads," sung by Don McLean. The lyrics and haunting melody help clients to get in touch with that part of themselves that is yearning for a relationship with a higher power and wish for forgiveness.

After listening to this song, clients would often comment that these lyrics reflected their prayer—that their higher power would heal them and take away their pain. Other clients would reflect on these lyrics to discuss how their feelings of shame and guilt prevented them from turning to their higher power for spiritual healing.

These are just a few examples of how songs that can be used to address psychoemotional and psychospiritual goals. Music therapists working in substance abuse treatment are encouraged to develop a song collection that includes music of varying genres and of styles reflective of 12-step principles and concepts.

IMAGERY

Imagery is incorporated into several receptive music listening experiences (see Murphy, 2013). The addition of imagery is indicated when addressing psychoemotional and psychospiritual goals. Imagery should be introduced when the clients are ready to have a "more direct, non-analytic encounter with [their] inner process" (Borling, 2012, p. 158). The use of imagery in

early recovery should be highly structured, therapist led, and goal directed. Supportive music that will not take a client too deeply into dynamic material is recommended (Borling, 2011).

Imagery is often incorporated into MAR experiences. In this instance the imagery serves to hold the client's attention, helping to minimize intrusion by distracting thoughts. For example, when working with women in a long-term recovery program, I often invited them to imagine themselves wrapped in a blanket, sitting/lying in a comfortable place and allowing the music to nurture their mind, body, and spirit. This nurturing imagery experience was used as a means of allowing the women to practice self-care. Initially many of the women felt guilty or self-indulgent. This reaction changed overtime as they came to understand the relationship between self-care and sobriety.

STRUCTURED IMAGERY

Structured imagery (Borling, 2011) is often used to address psychoemotional and psychospiritual goals. The imagery directives for this type of experience should be clear and direct and related to the intention of the group or client need. Imagery suggestions may be related to increased self-awareness, exploration of emotions, or relationship with a higher power. Music for these types of experiences should be supportive and stable, with some variations in tempo and dynamics to help stimulate imagery. The imagery experience may be followed with mandala drawing or writing to help clients consolidate their experience. The verbal discussion that follows helps clients to find personal meanings and make connections between the images and their recovery journey.

CLINICAL EXAMPLE

In one session I led, a client was not able to understand why an image of her dog appeared in response to the directive: "Let the music bring you an image that reflects a personal quality you possess that will be helpful in your recovery." During the discussion she reported that her dog loved her whether she was sober or drunk, and she wondered if her dog was a reminder that she needed to love herself in that same nonjudgmental way.

In another session focusing on one's higher power, a client came to the realization that his relationship with his higher power was a one-way street; that he did all the talking but never did any listening. In the following session, he reported a change in how he prayed, in that he took time to listen and just be in the presence of his higher power. This change from talking at, to being with, represented a shift in his understanding of the 11th step. He was able to share the impact this shift had in his daily work toward recovery.

Imagery work is not appropriate for all clients in that it involves moving into a non-ordinary or altered state of consciousness. Not all clients in substance abuse treatment have the ego strength or cognitive abilities to work in this way. Music therapists who want to use imagery should work under the supervision of a qualified supervisor. More advanced imagery techniques, including the Bonny Method of Guided Imagery and Music (BMGIM or GIM), should not be used unless the music therapist has completed the appropriate training and is receiving supervision.

Improvisational Methods

Instrumental (using untuned and tuned percussion instruments) and vocal improvisations are used to work on psychoemotional and psychospiritual issues. Typical goals include (1) exploration and communication of feelings/emotions, and (2) development of relationships, support, and opportunities for creative self-expression. Improvisations can be nonreferential (organized according to musical considerations) or referential (the music represents a given theme; Bruscia, 1987). Nonreferential improvisations often begin with a basic beat. Once the beat is established, one client can take a solo, while the rest of the group supports; rhythmic, dynamic, and temporal elements can be directed by the therapist or added in spontaneously by the clients. Referential improvisations can reflect such themes as acceptance, grief/loss, unmanageability, and "my recovery journey."

Improvisations require clients to observe, listen, respond, and give and receive feedback—behaviors that are not seen in active addiction, but that are necessary for long-term recovery. Improvisations can be used to identify or work through therapeutic issues. For example, when group members seem to be reluctant to verbally share what is going on, the session can begin with a free improvisation. When the music comes to its natural end, the therapist can ask clients for feedback on their playing, the group sound, feelings or images that came up, or to give the improvisation a title. During the discussion, the therapist should look for opportunities to make connections between the client's experiences and 12-step principles.

Improvisation can be used to help clients explore a range of emotions. One improvisation exercise I have found successful for this purpose incorporates poetry. The diamante (see Figure 28.1) works well, as this poetic form begins and ends with words that could be found on either end of a continuum, such as *relaxed* and *stressful*, or *calm* and *tense*. When the poem is completed, one group member reads it, while the remaining participants create an improvisation that reflects the movement from the opening word to its opposite.

Drumming can be used in early recovery to help manage withdrawal symptoms, especially restlessness and agitation. In all stages of recovery drumming can be used to release energy and help clients connect, or stay connected to, their physical body (Borling, 2011). The drumming experience can be highly structured by the therapist (e.g., call and response, variations on

A *diamante* is a seven-line poem that is arranged in a diamond pattern. It is a creative way to explore contrasts, opposites, and to identify solutions to problems. You will be working with your group members to create a diamante that identifies a common obstacle to recovery experienced by them and its opposite. Use the following format in creating your group's diamante:

- Line 1: One word to describe the obstacle
- Line 2: Two vivid adjectives describing the obstacle identified in line 1
- Line 3: Three interesting *-ing* action verbs that describe the obstacle in line 1
- Line 4: Two concrete nouns about the obstacle and two concrete nouns about the opposite of the obstacle
- Line 5: Three interesting *-ing* action verbs that describe the opposite of the obstacle identified in line 1
- Line 6: Two vivid adjectives describing the opposite of the obstacle identified in line 1
- Line 7: One word to describe the opposite of the obstacle

Create one or two sentences linking the obstacle to the solution, using the words from your diamante.

Example:
Stress
Useless, Persistent
Intruding, Interfering, Tantrumming
Gyro, Spiral, Sky, Ocean
Calming, Affirming, Energizing
Helpful, Grounded
Calm

Sentence:

Persistently stressing is useless. It is like a tantrum that intrudes and interferes, making me feel like my thoughts are like a gyro spiraling out of control. Focusing on the sky or the ocean is helpful in affirming, energizing, and grounding me, which leads to a feeling of calm.

FIGURE 28.1. Diamante guidelines.

a steady beat) or unstructured (e.g., clients play freely, entering, playing, and stopping as they see fit). For example, Dijkstra and Hakvoort (2010) use a highly structured sequence of drumming exercises to assess their clients' development of coping skills. On the other end of the spectrum, the drum circles tend to be less structured. They provide a music-making opportunity in which clients can give and receive support and give voice to feelings and emotions. Each client's musical contribution is accepted, similar to what happens in an AA meeting where each person who is seeking recovery is accepted. The various sounds and rhythms add to the richness of the music and also serve as a metaphor for living in community with others.

It is not uncommon for clients to experience a "high" or have a spiritual experience while drumming. Individuals who use drugs and alcohol often do so to change their conscious experience (Frye, 1990). Drumming (as well as other music therapy methods, such as structured imagery) can have the same effect on conscious experience as the use of illicit substances. These types of experiences provide an opening for the therapist to talk about healthy ways of changing consciousness and releasing tension and stress.

Compositional Methods

Compositional methods, in which the client creates a musical product (e.g., lyrics for a song), are used to address psychoemotional and psychospiritual goals. Songwriting is used to address goals such as creative self-expression, identification and exploration of therapeutic issues, collaboration and cooperation, frustration tolerance, and perseverance (working on the composition until it is completed). Typical methods of facilitating songwriting include lyric substitution, creating a new verse, setting newly composed lyrics to a precomposed melody, or creating both the lyrics and music. Regardless of which format is used for songwriting, clients should be encouraged to write lyrics related to their recovery journey and to share the newly created songs with the group. In the following example, group members identified the biophysical (body aches) and psychoemotional (feeling confused and lost) symptoms related to loss and grief as well as addictive behavior patterns (isolating) and fears (relapse):

> I'm feeling lost, like I'm no good to anyone
> My body aches and I'm so confused
> I'm isolating because it hurts so much
> I'm grieving; I'm afraid I'll relapse

Songwriting and subsequent sharing give clients the opportunity to practice honesty and risk taking in a supportive environment, as they authentically share their thoughts and feelings with others (Borling, 2011).

Putting It All Together

Within a music therapy group, it is likely that each member will be at a different place in his or her recovery, so choice of method should be based on the presenting needs of the group members in the present moment. The use of a *check-in* at the beginning of group can help inform the music therapist as to which music experiences will be most beneficial for the clients. Common check-in procedures include asking clients to identify (1) how they are feeling physically, mentally, emotionally, and spiritually in the moment,

or (2) what is getting in the way of their recovery. Clients can also be asked which type of music experience would be most helpful (e.g., "Which do you think would be most helpful for you today—songwriting or music and imagery?") or to pick a song that reflects their mood or that of the group. It is the responsibility of the therapist to make an in-the-moment determination of which music therapy method(s) will meet the needs of the group. Although scripted or manualized approaches may be useful in research, use of a decision-tree model (Eyre, 2008; Thompson, 2013) is recommended in real-world contexts, because it supports the immediate needs of the group and is congruent with client-centered treatment.

CLINICAL EXAMPLE

I led a music therapy session that incorporated drumming (improvisation), singing (re-creative), and verse completion (composition). The group members were having difficulty focusing on their treatment because they were distracted by outside concerns. The drumming was used to bring their attention into the present moment and to focus restless energy. The song "Three Little Birds" by Bob Marley was introduced when the group had established a groove, and clients were invited to sing along. Eventually, in a round robin style, each member was asked to fill in the phrase "I won't worry about _____," to which the group responded, "cuz every little thing will be alright." The music making was brought to an end with a rumble. At the conclusion of this experience, clients commented on how much better they felt and their surprise that "such a simple song" could turn their mood around.

Verbal processing of music experiences is used to integrate the client's experience, with recovery principles or themes from the 12 steps. This discussion can happen on three levels, depending upon the functioning level of the client and skill level of the therapist. The first level focuses on the music experience itself. At this level, the clients can be asked to comment on what stood out for them or what they noticed. Also at this level, they may be asked to notice any changes in physical tension, mood, or affect. The second level focuses on personal meanings or connections the clients may have found in relation to the music experience. The third level connects the thoughts, feelings, and actions seen in the music experience to healthy or addictive behaviors and/or to 12-step principles.

Applications to Other Disciplines

Individuals in substance abuse treatment often have an affinity for music, both live and prerecorded. Within residential substance abuse treatment facilities, opportunities should be made available for patients to listen to/create music. Both passive and active participation in recreational music can alleviate stress and improve mood. It is important for those in recovery to practice healthy coping skills during treatment, and scheduled times for recreational music making provide that opportunity. Addictions counselors are also encouraged to consult with music therapists for suggestions on how to incorporate music into relaxation and stress management sessions. Additionally, music therapists can assist in the development of listening libraries that can include music for relaxation, sleep, exercise, or leisure.

As in other clinical settings, music therapists function as a member of the multidisciplinary team and often are addressing similar goals as other team members. This offers opportunities for collaboration and co-treatment. Music experiences facilitated by the music therapist can be designed to uncover and explore issues related to addiction and recovery that could then be verbally processed further by the addiction counselor/social worker during group therapy. The opposite could also occur. In my experience, group therapists would often bring issues that came up in their verbal therapy groups and ask that they be explored further within the context of music therapy. Lastly, groups can be co-facilitated by a music therapist and other team member. Within this type of group, music experiences and verbal processes would be used to best meet the needs of the clients. As an example, when I was co-facilitating a group with the social worker, several of the group members identified having difficulties with "self-nurturing." I facilitated a structured imagery experience during which patients were guided through a "nurturing experience." The social worker and I then co-facilitated the discussion that followed the imagery experience.

Conclusions

As has been discussed, music therapy has a significant role in the treatment of substance use disorders. However, music can also have negative effects and lead to relapse (Horesch, 2010). Music evokes emotional and physical responses that may be related to actual drug use, negative experiences or emotions, or euphoric recall of intoxication (Horesch). For those in recovery, these responses can lead to cravings or feelings of shame, guilt, depression, or, in the case of euphoric recall, a sense that their use was not so bad after all.

Music listening can lead to self-isolation and withdrawal from a social network than can help support recovery. A recent study (Baker, Dingle, & Gleadhill, 2012) suggests that individuals with substance use disorders tend to view music listening as a private experience. Using music as a barrier or as a means of preventing meaningful connection with others can lead to a deepening of negative feelings and emotions or trigger cravings, both of which have the potential to lead to a relapse.

Therefore, the relationship between music and relapse needs to be addressed in treatment, and music listening habits may also need to be rehabilitated (Horesch,

2010). Horesch suggests that individuals in recovery pay attention to the music they listen to, as their choices may signal a relapse. In addition to addressing issues related to addiction, music therapists may also want to help their clients understand the benefits and dangers of music listening in recovery.

Music therapy, as an experiential therapy, offers individuals with substance use disorders a means to reconnect with their body, mind, and spirit. In order to do this, music therapists must be prepared to address treatment needs in each of these areas based on the presenting needs of the clients, understanding that each person's recovery journey will be different. Familiarity with AA/NA and the 12 steps provides a foundation for music therapists to develop meaningful music experiences that can help to facilitate recovery on physical, emotional, and spiritual levels.

REFERENCES

Alcoholics Anonymous World Services. (2001). *Alcoholics Anonymous* (4th ed.). New York: Author.

American Psychiatric Association. (2013). *Diagnostic and statistical manual of mental disorders* (5th ed.). Arlington, VA: Author.

Baker, F. A., Dingle, G. A., & Gleadhill, L. (2012). *Music preferences and music listening experiences of people with substance use disorders*. Unpublished manuscript.

Borling, J. (2011). Music therapy and addiction: Addressing essential components in the recovery process. In A. Meadows (Ed.), *Developments in music therapy practice: Case study perspectives* (pp. 334–349). Gilsum, NH: Barcelona.

Borling, J. (2012). Considerations in treatment planning for addictions. In A. L. Gadberry (Ed.), *Treatment planning for music therapy cases* (pp. 144–163). Denton, TX: Sarsen.

Bruscia, K. E. (1987). *Improvisational models of music therapy*. Springfield, IL: Charles C Thomas.

Bruscia, K. E. (1998a). *Defining music therapy* (2nd ed.). Gilsum, NH: Barcelona.

Bruscia, K. E. (1998b). An introduction to music psychotherapy. In K. E. Bruscia (Ed.), *The dynamics of music psychotherapy* (pp. 1–15). Gilsum, NH: Barcelona.

Center for Substance Abuse Treatment. (2006). *Detoxification and substance abuse treatment* (Treatment improvement protocol [TIP] series, Number 45, DHHS Pub. No. [SMA] 06-4131). Rockville, MD: Substance Abuse and Mental Health Services Administration.

Center for Substance Abuse Treatment. (2010). Protracted withdrawal. *Substance Abuse Treatment Advisory, 9*(1). Available at *www.kap.samhsa. gov/products/manuals/advisory/pdfs/SATA_Protracted_Withdrawal.pdf*.

Dijkstra, T. F., & Hakvoort, L. G. (2010). "How to deal music"?: Music therapy with clients suffering from addiction problems: Enhancing coping strategies. In D. Aldridge & J. Fachner (Eds.), *Music therapy and addictions* (pp. 88–102). Philadelphia: Jessica Kingsley.

Eyre, L. (2008). Medical music therapy and kidney disease: The development of a clinical method for persons receiving haemodialysis. *Canadian Journal of Music Therapy, 14*(1), 55–87.

Frye, R. V. (1990). Affective modes in multimodality addiction treatment. In H. B. Milkman & L. I. Sederer (Eds.), *Treatment choices for alcoholism and substance abuse* (pp. 287–307). Lexington, MA: Lexington Books.

Gardstrom, S. C., Carlini, M., Josefczyk, J., & Love, A. (2013). Women with addictions: Music therapy clinical postures and interventions. *Music Therapy Perspectives, 31*, 95–104.

Gray, M., & Gibson, S. (2004). Relapse prevention. In S. L. A. Straussner (Ed.), *Clinical work with substance-abusing clients* (2nd ed., pp. 146–168). New York: Guilford Press.

Horesch, T. (2010). Drug addicts and their music: A story of a complex relationship. In D. Aldridge & J. Fachner (Eds.), *Music therapy and addictions* (pp. 57–74). Philadelphia: Jessica Kingsley.

Miller, A. S. (1970). Music therapy for alcoholics at a Salvation Army Center. *Journal of Music Therapy, 7*, 136–138.

Murphy, K. M. (2010, November). *The role of music therapy in substance abuse detoxification services.* Paper presented at the annual conference of the American Music Therapy Association, Cleveland, OH.

Murphy, K. M. (2013). Adults with substance use disorders. In L. Eyre (Ed.), *Guidelines for music therapy practice: Mental health for adolescents and adults* (pp. 449–501). University Park, IL: Barcelona.

National Institute on Drug Abuse. (2012). *Drugs, brains, and behavior: The science of addiction.* Bethesda, MD: National Institutes of Health.

Sandoz, J. (2001). The spiritual secret to alcoholism recovery. *Annals of the American Psychotherapy Association, 4*(5), 12–14.

Straussner, S. L. A. (2004). Assessment and treatment of clients with alcohol and other drug abuse problems. In S. L. A. Straussner (Ed.), *Clinical work with substance-abusing clients* (2nd ed., pp. 3–35). New York: Guilford Press.

Substance Abuse and Mental Health Services Administration. (2012). *Overview of findings from the 2011 National Survey on Drug Use and Health* (Office of Applied Studies, NSDUH Series H-32, DHHS Publication No. SMA 07-4293). Rockville, MD: Author.

Thompson, S. (2013). Decision making in music therapy: The use of a decision tree. *Australian Journal of Music Therapy, 24,* 48–64.

CHAPTER 29

Music Therapy for Older Adults

Hanne Mette Ridder
Barbara L. Wheeler

Growing older is not a diagnosis. Old age is a period of life, with the potential of healthy and successful aging, despite the fact that normal aging processes lead to changes in the nervous system, the sensory apparatus, and attention. Our focus for this chapter is how music can play a role in facilitating healthy aging, including a perspective on music therapy applied when aging processes are complicated by disease, as when a person develops dementia.

In the science of *gerontology*, professionals from various fields collect knowledge about what it means to become old. In fact, *geron* means *old man*. Gerontology represents a broad interdisciplinary perspective on the biological, psychological, and social aspects of aging and seeks to understand normal and pathological aging processes. Gerontologists are interested in providing the field of developmental psychology with knowledge regarding lifespan development into old age. One of the first gerontologists, Stanley Hall, in his 1922 book, *Senescence: The Last Half of Life*, formulated the perspective that old age is not a good-bye to life but

rather an opportunity to embrace life with gratitude and love, even when confronted with biological aging and death. The word *geriatrics* is related to gerontology. It also refers to the science of aging but is focused more on medical treatment and prevention of age-related diseases.

Clientele

In 2000, the world's population of those who were 60+ years of age was 600 million. The World Health Organization (2011) expects this number to reach 2 billion by 2050, more than tripling the current number of older adults. This means that one in five persons will be 60+ years old in 2050. In the normal aging process, people lose aspects of their physical functioning as the body grows older, leading to problems with vision, hearing, and mobility and adding other health issues such as heart disease, arthritis, and so forth. People often lose some social functioning and become more isolated as spouses and friends pass away, and they may have new psychological problems as they deal with loneliness or loss of social stature after retirement.

According to the World Health Organization (2011), this projected substantial increase in older adults represents great challenges but also great opportunities. Though increased life expectancy is a triumph, it is challenged by disease and frailty. Those who become the oldest-old may grow frail and experience social isolation, limited mobility, and physical or cognitive decline sufficient for them to require long-term care. However, in order to prevent deleterious outcomes resulting from social isolation, the World Health Organization has formulated a policy framework for *active aging*, in which mental health and social connections are considered as important as improved physical health status. These connections are not only important for feeling good but are also related to reducing the risk of neurodegeneration and the development of dementia.

Dementia and Cognitive Reserve

One of the major causes of cognitive decline in old age is dementia. It is estimated that 36 million people live with a dementia disease (Alzheimer's Disease International, 2011) and that the majority (61.5%) of residents in nursing homes have dementia (Huber et al., 2012). According to the fifth edition of the American Psychiatric Association's (2013) *Diagnostic and Statistical Manual of Mental Disorders* (DSM-5) and the 10th revision of the World Health Organization's (1992) *International Classification of Diseases* criteria (ICD-10), the essential feature of dementia (also called a *neurocognitive disorder* in DSM-5) is a progressive development of multiple cognitive deficits, such as memory impairment or a change in executive functioning.

The most common dementia diagnoses include Alzheimer's disease, vascular/mixed dementia, Lewy body dementia, and frontotemporal dementia, but a precise diagnosis can only be confirmed at postmortem examination. Researchers suggest that scanning the brain may assist in the early diagnosis of dementia or in tracking disease severity, and it is expected that diagnostic techniques will improve in the years to come. Epidemiological studies purport that certain persons have a *cognitive reserve* that is associated with adult life work complexity and education, social network, and complex leisure skills that compensate for the brain abnormalities that lead to dementia (Meng & D'Arcy, 2012). Some researchers explain cognitive reserve as the brain's ability to actively cope with structural changes to compensate for brain damage, or because the brain's reserve capacity allows some persons to maintain cognitive function.

Research shows that inactivity is a risk factor for dementia and that engagement in leisure activities influences working memory and changes brain function across the lifespan. The positive effects of cognitive reserve may be explained by learning and stimulation in early life that increases cortical volume in certain areas of the brain (Robertson, 2013). In addition, the cognitive stimulation inherent in higher education, complex work, and leisure activities, along with social interaction, directly influences brain processing to create intricate pathways that allow for compensation and the ability to bypass pathologies. The elements of cognitive reserve are therefore defined by cognitive stimulation that not only includes education/IQ, mental activity, and previously learned skills but also enriched/novel environments and social interaction. With this understanding, we should be encouraged to look at how we increase cognitive reserve across the entire lifespan with the goal of assuring a process of positive and healthy cognitive aging.

Finally, some research demonstrates that less mental stimulation and poor social interaction with others directly impact the deterioration process of dementia itself, not just the brain's capacity to compensate for the disease. Consequently, social engagement, as well as physical exercise and cognitive stimulation across the lifespan, might act to prevent or delay the onset of dementia. Important cognitive stimulation can come from a range of sources, including social interaction.

When dementia leads to memory impairment, aphasia, apraxia, agnosia, or a change in executive functioning, social interaction becomes very challenging. Therefore, it is important to find ways to enhance social interaction that is adjusted to the cognitive function of the person with dementia or before the onset of dementia. From research, we know that activity programs improve quality of life, and that positive engagement leads to positive affect, interest, and pleasure in agitated nursing home residents with dementia (Cohen-Mansfield, Dakheel-Ali, Jensen, Marx, & Thein, 2012). Persons with dementia are described as being able to express themselves and to respond to social interactions regardless of the level of cognitive impairment, and music significantly increases the duration of engagement in an activity. Compared to other psychosocial interventions, music is suggested as the best technique for ensuring active involvement (Ferrero-Arias et al., 2011). We therefore explain how music can help older adults to engage, or reengage, socially with one another.

Music and Healthy Aging

Evidence indicates that singing in a choir or participating in group singing activities can improve health and well-being in older adults, that choir singing leads to positive physiological changes, and that social relationships develop when opportunities for choral bonding are offered through participation in choral singing (see Clift, 2012). Active participation in music has powerful influences on health and well-being because of the motivational and emotional role of music. Neuroscientists explain the positive health effects from music as natu-

ral rewards that are received through music experiences and positive social interactions that trigger certain activating processes in the brain to release dopamine, the *feel-good* neurotransmitter (Altenmüller & Schlaug, 2012).

Involvement in active music making or music listening, along with social engagement, is important to older adults who like music, are motivated by it, and desire social engagement. Still, little is known about the function of music in older adults in affecting cognitive function and subsequent prevention or postponement of dementia. There is, though, evidence of positive life quality outcomes in older persons who value cultural events and activities where music is included and who enjoy social engagement through participation in these activities (Theorell & Kreutz, 2012). What happens to older adults who do not value music and musical experiences is not known. Further research is needed to understand the relationships.

Music and Dementia

Although music activities in general hold promise for positive experiences as part of healthy aging, little is known about the perceptions and experiences of music in people with neurodegeneration and cognitive decline, such as occurs in dementia. Persons in early stages of dementia still perform skills, including music skills, learned early in their lives; however, the loss of procedural memory in late-stage dementia results in loss of previously learned skills. Consequently, persons who have played musical instruments throughout their lives lose the ability to play them.

As mentioned in the first part of this chapter, various dementia diseases exist and have very different symptoms. Some persons may, for example, lose the ability to name familiar songs at an early stage, whereas others, even in later stages, can name songs and still process basic pitch and novel melodic information, enabling them to actively participate in singing and rhythm playing (Clair & Memmott, 2008; Johnson et al., 2011).

Clinical Work

Literature on Music Therapy in Dementia Care

Several descriptions of the use of music therapy in dementia care exist. Books by Bright (1997), Aldridge (2000), Clair and Memmott (2008), and Belgrave, Darrow, Walworth, and Wlodarczyk (2011) serve as resources for clinical applications of music therapy in dementia care. Abbott (2013) provided extensive information on older adults in nursing facilities, and Young (2013) did the same for those with Alzheimer's disease and other dementias. In addition, several research literature reviews provide evidence of the benefits of music therapy clinical practice for persons with dementia.

In a comprehensive literature review in the *British Journal of Nursing*, the aim was to determine influences of music therapy on behaviors of older people with dementia (Wall & Duffy, 2010). Thirteen music therapy studies were identified and analyzed, and the authors accentuated positive effects on communication and agitation:

> Music therapy has been shown to promote communication between carers and patients with dementia, with evidence highlighting that it has a positive effect on agitated patient behaviour, reducing anxiety and aggressive behaviour, restoring cognitive and motor function and overall improving patients' quality of life. (p. 113)

The authors added that most of the included studies used a quantitative methodology and therefore called for further qualitative research to achieve a cross-professional and integrated view of the effects of music therapy.

In a metareview (a review of review articles) in the *International Journal of Geri-atric Psychiatry*, 33 systematic reviews that included as a minimum one randomized controlled trial of a "non-drug intervention" were identified. The aim of the review was to provide a source of evidence for family caregivers about approaches that they could make use of in daily living (Hulme, Wright, Crocker, Oluboyede, & House, 2010). The researchers identified 10 systematic reviews where music and/or music therapy was included among the nondrug interventions. They found evidence that music interventions and music therapy improved food intake and reduced behavioral and psychological symptoms of dementia, such as agitation, aggression, wandering, restlessness, irritability, and social and emotional difficulties. Preferred music was emphasized for reducing agitation. It was concluded, though, that the study designs generally were weak and included too few participants. The researchers also reviewed interventions such as light therapy, physical exercise, animal-assisted therapy, aromatherapy, massage/touch, and reminiscence therapy and concluded that it was possible for carers to use some of these interventions, but that they would need training or instruction for certain interventions. They suggested exploring "the provision of group music therapy and group exercise activities that meet the needs of both the person with dementia and their carer" (p. 756).

Since this review, a Cochrane review by Vink and colleagues was updated to include 10 controlled studies (Vink, Bruinsma, & Scholten, 2011), and, as part of her doctoral research, McDermott (McDermott, Crellin, Ridder, & Orrell, 2013) carried out a narrative synthesis, a type of systematic review, published in the *International Journal of Geriatric Psychiatry*. It focused specifically on music therapy, whereas previous reviews had included a mixture of music therapy and various other types of music interventions. In order to differentiate between music interventions and music therapy, McDermott et al. selected studies that followed a clear definition of music therapy, including (1) theory, (2) a practice/operational definition, and (3) evidence. Out of 70 studies, 15 quantitative and three qualitative or mixed methods studies met the full inclusion criteria. It was found that the studies could be divided into three groups in relation to which overall changes or aspects of music therapy were investigated: (1) behavioral and psychological (eight studies), (2) hormonal and physiological (five studies), and (3) social and relational (five studies). The studies primarily investigated the use of group music therapy. This was either improvisation-based group music therapy or group music therapy based on singing or listening to well-known songs, listening to live music, or a combination of various music activities such as song request and active reminiscing. Individual active or receptive music therapy was investigated in three studies. Overall, singing was featured as an important medium for change (McDermott et al.).

Clinical Applications of Music Therapy in Dementia Care

In the description of the application of music therapy for people with dementia at Beth Abraham Hospital, where he has worked as neurologist for much of his career, Oliver Sacks suggests that "music is no luxury to them [the patients], but a necessity" (Sacks, 2007, p. 347). Nevertheless, music therapy is not offered as a primary treatment in dementia care in general and is only slowly gaining a footing in the field. We have described the positive effects and evidence for using music with a focus on social engagement as important for well-being and the hope of preventing cognitive decline in healthy older adults and persons with dementia. Here, we focus on how we achieve this positive effect in dementia care. From the many studies and reviews, there is no consensus on best practice, and guidelines on how to implement music therapy in dementia care are missing. Further research is needed to learn more about whether individual or group music

therapy is most helpful or if the therapist should prioritize singing, improvising with instruments, or listening to favorite music, and how this is best implemented according to each client's personal needs and preferences. We expect best-practice research to advance in the years to come. However, several studies give new information on the clinical applications of music therapy.

Ridder (2005) conducted a literature review to gather information on the clinical use of music and music therapy in dementia care. In the review of clinical strategies, 92 publications were included, and, from this material, 18 therapeutic initiatives were identified, including social dancing, songwriting, music listening, music therapeutic care, assessment, and vibroacoustic therapy (the transmission of music vibration and sound waves through loudspeakers or soundboards to the body). It is suggested that some of these initiatives should be carried out by a professional music therapist, others by professional or informal carers or relatives. Based on the review, it is recommended that when nonmusic therapists use these interventions, a professional music therapist be involved as an instructor and/or supervisor to assure that the initiatives/activities do not lead to overstimulation or social isolation.

McDermott et al. (2013) categorized music therapy methods as follows:

- Group music therapy, including song requests, singing well-known songs, and listening to live music
- Improvisation-based group music therapy
- Group music therapy based on the Clair and Bernstein protocol, incorporating a vibrotactile response, defined as drum playing with the drum held in the client's lap
- Music listening
- Individual play-along sessions
- Music reminiscence
- Individual music therapy
- Group music therapy, including caregivers

Rather than describing these diverse ways of applying music therapy, later in the chapter we present a theoretical understanding of the therapeutic use of music in dementia care that is based on a person-centered care (PCC) approach and includes the theory of personhood (Edvardsson, Winblad, & Sandman, 2008). This understanding of dementia and therapy is rooted in a humanistic and psychodynamic tradition, but in our view requires an integrated understanding. PCC is being increasingly incorporated into dementia care around the world and provides a theoretical basis as to why music is such an important medium for persons with dementia who lose those cognitive abilities that play an important part in human communication and social interaction.

The Theory of Personhood and PCC

Music therapists working in dementia care need to be aware of how they understand dementia. In the first part of this chapter, we touched upon the following questions: Is dementia a condition that all old people can anticipate, or is dementia a disease? Or can humans expect healthy aging? Another essential question is whether a person with severe dementia loses personhood—loses his or her perception of *self*, and thus, so to speak, ends up as an empty shell. A person adopting a PCC approach would answer *no*, and, with reference to the theory of personhood, the explanation would be that even in late stages of dementia we are able to be with or meet the person. According to this theory, *personhood* is a social construction and persons with dementia still show emotions and awareness, although sometimes only for short moments (Edvardsson et al., 2008).

Traditionally in dementia care, the associated behavioral and psychological symptoms are described as disturbing behaviors that are to be treated with diverse interventions, primarily medication. However, with a person-centered understanding, these behaviors are seen as closely related

to needs. Dementia researcher Kitwood (1997) describes a cluster of psychosocial needs—comfort, attachment, inclusion, occupation, identity, and love—and suggests that these needs are grounded in our evolutionary past and mediated by basic nervous system functioning. If psychosocial needs are met, the person "may be enabled to move out of fear, grief and anger, into the domain of positive experience" (Kitwood, p. 20). Behavioral and psychological symptoms, such as agitation, are thus seen as reactions to unmet psychosocial needs and as attempts to communicate these needs. Kitwood describes 12 types of positive interactions that carers and therapists can use to meet the psychosocial needs of persons with dementia that enhance the experience of personhood. These interactions are recognition; negotiation; collaboration; play; timalation;[1] celebration; relaxation; creation; giving; and validation, holding, and facilitation. Kitwood defines the latter interactions—validation, holding, and facilitation—as psychotherapeutic techniques. Music therapy holds rich possibilities for applying these positive interactions or techniques with music as a meaningful media for exchange.

Music Therapy and Psychosocial Needs

Based on the theoretical understanding of PCC, the goal of music therapy in dementia care is to meet psychosocial needs and to understand the person with dementia on a feeling level. The question is how this is possible, when we know that in advanced dementia, the person will not understand that music therapy is going to take place or what the therapeutic intentions and goals for the setting are. As an answer to this, we therefore see it as the therapist's responsibility to create a safe setting so that the person with dementia understands what is

---

[1] *Timalation* occurs when a person encounters sensory experiences, as may be offered by multisensory environments where people can experience a range of sensory stimuli.

going on and is able to focus attention on the mutual interaction.

Acoustic cuing is an effective way of attracting the attention of the person with dementia. Instead of words and explanations, the therapist uses music and voice to signal what is going to happen. The musical cues trigger memory, which helps the person connect certain music with certain events, as occurs with jingles or sound themes in advertising. With this cognitive understanding of memory and cuing, integrated into the PCC approach, the music therapist uses music in various ways to structure a music therapy session (Ridder, 2011).

When a person with severe memory deficits, over time, becomes familiar with and starts to (at some level) understand the cues that signal the structure, the music therapist can use music with the goal of regulating the arousal level of the person with dementia. Psychophysiologically, a person who is highly aroused will not be able to pay attention to the interactions occurring in the therapy session. Through musical entrainment, the therapist can create a process where physiological rhythms of the body are synchronized with music elements such as dynamics, tempo, and pitch (Ridder, 2011). People vary in their reactions to music and in their preferences. The music therapist therefore carefully selects music and observes reactions. In addition to using music with the goal of regulating arousal level, either by actively playing music or by listening to music with the client, the therapist uses social interactions. Consequently he or she is aware of his or her own use of eye contact, proximity, facial expression, gestures, and tone of voice, all of which influence the physiological state of the person with dementia.

With the use of acoustic cuing and arousal regulation, the therapist can create a safe setting, and, with this as the basis, can work at a personal level to create situations in which the person with dementia can engage in social communication. The therapist uses positive interactions, with validation, holding, and facilitation as par-

ticularly useful, to meet psychosocial needs in the person with dementia. The sharing of music experiences and a mutual understanding created through communicative musicality make it possible to move out of negative experiences and to enhance personhood. This integrated understanding of PCC and music therapy may be implied in voice work (Ridder, 2011) or in any other of the previously described music therapy methods (see McDermott et al., 2013), and challenges the music therapist to integrate theoretical perspectives based on cognitive psychology, psychophysiology, and psychodynamic theories. This approach was applied by Ridder, Stige, Qvale, and Gold (2013) and led to positive effects on agitation and prescription of medication. In the following, we give an example of how singing can be used to meet psychosocial needs, focusing on validation, improvisation, and vitality forms (Daniel Stern describes vitality forms as part of our episodic memories [2010, p. 11] and the "most fundamental of all felt experiences when dealing with other humans in motion" [2010, p. 8]).

Therapeutic Singing

Singing is useful when there is a need to distract a person, to create a good atmosphere, or to entertain. A song can bring forward memories and bring a group together. But singing is more than that. Expressing sounds with the voice is a fundamental means of communication. Such basic communicative musicality is still present in persons with severe dementia, although they have lost the ability to communicate through words. They may not understand what is said, but they know how it is said and the intentions and emotions that are communicated through the expressiveness of the voice. An intense sharing of emotions can occur through the sharing of a simple melody. It seems that the recognition of a familiar song brings safety and structure.

An interaction between Naomi Feil, founder of the validation method for communicating with older adults with dementia (Feil, 2012), and a woman named Gladys Wilson[2] is an excellent example of how singing is used therapeutically (Feil, 2009). The focus of validation therapy is to understand what a person with dementia is expressing through his or her behavior, so the behaviors are valued instead of being seen as disturbing. This example is not from a music therapy session, and a music therapist might have replaced the verbal interactions with musical interactions. But it illustrates the use of music as a way of enhancing personhood and shows the core of therapeutic work where psychosocial needs are met.

CLINICAL EXAMPLE: Therapeutic Singing Helps to Draw a Woman Out of Her Private World

Mrs. Wilson is sitting with closed eyes in a chair, with Feil in front of her. Feil explains that when people are old and deteriorated and no one enters their world, they withdraw inward more and more. Still, inside there is a desperate need for connection and a longing for closeness. Feil shows that she is attentive to these needs of Mrs. Wilson, who expresses her needs through her movements. Feil puts into words what she sees, for example, that Mrs. Wilson is crying and that there is a tear on her cheek. Feil asks if there is a pain, if she is sad or afraid. The pace is slow, and she waits for Mrs. Wilson to answer. She touches Mrs. Wilson's cheek, like a mother would touch her child, and afterward explains that this use of touch opens up communication. Mrs. Wilson relates to religious songs, as church music is tied to emotion and safety for her. Feil sings "Jesus Loves Me," and, almost immediately, Mrs. Wilson follows the rhythm of the song by tapping her hand at her armrest. She opens her eyes and looks directly at Feil. Mrs. Wilson's hand tapping increases in tempo and dynamic, and Feil follows her in the song. She matches the intensity of her

voice with the intensity of Mrs. Wilson's movements and describes that, for a split second, when they share the music, they become one person. After this Mrs. Wilson appears peaceful and her breathing slows down. She gently grabs Feil and pulls her close. Their foreheads touch. Feil says that, in this moment, she believes that she is a symbol of Mrs. Wilson's mother.

The example illustrates how Feil acknowledges the reality of Mrs. Wilson and uses her voice and the tempo, volume, and intensity of her singing to match what Mrs. Wilson is expressing. She is empathically attentive to Mrs. Wilson and seeks to understand what she is communicating. She suggests that it is necessary that the therapist be centered and attentive in order to bring forth communication. This type of nonverbal communication and intersubjective exchange parallels Wigram's (2004) description of *mirroring*, wherein the therapist imitates the vitality form (Stern, 2010), rhythm, or melody in what the client does. Feil mirrors Mrs. Wilson in the example. She also matches Mrs. Wilson by maintaining the dynamic features of what Mrs. Wilson does, like a musically based affect attunement. This is described by Wigram (2004) as "one of the most valuable improvisational methods that can be applied in therapy" (p. 83), and this way of improvising is an important feature of singing a well-known song. Certain elements, such as melody, are predefined and fixed, but within the structure of the song, Feil matches the movements, the expressions, the dynamics, in short, the vitality forms of Mrs. Wilson, and in this way these are "sculptured in the nature of the relatedness" (Stern, 2010, p. 138) between Mrs. Wilson and Feil.

Feil sings one more song, and Mrs. Wilson joins in singing. The video clip shows how turn taking occurs, each of them singing alternately, and how they sing together. Finally, Feil asks if she feels safe, and Mrs. Wilson whispers, "Yes."

---

[2]This interaction can be viewed in the following link: *www.memorybridge.org/video9.php* (Feil, 2009), but can also be read and understood without viewing the link.

Here we see that singing is not only the reproduction of predefined musical patterns, but that certain elements, such as tempo, can be modified to open up reciprocal communication. These improvisational techniques are important means of breaking social isolation. With the method of therapeutic singing, basic psychosocial needs are expressed and met, and the person is comforted and understood. The validation method is a psychotherapeutic technique, where the "heart of the matter is acknowledging the reality of a person's emotions and feelings, and giving a response on the feeling level" (Kitwood, 1997, p. 91). The musical communication is the use of vitality forms whereby experience is shared or interchanged (Stern, 2010).

We conclude the chapter with three short clinical examples of music therapy that include instrument playing, moving/dancing, and music listening.

Instrument Playing

The following clinical example supports the research results of Clair and Bernstein (1990), who found that people with dementia were more engaged with vibrotactile (e.g., when having a drum placed on the lap whereby sound and bodily sensations are merged) responses than with nonvibrotactile responses. It occurred when I (Barbara Wheeler) worked in a day program for people with Alzheimer's disease. The people spent the day at the center, allowing their caregivers to work or pursue other aspects of their lives. The music therapy group included as many of the attendees as wanted to attend, generally about 20 people.

CLINICAL EXAMPLE: Effectiveness of Instrument Playing Varies by Type of Instrument

One man, approximately 85 years old, was an enthusiastic participant in the group. However, he had fairly advanced dementia and was quite confused, usually requiring the assistance of a staff member to play the instrument that he was given at the designated time. During a sequence of musical activities in which participants were playing instruments, his dramatically different responses to two different instruments were observed. During a song where group members held different resonator bells, and I would point to each when his or her bell/note fit into a familiar melody, he was not able to play his bell just one time. Even with a staff member helping him play at the right time, once he began playing, he perseverated in hitting the bell. It was clear that he had no comprehension of his part in the song, and his repeated notes confused the others by making the melody unclear.

In contrast, when he was given a hand drum and encouraged to play it as part of a musical ensemble, he played and seemingly comprehended what he was doing. He still required the assistance of a staff member, but he played individual notes, and they were in time with the rest of those playing.

Moving/Dancing

Movement can range from the movement of the diaphragm in the process of relaxed deep breathing, to sitting dances where swaying and rhythmic gestures are shared, to social dancing where the entire dance floor is used. This example is with Mrs. C, who suffered from severe vascular dementia, lived in a nursing home, and was offered group music activities as well as individual music therapy.

CLINICAL EXAMPLE: Rhythmic Movement to Help a Woman Join the Group

When Mrs. C took part in activities, she would either sit with her eyes closed or a stream of words would come out of her mouth as if she were talking to an imagined person. She did not seem engaged in any activities and never joined in singing or playing the instruments given to her. She seemed to be in her own distant world. However, this detachment was completely absent when she took part in the weekly folk dancing group. When someone took her hand and led her to the dance floor, she smiled, followed the rhythm with her movements and gestures, and made intense eye contact. The same pattern occurred in our individual music therapy sessions. She never joined in, unless I took her hands or put my arm around her and clearly marked the rhythm of the music. This would wake her up, and she would take part in the music for several minutes, but as soon as the rhythmic swaying or sitting dances stopped, she drew back into her own world again.

Music Listening

Music listening can be a rich experience that brings forth memories that are related to one's identity and to important relations. This example comes from Ridder's clinical work at a psychiatric nursing home for 24 residents.

CLINICAL EXAMPLE: Listening to Music to Calm a Woman with Dementia

Mrs. K suffered from severe dementia and often seemed to hallucinate. She yelled in great panic about the children she could see outside the room. She could see fires and how the children were burning. Mrs. K clearly experienced immense suffering, and it took a long time to calm her down. I (Hanne Mette Ridder) would sing to her, acknowledging her panic, but then slowly trying to guide her to a calmer and safer place. When she was calm, we would listen to the tenor Plácido Domingo, especially the recordings of *The Three Tenors*. She then closed her eyes, leaned back in her chair, and sighed deeply with relief. I imagined that the voice of Domingo reminded her of those moments she shared with her now long-deceased husband. He once gave her a gramophone, and I understood from her children that they often listened to records together.

Applications to Other Disciplines

Music is unique for ensuring social engagement and active involvement for healthy older adults as well as for persons with de-

mentia. Music therapists play an important role in implementing the use of music in activities, in daily care, and in therapy. Music therapists know the importance of music in facilitating social cohesion, of personalized music, of how music can function as a trigger of memory, and its entraining function. They can integrate this knowledge in the prevention of social isolation and in a PCC approach by guiding and instructing carers and relatives.

At present in dementia care, music listening activities, live concerts, sing-along sessions, social dancing, and music groups are carried out with good intentions and seemingly with good results, but often lacking professional expertise, with the risk of leading to overstimulation and/or social isolation. Some of the initiatives described in this chapter are to be carried out by a professional music therapist, others by professional or informal carers or relatives. However, a professional music therapist should be familiar with the use of music interventions in various forms and be able to train, instruct, and guide carers and relatives to use music in relevant ways. The music therapist ideally works as part of an interdisciplinary team, taking a leading role in training, guiding, and supervising staff and relatives in best-practice techniques involving music and communication through music to be used in daily living and care. In addition, the music therapist possesses the competencies to offer the necessary therapeutic treatment to those persons who are referred to music therapy.

Conclusions

Old age does not need to be a time of illness, although it does typically involve decreased functioning and increased challenges. Seeing music not as a luxury but as a necessity, music therapists can play a role in assuring a high level of professional care. Along with this role, music therapists are qualified to carry out individual and group treatment for persons with neuropsychiatric symptoms of dementia and to initiate preventive activities and procedures.

There is a need for more research on music therapy. Additional research in support of music therapy can lead to increase awareness of music therapists as important contributors to the field of gerontology and to a PCC that is informed by evidence-based treatment, best practice, clinical insight, and high-level academic professionals.

ACKNOWLEDGMENTS

We would like to thank Alicia Ann Clair and Shannon Bowles for assistance with and feedback on this chapter.

REFERENCES

Abbott, E. A. (2013). Elderly residents in nursing facilities. In L. Eyre (Ed.), *Guidelines for music therapy practice in mental health* (pp. 685–717). University Park, IL: Barcelona.

Aldridge, D. (Ed.). (2000). *Music therapy in dementia care*. London: Jessica Kingsley.

Altenmüller, E., & Schlaug, G. (2012). Music, brain, and health: Exploring biological foundation of music's health effects. In R. MacDonald, G. Kreutz, & L. Mitchell (Eds.), *Music, health, and wellbeing* (pp. 12–24). New York: Oxford University Press.

Alzheimer's Disease International. (2011). *World Alzheimer report: The global economic impact of dementia*. Alzheimer's Disease International (ADI). Retrieved from *www.alz.co.uk/research/world-report-2011*.

American Psychiatric Association. (2013). *Diagnostic and statistical manual of mental disorders* (5th ed.). Arlington, VA: Author.

Belgrave, M., Darrow, A.-A., Walworth, D., & Wlodarczyk, N. (2011). *Music therapy and geriatric populations: A handbook for practicing music therapists and healthcare professionals*. Silver Spring, MD: American Music Therapy Association.

Bright, R. (1997). *Music therapy and the dementias: Improving the quality of life*. St. Louis, MO: MMB.

Clair, A. A., & Bernstein, B. (1990). A comparison of singing, vibrotactile and nonvibrotactile instrumental playing responses in severely regressed persons with dementia of the Alzheimer's type. *Journal of Music Therapy, 27*(3), 119–125.

Clair, A. A., & Memmott, J. (2008). *Therapeutic uses of music for older adults* (2nd ed.). Silver Spring, MD: American Music Therapy Association.

Clift, S. (2012). Singing, wellbeing, and health. In R. MacDonald, G. Kreutz, & L. Mitchell (Eds.), *Music, health, and wellbeing* (pp. 113–124). New York: Oxford University Press.

Cohen-Mansfield, J., Dakheel-Ali, M., Jensen, B., Marx, M. S., & Thein, K. (2012). An analysis of the relationships among engagement, agitated behavior, and affect in nursing home residents with dementia. *International Psychogeriatrics, 24*(5), 742–752.

Edvardsson, D., Winblad, B., & Sandman, P. (2008). Person-centred care of people with severe Alzheimer's disease: Current status and ways forward. *Lancet Neurology, 7*(4), 362–367.

Feil, N. (2009). *There is a bridge: Naomi Feil and Gladys Wilson share a breakthrough moment in communication*. Retrieved from *www.memorybridge.org/video9.php*

Feil, N. (2012). *The validation breakthrough: Simple techniques for communicating with people with Alzheimer's-type dementia* (3rd ed.). Baltimore: Health Professions Press.

Ferrero-Arias, J., Goñi-Imízcoz, M., González-Bernal, J., Lara-Ortega, F., da Silva-González, A., & Díez-Lopez, M. (2011). The efficacy of nonpharmacological treatment for dementia-related apathy. *Alzheimer Disease and Associated Disorders, 25*(3), 213–219.

Hall, G. S. (1922). *Senescence: The last half of life*. New York: Appleton.

Huber, M., Kölzsch, M., Rapp, M. A., Wulff, I., Kalinowski, S., Bolbrinker, J., et al. (2012). Antipsychotic drugs predominate in pharmacotherapy of nursing home residents with dementia. *Pharmacopsychiatry, 45*(5), 182–188.

Hulme, C., Wright. J., Crocker, T., Oluboyede, Y., & House, A. (2010). Non-pharmacological approaches for dementia that informal carers might try or access: A systematic review. *International Journal of Geriatric Psychiatry, 25*, 756–763.

Johnson, J. K., Chang, C.-C., Brambati, S. M., Migliaccio, R., Gorno-Tempini, M. L., Miller, B. L., et al. (2011). Music recognition in frontotemporal lobar degeneration and Alzheimer disease. *Cognitive and Behavioral Neurology, 24*(2), 74–84.

Kitwood, T. (1997). *Dementia reconsidered: The person comes first*. Buckingham, UK: Open University Press.

McDermott, O., Crellin, N., Ridder, H. M., & Orrell, M. (2013). Music therapy in dementia: A narrative synthesis systematic review. *Interna-*

tional Journal of Geriatric Psychiatry, 28(8), 781–794.

Meng, X., & D'Arcy, C. (2012). Education and dementia in the context of cognitive reserve hypothesis: A systematic review with meta-analyses and qualitative analyses. *PloS One, 7*(6).

Ridder, H. M. O. (2005). An overview of therapeutic initiatives when working with people suffering from dementia. In D. Aldridge (Ed.), *Music therapy and neurological rehabilitation: Performing health* (pp. 61–82). London: Jessica Kingsley.

Ridder, H. M. O. (2011). How can singing in music therapy influence social engagement for people with dementia?: Insights from the polyvagal theory. In F. Baker & S. Uhlig (Eds.), *Voice work in music therapy* (pp. 130–145). London: Jessica Kingsley.

Ridder, H. M. O., Stige, B., Qvale, L. G., & Gold, C. (2013). Individual music therapy for agitation in dementia: An exploratory randomized controlled trial. *Aging and Mental Health, 17*(6), 667–678.

Robertson, I. H. (2013). A noradrenergic theory of cognitive reserve: Implications for Alzheimer's disease. *Neurobiology of Aging, 34*(1), 298–308.

Sacks, O. (2007). *Musicophilia: Tales of music and the brain.* New York: Knopf.

Stern, D. N. (2010). *Forms of vitality: Exploring dynamic experience in psychology, the arts, psycho-therapy and development.* Oxford, UK: Oxford University Press.

Theorell, T., & Kreutz, G. (2012). Epidemiological studies of the relationship between musical experiences and public health. In R. MacDonald, G. Kreutz, & L. Mitchell (Eds.), *Music, health, and wellbeing* (pp. 424–435). New York: Oxford University Press.

Vink, A. C., Bruinsma, M. S., & Scholten, R. J. P. M. (2011). Music therapy for people with dementia. *Cochrane Database of Systematic Reviews, 2003*(4), CD003477.

Wall, M., & Duffy, A. (2010). The effects of music therapy for older people with dementia. *British Journal of Nursing, 19*(2), 108–113.

Wigram, T. (2004). *Improvisation: Methods and techniques for music therapy clinicians, educators, and students.* London: Jessica Kingsley.

World Health Organization. (1992). *International classification of diseases* (10th rev.). Geneva, Switzerland: Author.

World Health Organization. (2011). *Global health and aging.* National Institute on Aging. Retrieved from *www.who.int/ageing/publications/global_health/en/index.html.*

Young, L. (2013). Persons with Alzheimer's and other dementias. In L. Eyre (Ed.), *Guidelines for music therapy practice in mental health* (pp. 718–766). University Park, IL: Barcelona.

CHAPTER 30

Music Therapy for Women Survivors of Domestic Violence

Elizabeth York
Sandra L. Curtis

Documentation of music therapy with women survivors of domestic violence in North America has appeared only sporadically in the music therapy literature (Cassity & Theobold, 1990; Curtis, 2000, 2006, 2008, 2013b; Curtis & Harrison, 2008; Fesler, 2007; Hahn, 2004; Whipple & Lindsey, 1999; York, 2006). This is not surprising given that, according to the latest workforce statistics reported in the American Music Therapy Association (AMTA) member survey (AMTA, 2013), only 24 of 1,184 professional members (2%) indicated that they worked with abused or sexually abused clients. In the same survey, only 79 music therapists reported that they worked with persons diagnosed with posttraumatic stress disorder. Other responders reported that they worked in community-based services, community mental health centers, or in general hospitals. Since services for victims of domestic violence are often provided through community-based agencies (including the legal system, shelters, and hospitals), one could surmise that the numbers of music therapists who have treated survivors of abuse are much higher than reported in the AMTA survey.

In terms of actual music therapy practice with survivors of domestic violence, neither the AMTA nor the Certification Board for Music Therapists (CBMT) includes specific standards or information in their *Standards of Clinical Practice* or *Scope of Practice*, respectively. Clinical practice in this area is considered to be emerging, and clinical music therapy models related to women's issues—specifically feminist models—are only beginning to be identified and disseminated (Curtis, 2013a; Hadley, 2006). Purdon (2006) has noted that the topic of domestic violence has not generated as much interest or research in the field of music therapy, speculating the lack of knowledge surrounding domestic violence or of a basic understanding of abuse-related issues. Subsequently, music therapists may overlook the reality of abuse (past or present) with their female clients, and inadvertently contribute to the revictimization of women who are already vulnerable.

The harsh reality is that violence against women is pervasive (Curtis, 2013b), with women accounting for 85% of those reporting abuse by significant others (National Coalition against Domestic Violence, 2012). In the United States, one in four women will become a victim of domestic violence in their lifetime, and an average of three women a day will be killed by their intimate male partner (Black et al., 2011). Domestic violence statistics reveal that worldwide, every 9 seconds, a woman is beaten, coerced into having sexual relations against her will, or killed by an intimate partner (Domestic Violence Statistics, 2012). Of women surveyed on the same website, 92% identified reducing domestic violence and sexual assault as their number-one concern. Abusive and controlling behavior is so prevalent that, according to Purdon (2006), "It is hard to imagine a music therapist who does not have firsthand experience as a witness to abusive behavior, as a victim or perpetrator, or as a helper" (p. 210).

In light of the high prevalence of violence against women, it becomes clear that music therapists—whether or not they work specifically with survivors—need to be familiar with the issues surrounding this violence as well as with music therapy best practices to support abused women. This chapter provides this essential information. Women's experiences of abuse are outlined, along with their strengths and challenges. An overview of the current music therapy practice in this area is then detailed, followed by clinical illustrations from each of our practices and research with abused women.

The Experiences of Women Survivors of Abuse

Multiple factors contribute to the experience of domestic violence, also referred to as *intimate partner violence*. The latter term has been expanded to include physical or sexual violence between spouses (or former spouses), as well as violence that occurs within heterosexual and homosexual dating relationships (Friedman & Loue, 2008). Cascardi, O'Leary, Schlee, and Lawrence (1995) described characteristics of women physically abused by their spouses. Among these are (1) low self-esteem, (2) the tendency for the woman to blame herself for the abuse and subsequent shame, and (3) perceived helplessness and feelings that she cannot escape from the abuse. Sociocultural factors may also affect women survivors. Many exhibit (1) strong traditional views on marriage, (2) emotional and economic dependence on the male spouse, (3) traditional gender roles that encourage passivity in women and lead to (4) putting the needs of others over their own needs, and (5) an unrealistic hope that the abuse will cease. Rubenstein (2004) identified three phases of the abuse cycle: (1) a building of tension around an issue or infraction of rules, (2) the acute violent event, and (3) a postabuse honeymoon phase that contributes to the woman's hope that the violence will never happen again.

The fifth edition of the *Diagnostic and Statistical Manual of Mental Disorders* (DSM-5; American Psychiatric Association, 2013) contains a subheading under posttraumatic stress disorder (PTSD) titled "Gender-Related Diagnostic Issues," stating that PTSD is more prevalent among women. "At least some of the increased risk for PTSD in females appears to be attributable to a greater likelihood of exposure to traumatic events, such as rape, and other forms of interpersonal violence" (American Psychiatric Association, p. 278). The diagnosis of PTSD is sometimes used in defense of a woman who has killed her abusive spouse. It must be stated that pathologizing trauma associated with domestic violence by using DSM criteria is, in itself, problematic from a feminist point of view.

These "symptoms" might just as easily be explained and understood from the perspective of one's own cultural context, and history and nature of the trauma. From this perspective, a client's "symptoms" may actually be a culturally appropriate, non-pathological management of cultural [and situational] conflicts. (Morrow, Hawxhurst, Montes de Vegas, Abousleman, & Castaneda, 2006, p. 240)

Music Therapy for Women Survivors of Abuse

With an understanding that abused women should not be pathologized for their response to such violence, attention is now directed to how they can be sensitively supported in music therapy in recovering from the harm. Within this emergent practice, a variety of music therapy interventions are used, most of which are used in combination, and many of which are commonly used across practices with divergent approaches (Cassity & Theobold, 1990; Curtis, 2000, 2006, 2008, 2013b; Curtis & Harrison, 2008; Fesler, 2007; Hahna, 2004; Whipple & Lindsey, 1999; York, 2006). These interventions fall generally into one of four categories: receptive, improvisational, re-creative/performance, and compositional music therapy methods (Curtis, 2013b). *Receptive Music Therapy* with abused women includes such techniques as music-centered relaxation, lyric analysis, and the Bonny Method of Guided Imagery and Music (BMGIM). *Improvisational Music Therapy* includes such techniques as individual and group music improvisation (vocal and instrumental, with or without a preset theme). *Re-Creative/performance Music Therapy* includes such techniques as reflective singing and music performance (within the therapy group or for a larger audience). *Compositional Music Therapy* includes such techniques as songwriting and recording (by the client alone, with the therapist, or by the therapist alone). Each

of these can be enhanced with the inclusion of such other media as artwork, poetry, theatre, and dance/movement elements (Curtis, 2013b; Hahna, 2004; York, 2006).

Although these music therapy methods are common to diverse music therapy practices with abused women, what distinguishes them is their application within a different approach, with a different understanding of abuse of women, and with different goals. While relatively new to music therapy, a feminist approach is increasingly being recognized for its better understanding of the complexities of violence against women as they play out in the sociocultural context (Curtis, 2000, 2006, 2008, 2013a, 2013b; York, 2006). It is a feminist approach to music therapy that has been identified as a component that is critical to the therapeutic effectiveness of our work with our clients. Prior to describing this work, it is important therefore to turn attention first to feminist approaches to music therapy as they relate to work with abused women.

Feminist therapy grew out of the second wave of feminist activism in the United States in the 1970s. Overall goals were twofold: to engage women in a process of political analysis geared to raising their awareness of how interpersonal and societal power dynamics affect their well-being, and to mobilize women to change the social structures contributing to these harmful power dynamics (Ballou & Gabalac, 1985). Subsequent goals have been identified by Worrell and Remer (2003) and include (1) assisting clients to trust their own experiences and intuition, (2) enabling clients to appreciate female-related values, (3) encouraging women to take care of themselves, (4) helping women define and act according to their own sexual needs, and (5) helping women to accept and like their own bodies.

Feminist music therapy involves the direct application of these feminist therapy goals and principles within a music therapy context. Thus informed by feminist therapy, feminist music therapy is a relatively recent development, with some music therapists gaining an understanding of the benefits it can offer their clients (see Curtis, 2000, 2006; Hadley, 2006; Hahna, 2004; York, 2006). To permit greater insight into this approach, attention is directed next to how it plays out in our work with abused women.

Clinical Work with Survivors of Abuse

I (Sandra L. Curtis) have been working with women and teen survivors of violence since 1993 in both clinical and research contexts. It has been my honor to join these strong and courageous women on their journey to recover from the harm—both physical and emotional—of violence. I have learned much from these women, who in the face of incredible adversity have shown such resilience of the human spirit. During the course of the past 19 years, I have worked with women survivors of violence at the hands of their intimate male partners, as well as adult and teen survivors of childhood sexual abuse. Although this chapter addresses survivors of domestic violence, it is important to understand that all forms of violence against women and girls are related, each rooted in a sociocultural context that has a long tradition of condoning this violence (Curtis, 2000, 2008; Curtis & Harrison, 2006). As a result, the underpinnings supporting these types of violence have much in common, as do the challenges facing women, along with the responses of others, including personal, familial, professional, and institutional responses. At the same time, women's experiences may differ because of the interaction of such multiple factors as racism, classism, ageism, and ableism; these factors are further differentiated by individual resources, social supports, and coping strategies (Curtis, 2000).

In a similar fashion, feminist music therapy for abused women is characterized by both commonalities and differences. The practice is informed by each individual

therapist's understanding of feminism and its meaning in the context of therapeutic practice (Curtis, 2000; Hadley, 2006; York, 2006). Consequently in describing my work with abused women, I first briefly describe my approach as a feminist music therapist. Starting in 1997, with my development of the first model of feminist music therapy (Curtis, 2000) and evolving from my ongoing work with abused women, for me:

> Feminist music therapy represents an approach to intervention that is rooted in a feminist belief system with its sociopolitical understanding of men's and women's lives as they are constructed within a patriarchal culture. It is unique among music therapy approaches with this understanding and in its twofold purpose—to accomplish personal transformation by individuals within their own lives and sociopolitical change within the community. (Curtis, 2007, p. 199)

This understanding translates into a few specific, hallmark goals of therapy: to empower women; to permit a sociopolitical understanding of women's experiences; to facilitate recovery from the harm of violence; and to bring about necessary social change (Curtis, 2007, 2008). These goals require work within therapy as well as outside of it, on the part of both the client and the therapist.

In my practice with abused women, I have worked independently and in collaboration with others at times—primarily with social workers (Curtis & Harrison, 2006). These collaborations have been particularly rewarding in offering unparalleled opportunities to model effective sharing of power as well as the give-and-take essential to egalitarian relationships aimed for in feminist music therapy. They also offer clients the opportunity to see their therapists in roles as both expert and learner, all geared toward laying the groundwork for women's empowerment.

Whether working alone or in collaboration, the music therapy has always been in the context of group therapy. Group work is critical for abused women—it makes it possible to break the social isolation established by the abuser. In seeing other women face similar experiences, sharing their challenges and their success stories, they are able to recognize their commonalities and that abuse, rather than being a personal phenomenon, has far-reaching sociopolitical underpinnings.

Sessions

Sessions typically last 2 hours and are held once or twice weekly. The sessions have been held in community centers (e.g., battered women's shelters, sexual assault crisis centers) or in music therapy clinics, led independently by myself or co-led with a social worker. Each of these locations ensured the necessary safety and confidentiality for these women and girls at risk. Groups were usually comprised of five to seven participants, with the same group meeting regularly for 8–15 weeks, depending on the constraints of a particular site. On occasion, some participants dropped out early or joined late, which is not unusual given the transitory nature of this population. All participants, regardless of length of stay in music therapy, provided informed consent in keeping with the research and clinical practice ethics guidelines of the particular facility/region involved.

Feminist Ways of Working

The techniques I used in this work evolved directly out of my own understanding of feminist music therapy and its specific goals. Those techniques unique to feminist music therapy practice encompassed (1) a feminist analysis of gender, power, and violence, including their sociocultural roots; (2) women's empowerment and gaining voice; and (3) women's self-nurturance (Curtis, 2007, 2008). For each of these, traditional music therapy techniques are used, but transformed within a feminist framework to achieve unique goals.

Feminist analysis can be accomplished through lyric analysis. In first listening to recorded music, then performing it live, women are able to move from hearing their stories in the voices of others to internalizing these as part of their own experiences and understanding. Music written and recorded by women can be particularly effective because it allows participants to more readily see themselves reflected in the music. A wealth of recorded music is available, because a gamut of themes can be explored in this feminist analysis, moving beyond women's experiences of violence to examine such issues as love, relationships, power, gender-role socialization, healing, strength, and empowerment. My collection of over 150 songs used in therapy (from pop, country, and rock to indie) has developed from my own listening, as well as from suggestions from many participants over the years. Bringing in their own music can provide women with a wonderful opportunity to experience themselves as experts of their own music and ultimately their own lives. Samplings of this music can be found in "Singing Subversion, Singing Soul" (Curtis, 2000) and in "Women Survivors of Abuse and Developmental Trauma" (Curtis, 2013b). These include a wide range of songs from indie to mainstream artists, such as Tracy Chapman's "Behind the Wall" and "Telling Stories"; Mary Chapin Carpenter's "He Thinks He'll Keep Her"; Saffire, The Uppity Blues Women's "Bitch with a Bad Attitude"; Cowboy Junkies' "Sun Comes Up," "It's Tuesday Morning"; Ani Difranco's "Not a Pretty Girl"; and the Dixie Chicks' "Goodbye Earl."

Women's empowerment can be accomplished through songwriting, performing, and recording; the recording can include final production and CD cover artwork (original art or selection of available, free artwork from the web). An experience common to many abused women and girls is that of being silenced—of not being heard, believed, or valued (Curtis, 2008). The opportunity to tell their own stories and reclaim their voices in songwriting and recording can be very empowering. The process of songwriting has to be presented very sensitively, providing as much support as is needed for the women who will enter therapy, each with her own individual level of self-esteem—esteem being one of the greatest casualties of abuse. Many of the participants in my music therapy practice have taken great delight in hearing their own voices in songs and in sharing these—not only with their supporters, but also with their abusers. In doing so, they begin their journey in truth telling and in social activism.

Women's self-nurturance can be accomplished through music-centered relaxation and imagery. It is first through lyric analysis, however, that participants gain a feminist understanding of women's experiences of violence, an understanding that underscores the importance of their own safety and self-nurturance as essential precursors to the safety and wellness of their children.

An exploration of techniques with abused women would not be complete without touching upon social activism, which is a unique and critical component of feminist music therapy. Social activism is expected on the part of both the client and the therapist; it takes place both within therapy and outside of it, and within musical and nonmusical contexts. It can start with truth telling in therapy, moves to witnessing in music recordings and performances, and expands to participation in social activism in the outside world. In reclaiming their own voices and in speaking for others without voices, women can greatly enhance their own healing and empowerment. Feminist music therapists have a responsibility, beyond their work in the therapy room, to advocate for change and work toward elimination of violence against women and girls in the outside world.

Women's Voices

Over the 19 years that I have been doing this work, whether within a research or clinical practice context, I have gathered measures of therapy outcomes, both quantitative and qualitative. These have included pen-and-paper tests such as the standardized Tennessee Self-Concept Scale (Curtis, 2000) and the Post-Traumatic Stress Disorder Checklist (Curtis & Harrison, 2006), as well as analysis of participant interviews and song lyrics. These have been remarkably consistent in documenting the effectiveness of feminist music therapy with abused women and girls (Curtis, 2000, 2007, 2008; Curtis & Harrison, 2006). There is, however, no more powerful reflection of this than women's own words and the music of their original songs. There were times when I wondered how it would be possible to recover from such harm and how I could connect with these women across such barriers as experience and culture; it was at these times that the music served as powerful cotherapist and catalyst for change. To see women move from insecurity, and at times skepticism of music therapy, to a place of remarkable transformation, as seen in their songwriting, never ceases to amaze me. The songwriting over the years has included powerful songs of resistance, resilience, transformation, and hope.

Research with Survivors of Abuse

The work described below as *Finding Voice* was informed by my (Elizabeth York) lived experience as a feminist, music therapist, musician, and my work as a writer, composer, and performer within the women's music network in the 1980s. (I have also enhanced my personal and professional growth by undergoing psychotherapy with a feminist therapist.) *Finding Voice* can also be described as *arts-based research*, since the clinical process involved multiple arts modalities (music, visual art, dance, and poetry). The project can be further defined as *participatory action research* because the women participants guided the research process and initiated new elements in the sessions, resulting in public performances to educate and inform the attendees as to the effects of domestic violence.

In 2002, I began a clinical research project with women survivors of domestic violence who were served in a community agency. The proposal was reviewed and approved by the appropriate boards and agencies. A complete description of this project can be found in York (2006). The overarching purpose of the qualitative study was to examine the efficacy of music therapy and creative/expressive arts approaches with women survivors of domestic violence through a feminist lens. A second purpose was to examine emerging themes of the work via a grounded theory approach to the data, and to document how women entered into the creative process. The metaphor of *finding voice* was used to describe the process of encouraging the women to give voice to their experiences, using the creative and musical arts as tools for empowerment and creative expression. As sessions progressed, the women decided that their creative work should be shared with a broader audience, and an ethnographic performance piece (including script and CD for recording), titled *Finding Voice: The Music of Utah Battered Women* (York, 2004), was created.

Participants

Forty women, members of an ongoing support group within a community agency, engaged in a total of 30 music therapy and expressive arts sessions. Case managers informed them all about the project, and all signed consent to participate. The women ranged in age from 18 to 58 years old and received additional services that included shelter, legal assistance, counseling, child care, and the drop-in support group. All were Anglo-American, and most self-identified as members of the Church of Jesus Christ of Latter Day Saints. Many of the women presented symptoms of PTSD, major depression, dependent personality,

and/or substance abuse. The most commonly displayed symptoms were low self-esteem, poor body image, hyperarousal/anxiety, and depressive symptoms.

Procedure

Weekly 2-hour sessions were held in a group room located at the facility. Sessions were audiorecorded and transcribed by Maureen Hearns, MT-BC, who served as research assistant and cotherapist (see York & Hearns, 2005). Barbara Scott, the group facilitator, brought me into the group as a participant observer in the early stages, to gain the women's trust and gradually introduce musical materials and creative arts interventions. Journaling and the sharing of journal entries were already ongoing components of the group. An informal means of attaining informed consent was agreed upon by group members, which allowed me to work with writings when women placed materials into a wicker basket that was prominently placed in the center of the circle.

Feminist Ways of Working

The methods and interventions used in *Finding Voice* (York, 2006) evolved over time with ongoing consultations and weekly meetings with the co-facilitators. In the beginning, the interventions corresponded to and enhanced the themes from an existing curriculum. They were also fashioned according to the cues provided by the women participants and their expressed needs and ideas. My first sessions as a participant and observer provided time for me to get to know the women, ascertain their creative urges, answer questions about the music therapy profession, and listen to their ideas about the potential for music and the creative arts as healing tools.

My initial connection to the group also involved sharing a recording of an original instrumental composition, entitled "Transformations," as a means of introducing myself. After listening to this piece, the women wrote and commented on what they thought I was attempting to express musically. This receptive music listening experience, paired with writing, bridged their familiar journaling with the new experience of integrating music into the sessions. In offering my own music, I became as vulnerable as they in seeking admittance to the group. Sharing my music provided the women with a way to assess a new member and come to consensus in regard to my intentions. From my point of view, this gesture was an intentional act of *power sharing*, a feminist concept indicating an egalitarian versus hierarchical approach.

Participants provided their creative intentions to the group by placing writings into a basket, signaling their consent to share with me and the other group members. The intentions were transformed into a variety of poetic forms, including choral readings, poetry, and songs. Women shared in reading each others' words and affirming their participation in the creative process.

Vocal Work

I gradually integrated breath work, vocal exercises, and warm-ups into the sessions, lengthening the duration of the musical/creative aspects of the group experience. A toning exercise (with hands placed over ears) allowed participants to hear the sound of their own voices without scrutiny or pressure to perform. Participants listened to the sounds of their own voices, gradually adding tones, extending breath. The *inner critic* was quickly identified as a theme. Judgments about the quality of voices came to the forefront of the experience, leading to verbal processing and insights into their experiences of verbal abuse of being criticized, of not being heard, acknowledged, or valued and how those messages were internalized. More traditional vocal warm-ups were introduced and integrated into the sessions, and women had the opportu-

nity to enter in at their own pace. A second stage of the vocal work expanded to simple chants with affirming lyrics that could be integrated into the sessions. Group singing was a second step toward being heard as participants exposed their negative self-evaluations and critiques and received support and goodwill in return.

Lyric analysis and songwriting were a means to question traditional gender roles and uneven power distribution between men and women. Comparing lyrics that perpetuate gender conformity to those from the genre of women's music that are intentionally empowering and comforting to women led to discussion about role expectations. Early messages about putting other people's needs first, about self-care, self-concept, and what constituted beauty emerged, as women brought other popular songs to discuss and analyze.

In subsequent sessions, a traditional American spiritual, "Sometimes I Feel Like a Motherless Child," was used to encourage each woman to express her feelings about being labeled a battered woman (e.g., "Sometimes I feel like a stormy day"). The blues form was a conduit for lyric writing about the women's day-to-day existence as they healed from abusive relationships. Women submitted complete poems into the basket, questioning power within their relationships: One poem described the self-centeredness of one woman's spouse and his expectation that she would always be there to do his will. Another posited the assertion, from the woman's point of view, that she hoped she would actually "matter" to her spouse. A poem cowritten by the participants and me began with the question "How did you get here?" and ended with the declaration "I just can't believe this is happening to me. I just can't believe my life has come to this. I just can't believe he could ever hurt me so" (York, 2004). Original lyrics became complete songs that were analyzed, processed, learned, and finally sung together.

Transformative Percussion Work

Although most music therapy interventions in *Finding Voice* focused on vocal work and poetry/creative writing, therapeutic drumming was gradually introduced. I insert an important contraindication here. The act of striking a drum can trigger past memories of being assaulted, hit, and otherwise abused. The dynamic sound of the drum (especially when played intensely and at high volume) can evoke the sounds of verbal abuse, yelling, and crying. Playing the drum with an open hand or a mallet are choices that should be carefully presented. When working with any drumming intervention, I suggest that elements be presented gradually and in stages, in order for women to maintain their sense of control and personal power.

First, a small frame drum can be passed around the circle, with each woman exploring the instrument in any way that she wishes. First contacts with a drum may be tentative, perhaps simply holding the instrument, rubbing hands or fingers over the drumhead, or playing softly for a short duration. The metaphor and irony of making the choice to strike an external object will not go unnoticed by women survivors; neither will the metaphor of power. A woman might request to play the drum softly while the others sing a nurturing chant. Another may choose a less percussive instrument such as the rain stick, which provides a softer, arrhythmic accompaniment.

As a group matures and the work deepens, it may be possible to bring a gathering drum into a session as a container to process more difficult feelings. A large gathering drum may facilitate the expression of anger, of power differences between group members using dyadic conversations, individual work, or quartets around the four quadrants of the instrument. The reminder of heartbeat as original drumbeat can serve to reframe the experience of the drum as container of all feelings; as womb, nurturer, and connection to women as creators of life. Safety in working with the drum is paramount as feelings of anger arise—feelings that are natural to the processing of violence toward women and to violence in general.

The construction of personal frame drums is metaphorically built on the theme of transforming the hierarchical *power over* (and potential to inflict harm) into *claiming personal power* (which I understand as empowerment). Square frames can easily be purchased at a hardware store and assembled. Women are encouraged to paint symbols of personal power on the inside of the frames. On the outside, symbols are painted that represent how personal power is shared with others—with family and in the community at large. Frames are wrapped with clear packing tape, with one woman assisting another. Together it is possible to affirm each other's creative process and redefine power. Incorporating the instruments and affirmations into a percussion ensemble (e.g., "I am beautiful and I am strong") reinforces and reframes the definition of personal empowerment. Poetry based on the theme of anger can also be created and read with percussive accompaniment.

Creative Arts Interventions Paired with Music

Besides creating the drums, visual and performing arts can be paired with music in a variety of ways. Women can draw mandalas to instrumental music based on the Bonny Method of Guided Imagery and Music (BMGIM) protocols provided by a trained therapist. Women with sewing skills can transfer mandalas to cloth and then into quilt squares that are sewn together and given as a gift to the shelter. Shawls representing the healing process can be created and worn during a dance within a performance. Mirroring, stretching, breathing exercises, and choreography can be incorporated as warm-ups to rehearsals. Women who identify with and reclaim performance skills on their personal instruments can offer to bring those musical elements in to accompany others.

Outcomes

Music therapy and creative arts interventions can be powerful tools for empowerment and creative expression for women survivors of domestic violence. Levels of involvement may vary in relation to personal circumstance, length of time in the group, and safety considerations. Creative arts interventions used during sessions enabled women to name and identify their abuse using an alternative language. They used these creative tools to move into and through the healing process. All 40 women in the *Finding Voice* project consented to have their creative materials included in a script, video, CD, and book of poetry. Twelve women became cast members and performed *Finding Voice* as a production in nine separate venues. Therapeutic outcomes gathered from an exit questionnaire included (1) claiming creative impulses, (2) the development of personal music skills, (3) increased self-esteem, (4) positive self-evaluation, (5) improved relationships with family members, and (6) perceived transition from victim to survivor to thriver to community advocate.

Conclusions

Given the pervasiveness of violence against women worldwide, and that many music therapists will find abuse survivors among their clients, regardless of where they work, we acknowledge the potential for an increase in clinical practice with survivors of domestic violence. It has been our experience that carefully chosen music therapy interventions, provided from a feminist perspective, can offer a means of empowerment for women survivors, most especially

by improving women's self-evaluation, assertiveness, and self-esteem, as well as by providing women with opportunities for creative self-expression that may support emancipation from an abusive environment. Music therapists have the potential to enhance the team of professionals who traditionally serves women survivors, adding an artistic component to support groups for women and their children.

As Purdon (2006) has asserted, it is not a simple matter to come to terms with violence in our society and combine that knowledge with the practice of music therapy. We can only speculate as to why the profession has been slow to fully recognize a clinical practice in this area. The work necessitates introspection through ongoing clinical supervision, undertaking personal therapy, and a gradual recognition that we cannot ignore the status of women: their oppression and victimization. A body of literature is developing on feminist music therapy (Hadley, 2006). It is our hope that educators will understand the importance of including this topic in their curricula. We would also encourage professional music therapy organizations to adopt standards of clinical practice that include work with women survivors and other survivors of trauma and violence.

REFERENCES

American Music Therapy Association. (2013). *A descriptive statistical profile of the AMTA membership*. Retrieved from *www.musictherapy.org/assets/1/7/13WorkforceAnalysis.pdf*.

American Psychiatric Association. (2013). *Diagnostic and statistical manual of mental disorders* (5th ed.). Arlington, VA: Author.

Ballou, M., & Gabalac, N. W. (1985). *A feminist position on mental health*. Springfield, IL: Charles C Thomas.

Black, M. C., Basile, K. C., Breiding, M. J., Smith, S. G., Walters, M. L., Merrick, M. T., et al. (2011). *The national intimate partner and sexual violence survey (NISVS): 2012 summary report*. National Center for Injury Prevention and Control, Centers for Disease Control and Prevention, Atlanta, GA.

Cascardi, M., O'Leary, K. D., Schlee, K. A., & Lawrence, E. E. (1995). Characteristics of women physically abused by their spouses who seek treatment regarding marital conflict. *Journal of Consulting and Clinical Psychology, 63,* 616–623.

Cassity, M. D., & Theobold, K. K. (1990). Domestic violence: Assessments and treatments employed by music therapists. *Journal of Music Therapy, 27,* 179–194.

Curtis, S. L. (2000). Singing subversion, singing soul: Women's voices in feminist music therapy (Doctoral dissertation, Concordia University, 1997). *Dissertation Abstracts International, 60*(12-A), 4240.

Curtis, S. L. (2006). Feminist music therapy: Transforming theory, transforming lives. In S. Hadley (Ed.), *Feminist perspectives in music therapy* (pp. 227–244). Gilsum, NH: Barcelona.

Curtis, S. L. (2007). Claiming voice: Music therapy for childhood sexual abuse survivors. In S. L. Brooke (Ed.), *Use of creative arts therapies with sexual abuse survivors* (pp. 196–206). Springfield, IL: Charles C Thomas.

Curtis, S. L. (2008) Gathering voices: Music therapy for abused women. In S. L. Brooke (Ed.), *Creative arts therapies and domestic violence* (pp. 121–135). Springfield, IL: Charles C Thomas.

Curtis, S. L. (2013a). Sorry it has taken so long: Continuing feminist dialogues in music therapy. *Voices: A World Forum for Music Therapy.* Retrieved from *https://normt.uib.no/index.php/voices/article/viewArticle/688/572.*

Curtis, S. L. (2013b). Women survivors of abuse and developmental trauma. In L. Eyre (Ed.), *Guidelines for music therapy practice: Mental health* (pp. 263–268). Gilsum, NH: Barcelona.

Curtis, S. L., & Harrison, G. (2006). Empowering women survivors of violence: A collaborative music therapy–social work approach. In S. L. Brooke (Ed.), *Creative modalities for therapy with children and adults* (pp. 195–204). Springfield, IL: Charles C Thomas.

Domestic Violence Statistics. (2012). *Domestic violence statistics: Let's put a stop to domestic violence and abuse.* Retrieved from *http://domesticviolencestatistics.org.*

Fesler, M. M. (2007). *The effect of music therapy on depression and post-traumatic disorder in a shelter for victims of domestic violence.* Unpublished manuscript, Radford University, Radford, VA.

Friedman, S. H., & Loue, S. (2008). *Intimate partner violence among women with severe mental illness.*

Retrieved from *www.psychiatrictimes.com/display/article 10168/1152781#.*

Hadley, S. (Ed.). (2006). *Feminist perspectives in music therapy.* Gilsum, NH: Barcelona.

Hahna, N. D. (2004). *Empowering women: A feminist perspective of the Bonny Method of Guided Imagery and Music and intimate partner violence.* Unpublished master's thesis, Radford University, Radford, VA.

Jacobson, N., & Gottman, J. (1998). *When men batter women: New insights into ending abusive relationships.* New York: Simon & Schuster.

Morrow, S. L., Hawxhurst, D. M., Montes de Vegas, A. Y., Abousleman, T. M., & Castaneda, C. L. (2006). Toward a radical feminist multicultural therapy: Renewing a commitment to activism. In R. L. Toporek, L. H. Gerstein, N. A. Fouad, G. Roysircar, & T. Israel (Eds.), *Handbook for social justice in counseling psychology: Leadership, vision and action* (pp. 231–247). Thousand Oaks, CA: Sage.

National Coalition against Domestic Violence. (2012). *Domestic violence facts.* Retrieved from *www.ncadv.org.*

Purdon, C. (2006). Feminist music therapy with abused teen girls. In S. Hadley (Ed.), *Feminist perspectives in music therapy* (pp. 205–226). Gilsum, NH: Barcelona.

Rubenstein, L. S. (2004). *DivorceNet. What is battered women's syndrome?* Available at *www.divorcenet.com/States/Oregon/or_art02.*

United States Department of Justice. (2012). *Office on Violence Against Women.* Retrieved from *www.ovw.usdoj.gov/index.html.*

Whipple, J., & Lindsey, R. (1999). Music for the soul: A music therapy program for battered women. *Music Therapy Perspectives, 17,* 61–68.

Worrell, J., & Remer, P. (2003). *Feminist perspectives in therapy: Empowering diverse women.* New York: Wiley.

York, E. (2004). *Finding voice: The music of Utah battered women* [CD]. Logan, UT: Fast Forward Productions.

York, E. (2006). Finding voice: Feminist music therapy and research with women survivors of domestic violence. In S. Hadley (Ed.), *Feminist perspectives in music therapy* (pp. 245–265). Gilsum NH: Barcelona.

York, E., & Hearns, M. (2005, July). *A music therapy research protocol with women victims of intimate partner violence.* Paper presented at the 11th World Congress of Music Therapy, Brisbane, Australia.

CHAPTER 31

Music Therapy for Survivors of Traumatic Events

Ronald M. Borczon

In a matter of moments, a person or community can be forever changed. When forces of nature or acts of human beings cause destruction and/or loss of life, a common result is a breaking of trust between the person/community and the earth or fellow humans. The myths that help people exist on a daily basis are shattered. Some of these myths might include that children should be safe in school, the wind should not blow so hard, the earth should not shake, and the waters from the river or ocean should not rise so high. A multitude of myths can be shattered by one significant event. The result of this destruction of the myth is that survivors might develop posttraumatic stress disorder (PTSD), and what was once a normal environment and life now becomes a place where people suffer on many different levels. This trauma can come into people's inner worlds and begin to disrupt their lives so that the previous experience of a normal life is forever changed. In order to move forward, people need to express what has happened to them as well as finding new ways to cope and live as their lives move to a new sense of what *normal* might look like.

We can experience many types of trauma. People survive natural events such as fires, earthquakes, hurricanes, tsunamis, floods, and tornadoes. Some traumas that are associated with accidents can involve cars, industrial sites, and loss of a loved one. (It should be noted that events such as physical and emotional abuse and war are not the focus of this chapter.) Although all of these categories can induce PTSD, to generalize music therapy techniques to such a wide range of causes could be difficult to cover in the scope of this writing. It is possible, however, to adjust some of the techniques that are discussed to meet various levels of clients' needs.

Clientele

The development of PTSD can have a dramatic effect on the quality of life and the overall functioning of an individual.

In PTSD a traumatic event is not remembered and relegated to one's past in the same way as other life events. Trauma continues to intrude with visual, auditory, and/or other somatic reality on the lives of its victims. Again and again they relive this life-threatening experience which they have suffered, reacting in mind and body as though such events were still occurring. (Rothschild, 2000, p. 6)

The fifth edition of the *Diagnostic and Statistical Manual of Mental Disorders* (DSM-5; American Psychiatric Association, 2013) cites symptoms, including having recurrent, involuntary, and intrusive distressing memories of the traumatic event; recurring distressing dreams related to the event; dissociative reactions (flashbacks), with the traumatic event reoccurring, as well as physiological reactions that occur because of reminders of the event. Because of the significance of the event, there can be lingering feelings of fear, sadness, helplessness, guilt, hopelessness, a feeling of detachment, and difficulty relating to others. There is often a period of time after a traumatic event when people think that they are functioning just fine, but on a deeper level there is a sense that something is wrong that they do not understand. They can't make sense of why unsettling feelings might be recurring. On a larger level, with communities that have undergone a trauma, the whole community can be feeling these things on an individualized level, yet people don't speak of it for fear of exposing their sense of inability to cope. An example of this was 4 months after the 1994 Northridge earthquake in a classroom at California State University, Northridge, when I, as the instructor, asked the class how many thought about the earthquake on a daily basis. Everyone in the class raised their hands, then we all proceeded to discuss that each person had thought that he or she was the only person who felt that way.

When a traumatic event occurs, those who are affected may go into a *survival mode*, which functions as a means to literally survive what has occurred, physically and emotionally. The survival mode is often accompanied by a sense of shock and numbness in relation to the event, as it can sometimes put a person in an altered sense of reality in order to survive. The event can become *frozen* within the survivor, both emotionally and physically, in that many survivors of trauma state that particular emotions, images, sensations, and muscular reactions related to the trauma are deeply imprinted on their minds (van der Kolk & Fisler, 1995). The stress of the event can have physical manifestations in the form of raised blood pressure, rapid breathing, increased heart rate, compromised immune system functions, increased muscle tension, a heightened state of alertness, and sleeplessness (Mitchell, 2007). Many of these symptoms might also be present when a survivor of trauma is reminded of the event, as they are the physical symptoms that have become imprinted in the body.

After large-scale events, the survivors are often afforded *psychological counseling* to deal with the immediate effect of the trauma. Later, though, when PTSD becomes a reality in one's life, music therapy can be an effective intervention for the survivor. Music therapy can be most powerful when the instinctual survival instincts have waned and the individual is faced with what to do with all that is held within. The fears, sadness, and reality of what happened begin to settle in and alter one's views of life. This emotional construct that lies within the survivor begins to affect him or her in many different ways. What is discovered through the music is processed, and what it brings to light can energize the spirit of hope and healing.

Clinical Work

I first started working with individuals with PTSD in the early 1990s as I co-led groups with Carolyn Braddock (*www.braddockbodyprocess.com*), who specializes in trauma work. Through this collaboration, I learned many non-music-related techniques that I then incorporated into musical interventions. I mentioned the Northridge earthquake above. Northridge was the epicenter of a 6.7 magnitude earthquake that devastated the campus and the area. From that experience, I learned firsthand about mass trauma and its effect on communities. My students and I developed musical interventions to take into grade schools to help the children process the event, have some fun time in music, and learn relaxation strategies for when they felt stressed.

Many goals can be addressed through music therapy experiences with those who have survived trauma. The goals and experiences that are decided upon must be within the scope of practice of the music therapist. In all instances, when working with those who have experienced a traumatic event, the music therapist must be clearly centered in his or her own sense of *self*. It is imperative to be aware of countertransference issues, as well as techniques that go beyond the scope of music therapy. The music therapist must be aware of "secondary traumatic stress" (Figley, 1995, p. 53), whereby the therapist develops symptoms of trauma from wanting to help the traumatized person. If the music therapist who is facilitating the music therapy experience has also been affected by a large-scale traumatic event, he or she must be even more keenly aware of his or her personal relationship with, and feelings about, the trauma. Although supervision is always suggested, the less experienced music therapist needs to be very active in seeking supervision and outside support.

Drumming Experiences

The experience of group drumming can address many goals, as well as creating various positive offshoots within the drumming experience. As individuals express what were previously regarded as feelings unique to them, a sense of cohesion may develop because many will report similar feelings; also, the physical act of playing a drum can reduce tension and, often, anxiety too (Borczon, 2013). Having good basic leadership

skills in structuring a drum circle is helpful, as the drum circle is the underlying framework from which therapeutic interventions can be integrated. Braddock (1995) states that the focus of using breath, sound, and movement intervention strategies is a central part of healing. By involving clients in drumming, the music therapist can bring attention to breathing to help regulate it and increase conscious awareness of the breathing cycle; using the voice in chant can help to install positive affirmations; and moving to the drumming can help release tension that has been held in the body following the trauma.

In leading the drumming experience, the music therapist must be aware of the power of the group sound. The dynamic level of the drumming and how it might affect the participants needs to be constantly monitored. Sometimes loud sounds are associated with the trauma, and on initial exposure to the drumming, individuals may be triggered to fall into a sense of reliving the trauma. When creating a large energized sound, one must vigilantly observe participants for any abreactions.

I have been successful in incorporating therapeutic drumming in both small and large groups, as well as with individuals. Some goals that can be addressed through drumming sessions include expression of feelings, development of group cohesion, an increased sense of community, a reduction in tension and anxiety, increased groundedness in participants, increased hope, and the creation of positive affirmations.

I generally place a 14-inch quartz toning bowl upon a gathering drum positioned in the center of the circle. To begin the session, I introduce the sound of the bowl to the group and invite the members to come up in groups of three and four to feel the vibration on the drum head and to hold the palms of their hands about 2 inches from the center of the bowl. Here they will feel the vibration of the bowl, and this experience can later be used as a metaphor for the vibrations that are created in the room among the participants, as well as going beyond the room to the vibrations that exist among people. After this initial experience, I do a simple call-and-response so that they can feel a sense of rhythm. I demonstrate through the call-and-response that there are beats within a basic beat. I give them a *heartbeat* (a constant beat without a sense of meter) that they all match, and, when they feel comfortable, they find their own rhythms within the beat. From that, several avenues that can be taken:

1. When the drumming comes to a stop, have the participants check in with their breathing. Instruct them to slow their breathing if it has accelerated. Have them also check in with their bodies to notice any signs of tension or relaxation.

2. In helping people begin to focus on emotional expression, first have them talk about what happened in the past week that was stressful. Have them find one word to describe that stressor, and teach them the rhythm of the word. Then, as a group, have them each play their word within a given rhythm, focusing on expelling the energy of that word through their sound. Next, have them focus on one word about how they would like to feel, and teach them the rhythm of that word. Have the group members drum their words in the rhythm of each of their words, supported by the feeling of the word. Have them discuss the different feelings between the musical expression of the two words. A chant can be developed to encompass what they want to feel. Rhythmic breathing to a slow drumbeat can enhance the experience of the chant.

3. Have participants repeat point 2, only instead of a word, ask them to create a body movement to the beat. The ending of the chant is the body motion that they would like to feel. This conscious effort helps the body learn a movement that is positive in character and through the rhythm becomes more entrained into the person's physicality.

4. A *home base* can also be created via positive words that come from the group. The rhythm of the words becomes a grounding metrical experience as well as being integrated into the psyche of the participants. Ending with a one-syllable (one-beat) word is recommended. Think of the rhythm of the following words: joy, comfort, rest, peaceful, energizing, lifted, strong. ♩♫ ♩♫ ♪ ♪ ♪ ♫ ♩

The session concludes with everyone playing a beat in unison, and, if the chant has been created, saying the chant together and then slowly taking the chant to a place where they are only hearing it inside their head. The following clinical example is an adaptation of this protocol.

CLINICAL EXAMPLE

After 9/11, much of the country felt helpless about how to help the victims of the event. Additionally, many people did not know what to do with their own feelings that had been stirred up through watching the event on television, as well as the emotional impact of knowing how many lives were lost. A week after 9/11, I did a collaborative community drumming event with Christine Stevens and Remo Drums. The event was advertised in local newspapers as well as around the campus of California State University, Northridge.

It began with asking people to just feel the rhythm that they were playing on their drum. They then were asked to play in rhythm with two or three people who were close to them. After a time, the Remo table drum was introduced, and people from various cultures were asked to come and play on the drum to symbolize a sense of universal community. A short time later the drumming came to a close, and I introduced the next experience. My idea was to try to make a connection between the drummers and those who had lost their lives on 9/11, so that in some way the participants could feel an even greater sense of meaning in their playing. Because so many people had lost their lives, it would be difficult to remember each one individually, so I decided to focus on those who were from California. I acquired a list of all of those Californians who had perished through the terror attacks of 9/11. Each name was printed on a small white piece of paper and randomly given out to the participants. The participants were taught how to play the rhythm of the name that they were given. The energy of the name and that person would be embodied through this rhythm. This was a very moving part of the day. After a time of drumming the rhythm of the name, the participants were instructed to fade out the drumming and quietly speak and focus on the name. The participants were then encouraged to find out as much as they could, in the following week, about the person whose name they played in rhythm. The session ended with my playing of a Shruti box (an instrument similar to a harmonium) and Christine Stevens leading the community in singing "Amazing Grace." To this day I have the name of the person I was given framed and sitting on my windowsill in my office.

Improvisation

Drumming can be a prelude to improvising with a number of percussion instruments, both pitched and unpitched. Limb and Braun (2008) discovered that during improvisation with jazz musicians, the prefrontal cortex essentially shuts down, allowing for improvisational material to come from "a combination of psychological processes required for spontaneous improvisation, in which internally motivated, stimulus-independent behaviors unfold in the absence of central processes that typically mediate self-monitoring and conscious volitional control of ongoing performance" (p. 1). This is important to recognize, because it implies that the improvised music might be coming from a deep place that is not consciously monitored, opening up the emotional aspects of the person to feel freely. Volkman (1993) states:

> The instrument/music acts as transitional object, bridging internal and external worlds as well as past and present. Although circum-

stances of the past may not be changed, a new way of relating is discovered. Musical improvisation gives the individual the power to respond. It is what was originally taken away from a traumatized person by perpetrators or circumstance. (p. 250)

Many of the same goals that are mentioned above in drumming can be addressed through improvisation. It is through the music that is created from the improvisation that there is a successful expression where words have failed. It is through that expression that the individual can begin to understand and process his or her feelings.

If group members are not familiar with the instruments, an orientation to how to play them and what they sound like is needed. I often begin similarly to how I begin group drumming, with a call-and-response. Once the members feel comfortable with their instruments and their rhythms, a number of different scenarios can take place:

1. They use their instruments as a way of expressing how they felt when the trauma occurred, how they currently feel, or what they want to feel in the future. In processing this experience, connections can be made between group members who share the same feelings.

2. Individuals can conduct the group in an improvised piece that depicts any number of scenarios, such as the trauma itself, feelings associated with the trauma, frustrations, or inspirations. If the improvisation is recorded, it can be listened to later and processed. The processing can be done not only by the conductor but also by the participants describing what it was like for them to follow the conductor.

3. A powerful improvisational experience by Carol Bitcon utilizes a simple chant: "There are two sides of me, one on the inside, and one on the outside. Here is my _____" (Bitcon, 1989, p. 22). During this improvisation the participants

take turns saying this chant and then playing for the group their *inside* or their *outside*. This experience can be processed in a couple of ways: the listeners can reflect on what they heard in the improvisation, giving feedback to the improviser; or the person who did the improvising can process what he or she wanted to depict in the improvisation. Recording and reviewing the recording can offer another avenue for processing.

4. An empathic improvisation can occur when the participants are asked to listen to one another and support each other though the music. This is best accomplished in small groups or in breakout sessions. Supporting group members will provide a sustained beat, allowing one of the members to play above the beat. This can be either a referential or nonreferential experience. In the referential experience, the soloist is asked to focus on a thought or feeling and portray that on the instrument(s) he or she has chosen. In a nonreferential experience, the soloist plays without reference to any outside thought or feeling, and then the experience is processed, focusing on the music and then transferring those ideas to a real-life experience. The role of serving as the supporter is also processed, reflecting on what was it like to be a genuine source of support for another person via the music.

CLINICAL EXAMPLE

The setting for this clinical example is the second day of a 3-day workshop for individuals with PTSD. The group consisted of 10 women and two men. I began with an introduction to the instruments and a short rhythmic improvisation. After a short time, I asked them all to return their instruments to the table. We then had a discussion about using verbal therapy to try to describe feelings that sometimes are very difficult to put into words. I explained to them the Bitcon experience (previously mentioned) and how they would be using the instruments to express how they feel on the inside or outside. They then chose an instrument to use as their "voice" in expressing these feelings.

We were all sitting on the floor as we began an improvisation in a slow and steady rhythm. When a person wanted to play, he or she cued the group by saying aloud, "There are two sides of me, one on the inside and one on the outside. Here is my _____." When the person was finished, he or she simply counted the group back into a rhythm by saying, "1–2–3–4–play." After everyone had finished playing, I brought the improvisation to a close, and it was time to process. The participants mainly described what it was like to play the instrument as their voice, and the content of what they were expressing also came through. The participants spoke of the power of the experience and the emotional release that they felt as they were able to use the instruments as their voice. This is in line with the idea that we can express through music what our words cannot describe.

Storytelling

I have used the art of storytelling with music since the early 1990s and have found it to be an important avenue of my practice. The rationale for storytelling can be found in Carl Jung's (1972) writings, as he speaks of the importance of fairy tales and myths: "In myths and fairy tales, as in dreams, the psyche tells its own story, and the interplay of the archetypes is revealed in its natural setting" (p. 217). Clarissa Pinkola Estés (1992), in *Women Who Run with the Wolves: Myths and Stories of the Wild Woman Archetype*, speaks of the power of stories as *medicine*, and that remedies for healing are within the stories. When stories are told to those who have PTSD, the relationship that occurs between the clients and the images and symbols of the story can be revealing for them. They will often project feelings as they interpret and discuss the morals and the characters of the story. The task of the music therapist, then, is to help the client see the connections between the projections, the symbols, and the self.

There are three components of storytelling: the musical drone, the telling of the story, and the story. The musical drone can be a zither or harp tuned to D–E–G♯–A–B, a guitar tuned to an open tuning such as D–A–D–F♯–A–D or D–A–D–G–A–D, a simple combination of hand drum sounds, a tamboura, or any instrument that provides a background of sound so that the voice can speak over it. The function of the music is to provide support for the words, to create atmosphere, and to entrain the listeners.

The story to be told must be practiced and practiced until a comfort level is achieved. The characters and situations must be described in such a way that the listeners can envision them in their minds. The clearer an image is for the listeners, the easier it is for them to resonate with the story. The tone of voice may, at times, change when different characters are talking. The rhythm of the voice must be slow enough for the listeners to grasp the scenes, but not so slow as to hamper the progression of the story. The story itself, for those who are suffering from PTSD, must have a moral that is couched in overcoming adversity, finding reasons for why things happen in life, strength, or anything that encompasses these themes.

Two levels of the story can be processed. With the first level, or the *moral* of the story, the clients process what they think they have learned from the story. I often relate this processing to the idea that ancient civilizations used story to teach the morals and values of the community. The second level is how the clients resonate with various symbols of the story. On this deeper level, the symbolic nature of the story comes to life. Jung (1969) stated, "The psyche contains all the images that have ever given rise to myths" (p. 7). The music therapist must understand how the client's relationship to symbols from the story can be explored, and thus must have some knowledge of symbols, dreams, and how Jung views these as important windows into one's psyche. However, this second level of discussion is not required for a client to prosper from hearing a well-crafted story to music.

I use a number of stories in therapy sessions, but the two that I use most often with those with PTSD are "Khdir and Moses" (Borczon, 1998) and "Grandma's Story." The story of "Khdir and Moses" finds them walking together, and Khdir asks Moses to not question what will happen that day, as Khdir seemingly instigates three acts that appear destructive to communities and a person. After each event Moses breaks his promise and questions Khdir. Khdir then sings to Moses a song that states, "The things that I do you may not understand, you promised not to question me." However, after the first two events, Khdir lets Moses walk with him, even though the promise was broken. After Moses breaks his promise a third time, Khdir lets him know that they can no longer walk together. Before Khdir leaves, he tells Moses that a greater good comes out of each one of the events that appears destructive. Through the processing of the story, clients often come to a point of acceptance that something good might come out of the trauma, or the theme of *everything happens for a reason*. The story is accompanied by a slow drumbeat of four, using a different attack on each beat and with the third beat being a half note.

I developed "Grandmother's Story" through various story creation experiences that I have done with clients. The synopsis of the story is that a grandmother is telling her two grandchildren a story about a young couple that lives through an extraordinary event and ends up surviving it because of their trust in one another. In the story, a piece of paper is given to the young man, but the listener is not told what was on the piece of paper. The grandmother tells the children to go down by the seashore and look inside all the seashells to find the paper. In the center of the room, I have a seashell with a piece of paper inside of it. On the piece of paper is the Chinese symbol that many believe to be the concept of *crisis = opportunity*.

危机

Each participant looks at the piece of paper, and from there processing begins. The musical background is that of the zither tuned to the scale mentioned earlier. A complete rendering of these two stories can be found at the following website: *http://mstcman.wix.com/stroy-page*.

An offshoot of telling established stories is creating a new story based on the images that come from the group as they listen to three selections of music. The first music selection is "Unseen Rain" by W. A. Mathieu. The group is instructed to listen to the music and let whatever images arise, come to their mind. They can allow the images to shift and change. After a brief relaxation exercise, the music is played. At its conclusion, each member is asked what he or she imaged, and the music therapist writes down the main parts of each person's image. Then the music therapist must adeptly use some part of each person's image to begin creating a story.

For example, if in a small group session the main images that come up are a young boy and girl, an old couple, a field, a piano, a dancer, someone leaving, and someone riding on a horse, the story might begin with an old couple reminiscing when they were young. It could go on to say that he played piano and she was a dancer, and they would often ride horses in the fields. Then there must be a turn in the story to set up for the second piece of music. The turn is how something is going to happen and a journey is going to take place—in this case, the young couple had parents and families who did not want them to be together, so they took their horses and ran away. This event sets up the second piece of music, "Fire Dance," by Manuel De Falla. The group is instructed to start with the same image of the young couple riding to get away from their parents. At the end of the selection, each person tells what happened to the young couple, and the music therapist puts the suggestions together into the story. The end of this section must be set up so that the characters are in danger from something. The group is instructed to all start at the same place again, where now the characters are in danger. The third and final piece of music is the "Overture to Jesus Christ, Superstar" by Andrew Lloyd Weber. This piece has very intense sections but ends with the main theme of the musical, which sounds like a glorious ending. Once all the participants have given their idea of how the story will end, the music therapist retells the whole story as if it were an old myth. I do this with the zither. At the end of the telling of the story, the morals of the story can be discussed as well as any relationship to symbols that came up form the story. It should be noted that the final theme in the "Overture to Jesus Christ, Superstar" is edited so that the theme is heard three times, thereby allowing a real sense of ending.

CLINICAL EXAMPLE

I was doing a music and trauma workshop and after the workshop, I was able to work bedside with a patient who had survived an extremely traumatic event. This was about 3 weeks after the event, and she had seen many different types of therapists but was particularly drawn to the music therapist in the hospital and music therapy. I was able to work with her twice on two different days. On the first meeting I told her the story of "Khdir and Moses." As I told the story, her eyes fixated on the drumming pattern that I was doing to accompany the story. When I finished the story, I asked her what its moral was. She had a difficult time finding the words, but eventually came out with, "Things happen and we don't understand why." At this moment she was smiling, and a tear came out of her eye. I asked her where the tear was coming from. She simply said that she was not crying. The hospital music therapist, who was also present, said that when this happens, they simply say that she is "leaking." Although we did not verbally process the story, and I had no idea what kind of effect the story had on her, I received a letter and drawing from her 3 weeks later, saying that through our interaction, she felt as if she had "a brand-new life."

Songwriting

Songwriting is a wonderful way for the participants in a group to bond together and be creative. I often use a progression on the guitar that moves like this:

> A-major chord,
> A-minor form on the third fret,
> A-minor form on the fifth fret,
> Back down to an A-minor form on the third fret,
> Back down to an A-major chord.

This simple progression in 4/4 time can open up many melodic possibilities. Once you have come to a place of defining your melody and how many syllables are in the line, you can open it up to the group to compose a song. I often use three verses with four lines per verse. I have the group first compose a verse about aspects of how the trauma first affected them; then the middle verse is about what they are going through now; and the last verse is what they want to happen in their future. After writing the song, it is orchestrated and recorded with those who wish to play instruments, with each member receiving a copy of the recording. There is a time of processing about the writing and the meaning of the song.

CLINICAL EXAMPLE

The following song came out of a small group that had a particularly difficult day processing their trauma with the primary therapist during a weekend retreat that focused on people who had undergone trauma. This session was with individuals who had a variety of initiating events as their source of trauma.

Some participants had undergone large-scale traumatic events, and others had survived traumatic occurrences in the form of emotional and/or physical abuse (unlike most of the focus of this chapter). The group worked together to come up with three verses, and the song was sung by one of the participants. Another participant played a program on the iPad that emulated a synthesized sound in the keyboard and was set up as a pentatonic scale. This participant had a solo between verses two and three and also played through verse three. The interaction between the participants was extremely positive, as they supported each other's ideas. The performance was recorded and each member was given a CD. It should be noted that there was no processing of the lyrics after the recording, only a time of support and a group feeling of accomplishment.

> *Sunset to a Long Day*
> The sun is setting here in the West
> The colors speak to my heart
> Each day prettier than the rest
> It paints the sky like a piece of art
>
> The stars are ready to come out and play
> They're like a flowing river up in the sky
> It's a perfect ending to a very long day
> It brings a joyful tear to my eye
>
> The moon rises golden bright
> Like my future yet to be
> Shooting stars running across the night
> They bring me home and serenity.

Applications to Other Disciplines

In working with groups and individuals after a large traumatic experience, the music therapist will often be in contact with other trauma team members. At times those affected are reluctant to try something new such as music therapy, but their apprehension may be alleviated with the support of team members. Collaborating with other team members allows for more individual attention in larger groups, and this is especially true if issues arise during the session. A therapist who has musical ability can conduct some of the experiences previously described.

Drumming has become very visible in the past 10 years as a way for people to connect, and training programs for becoming a drum facilitator are held across the country. Many drum facilitators want to be of assistance in the wake of disasters, but although they can lead the survivors in the experience of group drumming, they may be unfamiliar with noticing and processing the therapeutic needs of the participants. A drum circle can accomplish many goals, but it takes on a different tone when conducted by a music therapist. Working in collaboration with drum facilitators in the wake of traumatic events can be beneficial as a way of combining physical resources such as drums with attention to individuals within a large group.

Improvisational experiences that are co-led with a primary therapist can be very effective. I have done "There Are Two Sides of Me" with a cotherapist, adding an enriched environment for processing. The music therapist can focus on the actual sounds and manner of playing in which the individual is engaged, and the verbal therapist can help in the processing of the experience. Together the two can offer complementary feedback and processing to those in the group experience.

Storytelling is not unique to music therapy. Numerous storytellers provide entertainment for young and old alike. Telling stories with therapeutic goals in mind is not practiced widely, and telling stories with a musical component is even less prevalent. Therapists can utilize very basic background music experiences to enhance the story by using various types of drones such as harps, zithers, and even some iPad applications to help create an atmosphere conducive to storytelling.

Songwriting requires the musical ability to be creative and to be able to accompany the voice with guitar, piano, or another accompanying musical instrument. Many nonmusic therapists have these musical abilities and could possibly lead a songwriting session. To be able to manage a group in the creative process can be challenging and requires sensitivity to the roles that many group members may take in the songwriting process. Thus the basic requirements for a songwriting experience are the musical ability to create the song, the understanding of how to create a song that has a therapeutic timbre, and the ability to guide the group through the creative process.

Conclusions

It is often said that the world is changing fast, and yet in many ways, this is not true. There will always be acts of nature that change the face of the land and how people live; there will be violence affecting from one person to thousands; and there will be unforeseen accidents and events that can affect communities of any size. When these things occur some of those affected will be able to cope with the event and return to a normal life, for not everyone is affected in the same way. But there will be others who will begin to suffer, and often that suffering will occur in silence so as to not show that they are different or can't *handle* things. The aftereffects of trauma can range from a mild disruption in someone's life to an all-encompassing and debilitating sense of fear. When those affected need to find a way to express these inner battles and feelings, they will often turn to a verbal therapy modality that can be helpful for them. But since music and its elements are at the core of being human, those who are struggling to find a voice to express their inner world may find this voice through the music experience. Through improvisation, composing, listening, and various creative experiences with music, the survivor can connect with what he or she could not express verbally and begin to rebuild a new sense of normal in life.

REFERENCES

American Psychiatric Association. (2013). *Diagnostic and statistical manual of mental disorders* (5th ed.). Arlington, VA: Author.

Bitcon, C. (1989). *Risk it: Express.* St. Louis, MO: MMB Music.

Borczon, R. (1998). *Music therapy: Group vignettes.* Gilsum, NH: Barcelona.

Borczon, R. (2013). Survivors of catastrophic event trauma. In L. Eyre (Ed.), *Guidelines for music therapy practice in mental health* (pp. 237–262). Gilsum, NH: Barcelona.

Braddock, C. (1995). *Body voices: Using the power of breath, sound and movement to heal and create new boundaries.* Berkeley, CA: Page Mill Press.

Estés, C. P. (1992). *Women who run with the wolves: Myths and stories of the wild woman archetype.* New York: Ballantine Books.

Figley, C. R. (Ed.). (1995). *Passion fatigue: Coping with secondary traumatic stress disorder and those who treat the traumatized.* New York: Brunner/Mazel.

Jung, C. G. (1969). *The collected works of C. G. Jung:* *Vol. 9i. Archetypes and the collective unconscious* (R. F. C. Hull, Trans.). Princeton, NJ: Princeton University Press.

Jung, C. G. (1972). *Four archetypes.* New York: Routledge.

Limb, C., & Braun, A. (2008). Neural substrates of spontaneous musical performance: An fMRI study of jazz improvisation. *PLoS ONE, 3*(2), e1679.

Mitchell, J. (2007). The psychological aftermath of large- and small-scale fires. In E. K. Carll (Ed.), *Trauma psychology: Issues in violence, disaster, health and illness* (pp. 231–254). Westport, CT: Praeger.

Rothschild, B. (2000). *The body remembers: The psychophysiology of trauma and trauma treatment.* New York: Norton.

van der Kolk, B., & Fisler, R. (1995). Dissociation and the fragmentary nature of traumatic memories: Overview and exploratory study. *Journal of Traumatic Stress, 8*(4), 505–525.

Volkman, S. (1993). Music therapy in the treatment of trauma-induced dissociative disorders. *Arts in Psychotherapy, 20*, 243–251.

CHAPTER 32

Music Therapy for Grief and Loss

Robert E. Krout

Phyllis was a 72-year-old woman whose husband had died of lung cancer with the help of a local hospice organization 8 months ago. She was having great emotional difficulty as the winter holidays approached and requested bereavement support from the organization where I worked. Facing these traditionally family-oriented holidays is often difficult for bereaved persons, especially the first time that such a holiday occurs after the death. When I first met with Phyllis, she asked to hear a song that might help her deal with her anxiety about the upcoming holidays. I told Phyllis that I would like to share a song I wrote that explores this issue, titled "Walking Together as Our Journey Starts" (more about this in a later section). I gave her a copy of the lyrics and invited her to just listen and read along as I played and sang. The song, sung in a slow but steady tempo, began, "As we near the holidays, times when families join together, we think back on all the days, when we have made it through stormy weather." Phyllis listened intently and nodded her head in apparent affirmation several times during the song. After the song finished, Phyllis said "That song really hit home—I am facing a dif-

ficult journey in my life this year with Fred [husband] not here for Christmas." In this first session, we began to explore this theme and ways in which she could find support from family and friends during this difficult time. The song and the music appeared to open the door for Phyllis to safely begin sharing her grief with me.

Clientele

In this chapter I discuss adults who have experienced one or more losses that have impacted their lives in a significant way and who are receiving grief support services. It is not necessarily the loss itself that determines the significance, but rather the significance of the loss and resultant impact on that person's life that usually brings the client to the attention of, and referral to, the music therapist. I do not discuss grief and loss in children and adolescents, although there are many parallels between the grieving processes in older adolescents and young adults (Dalton & Krout, 2014).

Definitions

Loss

Many types of personal losses can be life-changing events (Attig, 2010). In addition, a new loss may renew the experience, memory, and grief from previous losses (Apollon, 2012). The loss event or events that lead to or result in a person experiencing grief may include the death of a family member, friend, loved one, or other person of significance. The term *bereaved* is often used to describe one who has experienced and is grieving the death of a loved one, including a family member or other person of significance (Diamond, Llewelyn, Relf, & Bruce, 2012). Although the death of a loved one or other significant loss is often the demarcation point for a person's grief and grieving processes to begin, the anticipation of an upcoming loss may also be a trigger point for what is often termed *anticipatory grief* (Johansson & Grimby, 2012).

Grief and Grieving

Although grief is sometimes considered a discrete event, it is more a process, and it is during this process of grieving that the music therapist can intervene. Grieving has been described as an active form of coping with a loss and its impact for the survivor in an effort to remake and adjust to current reality (Friedman, 2013). After a significant loss, a person may question his or her existence and the value and meaning of life (Attig, 2010). It is important to note that each bereaved person's grieving experiences are unique, and there can be enormous variation in individual responses to loss. However, some common tasks, aspects, and phases of grieving have been frequently described in the bereavement literature (Hirsch, 2010).

One foundational model of grieving that was outlined by O'Toole (1987) and is still in use describes the grief process as a wheel in motion. This model includes five phases following the death of a significant person

in one's life. In this model the bereaved person enters this process in transition from his or her life before the loss and exits into or returns to the resumed and adjusted life following the grieving process. O'Toole's grief wheel processes and phases include loss, shock, protest, disorganization, and reorganization. Worden (2001) presented another commonly used model in which he described four main tasks for persons experiencing grief. These tasks include (1) accepting the reality of the loss, (2) experiencing the pain of the grief, (3) adjusting to an environment in which the deceased is missing, and (4) withdrawing emotional energy from the deceased and reinvesting energy in new relationships without guilt. A third relevant model was developed by Rando (1993), in which she delineated the "six R's" of grieving: (1) recognizing the loss, acknowledging the death, and understanding its ramifications; (2) reacting to the separation of both the primary and resulting secondary losses; (3) recollecting and reexperiencing the deceased and the relationship by reviewing and remembering; (4) relinquishing attachments to the deceased and the old assumptive world; (5) readjusting and moving adaptively into the new world without forgetting the deceased; and (6) reinvesting the freed-up energy in a new life or identity.

Although these and other models describe processes that allow the bereaved person to experience and move through his or her own grief in a natural and healthy way, bereaved persons are not always able to access, experience, or move through these processes unassisted or with the support of only family and friends. They may become what is termed *stuck* in their grieving, and they may experience feelings of hopelessness and despair and not be able to continue in their lives in an adaptive and healthy manner. This state has been termed *complicated* or *disenfranchised grief* (Doka, 2008; Wlodarczyk, 2013). In this case, grief counseling and support services that include music therapy may be warranted.

Challenges

There are several unique challenges in providing music therapy for adults who are grieving. One challenge is the varied nature of the losses and the relationship of the client to the deceased. For adults, these losses and relationships can include the death of an older parent, a spouse, sibling, child, grandchild, or other significant people. Whereas the death of a friend or coworker can also be difficult to deal with, it is often a family member's death and the resultant grief that brings the person to the attention of a music therapist.

A second challenge is whether or not a death was expected or anticipated. A best-case scenario, one that I experienced many times in my work with a hospice and bereavement organization, is one in which family members had time to process feelings of anticipatory grief while the patient was still alive and able to communicate. In this case, music therapy could also help the adult patient process the grief regarding his or her own impending physical decline and death. A more challenging scenario is when a death is unanticipated or sudden, as the result of a heart attack or other medical event, an accident, suicide, homicide, and so forth. A sudden death and the inability of the person to say good-bye to his or her loved one can lead to the complicated or disenfranchised grief previously discussed (Doka, 2008).

A third challenge arises when an adult has experienced the death of a child—whether a loss from a miscarriage, a still-birth, a disease such as cancer, an accident, or sudden infant death (such as one from sudden infant death syndrome [SIDS]). The death of a child can be one of the most difficult losses for adults to adjust to. Even when a child has a life-limiting illness such as a terminal cancer and is expected to die, few adults know what to do when that death actually occurs. Adults are challenged as to how to help themselves and may not allow themselves to grieve if they need to focus their energy and attention toward surviving children or a spouse (Krout, 2006; Krout & Jones, 2005).

As mentioned previously, a new loss often triggers a grief cascade that may cause the person to reexperience and grieve previous losses. As such, the therapist may have to work with the client in exploring feelings and thoughts regarding other losses, which the person may have thought to be *over*. A significant loss history can cause a person to feel as if there is no hope and question his or her very existence or reason for living (Hepburn & Krout, 2004).

Clinical Work

The music therapy models, intervention techniques, and clinical examples I share come from my experiences with hospice and bereavement organizations in the United States and abroad. They represent a range of applications and are representative of many of the ways that music therapy has been reported to address grief and loss worldwide.

Music Therapy in Anticipatory Grief Work

When working with a person who is expected to die, grieving may begin as early as the initial diagnosis of a life-limiting condition (Friedman, 2013). For the clinician, beginning to interact with the patient and loved ones as soon as possible is important. The music therapist who is a member of a hospice or palliative care interdisciplinary care team may have an excellent opportunity establish a therapeutic relationship with the person and his or her loved ones prior to the death, which can enable the music therapist to be more effective in bereavement work with the loved ones after the death. The music therapist may also be in a better position to help identify loved ones who may not be coping well and may be at risk for complicated grieving (Krout, 2004).

When working with a patient prior to death, it is important to realize that grieving is a multifaceted process that is unique to each individual. In addition, as previously mentioned, grieving over the death of a loved one or other significant loss may go on throughout a person's lifetime. Bertman (1999) pointed out ways that creative arts therapists can help allay anxiety, emptiness, and meaninglessness in these situations by enabling patients and clients to connect with their wholeness. Patients can also make peace with, discover, and respect the coherence of their life's story; seek reconciliation with alienated family and friends; give and receive love, forgiveness, appreciation, and expression of affection; say good-byes; complete relationships with others; and assure continuity, relationship, and meaning beyond death.

As previously mentioned, music therapy may help address the anticipatory grief needs of the patient's family and loved ones. When the grief needs of the family are addressed, the patient and family can interact in a more meaningful manner, possibly even after the patient, in the case of a person with a terminal illness or condition, dies. Adult family members often are faced with the challenge of expressing their feelings to the patient and to each other. The patient may also not able to communicate with, or respond to, family members due to the medical condition, which can make this sharing difficult.

The active expression of feelings of grief by loved ones during this difficult time is often considered to be both normal and healthy (Krout, 2003). When adult family members are present in a session, the music therapist can engage them in meaningful music-based experiences. Music therapy experiences can involve passive or active participation by the family. As one example, the intervention often called *song choice*, in which clients select, sing, or listen to requested songs, may stimulate discussion relating to life memories, reminiscence, and life review. Here, family members may request a specific song, listen to or sing with the therapist, and then reflect on the significance of that song to them and the patient. The music may also elicit or stimulate emotional or grief-related feeling responses. These feelings can then be validated, normalized, and explored by and with the therapist. For families with a strong spiritual base, hymns or sacred songs may be helpful in addressing grief needs.

Grief and Spirituality

Music therapy can provide spiritual support both for patients and for loved ones and caregivers who become survivors, especially through the use of familiar spiritual music, hymns, and songs. Magill (2011) investigated the spiritual meaning of music therapy for caregivers of cancer patients after those patients had died. In her study, caregivers who were present during music therapy sessions reported experiencing feelings of autonomous joy (sessions affected the caregiver directly), empathic joy (seeing the patient happy in music therapy), and empowerment by contributing to care of the patient through participation in music therapy. Caregivers also engaged in reflection on the past (remembrance), reflection on the present (connectedness), and reflection on the future (hope). Finally, caregivers shared that music therapy helped them find connection within themselves, with others, and beyond (Magill, 2011).

Music of a spiritual nature can help patients and loved ones validate their spiritual faith- bases and strengths. Spiritual suffering, when part of the grief experience, can be palliated by spiritual music when used to provide comfort and reassurance. Music experiences can also provide opportunities for patients and families to explore and work through spiritual conflicts. Music and spirituality are often intertwined. Music therapy can meet spiritual needs by providing a means of expressing spiritual feelings, as well as providing an avenue for expressing doubts, anger, fear, and questions (Hepburn & Krout, 2004).

Bereavement Work

Music therapy following a loss can be a beneficial part of the bereavement process that meets a number of grief goals for the survivors. To begin with, after the death the music therapist can participate in a funeral or memorial service that offers reassurance and support to the bereaved. Music therapy may also facilitate the expression of grief and reintegration of the bereaved into their ongoing lives and community. It can help bereaved individuals to use their existing support systems and to develop additional support mechanisms and strategies if needed.

After a death, music therapy can aid in what we might term *healthy grieving* for survivors. Music can function as a catalyst for healing grief and thereby facilitate a sense of wholeness. In music-therapy-related bereavement, we can consider music as an enhancer and resonator of the grief, not as a medium to mask or distance it. For example, interventions such as songwriting may allow survivors to create songs that become safe vessels for their feelings, emotions, and memories. Although survivors may have a natural reaction to distance themselves from their grief, music can help them experience, free, release, and express grief on a deep level. Music can thus serve to bridge the distance between the grieving survivor and his or her deceased loved one, thereby facilitating a healthy healing process.

When working with clients who do not display what was previously described as complicated or disenfranchised grief, the music therapist can support the healthy and natural grieving process in through an approach that has been described by the acronym *VINE*: facilitating the validation, identification, normalization, and expression of feelings and emotions through the use of music therapy (Teahan, 2000).

More about Music Therapy Interventions and Techniques

No single intervention is appropriate for use with every patient, family, or clinical need. Music therapists often use a treatment strategy that combines receptive and active modalities to address grief needs. Techniques may include music listening, improvisation, singing, songwriting, music playing (structured), composing music, song choice, music and imagery for relaxation, music with progressive muscle relaxation and deep breathing, Guided Imagery and Music (GIM; Bonny Method of Guided Imagery and Music), and lyric analysis, including music-assisted cognitive reframing.

Bright (2002) described a number of useful techniques that she termed *supportive eclectic music therapy for grief and loss*. She considers the many and varied uses of music therapy to address grief and loss needs across a broad range of client and patient populations. Her approach embraces an eclectic attitude in considering a variety of treatment approaches and clinical interventions. In an interview describing this practical approach (Krout, 2009), Bright stated:

> To describe my approach as "eclectic" ensures that readers know that I shall be describing the results achieved through a range of different methods, depending on the needs of the individual concerned. I have always used an eclectic approach, and there were various reasons for this. I realized very early on that individuals are different, and that a particular approach that works for one person does not necessarily work for everyone. In other words, one approach doesn't suit everybody. I also realized that a single individual may need different approaches at different stages in the management or treatment of their condition. Someone who is coping with a difficult grief may need initially to explore all the reasons why the loss has hit so hard—the relationship with the person, their own self-esteem and whether this has been impaired in some way, and so on. But for many people there comes a

stage when the analytical approach is no longer appropriate because the person is at risk of getting stuck in introspection, and needs to "put things in the cupboard" intellectually, allowing full expression of feelings—but then start to work out new ways of living and relating to others. At this point, the cognitive, practical method is more useful.

Songwriting

Songwriting (by the music therapist and/or participant) and the use of lyrics and metaphors in providing a focus for grief work been widely reported in the music therapy and grief literature (Krout, 2005). The word *metaphor* is from the Greek word *metapherein* and means to carry or transfer between places or settings. In grief work, this transfer may happen between the images in the songs and the feelings of the bereaved toward their loved one who has died. As such, songs may create a safe, shared music space for this transfer. The use of metaphors in the shared space of song may help participants in grief programs connect the songs with their own lives. Furthermore, experiences to which the song-based metaphors refer may be the death(s) of their loved ones and the processes of grieving and healing for the participants.

With many available popular and sacred songs, one may question the need to compose original songs. For example, there are music therapy texts and resources that contain lists of songs appropriate for use with persons who are bereaved. However, composing original songs may offer advantages for the music therapist. For example, original songs offer flexibility and opportunity to use planned metaphors for specific purposes or for the needs of particular participants and types of losses. The song that is written can be thereby individualized to more personally address the needs of that individual or group at that time. In addition, participants will not have existing associations with unfamiliar songs and so

may be less prone to respond to or interact with the songs in habitual ways.

In my work with grieving clients, I have found songwriting to be particularly valuable in allowing individuals to examine and express their feelings as part of their grief processes. There are various methods for writing songs for, and in, music therapy (Baker & Wigram, 2005). I see the therapist using songwriting techniques to reflect the orientation and approach that he or she is using with any given client at that time based on the client's needs. I have used songwriting in both individual and group music therapy to meet the grief needs of clients.

These interventions have included facilitating songwriting by or with the clients, as well writing songs ahead of time (precomposing songs) to be used and adapted in both individual and group music therapy grief work. Using songs that the therapist has precomposed for use in grief interventions may be an option for the clinician, depending on the needs of the clients at that time. Precomposing a song allows the therapist to incorporate the song in one or more sessions without using session time to actually write the song. The song may also be used as a springboard for discussion and verbal processing and for related arts activities such as drawing, painting, writing poetry, collage making, and movement.

Choices and options are available in the actual songwriting process. These include writing the lyrics first, composing the music first, or writing them together as the song evolves and progresses (Baker & Wigram, 2005). If writing the song with contributions from the client(s), then these options may all be available and equally valid. In fact, the clients may want to have input as to how and in what order (lyrics, music) the song itself is created.

There are many possible applications for original songs when working with persons who have experienced the death of a loved one. Music therapists working as a member of a grief counseling team may have a number of creatively challenging opportunities to compose and make use of such songs. Working with team members such as social workers, grief counselors, art therapists, mental health counselors, and others has given me many occasions to be inspired to craft songs for specific programs and events. It can be a very powerful experience for the music therapist to be part of such a team, especially during the actual grief programs as they take place. By writing original songs for such purposes, the therapist can craft them to best support and facilitate the goals of the programs, and to enable the participants to work and move through their grief journeys in meaningful and healthy ways.

Music-Therapist-Composed Songs in One-Time Grief Rituals and Programs

In addition to music therapists' role in designing and facilitating ongoing support groups and services for those who have experienced the deaths of loved ones, they may also have a role in contributing to the creation of one-time grief programs that take place in health, community, and other professional settings. Regardless of whether or not bereaved persons feel they are progressing through their grief processes in healthy ways, one-time group grief-oriented programs and events can be beneficial. These one-time programs can be used to supplement ongoing grief counseling or stand on their own (Krout, 2005). Bereaved persons who are not experiencing complicated grief may attend such programs to *check in* with how they are doing. They may want reassurance that they are grieving *normally* and feeling or doing the *right* things. These one-time programs may also offer opportunities to assess whether the bereaved person is adapting to life after the loss in a healthy way and to offer further grief services if such needs are identified.

These one-time grief programs often use ritual as a way to bring participants together and to foster sense of community, group validation, and expression on an individualized and personalized level within the group. A ritual is a specific activity that gives symbolic expression to certain feelings and thoughts of the actor or actors, individually or as a group. It may be habitually repeated or a one-time occurrence. In addition, the ritual can take place at a key point in the program, such as toward the culmination. Here, participants can join together and contribute to the ritual individually in memory of their loved one. Bereavement rituals, which are practiced by many societies in a variety of ways, have one common benefit: They have tremendous therapeutic value in helping participants cope with areas of transition or moving on with their lives. Rituals can provide healing, a sense of continuity, and balance if the griever believes there is meaning in them.

Group Bereavement Intervention for Adults with Uncomplicated Grief

I'd like to share an example of how a song I wrote as a music therapist working as a team member in a bereavement center was used in a one-time grief program to help create participant connections with adults who had experienced the death of a loved one (Krout, 2005). The song also served as a program focus and structure for the group ritual. I composed the song myself to accommodate the one-time nature of the program, program time limitations, and the large size of the group. I was not attempting to guide any participant's grief process in a particular direction. Rather, the song and ritual were designed to allow participants to come together as a community and also check out how their own grief processes were progressing. It should be stressed that this one-time program was not designed to replace ongoing individual or group counseling or grief therapy. It was designed as group bereavement intervention for adults with uncomplicated grief needs.

The program was planned and facilitated by an interdisciplinary team of bereavement counselors and therapists, which included a social worker, art therapist, mental health counselor, pastoral counselor, and me as the music therapist. Before the event, the team met to discuss how to best structure the program, especially the ritual to be used. The song was written for a program titled "Coping with the Holidays and Special Days." This was an annual event to precede fall or winter holidays such as Thanksgiving, Hanukkah, Christmas, Kwanzaa, and New Year's. Facing family-oriented holidays is often difficult for bereaved adults, especially the first time that such a holiday occurs after the death. The song was used at the opening of the program, as well as before and during the ritual. The purpose of writing the song was to help structure the theme for the program, as well as for framing and structuring the group ritual near the conclusion.

After welcoming participants to the program, we (staff) shared the program theme. I sang the song, and participants were invited to listen and to read along in their booklets if they wished. The metaphors in the song were not directly addressed at this point. Thus, the song was intended to begin to connect participants with the phrase, "as we near the holidays." The full lyrics of the song can be seen in Figure 32.1. Later in the program, which included readings, educational components presented by staff, and sharing by participants of concerns and experiences, the ritual for the program was introduced. The ritual project for this program included participants, as a group, writing the names of loved ones on smooth river rock stones and placing them to make a connected path.

After the ritual was introduced and briefly described, I shared that words for the song to accompany the ritual were in participants' booklets. I read the words of the song, emphasizing the metaphors with vocal inflection. Participants were next invited to listen

---

> As we near the holidays
> Times when families join together
> We think back on all the ways
> That we have made it through stormy weather
>
> But now our path is growing clear
> As the skies grow light before us
> These are times we feel you near
> We know your presence will help assure us
>
> We'll find our strength with your memory beside us
> We'll light our path with the light in our hearts
> We will allow one hand to touch the water
> Walking together as our journey starts

FIGURE 32.1. Lyrics to "Walking Together as Our Journey Starts," by Robert Ellis Krout. Reprinted with permission.

---

to the song. After the song, the development phase of the ritual was begun, which involved handing out materials to the participants and guidelines or instructions. Questions about the ritual and what participants were to do were answered, the metaphors were verbally explored by staff and participants based on participant interest, reaction, or feedback, and staff assisted participants during the creation of the ritual project. Reactions to the metaphors were positive.

Once participants completed their ritual project, which took approximately 15–20 minutes, they were invited to engage in the next phase of the ritual, which was placing the painted rocks together to form a connected path while the song was sung again. Participants were invited to sing during the chorus or as they felt comfortable. I continued playing the song (instrumentally) after the words were sung until the last participant completed their contribution. Following the ritual, participants were invited to share how they experienced it and any feelings that they wanted to voice to the group. The metaphors were reexplored based on participant feedback and comments.

Informal responses and feedback from participants about the programs, songs, and rituals were positive, with participants making comments such as (paraphrasing),

"My grief has certainly felt like a journey," and "I don't feel so alone on this journey with everyone here with me" (Krout, 2005).

Individual Intervention for Adults with More Complicated Grief Needs

A music therapist colleague with whom I was working at a hospice organization abroad was providing music therapy for a 60-year-old woman dying from mesothelioma (Hepburn & Krout, 2004). The sources of loss and grief were many in her life. She had a childhood history of abuse and had experienced spousal abuse as an adult. The psychosocial assessment shared by the social worker indicated that the patient had significant abandonment and grief issues. These appeared to be exacerbated by the fact that her only daughter had recently moved overseas.

The initial goal was to establish a therapeutic relationship with this woman who felt so isolated. The therapist initially used song choice and offered popular songs for her to select and listen to. The therapist was able to share and use these songs as entry points for talking about the patient's present situation and various aspects of her loss history. When asked by the therapist what she most wanted in life at this time, she said, "I want peace and happiness," and she asked the therapist to play "something spiritual." The music therapist asked her to close her eyes and imagine herself at peace. She then sang the spiritual "Peace Like a River," adding the patient's words:

I want peace and happiness, I want peace and
    happiness,
I want peace and happiness today.
I want peace and happiness, I want peace and
    happiness,
I want peace and happiness all my life.

Through the developing relationship with the therapist, the patient explored aspects of meaning and purpose in her life, as well as expressed feelings of grief, loss, and hope. She shared that she accepted her present situation and was at peace (Hepburn & Krout, 2004).

Applications to Other Disciplines

The use of music in grief counseling offers opportunities to a broad spectrum of mental health practitioners, from thanatologists to hospice staff (Berger, 2006). Music therapists working in the context of an interdisciplinary bereavement or grief counseling team may have a number of opportunities to work with other team members, such as social workers, grief counselors, art therapists, and/or mental health counselors. It has been a very powerful experience for me to be part of such a team, especially during the actual grief programs as they take place. Music experiences that are created and designed for such purposes can be crafted to best support and facilitate the goals of the programs, thereby enabling the participants to work and move through their grief journeys in meaningful and healthy ways.

Music therapists can also facilitate the grief processing of team members who experience the losses of patients who die in environments such as hospice organizations and cancer programs. For example, Popkin et al. (2011) described a music therapy intervention developed by an interdisciplinary inpatient team at a comprehensive cancer center, with the aim of facilitating the processing of staff grief in a group setting. The experience and ritual for the staff included live reflective music, a ceremony to bless the healers' hands, readings, and an opportunity to express feelings of loss and grief.

The mutual significance and effectiveness of joint interventions with team members may be enhanced partly due to the power of music to hold and connect everyone present in the shared time and space (Krout, 2013). For example, when a pastoral counselor and I worked together with a client and family, the spiritual aspects of the music seemed to have been intensified. In addition, I observed the pastoral counselor being able to take the discussions or exploration of spiritual issues deeper than I alone as a music therapist would feel comfortable doing.

Our colleagues in counseling, psychotherapy, social and pastoral work, grief and bereavement therapies, and other creative arts therapies can also use music in creative ways, even when a music therapist is not present or part of that team. Listening to songs that are significant to grieving adults, lyric analysis and discussion, music and relaxation with or without imagery, drawing and painting feelings to background music, and other music-based experiences may be beneficial. If the organization providing services does not have a credentialed music therapist on staff, one can be consulted on either a long- or short-term basis.

Conclusions

Grief and loss can affect adults in a number of ways, and they are often unable to verbally identify or express their feelings and emotions in ways that help them in their grief journeys. Verbal therapies can be helpful for some adults, but others may not be able to express what they feel with words. Music is processed in a unique way by the brain (including the limbic system, which may stimulate and modulate emotions) and nervous system. In addition, music may trigger long-term memories, and these memories may also be useful when helping adults identify and process sources of their grief. Music and expressive arts therapies also offer opportunities for the shared ownership of grief and loss, and they provide necessary structures and modes of expression for creative experiences that may be hard to convey in conventional language or for which there are no words (Thompson & Berger, 2011).

Music may stimulate conscious thought, reflection, and verbalization in the client.

As such, music therapy interventions in grief and loss work can assist bereaved persons (or those anticipating a loss) to identify feelings, express emotions, and alter mood in a positive direction as part of the grieving process (Sekeles, 2007). Music therapy therefore has a unique position in its possible applications with adults in grief therapy.

REFERENCES

Apollon, S. (2012). Grief and loss. *Personal Excellence, 17*(3), 7.

Attig, T. (2010). Existential suffering: Anguish over our human condition. In D. L. Harris (Ed.), *Counting our losses: Reflecting on change, loss, and transition in everyday life* (pp. 119–125). New York: Routledge/Taylor & Francis.

Baker, F., & Wigram, T. (Eds.). (2005). *Song writing methods, techniques and clinical applications for music therapy clinicians, educators and students.* London: Jessica Kingsley.

Berger, J. S. (2006). *Music of the soul: Composing life out of loss.* New York: Routledge/Taylor & Francis Group.

Bertman, S. (1999). *Grief and the healing arts: Creativity as therapy.* Amityville, NY: Baywood.

Bright, R. (2002). *Supportive eclectic music therapy for grief and loss: A practical handbook for professionals.* St. Louis, MO: MMB Music.

Dalton, T. D., & Krout, R. E. (2014). Integrative songwriting. In B. Thompson & B. Neimeyer (Eds.), *Grief and the healing arts: Practices for the creation of meaning* (pp. 222–225). New York: Routledge, Taylor & Francis Group.

Diamond, H., Llewelyn, S., Relf, M., & Bruce, C. (2012). Helpful aspects of bereavement support for adults following an expected death: Volunteers' and bereaved people's perspectives. *Death Studies, 36*(6), 541–564.

Doka, K. J. (2008). Disenfranchised grief in historical and cultural perspective. In M. S. Stroebe, R. O. Hansson, H. Schut, & W. Stroebe (Eds.), *Handbook of bereavement research and practice: Advances in theory and intervention* (pp. 223–240). Washington, DC: American Psychological Association.

Friedman, R. (2013). *The best grief definition you will find.* Available at *www.griefrecoverymethod.com/2013/06/grief-definition/#.*

Hepburn, M., & Krout, R. E. (2004). Meaning, purpose, transcendence and hope: Music therapy and spirituality in end of life hospice care. *New Zealand Journal of Music Therapy, 2,* 58–82.

Hirsch, M. (2010). *Coping with grief and loss: A guide to healing*. Cambridge, MA: Harvard Health Publications.

Johansson, A. K., & Grimby A. (2012). Anticipatory grief among close relatives of patients in hospice and palliative wards. *American Journal of Hospice and Palliative Care, 29*(2), 134–138.

Krout, R. E. (2003). Music therapy with imminently dying hospice patients and their families: Facilitating release near the time of death. *American Journal of Hospice and Palliative Care, 20*(2), 129–134.

Krout, R. E. (2004). A synerdisciplinary music therapy treatment team approach for hospice and palliative care. *Australian Journal of Music Therapy, 15*, 33–45.

Krout, R. E. (2005). Applications of music therapist-composed songs in creating participant connections and facilitating goals and rituals during one-time bereavement support groups and programs. *Music Therapy Perspectives, 23*(2), 118–128.

Krout, R. E. (2006). Following the death of a child: Music therapy helping to heal the family heart. *New Zealand Journal of Music Therapy, 4*, 6–22.

Krout, R. E. (2009). Exploring contemporary aspects of supportive music therapy in addressing client grief and loss: Reflections with Australian author Ruth Bright. *Voices: A World Forum for Music Therapy*. Available at *www.voices.no/main-issues/mi40009000324.php*.

Krout, R. E. (2013). Music-mediated strategies for the integrative management of pain in end of life care. In J. Mondanaro & G. Sara (Eds.), *Music and medicine: Integrative models in pain medicine* (pp. 403–417). New York: Satchnote Press.

Krout, R. E., & Jones, L. (2005, November). *When a child dies: Music therapy in facilitating family grief processing*. Paper presented at the annual conference of the American Music Therapy Association, Orlando, FL.

Magill, L. (2011). Bereaved family caregivers' reflections on the role of the music therapist. *Music and Medicine, 3*(1), 56–63.

O'Toole, D. (1987). *Healing and growing through grief*. Burnsville, NC: Rainbow Connection.

Popkin, K., Levin, T., Lichtenthal, W. G., Redl, N., Rothstein, H. D., Siegel, D., et al. (2011). A pilot music therapy-centered grief intervention for nurses and ancillary staff working in cancer settings. *Music and Medicine, 3*(1), 40–46.

Rando, T. A. (1993). *Treatment of complicated mourning*. Champaign, IL: Research Press.

Sekeles, C. (2007). *Music therapy: Death and grief*. Gilsum, NH: Barcelona.

Teahan, M. (2000, October). Grief interventions. In M. Teahan & T. Dalton, *Helping children and adolescents cope with grief and bereavement*. Symposium at the alumni conference of the Barry University School of Social Work, Miami, FL.

Thompson, B. E., & Berger, J. S. (2011). Grief and expressive arts therapy. In R. A. Neimeyer, D. L. Harris, H. R. Winokuer, & G. F. Thornton (Eds.), *Grief and bereavement in contemporary society: Bridging research and practice* (pp. 303–311). New York: Routledge/Taylor & Francis Group.

Wlodarczyk, N. M. (2013). The effect of a group music intervention for grief resolution on the disenfranchised grief of hospice workers. *Progress in Palliative Care, 21*(2), 97–106.

Worden, W. (2001). *Grief counselling and grief therapy: A handbook for the mental health practitioner* (3rd ed.). London: Tavistock/Routledge.

SECTION C

Medical Music Therapy

CHAPTER 33

Music Therapy in the Neonatal Intensive Care Unit

Helen Shoemark
Deanna Hanson-Abromeit

Music therapy for hospitalized newborn infants is a relatively new area of practice. Early research in the 1970s focused on the preterm infant's need for stimulation, but by the early 1990s attention had split, with one strand still dedicated to recorded music as stimulation and the other concentrating on the need to sustain a stable physiological state or homeostasis. The subsequent refinement of research has produced an emphasis on more specific effects, such as recovery from procedures (Bo & Callaghan, 2000) and attainment of developmental goals such as self-regulation and feeding (Hanson Abromeit, 2003; Standley, 2012a), neurodevelopment (Malloch et al., 2012; Walworth et al., 2012), and good quality of sleep (Olischar, Shoemark, Holton, Weninger, & Hunt, 2011).

The greatest benefits for music therapy in the neonatal intensive care unit (NICU) are reported to be live music therapy and use early in the infant's admission (Standley, 2012b). However, it has also been suggested that there is too much heterogeneity in the population, interventions, and measures to render useful results (Hartling et al., 2009).

More detailed reporting (Hodges & Wilson, 2010) is necessary, as well as research that involves parents, active music making, and longitudinal studies (Haslbeck, 2012). Although the need for evidence continues, music therapists are already being employed in NICUs, which is an indicator that music is meeting key needs of medically fragile newborn infants.

It is increasingly understood in the NICU that the care must address the infant in the context of family to ensure healthy development into the future. For the music therapist, the application of music as treatment (sometimes called *music medicine*) remains key in facilitating the physiological stability and sensory development of the preterm infant, but the discourse has now widened to promote live music making (also called *Active Music Therapy*) as a vehicle for attachment between parent and infant and for the neurodevelopment of the infant. A range of factors, including the culture of the unit, the published evidence, and the clinical skills of the therapist, as well as the individual needs of the premature infant, drives the potential of a clinical service.

The rise of evidence-based practice compels all clinicians to make more effective use of the literature and requires researchers to reconsider the feasible application of research outcomes to clinical practice. Clinicians are ethically and professionally bound to use proven and safe methods, although the evidence is still emerging. Therefore, music therapy for hospitalized newborn infants is reliant on emerging and hybrid evidence from closely related fields.

Characteristics of Preterm Infants

Classification of Premature Birth

Because premature infants do not have fully developed biological, physiological, or neurological systems that allow for competent transition to life outside of the womb, their neurological development differs from that of full-term infants (van Soelen et al., 2010). Preterm infants rely on medical and developmental intervention to appropriately support their at-risk systems. Prematurity can have lifelong implications for biological, physiological, sensory, and neurological development, as well as social and emotional well-being and school readiness (Rais-Bahrami & Short, 2013).

Gestational age, weight, and physical and behavioral characteristics are key to assessing the risk of medical and developmental complications and survival, as well as appropriate treatment and intervention for the preterm infant. At birth a baby will be classified as term (born between 38 and 42 weeks), postterm (past 42 weeks), or preterm (born before 37 weeks gestation). Subcategory classification of premature infants include extremely preterm (less than 28 weeks), very preterm (28 to less than 32 weeks), and moderate to late preterm (32–37 weeks). Infants are also categorized based on their weight at birth. Those born weighing less than 2,500 grams (5.8 pounds) at birth are described as low birthweight (LBW), infants weighing 1,500 grams or less (3.5 pounds) are described

as very low birthweight (VLBW), and those born at less than 1,000 grams (2.3 pounds) are labeled extremely low birthweight (ELBW; Rais-Bahrami & Short, 2013).

Combined classification of infants by birthweight and gestational age include small for gestational age (SGA) (birthweight that is less than 10% of the normal weight for a baby at that gestational age), large for gestational age (birthweight > 90% for age), or appropriate for gestational age (birthweight between 10 and 90% for age; Kelly, 2006). The premature infant looks different than a full-term infant, most notably due to an absence of ear cartilage, breast buds, and skin creases; a reddish tone to the skin; and the presence of body hair, known as *lanugo*. Neurological development is also initially assessed in relation to gestational age, weight, physical appearance, and observable motor–muscular abilities that predict both short-term and long-term developmental consequences (Rais-Bahrami & Short, 2013).

Biological and Physiological Systems

Infants born prematurely have underdeveloped biological and physiological systems. Before any intervention, attention must be given to the infant's major systems (respiratory, heart, brain, and gastrointestinal), which inform his or her biological and physiological prognosis. An infant's respiratory status, heart rate, and oxygen saturation are continuously monitored in the NICU and form the commonly collected triad of *physiological signs*.

Respiratory Function

Infants born before 34 weeks gestational age (GA) will have immature lungs and insufficient production of surfactant. Surfactant is a chemical produced by the body that keeps the alveolus—clustered air-filled sacs in the lungs—expanded for the steady exchange of oxygen and carbon dioxide. A deficiency of surfactant will contribute to respiratory distress syndrome (RDS). Most preterm infants will receive synthetic surfactant and require additional or supplemental respiratory or ventilator support. Infants requiring prolonged use of supplemental mechanical ventilation may be diagnosed with chronic lung disease (CLD) and are at risk for lifelong respiratory diseases. A common respiratory response of premature infants is apnea, which is a pause in breathing that can be short or prolonged, but is effectively treated with caffeine. Apnea is an indicator of an immature central nervous system in which the brain is unable to control respiration (Rais-Bahrami & Short, 2013).

Heart Rate

Premature infants may experience increased heart rate or bradycardia, or a heart rate that is too low. Bradycardia, combined with apnea, can negatively affect the level of oxygen (oxygenation) in the brain, causing subsequent complications such as CLD. A more serious condition is patent ductus arteriosus (PDA). The ductus arteriosus is a fetal blood vessel that prevents blood flow to the lungs. It typically closes at birth so that blood flow can move to the lungs for oxygenation and proper respiration, but often does not close in preterm infants. This can create hypoxia, in which there is not enough oxygen to the blood and body organs, including the brain, and can potentially cause heart failure (Rais-Bahrami & Short, 2013).

Brain

The preterm infant is at risk of several neurological conditions. Reduced oxygen or blood flow to the brain can cause periventricular leukomalacia (PVL), a condition in which small cysts develop in the white matter in the brain, or intraventricular hemorrhage (IVH) in which there is bleeding in the ventricles (open spaces that connect fissures in the brain). There are four grades or types of IVH, with grades III and IV likely to cause severe neurological damage (Rais-Bahrami & Short, 2013).

Gastrointestinal Problems

Premature infants can have a greater difficulty processing food, resulting in reflux or vomiting. Gastrointestinal problems often develop with the onset of feeding. Preterm infants are at high rate of risk for necrotizing enterocolitis (NEC), a serious condition in which infection causes inflammation in the cell lining of the bowel that can lead to the death of bowel segments. Significant medical treatment or surgery is required for repair (Kelly, 2006). Infants with NEC will take much longer than low-risk preterm infants to establish feeding.

Neurodevelopmental Functioning

The survival and development of the preterm infant is also dependent upon the preservation and adequate development of the infant's sensory and neurobehavioral systems. Neurobehavioral functioning is on a continuum with gestational age (Mouradian, Als, & Coster, 2000). Stimuli that are too complex and intense can have a negative impact on neurobehavioral development (Als, 1986); therefore an understanding of the neurobehavioral and sensory systems of fetal development must guide music therapy interventions.

Sensory systems develop in a sequential order of tactile, vestibular, gustatory/olfactory, auditory, and visual, and are dependent on reciprocal interaction (Gottlieb, 1983; Lickliter, 1993). The sensory environment of the NICU differs greatly from that of the womb. Supporting sensory system organization with careful introduction and adaptation of sensory stimuli may in turn support the organized and competent development of the preterm infant's neurobehavioral subsystems (Hanson Abromeit, 2003). Although music might be a predictable and controllable stimulus, it is nonetheless a complex stimulus and must also be considered potentially harmful.

Similar to sensory system development, the behavioral subsystems (autonomic, motor, state, and attention/interaction) develop in a sequential and reciprocal manner and are responsive to environmental stimuli. The behavioral subsystems begin development early in gestation, gaining greater competence in organization and integration throughout gestation. Observable behavior markers indicate the infant's competence to self-regulate and appropriately respond to stimuli. Behavioral markers include respiration patterns, motor movements, and attention cues (Fischer & Als, 2004). For the preterm infant, the ability to organize and integrate sensory stimuli is often compromised due to exposure to the dramatic and unprotected environment of the NICU.

Clear identification of the individual preterm infant's biological, physiological, neurological, and sensory system characteristics, and consideration of the impact of those characteristics on the infant's developmental competence, support the identification of appropriate music therapy intervention. The ability to recognize and interpret the idiosyncratic stress and self-regulatory cues of the infant is critical to the use of sensory stimuli to support neurobehavioral development. Careful ongoing assessment of the infant's behavioral responses to neurodevelopmental music-based interventions is complex and requires training, mentoring, and experience (Hanson Abromeit, 2003). The infant's developmental status will change frequently, and a multisystem assessment should take place prior to, during, and immediately following each session (Hanson-Abromeit, Shoemark, & Loewy, 2008).

Social and Emotional Well-Being

The immediate context of the infant in the NICU remains the presence and availability of the family. From a family-centered perspective, the infant is the center of his or her immediate family, supported by family and friends, and then served by a wider community of professionals. The family context in the NICU focuses on the parents and even more specifically on the mother because she remains the primary caregiver in most cases.

Parenting the Preterm Infant in the NICU

Parents in the NICU feel stress, strain, separation, depression, despair, disappointment, ambivalence, and lack of control over the situation, as well as vacillation between hope and hopelessness (Obeidat, Bond, & Callister, 2009). The intense emotional journey of the parent should be considered as the music therapist attempts to engage with the family (Shoemark & Dearn, 2008). Across cultures, the perceived role of parents on the unit varies greatly, based on the theoretical orientation and culture of the unit. Some NICUs may still consider the family as visitors who attend the infant briefly and consult with doctors and nurses to consent for treatment. However, most NICUs practice family-centered care and consider the role of the family integral to every aspect of the infant's day.

The music therapist may be required to work with the family in line with the unit's view or may have the opportunity to make a decision based on his or her own theoretical stance. A family-centered perspective assumes that the infant is inextricably bound to the culture, musical heritage, and context of family both now and into the future. It assumes that the infant is at the center of a family who potentially thinks about, cares about, and protects him or her. The family may or may not be physically present each day, but their role in the psychological well-being and progress of the infant is always present.

Music Therapy as an Intervention in the NICU

The newborn music therapy model describes, classifies, and categorizes the current literature and known practice to provide a comprehensive representation of music therapy for hospitalized newborn infants (Shoemark, 2011). The model broadly conceptualizes theory, practice, and evidence into infant-focused or family-centered frameworks for preterm, full-term, and older hospitalized infants. In addition, the application of recorded music and live music making as modalities to achieve efficacious outcomes are established within those frameworks.

Recorded music is a static stimulus that is not responsive to changes in the infant but serves as a source of consistent external regulation to support the stability of heart rate, oxygen saturation, and the state known as quiet sleep state (also known as *homeostasis*), and to modify response to painful stimuli. Recorded music has been used in more research than live music, because it provides a consistent stimulus that is more readily applied by nonmusic therapists (see Application to Other Disciplines). Most commonly recorded music is lullaby-like, sedative music. The parameters of the music encompass the musical elements, presentation, and assessment of effect (Standley & Walworth, 2010).

Live music usually entails live singing of familiar songs, or contingent singing. Familiar songs offer the advantage of being easily reproduced and potentially available to several caregivers. The family can be consulted for their preferences to establish a repertoire of favored songs. In contingent singing, the music is improvised in the moment and is often stimulated by pitches and words favored by the infant and responsive in the moment to the infant's behaviors. The music therapist can select either method easily, but parents may feel more comfortable beginning with familiar songs.

All the music used with preterm infants is constrained by each infant's fragile capacities to process stimulation. Careful consideration of the specific characteristics of the music in relation to the infant's developmental competence to process and respond to the stimulus is critical for effi-

cacious music-based intervention, and may be contraindicated based on the age and medical stability of the infant. The music therapist's selection of recorded or live music-based stimuli is supported by careful consideration of how the characteristics of the musical elements affect and support the intended therapeutic outcomes (Hanson-Abromeit, in press).

Clinical Work

The above sections have discussed the myriad issues that are faced by preterm infants. Much of their development has to occur in an environment that is not naturally suited for the complex development of the human infant. In this section, clinical practice is outlined through three scenarios that have been written to represent common referrals and situations that allow for the presentation of key issues. Although informed by clinical practice, the cases presented here are not real cases but are constructions to demonstrate real-world decision making and implementation of music therapy in the NICU.

CLINICAL EXAMPLE: "Mother Would Like to Play Recorded Music for Her Preemie"

The nurse left a message asking the music therapist to see a parent who would like to play some recorded music. When Sandra, the music therapist, read baby Selaya's medical file, she learned that Selaya was born at 24 weeks gestation and was transferred immediately from the women's hospital next door to the tertiary level NICU in the pediatric hospital. By 32 weeks GA, Selaya had shown herself to be physically strong and resilient. After 7 weeks on the ventilator, she had been on the simpler CPAP (continuous pressure air pathway) for the last week. Selaya had incurred bleeding on both sides of the brain (bilateral grade II IVHs) and had received a 5-day course of gentamicin (an antibiotic) for sepsis (systemic infection). Gentamicin (an ototoxic medication) is known to damage hearing, but Selaya's hearing could not be tested until she was off CPAP. The care manager told Sandra that Selaya's mother, Jenna, had wanted to use music during her pregnancy and thought that now she would like to play music to Selaya in her isolette.

Because the referral came from the mother, Sandra considered the mother to be as much the client as the infant. After discussion with the care manager and her first meeting with Jenna, Sandra knew Jenna's age and education level and that Selaya was her first baby. Jenna had played clarinet in school and listened to music every day, which confirmed that music was part of her heritage. When Sandra asked why Jenna wanted to play music for Selaya, Jenna revealed that she was worried that Selaya was not getting positive stimulation, only the random noise of the equipment and the unit. Sandra confirmed that she could measure the sound levels in Selaya's isolette as a first step. Sandra explained that recorded music can be a useful static stimulation for supporting behavioral state regulation and that Jenna talking, singing, or reading would offer Selaya age-appropriate auditory stimulation. Jenna decided she would like to know how loud the environment really was and how Selaya responded to the recorded music.

Sandra only had a handheld sound-level meter (SLM) that measured but did not store data. After cleaning it, she put the SLM through the porthole at the back of the isolette and closed the opening around her arm. She held the SLM so that the microphone was near Selaya's ear and documented the lowest and highest sounds every 20 seconds for 5 minutes. She repeated this procedure at other times of the day to create data on the noisiest and quietest times to inform the most likely times for music to be played.

Sandra then completed an assessment of Selaya's physiological and behavioral responses to a brief exposure to her choice of recorded music. The speakers were set up 20 centimeters (almost 8 inches) on either side of Selaya's head inside the isloette, and the player was located outside in a place where Sandra could activate it while still able to see Selaya and the monitor. This setup was completed prior to the commencement of the assessment.

The assessment had three 10-minute periods (Standley & Walworth, 2010): no music (Selaya's spontaneous presentation), music (the effect of music on her presentation), and then another period of no music (her ability to maintain regulation after the music is stopped). Sandra documented Selaya's underpinning state, and every 30 seconds documented her heart rate, respiration rate, and oxygen saturation, including any episodes of bradycardia or apnea. She continuously documented Selaya's behaviors to note any patterns. Selaya tolerated the music, with her physiological presentation remaining within the limits set by the nurses, and her behavioral presentation indicated no rise in stress with the addition of music. On this basis, music could be included in Selaya's care. Sandra and Jenna listened to the playlist that Sandra had prepared from Jenna's preferences. As they listened, Sandra shared the positive and negative features of the music so that Jenna could learn to identify the qualities of the music too. Jenna chose one quiet and slow piece to offer Selaya for her 5 minutes of stimulation. In Selaya's medical record, Sandra wrote instructions for nurses to allow Jenna and her husband to be the ones to implement the music for the first 3 days, when Selaya was in a quiet alert or quiet sleep state, to confirm the presence of music as a part of nurturing care. After 1 week, Sandra returned and met Selaya's father, Jeremy, who reported that Selaya looked toward the music when he turned it on, and then just drifted to sleep. They planned to meet the next day to listen to more music so they could build Selaya's library of music.

CLINICAL EXAMPLE: "Baby Does Not Tolerate Any Stimulation; Mother Not Attuned"

Chrissy is the obstetric and intensive care music therapist providing continuity of care to families across the outpatient clinics and inpatient units. Chrissy received a referral from Lucy's primary nurse when Lucy was 29 weeks GA, because he was concerned about Lucy's adverse response to any stimulation. He was also concerned about Lucy's mom, Darla. Because of Lucy's distress when stimulated, Darla was beginning to avoid interacting with her.

Chrissy reviewed Lucy's chart and medical history and then spoke to the primary care nurse, who had made the referral, at the bedside. Chrissy conducted an initial assessment at Lucy's bedside, but outside of her visual range, to observe Lucy's behavioral cues in response to typical environmental stimuli. During this 20-minute observation period, Chrissy noted that Lucy demonstrated disorganized stress responses, such as arching her back, extended arms and legs that never fully relaxed, and startle responses such as twitching and finger splays. Lucy also exhibited high and erratic heart and respiratory rates.

The following day, Chrissy observed Lucy during scheduled clustered nursing cares. Chrissy noticed that Lucy demonstrated similar stress behaviors as the nurse touched and moved her; however, Lucy briefly raised her eyebrows in a "face open" self-regulatory response if the nurse spoke to her as he performed the cares. As cares were ending, Lucy's mom, Darla, arrived at the bedside. Chrissy quietly greeted Darla, briefly told her about music therapy on the unit, and asked Darla to tell Chrissy about Lucy. Darla began to cry and shared her concern that Lucy did not like to be touched, and that she was unsure of how to help her daughter.

Chrissy knew that it was equally important to foster bonding with Darla and to empower her confidence in her mothering, as it was to support Lucy's integration and organization of sensory stimuli. Therefore, Chrissy focused the treatment plan on co-treating Lucy with Darla. Specifically, Chrissy helped Darla to recognize and interpret Lucy's behavioral cues, use her voice to bond with and support Lucy's development, and to develop confidence in her role as a mother.

At the start of each music therapy session, Chrissy stood at the end of the warmer bed, out of Lucy's visual range, and Darla stood at the side. They observed Lucy for a few minutes to understand her specific behavioral cues and responses to the current environmental stimuli. Then Chrissy cued Darla to vocalize an "ah" sound in a downward melodic contour with a tempo matched to Lucy's respiration rate. If Lucy's respirations were too fast, they used the iso principle to match the rate and then gradually slowed the elongation of the vocalizations to support a slow-ing of the respirations. Chrissy's role was to guide Darla and to support her recognition of Lucy's behavioral cues: When she observed a positive response, the vocal stimulation was continued; when she noticed a subtle disengagement cue, the most recent change in the stimulation was removed. Gradually, supportive touch was added to the vocalizations, with Darla being cued to add a cupped hand simultaneously over Lucy's head and her feet or to place her finger in Lucy's palm.

Over the course of several weeks, Chrissy noted that Lucy's self-regulatory responses were increasing in response to her mother's vocalizations and touch. She also noticed that the process of vocalizing was helping Darla to relax and be more in tune with Lucy's responses than with her own fears. The nurses also stated that Lucy seemed less agitated during cares. By the time Lucy was 36 weeks GA, Darla's vocalizations had progressed from "ah" to humming short phrases and familiar melodies. Nursing staff noted that Darla was also using this type of phrasing and contour with Lucy when speaking to her and was using more touch while talking or singing. Lucy's primary nurse had suggested kangaroo care (skin-to-skin contact), so Darla was holding Lucy several times a day.

Chrissy continued to monitor Lucy's development and to suggest and model modifications to the sensory stimulation to support Lucy's developmental competence. As Lucy moved closer to discharge, Chrissy also started educating Darla and her husband on how music could be incorporated into parenting at home.

CLINICAL EXAMPLE: "Baby Is Bored; Family Lives Far from Hospital"

Amy worked as part of the developmental therapy team in a pediatric NICU. The nursing team was concerned that when his mother was not there, Joshua was bored and would start crying and pulling out his nasal prongs and nasogastric tube (used for feeding him), all for attention. From his medical record, Amy knew that Joshua was born at 34 weeks GA and had experienced significant respiratory issues and that there were some cardiac concerns. Tests had shown that he had a chromosomal deletion consistent with a syndrome likely to result in an intellectual impairment.

At the start of the music therapy program, Joshua was 10 weeks old, or 4 weeks corrected age (CA), and he was awake for several hours each day. His family included three other children, but they all lived 4 hours away on a farm. His mother, Ellen, journeyed down by train each Friday morning to be with Joshua, and the whole family drove down on Sunday to visit with Joshua and take Mom home. The music therapist, Amy, did not work on Fridays so had no opportunity to meet face-to-face with Joshua's mother. Amy telephoned her to introduce herself, explain the music therapy service, and gain consent from Ellen to work with Joshua. Ellen was delighted and decided on two aspects of the service. First, Amy left information at the bedside on how the family could produce recordings of their voices and sounds from home to comfort and support Joshua. They also talked about having his sisters and brother create a songbook (with lyrics and pictures), so that each week when they visited they could add a song and matching picture to the book and sing the song with him. This encouraged a family musical heritage that also incorporated family voices as meaningful stimulation. Ellen had been worried about Joshua's unhappiness, so she readily agreed to the second part of the program: live interactive music therapy with Amy to engage Joshua in an opportunity for cognitive and social development.

The music therapy sessions were held twice a week, about 30 minutes after Joshua's feeding, when most of his digestion had occurred and he was still awake. Amy only used voice to begin with so that Joshua's visual focus remained on her face. Once they had established rapport, she introduced other sources of visual and auditory stimulation to offer him a range of sensory experiences, such as different frequencies to hear. When she began, she checked his availability for interaction, and was mindful that he might tire quickly and be ready for sleep. She used contingent singing (Shoemark, 2013) to stimulate active participation. Amy noted that Joshua responded with smooth movements and raised eyebrows, indicating interest. She continued to sing the four-bar phrase that he seemed to enjoy. He remained focused on her face for about 4

minutes, then looked away for a moment to self-regulate the stimulation and returned to focus on her for another 3 minutes. After this he looked away for a longer period, and his eyes began to flutter closed. Amy knew that he had received enough stimulation and was ready for sleep, so she moved into a lullaby and Joshua fell asleep.

Amy wrote in the little notebook at Joshua's bedside, which she and the family used to stay in touch. Amy saw that on their last visit, Joshua's brother and sister had written to ask Amy to find the lyrics to a song they once knew but now could not remember. Amy smiled, knowing that she was part of their team too.

Applications to Other Disciplines

The use of recorded music in the NICU has been adopted by nursing researchers and is used informally in many units around the world. Frequently, music is employed by nonmusic therapists in the NICU as a developmental stimulus to support state regulation, such as sleep, or non-nutritive sucking, a behavior necessary for competent feeding. Music to support sleep is generally referred to as *sedative* music. Lullabies are the commonly accepted form of sedative music for infants. Many commercially produced CDs of lullaby music have no therapeutic basis and should not be used without verifying that the music meets suitable parameters. Recorded music can also support non-nutritive sucking, such as with the pacifier-activated lullaby (PAL) (Standley & Walworth, 2010). Live singing as the auditory stimulus is a multimodal stimulation. As a multisensory modality, music alone or in tandem with other sensory stimuli (e.g., touch, rocking, eye contact) should be carefully introduced and monitored with consideration for overstimulation of the infant's sensory system.

When used inappropriately, music can become an extraneous and detrimental sensory stimulus. All professionals employing music must be aware of the sensory processing capacities of the infant for whom the music is intended. Professionals using music in the NICU should be adept at selecting music to match the therapeutic intent. In addition, they must be able to simultaneously monitor and adapt the music stimulus to the infant's behavioral and physiological responses. All professionals should proceed cautiously with the use of music in the NICU and seek the consultative services of a knowledgeable music therapist.

Conclusions

Music therapy in the NICU requires a significant understanding of the developmental trajectory in fetal and newborn development of physiological, behavioral, and social capabilities, and an engagement with the infant as part of the family unit. A strong understanding of the characteristics of premature infants is necessary for efficacious practice. The preterm infant's behavioral and physiological responses are indicative of neurobehavioral and sensory system development, and therefore serve as important indicators of the most relevant problems to be addressed through music therapy. The newborn music therapist (Shoemark, 2011) must be knowledgeable about measurement and control of the auditory environment and the role of music as both a stimulus and lived experience. In practice, the music therapist will consider music at its foundational elements and reconstruct the music using conceptual frameworks such as the newborn music therapy model (Shoemark, 2011) and the therapeutic function of music (Hanson-Abromeit, in press).

REFERENCES

Als, H. (1986). A synactive model of neonatal behavioral organization: Framework for the assessment of neurobehavioral development in the premature infant and for support of infants

and parents in the neonatal intensive care environment. *Physical and Occupational Therapy in Pediatrics, 6*(3/4), 3–55.

Bo, L. K., & Callaghan, P. (2000). Soothing pain-elicited distress in Chinese neonates. *Pediatrics, 105*(4), e49–e49.

Fischer, C. B., & Als, H. (2004). Trusting behavioral communication. In M. Nocker-Ribaupierre (Ed.), *Music therapy for premature and newborn infants* (pp. 1–32). Gilsum, NH: Barcelona.

Gottlieb, G. (1983). The psychobiological approach to developmental issues. In P. H. Mussen (Ed.), *Handbook of child psychology* (4th ed., pp. 1–26). New York: Wiley.

Hanson Abromeit, D. (2003). The newborn individualized assessment program (NIDCAP) as a model for clinical music therapy interventions with premature infants. *Music Therapy Perspectives, 21,* 60–68.

Hanson-Abromeit, D. (in press). A conceptual methodology to define the therapeutic function of music. *Music Therapy Perspectives, 1*(33).

Hanson-Abromeit, D., Shoemark, H., & Loewy, J. (2008). Music therapy in the newborn intensive and special care nurseries. In D. Hanson-Abromeit & C. Colwell (Eds.), *Medical music therapy for pediatrics in hospital settings: Using music to support medical interventions* (pp. 15–69). Silver Spring, MD: American Music Therapy Association.

Hartling, L., Shaik, M. S., Tjosvold, L., Leicht, R., Liang, Y., & Kumar, M. (2009). Music for medical indications in the neonatal period: A systematic review of randomised controlled trials. *Archives of Disease in Childhood: Fetal and Neonatal Edition, 94*(5), F349–F354.

Haslbeck, F. B. (2012). Music therapy for premature infants and their parents: An integrative review. *Nordic Journal of Music Therapy, 21*(3), 203–226.

Hodges, A. L., & Wilson, L. L. (2010). Preterm infants' responses to music: An integrative literature review. *Southern Online Journal of Nursing Research, 10*(3). Retrieved from *www.resourcenter.net/images/SNRS/Files/SOJNR_articles2/Vol10Num03Art05.html.*

Kelly, M. M. (2006). The basics of prematurity. *Journal of Pediatric Health Care, 20*(4), 238–244.

Lickliter, R. (1993). Timing and the development of perinatal perceptual organization. In G. Turkewitz & D. A. Devenny (Eds.), *Developmental time and timing* (pp. 105–123). Hillsdale, NJ: Erlbaum.

Malloch, S., Shoemark, H., Črnčec, R., Newnham, C., Paul, C., Prior, M., et al. (2012). Music therapy with hospitalized infants: The art and sci-ence of communicative musicality. *Infant Mental Health Journal, 33*, 386–399.

Mouradian, L. E., Als, H., & Coster, W. J. (2000). Neurobehavioral functioning of healthy pre-term infants of varying gestational ages. *Devel-opmental and Behavioral Pediatrics, 21*(6), 408–416.

Obeidat, H. M., Bond, E. A., & Callister, L. C. (2009). The parental experience of having an in-fant in the newborn intensive care unit. *Journal of Perinatal Education, 18*(3), 23–29.

Olischar, M., Shoemark, H., Holton, T., Weninger, M., & Hunt, R. W. (2011). The influence of music on EEG activity in neurologically healthy newborns ≥ 32 weeks' gestational age. *Acta Pae-diatrica, 100*(5), 670–675.

Rais-Bahrami, K., & Short, B. L. (2013). Premature and small-for-dates infants. In M. L. Batshaw, N. J. Roizen, & G. R. Lotrecchiano (Eds.), *Children with disabilities* (7th ed., pp. 87–104). Baltimore: Brookes.

Shoemark, H. (2011). Frameworks for using music as a therapeutic agent for hospitalized newborn infants. In N. Rickard & K. McFerran (Eds.), *Lifelong engagement with music: Benefits for mental health and well-being* (pp. 3–22). New York: Nova Science.

Shoemark, H. (2013). Working with full-term hos-pitalized infants. In J. Bradt (Ed.), *Guidelines for music therapy practice: Pediatric care* (pp. 116–151). University Park, IL: Barcelona.

Shoemark, H., & Dearn, T. (2008). Keeping par-ents at the centre of family centred music ther-apy with hospitalised infants. *Australian Journal of Music Therapy, 19*, 3–24.

Standley, J. M. (2012a). A discussion of evidence-based music therapy to facilitate feeding skills of premature infants: The power of contingent music. *Arts in Psychotherapy, 39*(5), 379–382.

Standley, J. M. (2012b). Music therapy research in the NICU: Updated meta-analysis. *Neonatal Net-work, 31*(5), 311–316.

Standley, J. M., & Walworth, D. D. (2010). *Music therapy with premature infants* (2nd ed.). Silver Spring, MD: American Music Therapy Associa-tion.

van Soelen, I. L., Brouwer, R. M., Peper, J. S., van Beijsterveldt, T. C., van Leeuwen, M., de Vries, L. S., et al. (2010). Effects of gestational age and birthweight on brain volumes in healthy 9 year-old children. *Journal of Pediatrics, 156*, 896–961.

Walworth, D., Standley, J. M., Robertson, A., Smith, A., Swedberg, O., & Peyton, J. J. (2012). Effects of neurodevelopmental stimulation on premature infants in neonatal intensive care: Randomized controlled trial. *Journal of Neonatal Nursing, 18*(6), 210–216.

CHAPTER 34

Medical Music Therapy for Children

Joanne Loewy

Admittance to the hospital in today's world is not an easy venture. Referring doctors and ER (emergency room) teams have a growing familiarity with the strict criteria that determine a patient's need for acute hospital services, or whether, in fact, he or she might be better treated in a less confining environment. With health care costs on the rise and insurance companies imposing restrictive sanctions, the recommendation for a continued stay in the hospital, or not, is subject to frequent evaluations by utilization review committees. Knowledge of and adherence to what requires hospital care and what does not places pressure on not only admitting doctors, but on hospital care teams as well, and this has changed the delivery of care within the past several decades. Efforts are underway to examine aspects of care to include substantiation of disease predictability and to define typical course of treatments related to the length of stay for patients.

This shift in strategy has influenced outcomes of care provisions for patients who require hospitalization. Formerly, patients who were admitted to the hospital would stay through the course of their disease, and the symptoms that were part of their presenting medical issue were not only diagnosed and treated, but were tendered toward resolution through observation and treatment. Currently, there is an urgency to stabilize patients in an effort to reduce hospital day stays and costs. As a result, a thorough and complete diagnosis and treatment course for a disease that was once diagnosed and treated in the hospital is now relegated to the outpatient setting and a referred physician (Kalra, Fisher, & Axelrod, 2010). There is indeed a pressure and trend to reduce the length of stay, the result of which is thought to yield large cost savings for hospitals and insurance companies.

One's first thought upon observing a decreasing length of stay for patients might seem to reflect that we are getting better at treating disease ailments more effectively and more quickly. Patients who were once hospitalized for a week might now perceive a shorter stay to mean that they are getting better faster. In current times, we alter our care delivery to focus more intently on the early stages of admission, where *diagnosis* and *assessment* are keys, and furthermore where "resource consumption is most intense" (Yu, Wier, & Elixhauser, 2011).

Issues related to length of stay do have a profound influence on how care is perceived and administered. A shorter length of stay calls upon music therapists to join other professionals in being clinically astute and succinct in our assessment, treatment planning, goal setting, and evaluation. We should also be forthright and accountable in collecting information and sharing our assessment findings with team members.

This chapter outlines a model of music psychotherapy for working with children, from neonates to adolescents, in a medical setting. The assessment and treatment strategies are based on my 20 years of experience in a medical setting, as well as extensive research of interventions and knowledge that have led to evidence-based clinical outcomes informing work with the pediatric populations.

Clientele

A critical aspect of working with infants, children, teens, and families is understanding the diagnosis and its medical implications. Pediatrics includes newborns through 18-year-olds, and in many hospitals, particularly when children have been *frequent fliers*–their stay may extend through age 21. Knowledge of common diseases such as FTT (failure to thrive), asthma, GAD (generalized anxiety disorder), PID (pelvic inflammatory disease), sickle cell anemia, and seizures is a must for the hospital-based therapist. The top 15 major diagnostic categories for hospital stays in children in 2009 were respiratory system; digestive system; nervous system; pregnancy; mental disorders; endocrine, nutritional, and metabolic; ear, nose, mouth, and throat; musculoskeletal system; skin and subcutaneous tissue; infectious and parasitic diseases; kidney and urinary tract; blood disorders;

circulatory system; injuries and poisonings; and neoplasms (Yu et al., 2011).

Many approaches to working with hospitalized children are based on treatment-specific populations or symptomatology such as recovery difficulties (O'Neill, 2002), anxiety (Wang, Kulkarni, Dolev, & Kain, 2002), burns (Edwards, 1994), stress and immune response (Avers, Mathur, & Kamat, 2007), asthma (Loewy, Azoulay, Harris, & Rondina, 2008), sedation for procedures (Loewy, Hallan, Friedman, & Martinez, 2005; Loewy, 2008), sedation complications (Loewy, 2013a), pain (Loewy, 1999, 2012; Mondanaro & Sara, 2013), and cancer (Brodsky, 1989; O'Callaghan, Sexton, & Wheeler, 2007).

It is important to approach children at their level, which requires familiarity with child development. The study of developmental milestones (Gesell, 1934; Greenspan, 2003), with an emphasis on play and musical development, should be prerequisite for the music therapist practicing in pediatrics. This education will guide assessment of what is *normal* or *delayed*, of what is *creative, avoidant, regressed,* or *defended,* and also what might reflect behavior that is secondary to being diagnosed with a disease.

Another essential ingredient to optimal care is knowledge of cultural customs and rituals. And then, along with having such knowledge, it is important to maintain the attitude that each patient and family is a culture onto him-/her-/itself, and that this culture can unravel and/or reformulate within the music to assist how a young patient is processing his or her understanding and thereby impacting the course of illness and wellness throughout the child's hospital stay.

Clinical Work

Theoretical Framework

Whatever one's approach to music therapy might be, the application and intervention are best served when it comes from a place of understanding and acceptance. Having the knowledge and belief in a theoretical model is important. However, the model needs to be integrated with the input and understanding of the physical, psychological, cultural, and spiritual aspects that distinctly intertwine with the medical issues at hand. This chapter describes an *integrative medicine* orientation, which ensures that music therapy will be part of the interdisciplinary plan of care. Figure 34.1 shows how an integrative approach to Medical Music Therapy compares and contrasts to the medical model of care. The areas under *Musical* (top) correspond with the polar opposite areas under *Medical* (bottom). For instance, *wellness* in the musical domain is related to *illness* in the medical domain, and further, *subjective experience* corresponds

to *clinical objective*, and so forth (Loewy & Scheiby, 2001).

Current music therapy approaches are based on the general development of science at large, and more specifically on the trends of research and practices that exist as an outgrowth of universities and trainings created and set forth by music therapy practices in the United States and internationally. A few of these approaches—a general behavioral approach (Standley & Whipple, 2003), a desensitization approach (Chetta, 1981), and a contextual support model (Robb, 2000)—are based on theories of motivation and engagement that include the effect of music to structure and provide autonomy, support, and involvement. Other approaches include, but are not limited to, biomedical orientations that incorporate music applications in the treatment

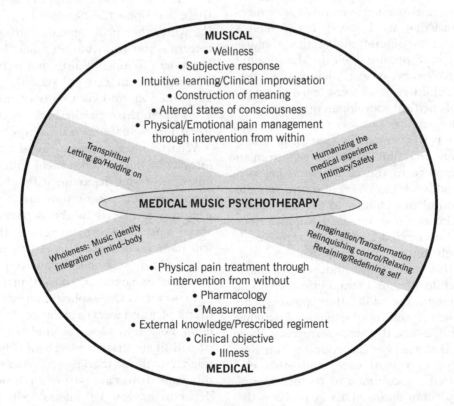

FIGURE 34.1. A model of integrative music psychotherapy. From Loewy and Scheiby (2001). Reprinted with permission of Satchnote Press.

of symptoms manifested in behaviors and sensations occurring "outside of the physical space of the brain" which implies that feeling and thought are not influencing the medical ailment, but rather, the condition is purely physical and concerning solely biological and physical function (Taylor, 2010, p. 14). Largely, a review of the music therapy literature reveals that pediatric music therapy approaches often stem from treatment strategies that have integrated music therapy into a child life perspective-which is based on developmental aspects of play, mastery, coping and achievement and learning (Ghetti, 2011; Hanson-Abromeit & Colwell, 2008).

The treatment approach undertaken by music therapists is critical to the way in which music therapy is perceived by patients, families, staff, and perhaps most importantly, by the therapist him- or herself. Psychological orientations and developmental knowledge are imperative parameters that affect the potency and quality of music therapy care provided within the hospital setting. Whereas most clinicians who treat infants, children, and teens learn about aspects of medical, developmental, and play-related domains that serve these areas of practice with children in a medical center, less knowledge and attention are given in the literature to the parameters that succinctly address the *therapy* of music. It is the intention of this chapter to provide theory and rationale for an integrative approach to music therapy that is psychotherapy-based. Although music therapists who practice within this model may be housed in a social work, child life, or therapeutic recreation department, the skills they possess and implement in serving the needs of patients and families are distinctly *therapeutic*. This means that therapy incorporates transference, countertransference, and other elements that are common to the practice of music psychotherapy. This is perhaps the strongest defining difference between a *specialist* and a *therapist*.

Location, Location, Location, and Space (the Final Frontier)

It is not uncommon for music therapists who work within a medical model in hospital or clinical settings to be part of a department that is not a dedicated music therapy department. Such departments include, but are not limited to, child life, recreation therapy, rehabilitation, social work, pastoral care, child and adolescent mental health services, and psychology departments. The location of a music therapy position or program placement may depend upon the philosophy of the institution, whereas other placements are based upon the developing interests of team members and/or the programmatic desires of the hospital's administration. There are pros and cons to being part of a department that is not exclusive to music therapy. Pros are that there are opportunities for daily interfacing with other professionals, during which referrals and team building may be easily instituted. Team building that is inclusive of co-treatment can enhance the timing, coordination, and continuity of care from assessment through discharge, extending toward home-based postdischarge plans.

What is most important is that the philosophy of the therapist meld with the orientation of the department in which one is employed. If you or your music therapy program is placed in the department of social work, you can be certain that you will have keen access not just to patients, but to families as well. If you are part of a child life department, you will presumably have access to the explicit interests of children's play and ways to incorporate medical equipment into play. You and the specialist will likely share a playroom, where you might run music therapy groups or community jams. If you are part of a pastoral care department, you will undoubtedly provide music in your medical institution's bereavement services and on spiritual holidays, in addition to standard music therapy care for patients.

In reality, any or all of the above constitute best care and community infiltration of music and therapeutic music, which will certainly enhance the way you—as a clinician, and also as a community builder—will ultimately be seen by your peers and allied health care professional team members.

In contrast, there may be some cons in working within a department whose members are not knowledgeable about, or open to becoming informed about, music therapy. These include, for example, working with a director of another discipline who does not understand the standards of practice in the music therapy profession and, as a result, may limit referral making or access to patients in need. This stance may impede the formation of a therapeutic alliance if the director simply tells a patient or parent about music therapy in a generic manner, rather than understanding that, when the music therapist provides an explanation, it is distinctly tailored to the referral. Limiting the music therapist's access to critical staff, such as doctors or nurses, can also impede integration and present communication challenges related to treatment, where continuity of care is imperative and best provided as directly as possible.

An ideal setting in which to work is within a music therapy department or a creative arts therapy department center that is linked with all of the aforementioned services. In this way, all referrals and patient care can be streamlined and served uniquely, according to the patients' needs and the music therapists' approaches (Nordoff–Robbins, Guided Imagery in Music, etc.) and/or subspecialty (e.g., release-oriented strategies, sedation effect, end of life, asthma initiative program).

Referral Solicitation and Confirmation

The development of a referral form and the institution of a referral process are critical factors in the provision of services to patients and contribute to the continued education and communication among staff. The referral form used in the Louis and Lucille Armstrong Music Therapy Program at Mount Sinai Beth Israel (see Figure 34.2) helps to identify patients who are in the greatest need of music therapy services. It also serves as a teaching tool for rotating residents and floating nurses that are a part of the modern-day hospital environment. Feedback on this form's use has indicated that it is particularly useful because areas of need can be checked off on the front, with corresponding identifiers and descriptors on the back. In this way, if a practitioner is able to identify an area of psychotherapeutic need and check it off, he or she can turn the form over and read about what a music therapist might offer to the patient who has the particular issue. This helps staff to learn about music therapy on an ongoing basis. Through the write-in comment section, staff members are challenged to provide details about a specific patient and provide their own handwritten account of what the music therapist might attend to when assessing the patient and family.

Referrals are generally made in person at rounds, in writing, or by page or voicemail, or they can be solicited, which tends to be the case when new staff rotates in or a new music therapy program is being developed or upgraded. The music therapist might ask questions that compel staff to think about how music can assist in addressing pain issues related to the care of a patient and family. For example, the music therapist might say to a child's physician, "This child is afraid of needles. Maybe we can warm her up for surgery tomorrow. I can contact the holding area nurse and anesthesiologist today about escorting her down to provide some music therapy in the holding area and operating room. What do you think?"

Upgrading of referrals may be necessary on a unit where staff has seemingly only referred one type of patient or treatment need. In such cases, the objective would be to increase the understanding of what music therapists do and how this service may expand and facilitate the depth and level of care provided by the team, particularly addressing the area of pain crises. Upgrading was needed at one time on our Family Medicine Unit when, during a 1-month period, there were 15 referrals, with each patient referred for "stimulation." Several of our patients with asthma, renal failure, and sickle cell disease had been admitted dur-

ing the month but were inadvertently overlooked by the team, who needed reminders that these patients were familiar with music therapy from our outpatient clinics. The staff needed explanations and cues from the music therapy team about how we work with breathing and pain management in music therapy, and the variety of options that could be provided musically during an asthma or pain crisis.

There was a brief period of time when it seemed that the nurses were limiting their writing in the comment section of the re-

---

MOUNT SINAI BETH ISRAEL
The Louis & Lucille Armstrong Department of Music Therapy

Name of Patient: _____

Diagnosis: _____

Floor & Room: _____

Primary Language of Patient: _____ English: ____ yes ____ no

Caretaker(s) Name: _____

Primary Language of Caretaker: _____ English: ____ yes ____ no

Relationship to Patient: ____ mother   ____ father   ____ sibling

                           ____ foster parent   ____ relative

                           ____ friend

Reason(s) for Patient's Referral for Music Therapy (definitions on reverse side)

Check areas that apply:

Anxiety/Fear: ( ) Separation anxiety   ( ) Pre- or postoperative anxiety

                          ( ) Generalized anxiety

Pain/Stress: ( ) Breathing difficulties   ( ) In need of tension release

Expressive Difficulties: ( ) Depression or nonverbal   ( ) Acting out or hyperactive

Coping: ( ) In facing the illness   ( ) Self-esteem

                          ( ) Communication/socialization

Loss of Consciousness: ( ) Increase awareness   ( ) Increase stimulation or use of imagery

Other

Specify: _____

Comments: _____

Person Referring: _____ Ext: _____ Date: _____

(continued)

FIGURE 34.2. Referral for General Pediatrics. Sample form for music therapy. Copyright 1994. Reprinted with permission of the Louis Armstrong Center for Music and Medicine.

Music Therapy Referral Criteria

I. Anxiety/Fear
Music therapy soothes, familiarizes, and/or activates:

A. Separation anxiety — Chanting, musical holding, and collaborative musical experiences create a feeling of safety in the hospital.

B. Pre/postoperative anxiety — Making music relaxes and eases the mind and body of tension and fear stimulated by hospital procedures.

C. Generalized anxiety — Musical experiences help patients make sense of their fears through a nonthreatening medium.

II. Pain/Stress
Clinical improvisation provides an alternative, non-verbal means of release for a patient in discomfort:

A. Breathing and vocalizing — Life rhythms and tonal intervallic synthesis help a patient synchronize and deepen the breathing process. Toning stimulates the connection between the body breath and feeling states.

B. Tension release — Opening channels of musical creativity stimulates the body's need to release tension.

III. Expressivity

A. Depression, nonverbal/inactivity — Structured and unstructured therapies help elicit feelings that may be "muted" or "blocked."

B. Acting out or hyperactivity — The implicit structure music therapy techniques such as African drumming, song sensation, and instrumental composition offer patients a safe means of channeling their excessive amounts of energy.

IV. Ego Strength/Coping

A. Facing the illness — The metaphorical use of music in song selection and composition offers patients a safe way into understanding and adjusting to their illness.

B. Self-esteem — Performing and tape creating strengthen a patient's feeling of worth during this fragile time.

C. Communication/socialization — Community singing, drumming circles, and collaborative free improvisations foster communications between patients and within families.

V. Loss of Consciousness/Coma/ICU

A. Awareness — The use of familiar melodies helps patients become oriented or tuned in to a state of grounded, familiarized awareness.

B. Stimulation — The use of music and guided imagery stimulates the healing process.

FIGURE 34.2. *(continued)*

ferral form to "has no visitors" or "needs to be distracted." At rounds, the music therapist explained how music therapy might work to expand a patient's ability to delve into a particular issue, say, relating to his or her pain and the anxiety and traumatic response to being hospitalized, rather than simply serving as a distraction to avoid working with something emotional that would most likely return hours after the distraction had worn off. In pediatrics, as in most hospital units, working with staff directly after they make a referral is invaluable to the integration of music therapy services. Thanking or reinforcing a good referral ensures that referrals will continue to be made and that they will occur at the most necessary times.

Checking in with a doctor or nurse and confirming that a referral led the music therapist to (provide brief description of music experience), which led to (provide description of changed medical and/or psychological outcome) may be the single most effective method of referral–team–program building—for example: "Thanks, Dr. Levin, your referral of Sarah for music therapy was invaluable. I noticed that the chart reflected that she hasn't eaten in 2 days. I invited her to the jam when I received your referral form, where you checked off *fear/anxiety*. After attending the music jam, she went back to her room and ate a yogurt and two pieces of toast. The drum helped her release her tension. Thanks, and please keep those referrals coming!"

Implementing Music Therapy Consult Services: Entry, Assessment, and Beyond

The way that the music therapist approaches patients and families is critical to how the therapy will be perceived and consequently its success. A gentle tap or knock on the door, followed by a firm handshake, with some reference or linkage to fellow medical staff and a direct statement about music therapy. The referral and an announcement for the patient and family, orienting them as to how long the initial assessment will take, is not only reassuring, but it is the culture that follows how virtually every other service is provided to patients. These simple and direct factors are often overlooked, leading to rejection of pain consult services and evoking misconceptions about what music therapy may, or may not, provide for patients during their pain crisis. Some common errors that are made in this part of the process include the following behaviors.

Forcefulness

Entering into patients' rooms too eagerly, too briskly, and too definitively does not show respect for their sense of space nor for their need of respect and privacy. Being too forceful about what music therapy provides does not always give patients and families the option to refuse the service.

Resistance is a meaningful aspect of music therapy assessment and treatment. The quality of a patient or family's resistance is worth exploration. Some of the most trusted working music therapy relationships have been initiated through numerous attempts met with allowance and acceptance of resistance and/or active and deliberate refusal of music therapy services. The music therapist should work to understand the quality of a patient's resistance, particularly on a day when pain has been exacerbated by procedures or disease symptoms.

There are many ways to work with resistance. The first and foremost may be to extend unconditional acceptance of the refusal of music therapy services. Rejection of the music therapy service should not be taken personally. Rather, the resistance can be used to understand and examine, countertransferentially, how the patient is working to maintain an avoidance of, and/or a pushing away of, a connection with life energy as he or she faces unexplainable illness and unpleasant unknowns.

Misrepresenting the Role of the Modality and the Therapist

Some music therapists think that introducing the provision of *music*, rather than music therapy, might influence patients and families to accept the modality. In actuality, an avoidance of the word *therapy* can misguide the patient and/or family. In fact, upon assessment, it may be that the patient does not want music, or that therapy is not something that would be beneficial to the patient at the time of entry or upon the first initial contact. It is an ethical responsibility to include the word *therapist* in introducing oneself or to include the word *therapy* upon introduction of the modality, if, in fact, one is providing music therapy services or if one's job title is, indeed, *music therapist*.

In working as a music therapist within an auxiliary department, the music therapist should clearly represent the music therapy modality and, furthermore, make clear distinctions, when necessary, between the department that he or she is a part of and the function that will be served in performing music therapy or a music therapy assessment. For example, "I am part of the Child Life team—I am a music therapist. . . ." "I am part of the Department of Social Work. Whereas the social worker will be assisting with your discharge planning, I am here to assist Kelly pre-op . . . using music for relaxation, if indicated. . . ."

Tentative Role/Service

It is especially useful for music therapists to announce themselves directly to patients and staff in a clear and concise way. Sometimes a music therapist will enter a patient's room showing anxiety. He or she might not make direct eye contact with the patient or might present the service but not explain what the goals or treatment areas of need might be. Because music therapy may be the most unfamiliar service offered, the music therapist should maintain a stance of confidence, yet not present as defensive. It is reasonable and likely that a patient will be skeptical and have no conception of what music therapy is or why it is being offered. The music therapist can anticipate questions of all kinds and be ready to answer in a way that provides clarity and comfort.

Reading the Chart Too Soon

It may be important to refrain from reading the details about a patient's medical condition as well as the family constitution and history until *after* the music therapy assessment has been performed. In this way, the therapist can learn about the patient and experience the illness from the patient's frame of reference. This is particularly important when assessing a patient in pain.

In reading the medical chart and discussing team opinions *after* the assessment session, the music therapist can combine three important sources of information before making a formal written assessment that will be completed within 24 hours of the evaluation. The first, most essential source is the therapist's impressions of the patient and how he or she presents in and out of the music during the assessment. The second is the chart (medical record), which provides a context for the patient's medical and psychosocial history. The third, the medical team, provides a host of opinions and impressions. At times, there is conflicting information, and this conflict provides a context for the treatment needs and goals that will follow.

Many patients think of the worst-case scenario regarding prognosis. Other patients may be in denial of a disease process that is life-threatening. Still others lack understanding about the medical treatment being offered because, at the time of diagnosis, for instance, there may have been a traumatic reaction, and the patient or family may have been unable to process information and may have become overwhelmed.

On the other hand, in intensive care units (ICUs), psychiatric wards, substance abuse units, and correctional facilities, delaying a reading of the chart may not prove useful. In such units, the music therapist may need to draw upon all sources of available information prior to performing the assessment. In this way, the therapist can work to avoid overstimulating the patient and also prepare some ways to safeguard him- or herself from unpredictable or unsafe behavioral conditions.

Some critical decisions must be made upon entry to the patient's room:

• *Where will the session will be held?*
The therapist must make the decision of
whether to come into the patient's room or
to encourage a patient to leave the room to
come to the music therapy room or separate space (e.g., lounge, office) that is available. Although working with a patient who
is mobile provides opportunities for attending sessions in a private, musically conducive environment, it can be advantageous to
come into a patient's space (room) if invited
and to work to absorb, assess, and perhaps
shift the energy or the patient's impression
of the hospital experience. The patient's
desire and the nurse's recommendation of
where the session would be most benefi-
cially conducted are among the factors that
should be taken into consideration.

• *Will the cart display of instruments be
shown or not?* Some patients (adults, children, especially teenagers) will be particularly turned off to the modality upon
seeing a cart full of instruments. It may
remind them of things that are *babyish* or
events they are missing in school. Musical
instruments (tambourine, organ) shown
prematurely to patients may remind them
of church, which could relate to their unconscious associations with death. It could
remind a patient of a grandparent whom
he or she has not visited, or who has not
been informed about the illness or hospitalization. At other times, the musical instruments may evoke potential or provide possibilities. They may encourage the patient
to take on a feeling of playfulness, thereby
taking him or her out of the *sick role*.

Music Psychotherapy Assessment

The Armstrong Music Therapy Program
is based on psychotherapeutic principles.
The assessment session itself is carefully
conducted and involves three layers of experiences: (1) entry and warm-up or opening, (2) process and tour of the room assessment, and (3) closing and distancing.
As the context of the music psychotherapy

assessment is so critical to a patient's willingness to trust, or a sense that a *guarded*
expression is more desirable (possibly related to mistrust), I explain a course of
music therapy assessment where a context
of trust might be developed through a musical relationship. The patient's willingness
or refusal to have music therapy can be
indicative of many factors. The therapist
who provides opportunities for a patient to
learn self-comforting strategies, and who
offers assurances by presenting a grounding and open introduction, usually through
the use of his or her own music, reflects a
feeling of safety and familiarity and such
a musical warm-up invites trust and open-
ings for self-expression. This may provide a
context where the expression of pain can be
co-evaluated in and out of the music.

The entry into a patient's room and noting the atmosphere therein are both critical
prephases of the assessment (Loewy, 2000).
The stance of the therapist—how he or she
introduces the modality as well as him- or
herself and the instruments and music—is
critical to how readily the service will be accepted or rejected by the patient and family.
The decision of whether to include family
members in a session is important, particularly when a pain music consult is considered. For the patients who seem smothered
by siblings or parents, the music therapy
time may be the perfect opportunity for
refuge, a time for family members to take
a break and have some personal space. For
the mother or father who seem emotionally
fragile or shut down, music may open some
avenues of communication through meta-
phoric play and the cues intrinsic to musical collaboration. Ideally, interviewing the
pediatric patient musically, both alone and
with significant family members, provides
valuable conditions through a variety of environments and circumstances (Greenspan,
2003). The opportunity to observe how a
patient reacts when he or she is alone versus
with a family member may reveal integral
components of who the person is, and how
this person functions differently with family

in the day-to-day experiences, and particularly within the moment of trauma (Loewy, 2011). Setting up the conditions that provide a stable, free-flowing invitation to the initial assessment and then the assessment itself are the most essential components that lead to effective treatment. Knowing the diagnosis and, in particular, what has led to a pain response will be especially helpful to the music therapist who will be devising interventions for treatment.

Implementation of service occurs after the completion of a clinical assessment. Critical information for the therapist, and particularly important in a pain assessment, is the gathering of information related to how the person who is hospitalized functioned *prior to the illness/hospitalization.* Wellness is an important prerequisite to ego support and emotional development of well-being, both in and out of music therapy. Once referred or identified (music therapists may draw their own referrals through observation, as well as through receiving written and verbal assessments from staff), the referral process leads the music therapist, with team input, to recommend an immediate music therapy treatment plan, a pending treatment plan (based on patient's prognosis, length of stay, treatment plan), to not recommend a treatment plan, or to refer to another modality.

A Medical Music Therapy assessment usually takes 30–45 minutes. At times, the assessment is achieved in several moments, as a patient will reveal an area of immediate need and attention. This may not be the case in music therapy assessments with other populations. As individuals who are medically fragile enter the hospital in perhaps the most vulnerable of states, the music provided and explored during an assessment may unlock many layers of emotional need. The music therapist's initial assessment session, therefore, should have enough structure to contain and provide a feeling of safety for the patient. At the same time, the assessment can provide space and a feeling of openness and exploration that

gives a patient the means to feel playful and empowered. It is likely that experiences during the hospital stay prior to having a music therapy assessment did not provide such opportunity. To simply be admitted to the hospital, one has to undergo a myriad of tests and several series of what may seem to be invasive questions. Many patients through the years have spoken about how music therapy provided nurturance, joy, and clarity amid what was, in other ways, a particularly frightening time.

The implementation of a music therapy intervention, for instance, for an infant with NAS (neonatal abstinence syndrome; a condition where a neonate is born with a dependency on opiate drugs, resulting from pregnancy) may be based on assessment of both parent and infant. A lullaby or song of kin can be offered to assist in calming or sedation if a procedure is necessary. A particular song of kin, or lullaby in this case, is best simplified into an intervalic, vowel-toned rhythmic response. That is, the lyrics are removed and a holding meter of 3/4 or 6/8 is set to the infant or child's rhythm of exhibiting symptoms (Loewy, 2008), which in this case would probably involve hyperstimulation or overactivity.

Tour of the Room Assessment Model

This model, which I developed (Loewy, 1995, 2000), does not assume that all patients want to engage in music immediately, or that the music is separate from the relationship between the patient and the therapist. Music may be a part of the relationship or not, but a person's relationship and associations with sound and music are best assessed before offering a music therapeutic experience. In this way, there are no assumptions. The tour will ensure that the particular music or sound used in treatment is indicated. This is particularly important when treating someone who has reported an experience of pain. The therapist conducts a tour demonstrating a broad range of instruments for the patient and watches the patient's physical, emotional, and cognitive responses and inquiries to the sounds. A free associational discussion may ensue. A patient's relationship with music, sound, and other elements may be easily revealed or subtly captured referentially, through the active and passive reactions (physical, emotional) that the patient has upon hearing the smorgasbord of sounds.

Once the tour is complete, the patient is asked to choose an instrument with which he or she wants to begin. He or she is invited to either play or to listen as the music therapist plays. The therapist's assurance about the acceptability of playing or not playing and his or her relationship with music and the comfort in playing for or with the patient create an atmosphere of trust and perhaps willingness in the patient to disclose pain and/or anxiety.

Usually music or talking is elicited through the exploration of sounds during the tour. Associations to the outside world and often to the impending hospitalization evolve through the patient–therapist exploration of music and collaborative play (Loewy, 2013a). The therapist's inquiry about a favorite song or type of music comes usually after the tour and may lead to a host of associational topics regarding family, school, religion, or significant others. The structure of the music can take the patient and/or the therapist to a playful place. The relationship is built, and often a significant amount of sharing occurs. The format of an assessment session is critical and combines structured and free-flowing experiences. A combination of these two types of experiences may provide for the optimal experience of assessing the therapeutic needs of a new client. The tour of the room is part of assessing these areas.

Unlike assessments with outpatient populations, the assessment of a patient in a hospital setting is completed in one session, rather than in several screenings. In the hospital, a patient can become emotionally engrossed in, and connected to, the music experience, so that the goals become apparent within the first moments of the evaluation. In such circumstances, the treatment might begin within the first few moments of the session. Examples of this include working with a patient who is having extreme pain or accompanying a patient who is undergoing a procedure or having a medical test. In such cases, the patient, often in crisis, will verbally alert the therapist to the problem and/or fear immediately. The traumatic reaction is addressed in the moment. At other times, the situation is not as observable, and the formal tour of the room, combined with team inquiry and chart review, will provide the therapist with the opportunity to combine a variety of experiences and opinions that will further substantiate the music therapy assessment. The treatment goals are developed from this knowledge.

Thirteen Areas of Inquiry

The 13 Areas of Inquiry instrument (Loewy, 2000, 2013b, p. 436) utilizes a music psychotherapy assessment context to evaluate 13 areas of functioning: (1) awareness of the self, others, and the moment; (2) thematic expression; (3) listening; (4) performing; (5) collaboration/relationship; (6) concentration; (7) range of affect; (8) investment/motivation; (9) use of structure; (10) integration; (11) self-esteem; (12) risk taking; and (13) independence. These 13 areas interconnect to address four core domains that are important because they integrate music and verbal evaluation within a music psychotherapy context: relationship, dynamics, achievement, and cognition. These domains are reviewed closely within the tour of the room assessment context.

Evaluation of Pain

A unique part of a hospital music therapy assessment is the evaluation of pain (Loewy, 1999). Using live music can help the therapist "understand and feel the pain of the patient" (p. 195), as it can be defined in a conjoint moment of interaction during music play. In addition to asking patients to comprehensively describe their pain, patients are encouraged to improvise music to convey their pain (Loewy, 2013a); these improvisations provide clues as how to address physical aspects of the tension. By playing with patients, we are able to assess the types of interventions that might serve to ameliorate their pain, such as toning (Loewy, 2011) or drumming (Loewy, 1999), and we can also define the therapist's role in doing so. My team and I use a CAS (Color Analysis Scale) in addition to the Wong-Baker FACES® Pain Rating Scale or 1–10 ratings (Loewy, 2011).

The CAS provides an evaluative rating that is dynamic and allows for the expression of pain through the patient's visual depiction using crayon illustrations marked on a sketch of a body figure that is provided (see Figure 34.3). The CAS is a usual part of our assessment battery and provides the

patient, therapist, and physician with information integral to enhance the pain evaluation experience. This type of creative pain assessment may open venues for a more comprehensive understanding of the pain experience than would a unidimensional scale rating. Gathering pain assessment evaluations prior to and after music therapy may provide useful information about the effectiveness of music therapy. In the CAS shown in Figure 34.3, the young female patient with sickle cell anemia said that the pain in her joints was "sharp, like a knife" and "hot." After drumming and releasing many rhythms with the music therapist, she said that she still had some pain, but that she "had more flow" and that "the heat is now cooler—I can breathe better."

Unlike other settings where the therapist may have months or even years of building connections with patients, the hospital is most often a quick and sharp-edged experience for patients. The traumatic feeling

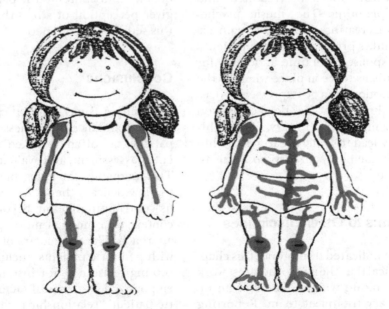

FIGURE 34.3. Color Analysis Scale. *Note*: The CAS is provided with front and back views of the body in order for patients to depict their pain experience with color. In this CAS (originally in color), the lines on the arms and legs were drawn (in red) by a young female patient (left) prior to music therapy and on the right were drawn (in blue) immediately after a music therapy pain intervention. The CAS is used in conjunction with a numeric rating of pain from 0 to 10, which is a typical part of the daily nursing flow chart. Copyright 1997. Reprinted with permission of Satchnote Press.

that one faces when hospitalized, no matter what the reason or suspected diagnosis, is often incomprehensible to the patient and/ or family.

Unlike therapists who work in other settings, the immediate depth and level of emotion that a hospitalist may unveil, particularly in a patient who has pain, within the initial moments of contact with the music therapist is often remarkable. This is due to the hefty amount of trauma and defense building that may occur within the experience of pain in the hours preceding the music therapy experience. When the therapist offers him- or herself in the music, the patient may feel trust for the first time since the pain occurred. Perhaps the patient has had no other place to release the fear, anger, or anxiety associated with the pain, as other personnel may not have made the space for such emotions to be shared and explored.

Other personnel may be addressing primarily medical aspects of treatment and discharge planning. The music psychotherapist, in creating a space for pain expression, makes provisions for the patient's negative response, with time and space for the mechanisms to be in place whereby the patient's emotions can be expressed and assistance to linkage of his/her connection to the body may occur (Loewy, 2011). This process may lead to better treatment within the current medical and psychosocial aspects of care.

Applications to Other Disciplines

As has been indicated throughout this chapter, it is critical that the music therapist work and communicate with members of an interdisciplinary treatment team. Reporting back to referral makers at rounds, including doctors and nurses in instances of sessions where the child may feel tension, and working together to solicit referrals and in devising a plan of care are integral to good care. Maintenance and upkeep of staff in-

clusion (such as through frequent inservice programs) provide assurances that music therapy will be called upon as an effective treatment modality. Although nurses and doctors typically do not have training to be therapists, there are ways in which they can be included in the care—and reap the benefits of both experiencing its benefits and observing its effectiveness as well.

Holding weekly *community jams, music meditations,* and *EMT* (environmental music therapy; Rossetti & Canga, 2013) can open opportunities where the music may filter into the medical or psychosocial care arenas and benefit treatment. For example, social workers who have experienced resistant parents have enhanced communication with families as a result of attending jams where successful musical interactions occurred. Doctors have spent nonmedical moments with patients in the ICU and commented that, when EMT was present, the intense environmental noise that so frequently contributes to the patient and caregiver perception of stress that is a part of this setting was softened.

Conclusions

The unique aspects of Medical Music Therapy care and its effectiveness with pediatric patients can often be linked to the referral, entry, assessment, and evaluation processes. This uniqueness includes, but is not limited to, how delicate the treatment of pain and its contributing factors become within the context of a medical music psychotherapy approach. The particulars of our approach with pediatric patients, inclusive of our accepting resistance, for instance, should be emphasized as a critical factor. The pediatric patient's relationships with others, particularly family members and staff, are easily and nonconfrontationally approached through music. From referral to entry, from the warm-up into the assessment, a music-based evaluation involving live associations with sounds and themes provides ample opportunities for goal planning. The plan of care is built carefully and playfully with the child's interest in mind. Whether an infant, toddler, latency-age child, or teen, Medical Music Therapy lends itself to a systematic, theme-oriented approach—one that is child-friendly and malleable, and one that will support the inner resources of the pediatric patient that are already in place.

REFERENCES

Avers, L., Mathur, A., & Kamat, A. (2007). Music therapy in pediatrics. *Clinical Pediatrics, 46*(7), 575–579.

Brodsky, W. (1989). Music therapy as an intervention for children with cancer in isolation rooms *Music Therapy, 8,* 17–34.

Chetta, H. D. (1981). The effect of music and desensitization on preoperative anxiety in children. *Journal of Music Therapy, 18,* 74–87.

Edwards, J. (1994). The use of music therapy to assist children who have severe burns. *Australian Journal of Music Therapy, 5,* 3–6.

Gesell, A. (1934). *Infant behavior: Its genesis and growth.* New York: McGraw-Hill.

Ghetti, C. (2011). Clinical practice of dual-certified music therapists/child life specialists: A phenomenological study. *Journal of Music Therapy, 48,* 317–345.

Greenspan, S. (2003). *The clinical interview of the child* (3rd ed.). Washington, DC: American Psychiatric Association.

Hanson-Abromeit, D., & Colwell, C. (2008). *Medical music therapy for pediatrics in hospital settings.* Silver Spring, MD: American Music Therapy Association.

Kalra, A., Fisher, R., & Axelrod, P. (2010). Decreased length of stay and cumulative hospitalized days despite increased patient admissions and readmissions in an area of urban poverty. *Journal of General Internal Medicine, 25*(9), 930–935.

Loewy, J. (1995). A hermeneutic panel study of music therapy assessment with an emotionally disturbed boy (Doctoral dissertation, New York University, 1994). *Dissertation Abstracts International, 55*(9), 2631.

Loewy, J. (1999). The use of music psychotherapy in the treatment of pediatric pain. In C. Dileo (Ed.), *Music therapy and medicine: Theoretical and clinical applications* (pp. 189–206). Silver Spring, MD: American Music Therapy Association.

Loewy, J. (2000). Music psychotherapy assessment. *Music Therapy Perspectives, 18*(1), 47–58.

Loewy, J. (2008). Musical sedation: Mechanisms of breathing entrainment. In R. Azoulay & J. V. Loewy (Eds.), *Music, the breath and health: Advances in integrative music therapy* (pp. 223–232). New York: Satchnote Press.

Loewy, J. (2011). Tonal intervallic synthesis as integration in medical music therapy. In F. Baker & S. Uhlig (Eds.), *Voicework in music therapy* (pp. 253–266). London: Jessica Kingsley.

Loewy, J. (2012). Music psychotherapy approaches for infants and children experiencing pain. *Painvew: American Society of Pain Educators, 8*(3), 13–17.

Loewy, J. (2013a). Music and medicine: Integrative models in the treatment of pain. In J. Mondanaro & G. Sara (Eds.), *Music therapy and integrative pain* (pp. 203–213). New York: Satchnote Press.

Loewy, J. (2013b). Respiratory care for children. In J. Bradt (Ed.), *Guidelines for music therapy practice in pediatric care* (pp. 403–441). University Park, IL: Barcelona.

Loewy, J., Azoulay, R., Harris, B., & Rondina, E. (2008). Clinical improvisation with winds: Enhancing breath in music therapy. In R. Azoulay & J. Loewy (Eds.), *Music, the breath and health: Advances in integrative music therapy* (pp. 87–102). New York: Satchnote Press.

Loewy, J., Hallan, C., Friedman, E., & Martinez, C. (2005). Sleep/sedation in children undergoing EEG testing: A comparison of chloral hydrate and music therapy. *Journal of Perianesthesia Nursing, 20*(5), 323–331.

Loewy, J., & Scheiby, B. (2001, May). *Developing the culture of music psychotherapy in the medical setting.* Paper presented at evening lecture series at NYU/Nordoff-Robbins Center for Music Therapy, New York.

Mondanaro, J., & Sara, G. (2013). *Integrative models in the treatment of pain.* New York: Satchnote Press.

O'Callaghan, C., Sexton, M., & Wheeler, G. (2007). Music therapy as a non-pharmacological anxiolytic for paediatric radiotherapy patients. *Australian Radiology, 51*(2), 159–162.

O'Neill O. (2002). The efficacy of music therapy on patient recovery in the post-anaesthetic care unit. *Journal of Advanced Perioperative Care, 1,* 19–26.

Robb, S. (2000). The effect of therapeutic music interventions on the behavior of hospitalized children in isolation: Developing a contextual support model of music therapy. *Journal of Music Therapy, 37*(2), 118–46.

Rossetti, A., & Canga, B. (2013). Environmental music therapy: Rationale for "multi-individual" music psychotherapy in modulation of the pain experience. In J. Mondanaro & G. Sara (Eds.), *Integrative models in the treatment of pain* (pp. 275–294). New York: Satchnote Press.

Standley, J., & Whipple, J. (2003). Music therapy with pediatric patients: A meta-analysis. In S. Robb (Ed.), *Music therapy in pediatric healthcare: Research and evidence-based practice* (pp. 1–18). Silver Spring, MD: American Music Therapy Association.

Taylor, D. B. (2010). *Biomedical foundations of music as therapy* (2nd ed.). Eau Claire, WI: Barton.

Wang, S. M., Kulkarni, L., Dolev, J., & Kain, Z. N. (2002). Music and preoperative anxiety: A randomized, controlled study. *Anesthesia and Analgesia, 94,* 1489–1494.

Yu, H., Wier, L., & Elixhauser, H. (2011, August). *Hospital stays for children, 2009.* Statistical brief #118. Healthcare Cost and Utilization Project (HCUP). Agency for Healthcare Research and Quality, Rockville, MD. Available at *www.hcup-us.ahrq.gov/reports/statbriefs/sb118.jsp.*

CHAPTER 35

Medical Music Therapy for Adults

Carol Shultis
Lisa Gallagher

The use of music in medicine can be traced to biblical times. Early writings document the historical use of music for medical purposes (Weldin & Eagle, 1991). Taylor (1981) described the use of music in general hospitals from 1900 to 1950, laying the foundation for modern music therapy in hospitals. In modern times, the use of music in medical settings can be traced to hospitals treating veterans after World War II. At that time, much of the application was focused on the psychological and rehabilitative needs of the patients.

The use of music therapy in the general hospital grew in the 1970s and 1980s. This growth included programs directed by Sr. Sandra Pelusi at Mercy Hospital of Pittsburgh, PA, Sr. Ruth Sheehan at Forbes Health System in Pittsburgh, and Dr. Deforia Lane at University Hospital's Rainbow Babies & Children Hospital in Cleveland, OH. I (Carol Shultis) worked in the medical setting in one of these early programs, taking the reins from Sr. Ruth Sheehan at Forbes in 1981. Forbes began their program because the administration and medical staff were committed to the value of music therapy to address the stress of hospitaliza-tion. From its inception the program took referrals from medical and surgical units and provided services to psychiatric, long-term care, and hospice patients.

Research into specific medical uses of music became more prevalent in the 1980s (Spintge & Droh, 1992). Investigation of music therapy interventions to address medical needs appeared in the literature (Rider, 1985; Standley, 1991). In the 1980s, music therapist Dale Taylor began to talk about the medical application of music and in 1997 first published his theory that "because music has observable effects on human brain functioning, its effects can be used therapeutically" (p. 15). He further discussed subtheories that dealt with the neural pathways responsible for the effect of music on pain, neural processing, physiological responses, and music's influences on anxiety and stress.

Other publications in the 1990s explored the use of music in medicine and music therapy. Maranto (1991) defined five categories of medical music therapy, including (1) music as medicine, (2) music in medicine, (3) music therapy and medicine, (4) music therapy as medicine, and (5) music therapy in medicine. More recently (Dileo & Bradt, 2005, p. 9), the distinction has been described as either (1) *music therapy*, involving interventions by a music therapist using specific methods; or (2) *music medicine*, involving listening to prerecorded music provided by medical personnel (nonmusic therapists). Reflecting the evolution of this area, Dileo (2013) found three categories of practice that result from the interface of music and medicine: (1) treatment of musicians by medical personnel and by music therapists; (2) music in medical and health education in medical humanities, medical education, and health education; and (3) music practices for medical patients and staff by musicians, medical personnel, and music therapists. She also includes foundational research that provides the basis for many of these practices.

Standley et al. (2005) published meta-analyses of research in medical/dental care, in pediatric specific studies, and with premature infants, identifying multiple benefits of medical music therapy, and Dileo and Bradt (2005) conducted a meta-analysis of 11 medical specialty areas in music therapy. Dileo and Bradt (2009) define specific clinical goals addressed in medical music therapy, including (1) improved physical functioning, (2) decreased pain perception, (3) decreased arousal and resultant relaxation, (4) enhanced social and psychological functioning, (5) increased cognitive functioning, and (6) behavior change. Medical music therapy may also provide spiritual support and a means to completion of relationships at the end of life for family and patient. Cochrane reviews relevant to general medical settings have investigated the medical music therapy research on mechanical ventilation (Bradt, Dileo, & Grocke, 2010), pain (Cepeda, Carr, Lau, & Alvarez, 2006), end-of-life care (Bradt & Dileo, 2010), coronary heart disease (Bradt & Dileo, 2009), cancer (Bradt, Dileo, Grocke, & Magill, 2011), preoperative anxiety (Bradt, Dileo, & Shim, 2013), and brain injury (Bradt, Magee, Dileo, Wheeler, & McGilloway, 2010), helping to identify the possible outcomes when addressing the above goals.

Clientele

Music therapy is frequently offered to patients via a referral system. Referrals may be made by medical staff (including doctors and nurses), interdisciplinary staff (social workers, occupational therapists, physical therapists, speech and language pathologists, dieticians), and, in some cases, services may be requested by family members or patients. Referral sources vary according to the policies and procedures established by the hospital and its medical staff. In most hospitals, patients receive treatment in their hospital room; however, some hospitals have space available on specialty units (especially rehabilitation units) for music therapy to be offered in a separate location. These locations usually have more space, and they are better able to accommodate group work.

Patients with many diagnoses are seen in medical facilities. Indeed, most patients in a hospital are potential candidates for music therapy. These patients may be seen in a variety of settings, including general inpatient units, specialized intensive care units, procedural rooms, operating rooms, delivery rooms, and waiting rooms. Treatment may also occur in outpatient waiting areas, procedural areas, rehabilitation units, clinics or outpatient locations, and patient homes, depending upon the policies, procedures, and preferences of the hospital.

Hospital Specialty Units

Most patients in the hospital are usually on general units, such as medical/surgical or general internal medicine units. However, hospitals are usually broken into many units specializing in specific types of medical issues. The Cleveland Clinic has the following inpatient units for adults:

hematology/oncology, nephrology/renal/ hypertension, urology, ReSCU, pulmonary medicine, gastrology/hepatology, transplant, bone marrow transplant, leukemia, colorectal surgery, colorectal telemetry, short stay, neurosciences, neurosurgery/ neurology, neuro-concentrated care, orthopedics, digestive disease, seizure monitoring, bariatric, bariatric surgery, palliative medicine, rehabilitation, and chronic pain rehabilitation. Patients with acute problems are often admitted to a unit where they are treated for a few days, then moved to a specialized unit, such as those previously listed. Patients may also be sent to a variety of different intensive care units (ICUs), including medical (MICU), surgical (SICU), cardiac (CICU), and neurological ICU.

Cardiac treatment may include progression through a variety of units. Some patients awaiting a heart or lung transplant may be admitted to a transplant unit, where they will stay until a new heart or lung becomes available. Then they, like other cardiac patients, will have surgery, go to an ICU, and move to a step-down unit prior to discharge from the hospital. The Cleveland Clinic, well known for its cardiac care, has an entire building dedicated to cardiac care, with over 20 cardiac and vascular care units, including postanesthesia care, intensive care, step-down, and transplant units.

Hospitals that offer transplants also utilize music therapy both prior to and after the transplant surgeries. The use of music therapy for patients in ICUs is becoming more common as research reveals the value of music therapy interventions, especially for mechanically ventilated patients (see Bradt et al., 2010). Terminally ill patients frequently receive music therapy as a part of palliative care, both in the hospital and in hospice programs, which often are extensions of hospital services (Gallagher, Lagman, Walsh, Davis, & LeGrand, 2006; Gallagher & Steele, 2001).

Some music therapists working in hospital settings are able to focus on one specific population, such as oncology, surgery, psy-chiatry, or rehabilitation; however, many music therapists are expected to see consults throughout the entire hospital. This leads to a different set of challenges, including working with patients of varied ages, diagnoses, lengths of stay, and treatments (Hanson-Abromeit, 2010). Medical music therapists also have to be skilled at working with patients from different cultural backgrounds and religions. This skill includes demonstrating respect for and knowledge of cultural traditions, coping with language barriers, and being comfortable with the discussion and/or expression of spirituality and/or religion (Aldridge, 1999, 2004; Hanson-Abromeit, 2010; Mondanaro & Sara, 2013).

Diagnoses and Patients

Patients in the hospital may have a variety of diagnoses, with some of the most common areas of treatment being cardiology (heart and vascular), oncology (cancer), neurology (brain-related disorders), and postsurgical complications. Other common diagnoses include leukemia, coronary heart disease, stroke, multiple sclerosis, dementia, Parkinson's disease, Alzheimer's disease, renal disease, hypertension, obesity, liver disease, cirrhosis, lung disease, epilepsy, traumatic brain injury, broken bones, knee or hip replacements, chronic pain, major depression, generalized anxiety disorder, substance abuse disorder, posttraumatic stress disorder (PTSD), and HIV/AIDS. Obstetrics patients, especially those experiencing ante-partum complications, are often referred to music therapy during prolonged pre-delivery hospital stays.

Patients may also be seen at different stages of their diseases, with cancer/oncology being the prime example. Patients who have just received a cancer diagnosis and are coping with the news may need to undergo surgery to remove the tumor, followed by radiation or chemotherapy treatments, or they may need to have a bone marrow transplant. Referrals to music therapy occur for a variety of needs. The psychological adjustments necessary after initial diagnosis, the onset of treatment, or repetitive admissions for treatment and late-stage cancers with complications all may trigger a referral. Outpatients receiving treatments that require long periods of idle time on a lounge chair or hospital bed may benefit from a consultative visit from the music therapist to learn about using music as a means to manage the time, the aftereffects, and the stress of treatment. Patients may become ill due to the treatment or as a side effect of the medication, they may no longer have treatment options but are in need of symptom management, or they may be actively dying. The music therapist needs to be prepared to deal with each stage and with the emotions or issues that may arise.

Cardiac unit patients are frequently referred for anxiety management, which may be addressed via music-assisted relaxation experiences, songwriting, or song discussion. Cardiac patients who have undergone surgery may be referred for pain management, as well as for music therapy to explore the changes in lifestyle that the future may bring. The interventions may include those listed above, as well as music-evoked imagery to work with the pain.

Challenges

There are many challenges related to working with patients in a medical setting. One of the biggest may be the large amount of knowledge that is needed to understand and speak the same language as the other health care professionals. This includes knowledge of medical terminology, abbreviations, procedures, and equipment; medications and their common uses; and various medical and mental health disorders and the characteristics of each (Hanson-Abromeit, 2010). It is also important to be aware of the latest medical and music therapy research, as well as of any advanced levels of training that would increase one's ability to work with specialized populations, such as hospice or neurological conditions (Hanson-Abromeit, 2010).

Hospitals are fast-paced and unpredictable environments, so music therapists must exhibit flexibility (Hanson-Abromeit, 2010; Wheeler, 2002). Patients are often unavailable due to such things as rounds, medical procedures, baths, being off the floor, nursing care, visiting with families, sleeping, talking on the phone, watching television or listening to iPods, and receiving treatments, thereby making it difficult to see those who have been referred to music therapy (Gallagher, Huston, Nelson, Walsh, & Steele, 2001). Even once a session is in progress, the therapist often has to deal with interruptions such as doctors making rounds, nurses giving medications, transporters arriving to take the patients for a test or procedure, the phone ringing, visitors arriving, and so forth. It would be ideal to have a schedule, but this is often not realistic in the hospital setting. Therefore, the music therapist must learn how to prioritize referrals so that the highest-priority patients are seen first. Even determining what makes a patient a priority may be difficult. It is usually based upon level of patient need, such as extreme pain or anxiety; however, it may also be based upon the most recently received referrals, patients who have not been seen yet, proximity to the last patient seen, and/or political requests such as being asked to see a VIP patient.

Another challenge is how often a patient is seen. The change in patient health status and ability can greatly affect the frequency and the duration of music therapy sessions. The music therapist may see some patients just once, whereas others may be seen for several months based on the severity of their illness and the use of music therapy in their treatment. Therefore, results may have to occur quickly, or progress may need to be demonstrated over time.

Other challenges facing the therapist revolve around music. Due to the wide variety of patient ages, cultures, religious backgrounds, and music preferences, the medical music therapist must have a huge repertoire. Even with a large repertoire, it is not possible to have everything, so the therapist needs to have a plan for what to do if he or she does not have the music the patient wants to hear. In order to please the listener, the music therapist needs to have excellent music skills, including the ability to sight-read (Wheeler, 2002). It is hard when a patient wants to hear a classical piece as it would sound with full orchestra when the therapist only has a guitar or keyboard on which to play the piece. Access to an iPad, hospital WiFi, and a cloud account with music loaded can be an asset in these situations.

Clinical Work

Song Choice and Song Discussion

Song choice and subsequent discussion can be very powerful interventions. The process of identifying a song that matches a mood, communicates a need, or tells a story about one's self, history, or current experience provides both a means of expression and communication for the client and assessment and evaluative information for the therapist. This song choice may lead to a discussion that provides a personal vocabulary for songwriting later in the session or may open the door to singing, improvisation, or the sharing of other songs/musical experiences that have meaning to the patient.

Song choices and the subsequent discussion can be very effective tools for drawing a patient into the music therapy process. The act of choosing a song is relatively easy, provides many options for a patient, and does not require much energy expenditure or initial emotional investment. The therapist might structure this experience to invite the patient to share something about him- or herself, or to invite the patient to choose a song that might help to make the day better. The patient might choose a song from a list provided by the therapist or request a preferred song, which the therapist will hopefully know. The therapist might sing the song for the patient or with the patient. The discussion after might be simple and address the patient's associations with the song, the impact of hearing or singing the song, or anything that the patient wishes to share. This process can also quickly move to a deep psychological intervention when the patient has a need for it to do so.

A man in his 50s with a love of music was asked to choose a song to begin the session. He chose a song and asked the therapist to sing it. After the song he proceeded to share personal information about his past and his current illness. He asked for additional songs, following each choice with a story about himself and his life before he became ill. The music therapist guided the discussion to help him explore his former understanding of himself, to look at what he was experiencing in the hospital at this time, and to ponder the future. He was feeling uncertain about what was to come and what he hoped would come. The song choices allowed him to consider his current state of mind in the context of his former concept of himself and to begin to explore options for the future.

Singing

Singing alone or with others is beneficial both physiologically and psychologically. The action of breathing deeply to sing has physiological benefits, especially for a patient post-op or someone with lung disease. The act of singing is very personal and may evoke a rainbow of emotions, depending upon the patient's previous experiences with singing. The music therapist must be vigilant to cues revealing the patient's response to singing. Are tears acceptable to this man when he begins to hum or sing along, or does he need to stop crying in order to maintain the stoic self that is familiar to his daily life? Does the smile during the song reveal pleasure or an attempt to please the therapist who is singing a preferred song? Is this a family who will benefit from staying with the patient and singing at bedside while sharing in the experience, or does this patient need the privacy to emote? Each patient has specific needs, which the music therapist must carefully assess.

A family with whom the music therapist had been working for several weeks was experiencing anticipatory grief as the husband neared death. The wife, who had previously chosen to leave the room during her husband's music therapy sessions, appeared relieved to see the music therapist. She spoke softly about her husband, expressing a feeling of powerlessness, of not knowing what to do for him, as he could no longer ask her to do anything. The music therapist suggested she choose a song for the therapist to sing that might be meaningful to the patient. She selected a song the patient had chosen many times before, and the therapist began to sing, inviting the wife to join in if she desired. Quietly, almost inaudibly, the wife began to sing along. The music therapist asked her to choose a second song and, as she did, she shared its importance in their life's journey. The wife proceeded to choose more songs, telling their life's story and singing softly to her husband with the support of the music therapist. After songs she would touch his hand or say a few words to him, "Honey, remember when we. . . ." This session provided a therapeutic intervention for the patient and his wife, movement toward relationship completion (as defined by Dileo & Bradt, 2009), and an opportunity for her to be the caregiver in a meaningful way.

Songwriting

Songwriting is used in music therapy in many forms with many different populations (Baker & Wigram, 2005). For medical patients, it provides an opportunity to put words to the feelings and experiences of being ill and hospitalized. The songwriting process engages creative thinking and invites the patient to approach the hospital experience from a different perspective. Songwriting can be an avenue to explore and address many needs for patients. A song may explore the trials of dealing with illness and hospitalization, identify coping skills available to the patient, or provide a medium for sharing a message with loved ones.

Songwriting can be very simple, with the patient filling in a few words to prepared lyrics; it can be a more involved experience of creating lyrics to a known tune; or it may involve creating a completely new piece of music with original lyrics, melody, and harmonies. The complexity of the experience is mediated by the needs and capacity of the patient in the session. The patient might be the author of the lyrics, while the therapist might guide the melody within the structure of the chord progression. Some patients will spontaneously create a melody when they hear the chords, but they may need guidance to fit the words to the melody. The therapist's role is to facilitate the process in order to allow patients to use this form of self-expression to create a meaningful musical product. In this case, both the process of creating the song and the end product may have therapeutic value. The therapist often creates a written copy of the song to be kept by the patient. In our experiences, patients are often proud of their creations and like to share them with family, friends, and staff members.

As discussed previously, songwriting takes many forms. Substituting words in a song to make it more reflective of the patient's thoughts and feelings can be a profound experience for a medical patient who is feeling overwhelmed by treatments and the hospital experience. For example, the traditional spiritual "Every Time I Feel the Spirit" can easily be altered by changing the words to "Every time I _____, I _____," allowing the patient to express important perceptions of the hospital experience. The verses can be altered to focus first on what the patient is experiencing and then to reflect on some of the coping skills the patient may use to manage the stressors related to being ill and hospitalized. Patients may also create completely new music, including lyrics and melody. For example, an original song about a topic discussed during the session might be created to a 12-bar blues progression. The therapist can play the harmonic progression and allow the patient to spontaneously create a melody, followed by fitting lyrics from the discussion to the music—or the lyrics may come first, with the therapist assisting the patient in their creation. The melody may then come from the patient or may be created by the therapist, who asks the patient questions in order to guide the melodic contour and its characteristics (e.g., stepwise movement or jumping to the next note or phrase). Songwriting affords the therapist many options for different approaches to the music experience, and it provides the patient not only with an experience in self-expression and discussion of coping mechanisms, but also a product (the song) to keep as a reminder of the experience.

A young man in his 30s, experiencing long-term chronic illness and multiple hospitalizations, was readmitted to the hospital. He was feeling frustrated and upset by the disruption of his daily life. He described his many stressors, and with some guiding questions, talked about things in his life that provided him with inner strength. The music therapist suggested that they create a song about his current situation and some possible responses to it. He agreed, and they began with the therapist playing various musical styles on the keyboard. The patient chose a moderate tempo blues progression as the framework for his song. The therapist offered a first line based on the earlier discussion and invited the patient to find a melody. He was reluctant to sing, so the music therapist offered three options for an opening melody line, and he chose the one he liked. They proceeded through the song, working together to find each new phrase of lyrics, harmonic progression, and melody line. At the conclusion, they had a song that reflected his frustration, his fears, and his hope that some specific beliefs

could "pull him through" this difficult time in his life. In addition to talking more positively about the future, his facial muscles held less tension. Nurses remarked that they had not seen him look so relaxed since admission. Following the session, the music therapist put the song on paper for the patient to keep as a reminder of his resolve to move forward in life, despite his current challenges.

Music-Assisted Relaxation

Using music to aid the relaxation response is a common intervention for medical patients. The music used may be recorded or performed live, and it may be coupled with specific relaxation techniques such as autogenic training, deep breathing, progressive muscle relaxation, or directed imagery. Directed imagery allows the therapist to create the structure for the imagery experience and maintain a safe container for the patient. Choosing the music for this process requires a critical listening ear. Music is most effective for relaxation when it is played at a slow tempo with few dynamic changes and with melodies that have few large interval skips and mostly stepwise motion. Preference also plays an important role in the effectiveness of music as a relaxation aid.

Music therapists may also use patient-generated imagery to facilitate relaxation. This approach allows the patient's psyche to choose the images that will be most helpful. It may include an exploration of issues related to the stressors of hospitalization and illness, evolving into a more in-depth psychotherapy approach to address an increased ability to relax. Music therapists often have additional training in this more complex use of imagery and music.

A young woman who was hospitalized for testing and diagnosis was experiencing pain. The pain was being addressed with medication, but the patient was getting only partial relief, and the pain intensified long before the next medication dose was permitted. The music therapist was consulted to teach the patient to use music-assisted relaxation as a pain management tool. The patient was receptive to the idea and chose keyboard for the music experience.

The music therapist helped the patient get comfortable in her bed, turned out the lights, and stood next to the bed with the keyboard on a bedside table. Beginning with some basic directions for breathing, the therapist began to play simple arpeggiated chords and give verbal directions for relaxation. The music therapist continued to improvise simple melodies over the chords, changing from arpeggios to slow rhythmic patterns and back again to arpeggios. After about 5 minutes, the patient was invited to create a place in her mind's eye where she might feel less pain and more comfort. The therapist continued to play on the keyboard while guiding the patient to explore her comfortable place. After about 15 minutes, and before the music was concluded, the patient was guided to create an associational cue to remember this place. After the music ended, the patient was asked to describe the feeling of being in her comfortable place, and she was asked if she could associate that feeling with her cue. She was able to do so and was instructed to practice using the cue to access the relaxed, comfortable feeling in her body, especially when her pain level was low. She agreed to practice and to use the techniques she learned in the session. The music therapist and the patient talked about possible recorded music for her to use independently at home. She was lent a CD player and CD for use while still in the hospital. As the session ended, the patient reported her pain had moved from a presession 7 (on a scale of 0–10, with 10 being the worst possible pain) to a 3. She was not pain-free, but she was more comfortable than before the music-assisted relaxation.

Improvisation (Instrumental and Vocal)

Improvisation in medical music therapy may utilize instruments or the voice. Vocal improvisation may be used to explore a symptom such as pain, or it may be used to engage the patient in spontaneous song lyric creation. When exploring a symptom,

the patient and therapist may use sounds to express the physical or psychological impact of the symptom.

A woman in her 60s was experiencing pain that was not responsive to medication. Unit nurses requested music therapy to attempt to address this pain. Upon approach, the patient was found lying in bed, moaning softly. The therapist attempted to talk with her, but she continued to moan. The therapist, with guitar at the ready, began to moan with the patient, gradually encouraging her to change her sound through nonverbal cues. The patient began to respond and allowed her sound to become louder and more expressive. This duet continued until the patient took a deep breath and sighed. The music therapist began strumming a chord progression on the guitar and invited the patient to make sounds to express how she was feeling now, drawing her attention to her body after the sigh and deep breath. The patient began to hum sounds that gradually became more song-like than her previous moaning. The music therapist supported her hum-singing with the guitar until the patient drew the music to a close. She was then able to talk about her pain experience. This opened the patient to exploring other ways to manage her pain, as the music therapist invited her to move into a relaxation exercise using music and imagery to begin to address her physical pain at another level.

Keyboard, guitar, electronic instruments, and handheld percussion instruments are also found in use with medical patients. Percussion instruments are used most often, as they are the easiest to play and require little or no musical experience or training. A drum may provide an outlet for the frustration of being *stuck in a hospital bed* for too many days, or a small glockenspiel may offer the opportunity to create a pleasing melody that might be incorporated into a relaxation experience or used in a songwriting project. Inviting the patient to provide rhythmic additions to a song or to therapist-improvised music serves to actively engage the patient in the music-making process.

Improvised conversations between the patient and the therapist can also be very powerful. Improvisation helps to create a new identity, to promote homeodynamic stability, to address the patient's specific issues, and to restore hope (Dileo, 1999). In addition, the give-and-take of making music with another person allows the patient to be expressive, to be in relationship with another, and to actively engage in the here and now.

A 15-year-old young man was brought to the hospital with injuries from a car accident, including physical and psychological trauma. He offered little verbal information about himself or the accident experience. Nursing referred him to music therapy in hopes that he could relate to the music and become more responsive and engaged in life. The music therapist met him and also found him to be minimally verbal. Attempts to learn about him yielded very little information. With this limited data, the music therapist invited the patient to join in an improvisation. Setting up an alto xylophone in a blues scale, the therapist began to strum a blues pattern on the guitar and invited the patient to join in. He tentatively struck a note or two, gradually becoming more involved in making music.

When this first improvisation drew to a natural close, the music therapist picked up a hand drum, invited the patient to begin playing, and followed him. The two played in a conversational duet for about 10 minutes, responding to one another's music in the moment. The patient became increasingly involved in making music and in the reciprocity of the duet. As the music concluded, he sighed and smiled. He was clearly more relaxed and less withdrawn, and, although he still had very little to say, his demeanor was changed.

Entrainment

Rhythm is involved in many music therapy interventions; however, one intervention in which rhythm is at the core is musical entrainment. One definition describes *musical entrainment* as a process of playing a musical rhythm at a different tempo from the personal tempo of the patient (Aldridge, 1996, p. 29). By doing so, the patient's rhythm adjusts to that of the music, thereby bringing about an unconscious, automatic response. Thaut (2005) refers to a similar concept, which he describes as *rhythmic synchronization*. Some may also know entrainment as the *iso principle*, which has been utilized to bring about changes in mood, anxiety, and physiological states (Dileo, 1999; Pinkerton, 1996). Psychological as well as some physiological pain can be improved utilizing entrainment techniques (Dileo; Pinkerton; Rider, 1985, 1997). Entrainment has also been used in the treatment of shortness of breath (Branson, 2013; Gerwick & Tan, 2010).

A young woman was readmitted to the hospital due to pneumonia and difficulty breathing. While she waited for assistance from her doctors, the first person she requested a visit from was her music therapist, as she believed she would be able to help her to improve her breathing. When the music therapist arrived, she assessed the situation and identified the patient's favorite music. As the therapist started playing the patient's favorite song on her keyboard, she focused on the patient's breathing, making sure that her tempo of playing matched the tempo of breathing. Then, very gradually, she began slowing down the tempo at which she was playing, and the patient's breathing entrained to her playing. This continued until the patient reached a comfortable tempo of breathing and was able to maintain it on her own.

Even though this patient could not explain the process of entrainment, nor did she even know how the music therapy intervention affected her breathing, she knew that it worked, and that is all that mattered to her. One of the advantages of this intervention is that it works even when the patient is confused, delirious, agitated, anxious, or unresponsive.

Instrument Playing

Patients can be encouraged to play instruments in many ways. Those who seem reluctant to participate, yet show some interest in what is happening, can be given small percussion instruments and asked to hold onto them for the therapist. In most cases, especially if the instrument is unique or interesting, the patient cannot resist playing it. Wind instruments can be used to help improve breathing, especially for patients with asthma, chronic obstructive pulmonary disease (COPD), and cystic fibrosis (Dileo, 1999). Rhythmic cuing, rhythmic stimulation, rhythmic entrainment, and functional use of limbs can all be accomplished through the playing of instruments (Standley et al., 2005; Thaut, 2005). Family members and patients can also be encouraged to play instruments together, along with the music therapist's accompaniment, giving rise to creativity and a new meaning for those involved (Aldridge, 1999). If the patient is a music teacher or professional musician, this intervention may take a different form, such as the revival of interest in playing a favorite instrument or once again being able to conduct music (Beggs, 1991, p. 611).

A music teacher who was in the hospital recovering after heart surgery assigned instruments to each of the individuals in his room, including the doctors and nurses. He demonstrated how he wanted each of them to play, and as the music therapist sang and played the patient's chosen song on her guitar, he conducted everyone in playing the instruments. He took them all through tempo and dynamic changes, and by the end of the song he was smiling and indicated that he once again felt good about himself.

Patients can also adjust their involvement in instrument playing as they adjust to different stages of illness.

A man who had once performed on piano at many famous music institutions throughout the world played the portable keyboard the therapist brought into his room. This continued throughout a number of visits until the patient became too ill to play. At that time he asked the therapist to play, and upon completion of the song he critiqued her playing, as he had many piano students prior to her illness.

It is also important to note that some patients who have been very involved in music throughout their lives may not want to participate in instrument playing or perhaps even music listening. This may be due to new medical problems such as broken bones, physical limitations or injuries, paraplegia, neuropathy, terminal illness, or a variety of other diagnoses. These individuals may not be able to play at the level at which they once played, and therefore become frustrated both with themselves and with the music. The memories of previous music performances make it too painful for them to currently participate in music. At these times it is important to try to redirect how they can still be involved in music, or to respect where they are emotionally and give them time to grieve and process their loss.

Applications to Other Disciplines

Counseling/Psychotherapy

Music is a powerful tool, and one never knows what effect the music might have on the patient. There are times that songs perceived as pleasant or happy could have a negative effect on the patient.

A woman in her 40s who had participated in music therapy sessions on several occasions had made it known that her favorite singer was Whitney Houston. One day at the start of a session she told the therapist to pick any Whitney Houston song to play. The therapist chose "I Will Always Love You" and began to play it and sing it. Halfway through the first verse, the patient started yelling at the therapist to get out of her room. The therapist stopped singing, assisted the patient in calming down, and investigated what had brought about the outburst. Through discussion and the use of verbal processing, it was discovered that "I Will Always Love You" was the song she and her husband had danced to at their wedding. Unfortunately, the day of the session was the anniversary of her husband's untimely death.

This example demonstrates the importance of the music therapist having empathy as well as skills in counseling and/or psychotherapy. If the music therapist in the example above had not had good counseling skills, she might have left when the patient told her to get out. If she had done so, she would have lost any therapeutic rapport she had previously had with the patient, and the patient would have been left in a state of emotional crisis. It is true that the patient could be referred to the social worker or psychologist for treatment; however, it is best if the music therapist is able to handle situations that arise due to the music used within sessions.

Musicians, Medical Personnel, and Music

The previous case example in which the patient told the music therapist to get out of her room is also an excellent example of why trained music therapists should treat patients rather than allowing untrained musicians to perform at patients' bedsides. Musicians often ask to perform at the hospital, stating that they would like to help people feel better. Therefore, if the hospital wants to have musicians perform, it is important that they be trained and that the locations in which they play are controlled. The Cleveland Clinic has developed a system in which three levels of musicians are utilized. *Musicians in the Environment* are those musicians who have been approved by the Performing Arts Committee and who perform in one of four public lobbies at the hospital. *Musicians in Residence* are those Musicians in the Environment who have given a lot of their time to perform at the

hospital, who have received training, and who have been hand-picked by the Performing Arts Committee. These individuals get a little closer to patients as they are invited to perform in specific waiting rooms or solariums on patient units. The third level is the *Board Certified Music Therapist* (MT-BC), the only ones who have enough training to work directly with patients and to deal with whatever issues may come from the music.

Similar work is being done in many other hospitals as well. This is due in part to a recent trend in the development of arts and healthcare programs. According to Sadler and Ridenour (2009, p. 4), some trends in health care that have been positively affected by the arts include patient satisfaction, quality of health care, and evidence-based practice. According to the Society for the Arts in Healthcare (2011; now the Global Alliance for Arts and Health), the areas where the arts can be utilized in the hospital include working with patients, families, and employees; creating environments that are healing; providing education; and conducting wellness programs for the community.

Medical personnel are often very supportive of music therapy, and at times they try to assist with providing recorded music to their patients. Although it is nice that they are supportive, they may not be aware of the patient's musical preferences, which could be problematic. One of the first things that most music therapists try to identify is the patient's preferred music. This should be done in order to provide music that the patient likes, that is culturally and religiously appropriate, and that has no unintentional negative attachments to it.

While the music therapist was on vacation for 2 weeks one December, the nurses on the floor decided to provide relaxing music to a patient who was actively dying. They knew that the patient had participated in music therapy, so they thought the patient would enjoy the music they provided. Unfortunately, they played a CD of Christmas music, and the patient was Jewish. When the music therapist returned from vacation and found out what they had done, she thanked them for thinking of providing music and gave them an in-service on patient preference and appropriateness of music choice.

It is also important to identify patient preferences because that individual's overall preferred music, as well as preferred relaxing music, is likely to be the most effective music to use with him or her (Dileo, 1999). Studies and literature have demonstrated that preferred music has decreased state anxiety, decreased perception of pain, increased positive emotions, and improved relaxation (Davis & Thaut, 1989; Pinkerton, 1996; Taylor, 2010).

Conclusions

Working with medical patients is an exciting, challenging, and rewarding branch of music therapy clinical work. Medical patients experience a vast array of emotional responses to hospitalization and illness, physical symptoms that may respond to musical intervention, and a whole person (mind–body) response that can be altered through musical experiences. Clinical music therapy addresses physical, psychological, social, cognitive, behavioral, and spiritual needs through assessment-based interventions delivered by a trained, credentialed music therapist. Music as an intervention, however, is not the purview of only music therapists but can be added to the medical environment by staff, family and friends, and the patient. Personal music players can bring comfort, help to decrease pain, and induce relaxation. Hospital staff may also provide music for patients; however, this might be most effective when chosen in consultation with a music therapist who can provide the needed consideration of patient preference. Ultimately, music and music therapy experiences will alter the patient's perception and memory of the hospital experience—an important benefit of music in medical environments. Music therapy can provide a relationship-based agent for change, and it can tap into the benefits of music's influence on mind and body.

REFERENCES

Aldridge, D. (1996). *Music therapy research and practice in medicine: From out of the silence.* London: Jessica Kingsley.

Aldridge, D. (Ed.). (1999). *Music therapy in palliative care: New voices.* London: Jessica Kingsley.

Aldridge, D. (2004). *Health, the individual, and integrated medicine: Revisiting an aesthetic of health care.* London: Jessica Kingsley.

Baker, F., & Wigram, T. (Eds.). (2005). *Songwriting: Methods, techniques and clinical applications for music therapy.* London: Jessica Kingsley.

Beggs, C. (1991). Life review with a palliative care patient. In K. E. Bruscia (Ed.), *Case studies in music therapy* (pp. 611–616). Gilsum, NH: Barcelona.

Bradt, J., & Dileo, C. (2009). Music for stress and anxiety reduction in coronary heart disease patients. *Cochrane Database of Systematic Reviews, 2009*(2), CD006577.

Bradt, J., & Dileo, C. (2010). Music therapy for end-of-life care. *Cochrane Database of Systematic Reviews, 2010*(1), CD007169.

Bradt, J., Dileo, C., & Grocke, D. (2010). Music interventions for mechanically ventilated patients. *Cochrane Database of Systematic Reviews, 2010*(12), CD006902.

Bradt, J., Dileo, C., Grocke, D., & Magill, L. (2011). Music interventions for improving psychological and physical outcomes in cancer patients. *Cochrane Database of Systematic Reviews, 2011*(8), CD006911.

Bradt, J., Dileo, C., & Shim, M. (2013). Music interventions for preoperative anxiety. *Cochrane Database of Systematic Reviews, 2013*(6), CD006908.

Bradt, J., Magee, W. L., Dileo, C., Wheeler, B. L., & McGilloway, E. (2010). Music therapy for acquired brain injury. *Cochrane Database of Systematic Reviews, 2010*(7), CD006787.

Branson, J. (2013). Measures of pain management and patient satisfaction as core factors in the development of medical music therapy programming at Norton Healthcare. In J. F. Mondanaro & G. A. Sara (Eds.), *Music and medicine: Integra-*

Medical Music Therapy for Adults

tive models in the treatment of pain (pp. 59–76). New York: Satchnote Press.

Cepeda, M. S., Carr, D. B., Lau, J., & Alvarez, H. (2006). Music for pain relief. *Cochrane Database of Systematic Reviews, 2006*(2), CD004843.

Davis, W. B., & Thaut, M. H. (1989). The influence of preferred relaxing music on measures of state anxiety, relaxation, and physiological responses. *Journal of Music Therapy, 26*(4), 168–187.

Dileo, C. (Ed.). (1999). *Music therapy and medicine: Theoretical and clinical applications.* Silver Spring, MD: American Music Therapy Association.

Dileo, C. (2013). A proposed model for identifying practices: A content analysis of the first 4 years of *Music and Medicine. Music and Medicine, 5*(2), 110–118.

Dileo, C., & Bradt, J. (2005). *Medical music therapy: A meta-analysis and agenda for future research.* Cherry Hill, NJ: Jeffrey Books.

Dileo, C., & Bradt, J. (2009). Medical music therapy: Evidence-based principles and practices. In I. Soderback (Ed.), *International handbook of occupational therapy interventions* (pp. 445–451). Stockholm, Sweden: Springer.

Gallagher, L. M., Huston, M. J., Nelson, K. A., Walsh, D., & Steele, A. L. (2001). Music therapy in palliative medicine. *Support Care Cancer, 9,* 156–161.

Gallagher, L. M., Lagman, R., Walsh, D., Davis, M. P., & LeGrand, S. B. (2006). The clinical effects of music therapy in palliative medicine. *Support Care Cancer, 14,* 859–866.

Gallagher, L. M., & Steele, A. L. (2001). Developing and utilizing a computerized database for music therapy in palliative medicine. *Journal of Palliative Care, 17*(3), 147–154.

Gerwick, J. S., & Tan, X. (2010). Intensive care unit (ICU). In D. Hanson-Abromeit & C. Colwell (Eds.), *Medical music therapy for adults in hospital settings* (pp. 97–160). Silver Spring, MD: American Music Therapy Association.

Hanson-Abromeit, D. (2010). Introduction to adult medical music therapy. In D. Hanson-Abromeit & C. Colwell (Eds.), *Medical music therapy for adults in hospital settings* (pp. 3–17). Silver Spring, MD: American Music Therapy Association.

Maranto, C. (1991). *Applications of music in medi-*

cine. Washington, DC: National Association for Music Therapy.

Mondanaro, J. F., & Sara, G. A. (2013). *Music and medicine: Integrative models in the treatment of pain.* New York: Satchnote Press.

Pinkerton, J. (1996). *The sound of healing: Create your own music program for better health.* St. Louis, MO: MMB Music.

Rider, M. S. (1985). Entrainment mechanisms are involved in pain reduction, muscle relaxation, and music-mediated imagery. *Journal of Music Therapy, 22*(4), 183–192.

Rider, M. (1997). *The rhythmic language of health and disease.* Gilsum, NH: Barcelona.

Sadler, B. L., & Ridenour, A. (2009). *Transforming the healthcare experience through the arts.* San Diego, CA: Aesthetics.

Society for the Arts in Healthcare (SAH). (2011). *What is arts and health?* Retrieved from *http://thesah.org/doc/Definition_FINALNovember2011.pdf.*

Spintge, R., & Droh, R. (1992). *MusicMedicine.* St. Louis, MO: MMB Music.

Standley, J. (1991). Long term benefits of music intervention in the newborn intensive care unit: A pilot study. *Journal of the International Association of Music for the Handicapped, 1*(1), 12–22.

Standley, J., Gregory, D., Whipple, J., Walworth, D., Nguyen, J., Jarred, J., et al. (2005). *Medical music therapy.* Silver Spring, MD: American Music Therapy Association.

Taylor, D. B. (1981). Music in general hospital treatment from 1900 to 1950. *Journal of Music Therapy, 18*(2), 62–73.

Taylor, D. B. (1997). *Biomedical foundations of music as therapy.* St. Louis, MO: MMB Music.

Taylor, D. B. (2010). *Biomedical foundations of music as therapy* (2nd ed.). Eau Claire, WI: Barton.

Thaut, M. H. (2005). *Rhythm, music, and the brain: Scientific foundations and clinical applications.* New York: Routledge.

Weldin, C., & Eagle, C. (1991). An historical overview of music medicine. In C. Maranto (Ed.), *Applications of music in medicine* (pp. 7–27). Washington, DC: National Association for Music Therapy.

Wheeler, B. (2002). Experiences and concerns of students during music therapy practica. *Journal of Music Therapy, 39*(4), 274–304.

CHAPTER 36

Music Therapy for Adults with Traumatic Brain Injury or Other Neurological Disorders

Jeanette Tamplin

Public interest and scientific research into the effects of music on the brain have increased considerably in the last decade. This interest has been fueled by recent advances in brain imaging technology and analysis and by the increasing availability and affordability of such resources for music neuroscience research. These developments continue to build a strong research foundation for music therapy intervention in neurorehabilitation and support the principles of evidence-based practice. Music therapy stimulates neuroplasticity and facilitates the repair of damaged neural processes through bypassing impaired neural connections and linking previously unrelated brain regions, as well as developing new neural pathways. Advances in brain imaging technology can now confirm cortical reorganization and verify structural and functional changes in the brain following intensive music therapy intervention (Rojo et al., 2011; Schlaug et al., 2010).

Publications on the use of music therapy in neurorehabilitation first began to emerge in the late 1980s as case studies and program descriptions. The field has grown significantly since then, as attested by books devoted entirely to this subject (Baker & Tamplin, 2006; Thaut, 2014) and the development of a specialized field of advanced training in Neurologic Music Therapy (NMT). A recent review of NMT interventions suggested that music making is a strong stimulant for neuroplastic changes in the brain and thus holds great potential for use in neurorehabilitation (Altenmüller & Schlaug, 2013).

Clientele

This chapter covers the treatment of people with either acquired (brain injury, spinal injury) or degenerative (Parkinson's disease, Huntington's disease, multiple sclerosis) neurological disorders. A brief description of each disorder is presented in the following section.

Brain injury can cause a wide range of impairments, with the potential to affect movement, speech and language, cognition, and affect. The three main causes of acquired brain injury are traumatic brain injury, stroke, and hypoxia. *Traumatic brain injury* (TBI) is caused by trauma, or an external cause, as distinct from brain injury caused from internal causes such as stroke or hypoxia. A *stroke*, or *cerebrovascular accident* (CVA), occurs when the supply of blood to the brain is suddenly interrupted. The cells in the affected area of the brain then do not receive enough oxygen to function and consequently die or become damaged. *Hypoxia*, or *hypoxic brain damage*, results from oxygen deprivation and may occur following heart attack, near drowning, attempted hanging, or electric shock. The heterogeneity within the brain injury population provides a challenging but stimulating clinical area in which to practice music therapy, but causes significant difficulties for conducting research. Further, traumatic injuries do not affect a representative cross-section of the population; they occur predominantly in young men, with a male to female ratio of 3:1 (Myburgh et al., 2008).

Motor impairments such as hemiplegia or hemiparesis are common following brain injury, as one side of the brain is typically damaged more than the other. Hence, improved physical function is a core goal for most patients in neurorehabilitation. Improvement of gait and upper limb function strongly correlates with functional independence. Cognitive impairments affecting awareness, attention, memory, and learning are also common, particularly for patients with TBI, who typically present with extensive frontal lobe damage due to the direction of impact. Communication impairments may affect speech and/or the ability to use or understand spoken and written language. The *acquired* nature of brain damage (as opposed to congenital brain damage) often causes the sudden imposition of severe and life-changing functional limitations, leading to significant and understandable effects on emotions and coping.

A *spinal cord injury* (SCI) is damage to the spinal cord, impeding the conveying of messages between the brain and muscles. Depending on the severity of injury, complete or partial loss of feeling and muscle control is experienced in the parts of the body below the injury level. Approximately half of SCIs occur at the cervical level (neck), resulting in reduction or loss of motor and/or sensory function in the arms, trunk, legs, and pelvic organs. This type of impairment is referred to as *quadriplegia* or *tetraplegia*.

Parkinson's disease involves progressive loss of dopaminergic neurons. Major symptoms are bradykinesia (slow movements), rigidity, resting limb tremor, shuffling gait, and gait instability. Other non-motor-related symptoms include cognitive difficulties, bowel and bladder problems, sexual dysfunction, depression, pain, and swallowing difficulties.

Huntington's disease is a genetic disorder that affects muscle coordination and leads to cognitive decline and emotional disorders. It is characterized by involuntary movements and abnormal voluntary movements (chorea) of any part of the body. This effect on the muscles can also affect speech, causing dysarthria, dysrhythmic bursts of speech, and difficulty initiating speech. Cognitive symptoms may include memory problems and difficulty with problem solving, initiation, and concentration.

Multiple sclerosis is an inflammatory disease in which the fatty myelin sheaths around the axons of the brain and spinal cord are damaged, causing demyelination and subsequent slowing of nerve impulses as they travel along axons. It commonly has a relapsing–remitting clinical course and occurs predominantly in females. Clinical symptoms can include gait disorder, spasticity, limb ataxia and weakness, impaired coordination, cognitive impairment, pain, bowel and bladder problems, and vision disturbances.

For each of the populations covered in this chapter, in addition to the numerous physical symptoms affecting functional independence, there is also much uncertainty about the future in terms of disease progression or potential for rehabilitation progress. This uncertainty produces a number of psychosocial concerns. Grief is commonly associated with the loss of physical functions and social roles, and anger at the unfairness of the situation is also frequently experienced. It is important to address emotional and adjustment-related issues during the rehabilitation process, as patients consumed by anger, anxiety, disbelief, or grief may be unable to participate in rehabilitation to their maximum potential, thus negatively affecting their functional outcomes.

Clinical Work

The efficacy of music therapy in neurorehabilitation stems from music's unique effect on behavior, brain function, motivation, and emotion regulation. The use of specifically composed songs as memory aids, and relearning to speak using the alternative neural processes involved in singing, are two clear examples of this effect. Music also offers a motivating medium for practicing repetitive tasks. This motivating quality can be used therapeutically to stimulate the repetitive physical movements required in neurorehabilitation, both to improve muscle strength and endurance and to stimulate neuroplasticity. As physical rehabilitation tasks are often difficult, tiring, and/or painful, the repetitive and predictable nature of music can provide valuable structure and motivation for neurorehabilitation training.

Music can be effective in the facilitation of muscle relaxation, which is important, as tense muscles may inhibit speech and physi-

cal movement. The music not only relaxes the patient but also acts as a distracter and encourages focus on something other than the cause of agitation. Similarly, music can be used in pain management, either as a distraction from pain or a means for regaining control over the rehabilitation experience. Breathing techniques and strategies for incorporating music in relaxation can enable patients to reframe perceptions or alter focus during painful rehabilitation experiences. The opportunity for control in music therapy is particularly significant for this population, for whom control has been removed in so many other areas of life, and may take the form of choosing songs to listen to or sing, choosing music activities, choosing an instrument to play, or simply choosing to participate.

The body of clinical research investigating music therapy treatment efficacy in neurorehabilitation is slowly but steadily growing. A recent Cochrane review of music therapy for acquired brain injury reported evidence (from two randomized, controlled trials) to indicate that rhythmic auditory stimulation (RAS) may improve gait parameters for stroke patients (Bradt, Magee, Dileo, Wheeler, & McGilloway, 2010). Other positive outcomes were only supported by single studies and thus need further research to confirm the findings. These positive results included improved upper extremity function using RAS, improved speech parameters for people with aphasia, and decreased agitation and increased orientation following listening to familiar music for people with posttraumatic amnesia.

Due to the potential for widespread impairment of function following neurological damage, a considerable array of effective music therapy techniques has been reported for this population. In general, active techniques predominate, given the need for active participation from the patient to stimulate neuroplasticity and practice of functional skills. Receptive music therapy techniques, such as song-based discussion or music-assisted relaxation, are more commonly used to address psychosocial goals. In degenerative neurological conditions, receptive techniques grow more appropriate as the disease progresses and voluntary movement becomes too difficult or painful (Steele, 2005).

The following section is divided according to area of neurorehabilitation focus: physical, speech and language, cognitive, and emotional. A brief literature review of music therapy techniques used in each area with various neurological populations is included. Composite case examples are provided to illustrate the application of a range of interventions.

Music Therapy in Physical Rehabilitation

There are a number of reasons that music-supported training approaches are beneficial in physical rehabilitation: (1) rhythm is a fundamental requirement for movement coordination; (2) music can elicit unconscious physiological responses (e.g., foot tapping); (3) the motivating qualities of music can increase level of engagement and extend participation length by energizing a patient for physically demanding exercise; (4) using music for physical exercise decreases perceived exertion; and (5) playing an instrument involves not only visual feedback, but also kinesthetic and aural feedback.

A recent systematic review of the effectiveness of music therapy in physical rehabilitation (Weller & Baker, 2011) found consistent positive and significant results for the rehabilitation of most gait parameters as well as fine and gross motor functioning. There are three main categories of music therapy intervention used in physical rehabilitation: (1) Rhythmic Auditory Stimulation, (2) playing musical instruments, and (3) movement to music. The role of the music therapist in physical rehabilitation is to assess level of function; engage patients in appropriate therapeutic musical activi-

ties; adapt interventions according to level of function; and provide musical stimulation, physical support, and verbal feedback.

A large body of research has demonstrated motor system arousal following the neural processing of auditory stimuli. This phenomenon results in an entrainment effect when walking or moving to auditory rhythm, where the internal rhythms of movement patterns synchronize with the external rhythms of the music. In addition, rhythmic music helps with movement timing. These effects have been applied therapeutically in RAS, where rhythm is used as an external timekeeper to organize and sequence complex movement. Application of RAS in rehabilitation has been demonstrated to improve motor function for patients with stroke (Thaut, McIntosh, Prassas, & Rice, 1993), TBI (Hurt, Rice, McIntosh, & Thaut, 1998), and Parkinson's disease (Thaut, McIntosh, McIntosh, & Hoemberg, 2001). Improvements have been found in gait parameters of velocity, cadence, stride length, and symmetry, as well as upper limb movement optimization. The role of the music in auditory stimulation is to act as "an anticipatory and continuous time reference for movements . . . and increase effect of rhythmic entrainment" (Weller & Baker, 2011, p. 52).

CLINICAL EXAMPLE: RAS for Gait Rehabilitation (Stroke)

Sarah, a 24-year-old woman, sustained a stroke and spent 7 months in rehabilitation to address her apraxic and dysarthric speech, hemiplegia, and high-level cognitive processing difficulties. RAS was used in music therapy to address her ataxic gait. In music therapy assessment, the introduction of musical pulse when walking (prior to any training with music) immediately made the timing of Sarah's steps more even. A program of gait training was commenced using live, beat-focused guitar strumming with a metronome pulse as the rhythmic stimulus. Initially, the tempo of the music was set at Sarah's comfortable walking pace (44 steps/minute). Tempo was gradually increased in 10% increments over the course of each session, and finally music was withdrawn at the end of each session. Assessments were conducted without music to determine carryover of these improvements. Sarah's physiotherapist was present in the sessions to provide physical assistance and verbal coaching to Sarah while she walked.

After only a few weeks of RAS training, Sarah's balance and walking speed had improved (66 steps/minute). This increase was accomplished primarily through improving gait speed and evenness, using music to cue step rate. At the completion of her program, Sarah had increased her gait velocity to 80 steps/minute and progressed from a four-wheeled frame to independent ambulation. Although this walking speed was still much slower than the average walking pace for women (117 steps/minute), it represented a considerable improvement and movement toward a more normal and functional gait.

Instrument playing to rehabilitate physical function has long been employed in music therapy. More recently this technique has been labeled as an NMT technique, *therapeutic instrumental music performance* (TIMP; Thaut, 2005). Randomized, controlled trials with stroke survivors (Schneider, Schonle, Altenmüller, & Munte, 2007) and those with Parkinson's disease (Pacchetti et al., 2000) found significant improvements in upper limb function following active music making. Therapeutic goals applicable to this technique include improving functional movement patterns; increasing bilateral coordination; and improving movement planning, execution, and sequencing. Depending on the movement to be targeted, different activities can be designed or applied. Patients receive immediate aural feedback if the movement has been performed correctly, acting as positive reinforcement for correct movement patterns.

Rhythmic and melodic patterns can help specific movement sequences be encoded in a type of memory in the nervous system called *motor memory* or *procedural memory*.

An example of motor memory is the ability of a pianist to play, sequentially and simultaneously, many notes in a few seconds without having to remember every individual note. On a simpler level, a patient can practice and eventually remember longer and more difficult sequences of movement, for example, combining the movement of different fingers or using the hands and arms in a coordinated way.

The therapeutic application of instrument playing in physical rehabilitation is really limited only by the imagination and creativity of the therapist. Instruments can be adapted and positioned in a way to maximize therapeutic value when playing. These adaptations may include enhancing the range of traditional playing motion, positioning the instrument in a planned manner, adding weights or padding, or attaching instruments to body parts. For example, a seated patient may be instructed to lift his or her foot in time with rhythmic music to contact a tambourine or drum positioned at knee height to improve the swing phase of the gait cycle. Weights might be attached to maracas to increase forearm strength and force during pronation–supination movements. Instrument playing activities should be designed to utilize a patient's current full range of movement and then extend this range. For example, the therapist could hold a drum at different positions, encouraging the patient to use shoulder, elbow, wrist, and/or waist movement, depending on the therapeutic goals. Directing the patient to play in time with the music can target the mobility and agility with which movements are performed. The speed of the music can then be increased or decreased, and the patient encouraged to play in time with the music. To increase fine motor control and motor planning, stickers can be placed on instruments as targets to aim for, in time with rhythmic music.

Rhythmic patterns in music facilitate a sense of structure and provide timing and anticipatory cues for movement sequencing and planning. These benefits are particularly relevant for patients with Parkinson's disease, as the rhythmic patterns in music can act as a sensory sequencer to bypass neural areas damaged by the disease. The rhythm thus provides movement command signals to overcome bradykinesia (slowness) and episodes of freezing (Thaut et al., 2001). The patient can be encouraged to sing along with the therapist while exercising or playing, if appropriate. In addition to the emotional benefits, singing provides an internal pace, helps the patient to maintain an upright posture, and assists efficient breathing.

CLINICAL EXAMPLE: Playing Instruments to Address Trunk Control (TBI)

Mark, a 35-year-old male, sustained a severe TBI in a motor vehicle accident. As is common following TBI, he presented with multiple areas of impaired function in speech, cognition, and movement. In addition to a mild hemiplegia, Mark exhibited decreased trunk control and difficulties with active balance. In music therapy, seated drumming activities (TIMP) were introduced to address these difficulties. During initial music therapy assessment, Mark was unable to achieve independent sitting balance. If his wheelchair armrests were removed and he tried to lean forward even slightly, he would lose his balance and fall forward or sideways. Initially when a drum was placed between Mark's legs to redevelop basic trunk muscle control and static balance, he was only able to play in this position for 5-second bursts. When playing with appropriately paced, preferred, rhythmic music, Mark became able to sit independently and play for increasing periods of time before tiring. After 8 weeks, his endurance had increased to the point where he could play for an entire song (2–3 minutes). Gradually, the drum was moved further away to challenge his active balance and further strengthen his trunk muscles, and later, additional drums were added to encourage his reach in different directions (side to side, or in front and behind). These improvements

made in music therapy transferred to other functional tasks, such as reaching to pick up a newspaper independently.

The use of music or musical elements to stimulate physical movement is another music therapy technique used in neurological rehabilitation. The NMT term for this technique is *patterned sensory enhancement* (PSE), and it is described as the translation of musical elements to match spatial, temporal, and force components of movement (Thaut, 2005). Rhythm and tempo can be used to drive the speed and timing of movement patterns, and spatial or directional cues may include ascending and descending melodic lines to indicate upward or downward movement. Dynamic changes and use of dissonance and harmony can cue the strength of muscle activation and contraction. Although PSE may improve the execution of movements, there is currently limited evidence that PSE increases exercise output (Clark, Baker, & Tayor, 2012).

Physical rehabilitation often involves painful procedures or interventions. Music therapy interventions can assist in calming the patient or distracting him or her from the pain, so that these interventions can be completed successfully. A patient with cognitive impairments may have difficulty understanding the need for these painful procedures, which can compound anxiety and/or resistance to therapy.

CLINICAL EXAMPLE: Active Music Participation as a Distraction from Pain (TBI)

David had sustained a severe TBI following a motor vehicle accident at the age of 19. The neurological sequelae following his injury were extensive, including hemiparesis, muscle spasticity and contractures, poor insight, impulsivity, and disinhibition. The increased muscle tone in his legs made stretching them out very painful. His poor insight meant that he had limited understanding of the need to stretch his legs in physical therapy, even though he wanted to walk again. The pain seemed to override everything, and his physical therapy program was eventually suspended due to his lack of cooperation and physical and verbal outbursts.

David was extremely motivated by music that he enjoyed. A combined music therapy–physical therapy program was introduced, in which David participated in singing and songwriting while undergoing physical stretches and standing in a tilt table. Music was an effective distraction, and his endurance for standing in the tilt table increased from 5 minutes to 40 minutes almost immediately when focusing on music therapy activities.

The use of music therapy techniques in physical rehabilitation is thus particularly effective due to the combined effect of rhythm on priming the motor system and the positive effects of music on motivation and the emotional centers in the brain.

Music Therapy in Speech and Language Rehabilitation

Music therapy has an important role in the neurological rehabilitation of speech and language impairments (Hurkmans et al., 2012). Research has demonstrated improvements in verbal intelligibility, word and phrase production, fundamental frequency variability (pitch range), rate of speech, vocal intensity (voice volume), speech naturalness, and reduction in pause time following music therapy intervention (Baker, 2000; Haneishi, 2001; Tamplin, 2008; Tamplin et al., 2013; Tomaino, 2012). Singing familiar song lyrics may elicit a priming effect on word retrieval, and rhythmic speech–motor entrainment may assist patients with verbal fluency disorders.

Singing shares many of the motor mechanisms used during speech, such as the use of respiratory muscles and the articulators. Other common elements shared by speech and singing include rhythm, pitch, dynamics, tempo, and diction. Therapeutic singing exercises use these musical elements in neurological rehabilitation to redevelop speech and language skills. Recent neuroimaging research has demonstrated shared neural pathways for the processing of speech and singing (Ozdemir, Norton, & Schlaug, 2006). This bihemispheric activation during musical processing (in comparison to left-hemisphere lateralization for language processing) may be the key to understanding why some patients with left frontal lesions can sing but not speak the lyrics of songs.

Melodic Intonation Therapy (MIT) utilizes this phenomenon in therapy to help people with aphasia (the loss of ability to produce and/or comprehend language, resulting from neurological damage) to learn to speak again. Simple phrases are translated into sung (intoned) patterns, exaggerating the normal accents and melodic content of speech. Higher pitch is used on syllables that would naturally be stressed during speech. While singing, each syllable is tapped out rhythmically using the patient's left hand. Three treatment levels increase incrementally in difficulty by extending phrase lengths and reducing the amount of support provided by the therapist. Hand-tapping assistance is provided at each step in traditional MIT:

1. Humming the phrase
2. Unison intoning (therapist and patient)
3. Unison intoning with fading (therapist fades out singing but continues tapping)
4. Immediately repeating the phrase (therapist models and patient repeats)
5. Responding to a probe question (immediately after the fourth step, therapist intones a question, for example, "What did you say?" (Norton, Zipse, Marchina, & Schlaug, 2009)

Many variations of this model have been used. Some use only two or three pitches, whereas some use many more pitches and write a different tune for each phrase (Baker, 2000). The goal in all applications of MIT is to use the inherent melody in speech to facilitate increased initiation and verbal fluency. Results of brain-imaging studies have suggested that singing, with concurrent tapping with the left hand, primes the sensorimotor and premotor cortices for articulation (Schlaug et al., 2010). MIT holds unique potential to engage both hemispheres of the brain through the simultaneous use of rhythm and melody. Rhythm is a fundamental component of speech production and perception; disruption of speech rhythm impairs speech perception. Singing provides the rhythmic and melodic cues for patients to organize their speech production and can subsequently be used to improve intelligibility and naturalness (Tamplin, 2008). Auditory rhythm has also been shown to enhance control for motor speech in patients with Parkinson's disease (Thaut et al., 2001).

Other music-based speech therapy techniques for patients with nonfluent aphasia have also been published recently (Tomaino, 2012). These include singing familiar songs, breathing into single-syllable sounds, musically assisted speech, dynamically cued singing, rhythmic speech cuing, oral motor exercises, and vocal intonation. The effectiveness of these techniques relies closely on the manipulation of tempo and rhythm to match and enhance the patient's verbal capability in terms of word retrieval, prosody, and articulation. In addition, the role of interplay between the patient and music therapist is important as it can "approximate a conversational exchange by allowing for pauses, or exaggerating dynamics, or melodic contour to convey meaning and facilitate expectation" (Tomaino, 2012, p. 316).

CLINICAL EXAMPLE: Singing to Improve Speech Intelligibility and Naturalness (Stroke)

Mary, a 51-year-old woman, presented with severe global dysarthria resulting from a stroke 2½ months prior to participation in music therapy. Dysarthria is a motor speech disorder resulting from neurological damage that causes disturbances in control of the muscles used for speech. It is often characterized by decreased verbal intelligibility, reduced vocal intensity or range, abnormal rate of speech and prosody, and the consequent impairment in speech naturalness. Mary's daughter described her speech as slower and more slurred after her stroke.

Mary attended 24 individual music therapy sessions over 8 weeks. This program consisted of oral motor respiratory exercises, rhythmic and melodic articulation exercises, rhythmic speech cuing, vocal intonation therapy, and therapeutic singing using familiar songs (see Tamplin & Grocke, 2008, for a detailed description of the music therapy protocol used). Standardized assessments of intelligibility were used, together with waveform analysis of pause time, to evaluate Mary's progress. On initial assessment, Mary achieved an intelligibility score of 82%, and her rate of speech was 51 intelligible words per minute. After 8 weeks of therapy, her intelligibility had increased to 93%, and her rate of speech was 70 intelligible words per minute (normal rate of speech is 190 words per minute). In addition, waveform analysis of Mary's speech revealed changes in speech rhythm and inflection between pre- and postassessments. Figure 36.1 shows waveforms of Mary's speech when reading a sentence prior to and after music therapy intervention. The top waveforms in gray (representing left and right audio channels) were recorded preintervention. There is a visibly regular rhythm where the words are evenly spaced, unlike the rhythm of natural speech. The bottom waveforms in white (postintervention) have more rhythmic variation and increased inflection and stress, demonstrated by the sections of increased amplitude on the waveforms. In addition, the inappropriate pauses and slower rate of speech visible in the top waveforms are not present in the bottom waveforms. The total length of pause time for this sentence decreased by 3.3 seconds.

The pauses initially present in Mary's speech may have occurred due to poor breath control, to assist the separation of words, and/or to improve articulatory clarity and intelligibility. However, they resulted

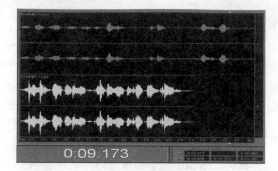

FIGURE 36.1. Spectrograph image of a sentence spoken by Mary before (top) and after (bottom) music therapy intervention: "He has made me feel that I am no different from before."

in stilted, robotic-sounding speech rhythms. Her decrease in the use of pauses in the postassessment and the use of more semantically appropriate placement of pauses suggest improvements in articulatory precision and better use of rhythm and stress to provide contextual cues for meaning. Following music therapy treatment, Mary's daughter described her mother's speech as "clearer now, with less slurring and better word formation . . . [it's] less gravelly, smoother."

Research has been conducted on the use of music therapy (in particular, oral motor and respiratory exercises and singing) to improve respiratory muscle strength for people with multiple sclerosis (Wiens, Reimer, & Guyn, 1999) and spinal cord injury (Tamplin et al., 2013). Respiratory muscle weakness is characteristic of both populations, often resulting in difficulty in clearing secretions and repeated episodes of pneumonia. Although improvements in respiratory function were not statistically significant in these studies, the sample sizes were small, and trends toward an intervention effect were indicated for both. Significant improvements in voice projection and mood were achieved in the study examining the therapeutic effects of singing for people with quadriplegia (Tamplin et al., 2013).

CLINICAL EXAMPLE: Singing to Improve Respiratory Function (SCI)

Peter sustained a fracture of the vertebral column with complete spinal cord injury at the cervical level (C6A) during a BMX bicycle accident. Ten years later, Peter participated in a therapeutic singing group practicing oral motor and respiratory exercises and therapeutic singing to improve his respiratory function and voice projection. The exercises included sustained voiced and unvoiced exhalations, tongue and lip trills, and pulsed rhythmic vocalizations, as well as gradual and sudden changes in pitch and intensity. A primary focus of the group was the incorporation of respiratory strategies for voice projection and endurance while singing familiar songs.

Peter attended this group three times a week for 12 weeks and also practiced at home with a practice CD and workbook. He made considerable improvements in both respiratory function and voice. Changes from pre- to postassessment indicated an increase in vital capacity (maximum amount of air a person can expel from the lungs after a maximum inhalation) of almost half a liter (2.33–2.71 liters), a 25% increase in maximum expiratory pressure (from 86 to 108 cm/H_2O), and a 12% increase in maximum inspiratory pressure (from 80 to 90 cm/H_2O). The sound pressure level of Peter's projected voice increased from 74 to 78 decibels, and his length of maximum sustained phonation increased by 12 seconds (from 7 to 19 seconds).

As can be seen, music can facilitate speech and language rehabilitation through a number of mechanisms: through strong timing mechanisms to entrain oscillatory circuits in the speech centers of the brain, rhythmic speech–motor entrainment to facilitate greater verbal fluency and rate control, a priming effect on word retrieval elicited by familiar song lyrics, and improvement of respiratory function. Further, in aphasia rehabilitation, singing can be used to stimulate neuroplasticity by activating undamaged parts of the left-hemisphere language network, language-capable regions in the right hemisphere, or a combination of both.

Music Therapy in Cognitive Rehabilitation

Music can be very useful in cognitive retraining activities. In particular, the efficacy of music as a mnemonic device has been well documented through research (e.g., Thaut, Peterson, & McIntosh, 2005). The rhythm in music provides a temporal ordering process that facilitates rhythmic attention control. In addition, rhythm and melody provide clear structures within which to organize, sequence, *chunk*, and recall verbal information. Daily music listening has been demonstrated to significantly improve focused attention and verbal memory for stroke survivors (Särkämö et al., 2008). In addition, translational research has found a strong effect for musical mnemonics on verbal learning both for healthy subjects and for patients with multiple sclerosis (Thaut et al., 2005). This effect has been demonstrated through increased synchronization of brainwave rhythms (measured on an electroencephalogram [EEG]), indicating music-induced neural plasticity. Information can be set to music and then rehearsed until it is encoded in memory. Musical cues can then prompt retrieval of this information until it is spontaneously recalled. Songs can be written to facilitate initiation, sequencing, and motor planning in activities of daily living (e.g., showering, dressing, cooking) or learning instructions (e.g., how to operate a remote control), directions (e.g., find directions from therapy office to ward), or lists of information (e.g., names of therapy team or family members, phone number, address). Short-term memory assessment can involve singing a song, then asking the patient questions regarding facts that were presented in the song lyrics, thus providing an indication of short-term memory difficulties. If the patient has trouble with this task, multiple-choice questions can provide aural cues to assist him or her in answering the questions.

Attention is a foundational skill necessary for all other cognitive and physical tasks. Attention can be addressed in music by modifying the length or difficulty of an activity. For example, the introduction of competing stimuli in a musical activity may challenge a person's capacity for sustained or divided attention. Improvisation can be useful in assessment of cognitive impairments. The improvised musical responses of patients with severe brain injury may initially be fragmentary, reflexive, perseverative, and/or stereotypical (e.g., repetitively playing five notes consecutively with one hand or playing all the notes on the piano in order, then stopping). These cognitive difficulties can sometimes be overcome by providing more structure and direction to improvisations—as, for example, playing question and answer phrases or playing only on the black notes. By encouraging creativity and engagement, the length of participation and concentration may also be increased.

The effect of therapeutic music techniques on executive function has received minimal research attention to date. Thaut et al. (2009) found significant increases in executive function in the form of mental flexibility following a single session of music therapy. These effects suggest that music provides an enriched environment for the brain and that "the inherent temporal structure in music and musical tasks provides strong self-regulatory and self-organizational constraints that cue and exercise reasoning, decision making, problem solving and comprehension processes in real time" (p. 413). They also posit that, similar to the entrainment effects of rhythm on motor control, music may help regulate the mechanisms of cognitive timing and mental flexibility, thus improving brain *agility*.

In summary, music therapy can be an effective tool in cognitive rehabilitation by using music to provide an enriched sensory environment for the brain and supply rhythmic timing cues and musical patterns that stimulate attention. The temporal and structural cues inherent in music can also be used therapeutically to assist memory formation, verbal learning, and executive function.

Music Therapy and Emotional Adjustment

Several music therapy methods are used in neurorehabilitation to address emotional needs and facilitate a greater sense of well-being (Nayak, Wheeler, Shiflett, & Agostinelli, 2000). These methods include music listening, improvisation, songwriting, and song discussion. Music is strongly connected to emotions and mood states and is a culturally appropriate way to express emotions. Writing a song, singing, or playing music may also represent a nonconfrontational way to express emotions.

In empirical studies, group therapeutic singing (Thaut et al., 2009) and self-directed music listening (Särkämö et al., 2008) have been demonstrated to significantly improve mood for TBI and stroke survivors, respectively. Särkämö et al. suggest that music has an *analgesic effect* in reducing anxiety and diverting attention from negative experiences, which can assist patients who have neurological difficulties to cope better with emotional stress. Emotional adjustment following severe trauma or debilitating illness can have a significant impact on rehabilitation outcomes. A patient needs to grieve the loss of future plans, the loss of confidence, and the perceived loss of status or authority. If the process of emotional adjustment becomes blocked and the patient is consumed by emotions such as anger, sadness, guilt, or denial, motivation is likely to decrease considerably, thereby negatively impacting the patient's participation in therapy and his or her rehabilitation outcomes.

Enjoyable and rewarding musical experiences can help promote relaxation, alleviate anxiety, and provide uplifting experiences. Musical improvisation can be cathartic and may provide an accessible emotional outlet for patients with severe communication problems, who may not be able to express their feelings verbally. Depending on the individual patient and the extent of the neurological damage, improvisation can serve as an outlet for expression. However, the abstract nature of improvisation makes it less effective for many patients with cognitive impairments, because they are unable to connect the music they create with the expression of their own feelings. In addition, physical impairments may limit patients' access to traditional forms of music making in this population.

For patients with intact communication skills, songwriting and song discussion are effective ways of working through emotional difficulties in music therapy. Patients can be supported by the music therapist to express how they feel and then organize these ideas into a song. Depending on the lyrical content, such songs can then serve to vent difficult emotions, act as a self-motivator, or communicate messages to others. A lyric analysis of 82 songs written in music therapy revealed that patients with TBI undergoing rehabilitation most commonly used songwriting for self-reflection and to communicate messages to loved ones. Other song themes included memories, reflections about significant others, expressions of adversity, and concern for the future (Baker, Kennelly, & Tamplin, 2005).

Music-assisted counseling can help the patient to work through issues of grief, pain, anger, and despair. Similarly, song discussion can be used to encourage the patient to identify with ideas presented in the lyrics and then discuss how these may be similar or different from their own feelings or situation. The beneficial effect of music therapy on mood also has positive implications for its use to improve social interaction, motivation for rehabilitation, and participation in therapy (Nayak et al., 2000).

Applications to Other Disciplines

The use of live music presented by a music therapist in a controlled clinical setting allows the music to be modified in the moment to match and drive patient behavior and thus maximize therapeutic effect. However, it may be possible for other therapists or nursing staff to utilize some of the potential therapeutic benefits of recorded music when informed about the indications and contraindications of using music with patients who have neurological disorders.

The blanket use of music in an attempt to improve care environments or enhance patient happiness should be cautioned against, though. Music is a powerful tool and can elicit a wide range of emotional responses. As such, the choice of music to be used in patient care must be considered carefully. In addition, the indiscriminate use of music can lead to sensory overload for patients with cognitive impairments, resulting in decreased cognitive performance or increased behavioral agitation. Therefore, the planned and considered selection of music is even more critical when working with people who have cognitive impairments secondary to neurological damage.

The potential for therapeutic benefit from music listening is closely linked to the characteristics of the music used. The distinction between patient-preferred versus therapist-selected music needs to be highlighted, and the qualities of the music itself must be taken into account when selecting music for this population. Bearing these requirements for music selection in mind, the music therapist can act as a consultant and *prescribe* recorded music based on therapeutic goals and patient preferences. For example, a selection of patient-preferred music with sedative or calming qualities (characterized by a slow tempo, with no abrupt changes or sharp timbres) might be collated with the aim of decreasing anxiety or promoting relaxation and sleep. These features of music can be particularly beneficial for patients with posttraumatic amnesia. These playlists could then be utilized by nursing staff when patients are agitated and a music therapist is unavailable.

Conversely, a music therapist can assess patients and collate individualized playlists of patient-preferred music with motivating or stimulating attributes (fast tempo; strong pulse/beat; and variation in pitch, instrumentation, and melody) that can then be used in physical therapy or at home with a physical exercise program to help increase physical activity levels. This education and facilitation can provide patients with a strategy for how to employ music therapeutically in their own rehabilitation. A music therapist can also assist patients in creating playlists at their current walking tempo, as well as modified versions of this playlist at incrementing tempos, to assist gait rehabilitation. Again, such playlists could be utilized by physical therapists in exercise sessions or used independently by the patient.

Interdisciplinary work is common for music therapists working in neurorehabilitation. Music therapists often work collaboratively with speech and language therapists to address communication disorders, and with physical therapists or occupational therapists when working on physical function and gait rehabilitation. Similarly, when addressing cognitive or emotional needs, music therapists will liaise closely with relevant members of the interdisciplinary team. For example, songs written as memory aids are usually recorded so that other staff can use them to prompt the patient's recall of information. The recorded version of a song written to cue the steps in a showering or dressing routine might be used with the patient by occupational therapists or nursing staff. Further, a song written by a patient in music therapy that expresses emotions and coping mechanisms might be used as a springboard for discussion in psychology or neuropsychology sessions.

Conclusions

There is a growing body of neuroimaging research and clinical studies examining the therapeutic use of music in neurorehabilitation. This research has demonstrated convincing evidence that music is able to stimulate changes in brain function that can be generalized to nonmusical, functional outcomes. This potential for music to be used therapeutically to influence nonmusical behavior has secured a future for music therapy in the neurosciences.

The temporal and structural cues in music can prime the motor system and entrain physical movement, stimulate attention, and assist memory formation. The melodic qualities of music engage the right hemisphere and can be used in speech and language redevelopment, memory retraining strategies, and emotional expression through therapeutic singing and songwriting.

Most people enjoy music participation, and therefore patients do not generally perceive involvement in music therapy as onerous. The motivational qualities of music can be harnessed in music therapy to promote greater participation in all therapies. Further, evidence for bihemispheric activation, stimulation of neuroplasticity, and the positive functional outcomes achieved indicate that music therapy can be as effective, if not more effective, than traditional therapies used in neurorehabilitation.

REFERENCES

Altenmüller, E., & Schlaug, G. (2013). Neurologic music therapy: The beneficial effects of music making on neurorehabilitation. *Acoustical Science and Technology, 34*(1), 5–12.

Baker, F. (2000). Modifying the melodic intonation therapy program for adults with severe non-fluent aphasia. *Music Therapy Perspectives, 18*, 110–114.

Baker, F., Kennelly, J., & Tamplin, J. (2005). Adjusting to change through song: Themes in songs written by clients with traumatic brain injury. *Brain Impairment, 6*(3), 205–211.

Baker, F., & Tamplin, J. (2006). *Music therapy methods in neurorehabilitation: A clinician's manual.* London: Jessica Kingsley.

Bradt, J., Magee, W. L., Dileo, C., Wheeler, B. L., & McGilloway, E. (2010). Music therapy for ac-quired brain injury. *Cochrane Database of Systematic Reviews,* (7), CD006787.

Clark, I., Baker, F., & Tayor, N. F. (2012). The effects of live patterned sensory enhancement on group exercise participation and mood in older adults in rehabilitation. *Journal of Music Therapy, 49*(2), 180–204.

Haneishi, E. (2001). Effects of a music therapy voice protocol on speech intelligibility, vocal acoustic measures, and mood of individuals with parkinson's disease. *Journal of Music Therapy, 38*(4), 273–290.

Hurkmans, J., de Bruijn, M., Boonstra, A. M., Jonkers, R., Bastiaanse, R., Arendzen, H., et al. (2012). Music in the treatment of neurological language and speech disorders: A systematic review. *Aphasiology, 26*(1), 1–19.

Hurt, C. P., Rice, R. R., McIntosh, G. C., & Thaut, M. H. (1998). Rhythmic auditory stimulation in gait training for patients with traumatic brain injury. *Journal of Music Therapy, 35*, 228–291.

Myburgh, J. A., Cooper, D. J., Finfer, S. R., Venkatesh, B., Jones, D., Higgins, A., et al. (2008). Epidemiology and 12-month outcomes from traumatic brain injury in Australia and New Zealand. *Journal of Trauma-Injury Infection and Critical Care, 64*(4), 854–862.

Nayak, S., Wheeler, B. L., Shiflett, S. C., & Agostinelli, S. (2000). Effect of music therapy on mood and social interaction among individuals with acute traumatic brain injury and stroke. *Rehabilitation Psychology, 45*(3), 274–283.

Norton, A., Zipse, L., Marchina, S., & Schlaug, G. (2009). Melodic intonation therapy: Shared insights on how it is done and why it might help. *Annals of the New York Academy of Sciences, 1169*(1), 431–436.

Ozdemir, E., Norton, A., & Schlaug, G. (2006). Shared and distinct neural correlates of singing and speaking. *NeuroImage, 33*, 628–635.

Pacchetti, C., Mancini, F., Aglieri, R., Fundaro, C., Martignoni, E., & Nappi, G. (2000). Active music therapy in Parkinson's disease: An integrative method for motor and emotional rehabilitation. *Psychosomatic Medicine, 62*(3), 386–393.

Rojo, N., Amengual, J. L., Juncadella, M., Rubio, F., Camara, E., Marco-Pallares, J., et al. (2011). Music-Supported Therapy induces plasticity in the sensorimotor cortex in chronic stroke: A single-case study using multimodal imaging (fMRI-TMS). *Brain Injury, 25*(7–8), 787–793.

Särkämö, T., Tervaniemi, M., Laitinen, S., Forsblom, A., Soinila, S., Mikkonen, M., et al. (2008). Music listening enhances cognitive recovery and mood after middle cerebral artery stroke. *Brain, 131*(3), 866–876.

Schlaug, G., Norton, A., Marchina, S., Zipse, L., & Wan, C. Y. (2010). From singing to speaking: Facilitating recovery from nonfluent aphasia. *Future Neurology, 5*(5), 657–665.

Schneider, S., Schonle, P. W., Altenmüller, E., & Munte, T. F. (2007). Using musical instruments to improve motor skill recovery following a stroke. *Journal of Neurology, 254*(10), 1339–1346.

Steele, M. (2005). Coping with multiple sclerosis: A music therapy viewpoint. *Australian Journal of Music Therapy, 16*, 70–87.

Tamplin, J. (2008). A pilot study into the effect of vocal exercises and singing on dysarthric speech. *NeuroRehabilitation, 23*(3), 207–216.

Tamplin, J., Baker, F., Grocke, D., Brazzale, D., Pretto, J. J., Ruehland, W. R., et al. (2013). The effect of singing on respiratory function, voice, and mood following quadriplegia: A randomized controlled trial. *Archives of Physical Medicine and Rehabilitation, 94*(3), 426–434.

Tamplin, J., & Grocke, D. (2008). A music therapy treatment protocol for acquired dysarthria rehabilitation. *Music Therapy Perspectives, 26*, 23–30.

Thaut, M. H. (2005). *Rhythm, music and the brain.* New York: Routledge.

Thaut, M. H., Gardiner, J. C., Holmberg, D., Horwitz, J., Kent, L., Andrews, G., et al. (2009). Neurologic music therapy improves executive function and emotional adjustment in traumatic brain injury rehabilitation. *Annals of the New York Academy of Sciences, 1169*, 406–416.

Thaut, M. H., & Hoemberg, V. (2014). *Handbook of neurologic music therapy.* Oxford, UK: Oxford University Press.

Thaut, M. H., McIntosh, K. W., McIntosh, G. C., & Hoemberg, V. (2001). Auditory rhythmicity enhances movement and speech motor control in patients with Parkinson's disease. *Functional Neurology, 16*(2), 163–172.

Thaut, M. H., McIntosh, G. C., Prassas, S. G., & Rice, R. R. (1993). Effect of rhythmic auditory cuing on temporal stride parameters and EMG patterns in hemiparetic gait of stroke patients. *Journal of Neurological Rehabilitation, 7*, 9–16.

Thaut, M. H., Peterson, D. A., & McIntosh, G. C. (2005). Temporal entrainment of cognitive functions: Musical mnemonics induce brain plasticity and oscillatory synchrony in neural networks underlying memory. *Annals of the New York Academy of Sciences, 1060*, 243–254.

Tomaino, C. M. (2012). Effective music therapy techniques in the treatment of nonfluent aphasia. *Annals of the New York Academy of Sciences, 1252*(1), 312–317.

Weller, C. M., & Baker, F. A. (2011). The role of music therapy in physical rehabilitation: A systematic literature review. *Nordic Journal of Music Therapy, 20*(1), 43–61.

Wiens, M. E., Reimer, M. A., & Guyn, H. L. (1999). Music therapy as a treatment method for improving respiratory muscle strength in patients with advanced multiple sclerosis: A pilot study. *Rehabilitation Nursing, 24*(2), 74–80.

CHAPTER 37

Music Therapy at the End of Life

Clare O'Callaghan
Lucy Forrest
Yun Wen

This chapter describes music therapy in end-of-life care across the lifespan, including its role in supporting family and staff caregivers. Following brief historical mention of music's role in supporting people through the end stage of life, palliative care definitions, which encompass end-of-life care, are delineated. Music therapy's application in palliative care is then discussed, including clinical contexts, assessments and goals, interventions, outcome evaluations, and research findings.

Throughout the ages, music has been pivotal in helping people deal with dying and bereavement. Traditional communities share worldviews about dealing with loss that incorporate ritualized and participatory music practices. In Western societies, audio technologies may aid people in using individualized, personal ways to cope with life-threatening illness and grief (O'Callaghan, McDermott, Hudson, & Zalcberg, 2013). Music can bring memories "back to life" (O'Callaghan, 2010) and elicit feelings of validation, joy, sadness, grief, or regret. Music may soothe, reduce distressing symptoms, and provide a contained vehicle for emotional expression. Patients and caregivers dealing with advanced illness and grief can feel supported and less alone through identifications with singers and song lyrics, or they can find strength and solace through resonating with music's non-discursive and emotive power (O'Callaghan et al., 2013).

The World Health Organization (2013) describes palliative care as

an approach that improves the quality of life of patients and their families facing the problem associated with life-threatening illness, through the prevention and relief of suffering by means of early identification and impeccable assessment and treatment of pain and other problems, physical, psychosocial and spiritual. (n. p.)

In the United States, palliative care is distinguished from hospice care in that hospice care is considered to be end-of-life care within the broader continuum of palliative, defined as a prognosis of 6 months or less to live. Settings can be inpatient, residential, home care, or long-term care facilities.

The focus is on the comprehensive needs of patients and families being identified and met by an interdisciplinary team, which is trained to tend the physical, psychosocial and spiritual needs of this population (J. Berger, personal communication, April 21, 2013). In Australia and many other countries, *hospice* is mainly used to designate a service or hospital setting that provides palliative care.

Palliative care provides relief from distressing symptoms, affirms life, and offers a support system to help the family cope (World Health Organization, 2013). In recent decades, pediatric palliative care has emerged as its own field of speciality, described by the World Health Organization as the "active total care of the child's body, mind, and spirit, and also involved giving support to the family. . . . Health providers must evaluate and alleviate a child's physical, psychological, and social distress" (n. p.). Palliative care in pediatric and adult settings requires a multidisciplinary approach and can be provided in acute care facilities, community health centers, patients' homes, day programs, residential care facilities for older adults, and even schools. Although palliative care principles are important throughout the trajectory of life-threatening conditions, they are especially significant in end-of-life care that contains a patient's final months, weeks, or days.

Clientele

Modern palliative care emerged under Dame Cicely Saunders's leadership in London in the 1960s, when it was provided primarily for people with oncological or malignant disease. Palliative care now increasingly supports those living with nonmalignant conditions such as neurodegenerative illnesses (e.g., motor neuron disease and dementia); coronary, renal, and multisystemic conditions; and people living with complex and life-threatening medical conditions and profound disabilities (World Health Organization, 2013).

Palliative care supports the patient, his or her significant others, including family members and friends, and sometimes the whole cultural community. For example, a patient living in a neurological unit with motor neuron disease, resulting in anarthria and quadriplegia, shared weekly music therapy sessions for 1 year with his wife before he died. Unexpected visitors either had to wait or were allowed to observe the sessions, in which the couple in their 50s chose songs that triggered memories from throughout their lives, bringing much laughter and validation of their meaning in each other's lives.

Community involvement is particularly apparent in home-based palliative care, where the patient may be part of and receive care from his or her social or cultural community. For example, an older woman invited her close friends and relatives to share her music therapy sessions with me (Lucy Forrest), using the time together to reminisce and prepare for her parting. In another instance, a Middle Eastern family whose young child was dying incorporated all of the female members of the cultural community and their children, so that his life celebration became a communal, shared activity through music therapy.

Patients and their families can choose where they would like to receive palliative care and may move between home, day care services, and inpatient programs as the illness alters. School-age children and adolescents with complex medical needs and profound disabilities may move freely and frequently between palliative care supports when they are unwell and other supports and services, such as school and community programs, when they are medically stable. Hence, palliative care services, particularly in the community, often work closely and in collaboration with special schools, disability support services, and community respite programs. As patients approach the need for end-of-life care, some may wish to receive this care at home, whereas others may wish to receive it in a hospital or through a hospice. Families may also, at times, access respite support through a hospice or hospital program. Increasingly, palliative home care services (e.g., Mercy Palliative Care, in Melbourne, Australia, Lucy Forrest's workplace) and pediatric inpatient hospice programs (Pavlicevic, 2005) provide care for dying children.

Music therapy in palliative care can be defined as the creative and professionally informed use of music in a therapeutic relationship with people who are living with life-threatening illnesses, and their close family and friends. Music therapy may be used to address the physical, psychosocial, or spiritual needs of the patient or family, or to facilitate increased self-awareness and enable increased life satisfaction and quality of life. The musical elements and the evolving therapeutic relationship provide a creative context and foundation for symptom alleviation, psychosocial adjustment, and existential contemplation, with the focus on the therapeutic process rather than the musical product (O'Callaghan, 2010). Sessions may include musical interaction, quiet reflection, conversation, and/or counseling. Music therapy can be a vehicle for nonverbal expression, meaningful interactions, and support. This is especially important when there are no words for unspeakable distress, fear, and loss, and for those who have difficulty using words to describe feelings, such as young children.

A Historical Perspective

Palliative care music therapy was inspired by pioneers Susan Munro (1984) and Lucanne Magill (2009). In 1975, Munro established the first music therapy program in a palliative care unit at The Royal Victoria Hospital in Montreal, and in 1973, Magill commenced the first oncology music (later, music therapy) program at the Memorial Sloan Kettering Cancer Center in New York City. Their groundbreaking writings

provide the foundation for music therapy in end-of-life care today. Publications from four international music therapy and palliative care symposia held between 1989 and 2004 (Dileo & Loewy, 2005; Lee, 1995; Martin, 1989; special issue in the *Journal of Palliative Care*, 2001, Volume 2, Issue 3) consolidated music therapy as an important part of the multidisciplinary team in palliative care contexts throughout the world (O'Callaghan, 2010).

Referral to Music Therapy

In both inpatient and community palliative care programs, patients/families may be referred to music therapy by members of the multidisciplinary team or through self-referral. Hilliard (2005) provides examples of referral and assessment forms used by palliative care teams. In inpatient settings, music therapists may offer music therapy to patients as time permits, a practice described as *case finding*. It can be helpful to tell patients that they do not have to have music backgrounds to be involved. Sometimes patients, families, and/or staff can be concerned that music will heighten distress in end-of-life contexts. In our combined experiences, when patients and families choose the scope of their music therapy involvement, including the music and songs to listen to or sing, adverse effects are rare.

Music Therapy Assessment and Goals

Music therapy assessment in palliative care is an evolving process. Alongside information received from team members, therapists may gently question patients and families throughout sessions, and watch and listen to evaluate strengths and vulnerabilities. Assessments may encompass the patient's physical state, mood, cognitive abilities, music background and preferences, cultural and spiritual backgrounds, social aspects, and how they and their family/close friends may or may not be coping. Toward the end of life, patients and their families may experience many needs that music therapists can assist in alleviating (see Table 37.1).

Music Therapy Interventions

Music therapists tailor music-based interventions to patients' capacities and desires, mindful that these may vary dramatically over time. Toward the end of life, patients may become increasingly drowsy, fatigued, and physically disabled, and they may also present in unconscious states. Although good palliative care can control or alleviate most symptoms, occasionally patients (1) report ongoing discomfort from difficult-to-relieve symptoms, (2) become delirious, or (3) experience existential distress stemming from factors such as anxiety and/or unresolved issues. Each patient's *total pain*

TABLE 37.1. Possible Areas of Need Addressed by Palliative Care Music Therapy

Psychosocial and existential needs of the patient and/or family

- Loss: anticipatory; personal control; self-image; relationships and roles; hope
- Fear and anxiety: how family will cope; dying process
- Grief, anger, frustration
- Communication difficulties (due to emotional issues and/or cognitive impairment)
- Sense of isolation; emotional and mood effects, including sadness, depression, guilt, regret; unresolved issues related to meaning
- Self-worth
- Unfinished plans and wishes related to music
- Desire for living (creating, learning, sharing) until dying
- Funeral plans and wish to leave legacy

Physical needs of the patient

- Pain
- Breathlessness
- Fatigue
- Tension
- Restlessness/agitation
- Neurologic symptoms, including sensory, motor, and/or cognitive systems
- Insomnia

experience is a manifestation of the physical components of the illness and the associated treatments, as well as his or her emotional, social, and spiritual concerns (World Health Organization, 2013). As patients deteriorate, therapists commonly shift from offering active, participatory interventions such as singing, songwriting, making recordings, and music improvisation, to more receptive interventions such as music listening, guided imagery, and music relaxation. Music therapy interventions are tailored to patients' energy levels, symptoms, and desires. Interventions that can be used in palliative care with children and adults are shown in Table 37.2.

Music therapists bring their idiosyncratic musical and therapeutic skills, as well as their life and educational experiences, to their therapeutic relationships with patients. Lee (1995) notes that although "a diversity . . . is at the heart of music therapy in palliative care . . . there is a core that connects all work . . . a belief that music can af-

TABLE 37.2. Methods Used in Palliative Care Music Therapy (O'Callaghan, 2010)

- *Replaying the music of their lives*: Live performance (by therapist and/or participant), music listening, lyric substitution in familiar songs
- *Exploring "new" music*: Therapeutic songwriting, improvisation, unfamiliar live or recorded music
- *Guided use of music*: Relaxation inductions with live or recorded music; guided imagery and music (GIM)
- *Music-based gift or legacy creation*: Song compositions, music-based audiovisual recordings
- *Music in the environment*: Live music providing opportunities for patients/families/staff to engage in individualized or connected levels; concerts involving patients/families
- *Verbal-based methods alongside the above*: Music-based counseling, lyric analysis, music and life review, adding verbal messages and stories to one's musical gifts and legacies, therapeutic music lessons

fect the expression of loss" (p. 6). The wide range of instruments used in this work can include keyboard, guitar, autoharp, harp, tuned and untuned percussion, and music software programs. The portability of instruments is integral, particularly in home-based palliative care and as patients deteriorate and become bed-bound. It is also necessary for music therapists to have extensive music knowledge and song repertoire to be able to meet the needs of people from as many age groups as possible and from diverse backgrounds. Patients and families may request music covering many different genres, styles, and eras, including classical, blues and jazz, musicals and theatre, popular music, country, folk, sacred, children's songs, and culturally specific music.

Sessions can be held with individuals or groups, the latter of which can include other patients and patients' families. Sensitivity to other patients' needs and musical likes and dislikes must be considered in multibed inpatient settings, and therapists should seek permission from neighboring patients to conduct music therapy sessions in shared spaces. In our experiences, patients in inpatient settings who are not part of sessions seldom object when the music is not loud and the session length is contained. There are many excellent illustrations of the applications of music therapy in palliative care, which readers are urged to explore to broaden their perspectives about the multifaceted ways that music therapists work with dying patients, including in pediatric (Lindenfelser, Hense, & McFerran, & 2012; O'Callaghan & Aasgaard, 2012; Pavlicevic, 2005) and adult care (e.g., Aldridge, 1999; Dileo & Loewy, 2005; Heath & Lings, 2012; Slivka & Bailey, 1986) populations.

Not everyone may desire music therapy, and this is especially applicable toward the end of life. Some patients may want quiet, and they may not want to develop unnecessary relationships with unfamiliar staff when preparing to withdraw from this life. Others may wish to use their own music, but without input from the music thera-pist. Occasionally musicians and music lovers do not want to play or hear live music, because it elicits sadness about what they can no longer do, and sometimes these patients choose to *play* or *sound* music in their minds.

The next section illustrates how we have addressed music therapy goals for patients. Many of these goals can also inform work with patients' families, who may share sessions with patients or have private sessions for specific purposes—for example, helping children to create and record a song as gift to a parent patient.

Goals for Adults and Their Families

• *Supportive validation of feelings and thoughts, life contributions, and existential perspectives.* Patients and families tend to choose music that reflects physical states, memories, images, people, feelings, or a spiritual place with which they want to be connected. Music therapists often encourage patients and families to choose the familiar music they would like in sessions. Through choosing their music, patients can control and moderate the evocation of feelings or memories. As such, music can support what is meaningful for participants at that time and yet also help to contain patients who are experiencing intense or overwhelming responses. When patients are tired, or their illness and/or medications affect their cognition, they may request that the therapist choose music for them. Therapists can sometimes be assisted in their decisions of what to play by asking patients about their preferred genres through offering multiple choice or yes–no questions.

In conjunction with playing music requests for patients, therapists may offer a supportive presence or an opportunity to talk about what the music elicited for them. Music therapist *artistry* is especially involved in deciding what to do here. For example, if a patient is looking away in apparent deep contemplation, the therapist may choose to remain a supportive presence. If the patient looks emotional, the therapist may say something like, "It seems that this is a meaningful song for you." If a patient chooses to reflect on what the music elicited, the therapist may offer supportive counseling to empathize with or validate the patient's story. Music therapy may also be a vehicle for patients to connect with their sense of what is important, including spiritual realms, and that which is existentially affirming for them, such as a loving God or a humanist perspective of living on through memories and physical matter. Using music that the patient finds spiritual, such as hymns, popular songs such as "You Raise Me Up," or a significant piece of classical music may be appropriate in these contexts.

• *Enabling a space for contemplation of "being" and reframing maladaptive patterns of thought.* Patients may prefer to listen to the music and not engage in conversation. One patient with advanced cancer, for example, requested that I (Clare O'Callaghan) play "Going Home" from Dvorak's *New World Symphony* repeatedly for as long as I could. In this way, music listening may transport people to a state of contemplation or sense of calm and peace, away from cognitive thought. In another example, I (Lucy Forrest) worked with a child patient whose mother held very negative self-beliefs relating to her child's illness, believing that the illness was the result of her being a bad wife and mother. Through targeted music therapy interventions, the mother was invited to engage in shared, interactive music activities with her child and encouraged to develop a new self-concept as a good and supportive mother who was able to share something very special and unique with her child.

• *Providing opportunities for increased self-awareness to aid coping.* Music therapy may elicit memories and thoughts related to unresolved concerns or regrets. Patients may find resolution in creative musical expressions or by engaging in supportive counseling with the therapist about arising issues. In the final weeks of life, for example, one patient composed a song questioning whether she had made the right choice of husband. As she composed the song lyrics and the therapist actively listened to her story, the patient stated her answer: She had made the right choice.

Through music therapy improvisation, clients can also musically express their creative selves, and the therapist's improvised musical mirroring can affirm and extend each client's musical and holistic way of being. These creative musical experiences can transform a patient's way of experiencing his or her world. The ongoing musical dialogue can affirm that the client has been heard and inspire further creativity that can transduce into adaptive self-awareness.

• *Symptom relief and relaxation.* Music therapists can offer patients different kinds of music and possibly guided inductions to assist with relaxation to alleviate symptoms (e.g., pain, dyspnoea, nausea, restlessness, insomnia). Whereas some patients find that preferred music helps them to relax and distract them from pain, other patients prefer unfamiliar music—so it is important to check. When patients are extremely ill, a short relaxation induction followed by 5–10 minutes of live music (improvised or familiar) can be helpful. Suggested music that may promote relaxation includes Enya's "Watermark," Saint-Saens's "The Swan," the first movement of Beethoven's *Moonlight* Sonata, Stanley Myers's "Cavatina" (from the film *The Deer Hunter*), and the second movement of Beethoven's *Sonate Pathetique*. Musical elements need to be balanced, without extreme variations in rhythms, dynamics, and tempo. Music therapists can use the iso principle to promote reduced tension and symptom relief through musically matching patients' emotional and physical states, then slowly shifting the musical elements as patients move into more desired states—for example, slowing the music as breathing rate slows.

• *Meaningful communication with family, staff, and other patients, and legacy creation.* When music relates to a shared memory between the patient and a family member or friend, it can enable validation of the importance each person has had in the other's life. Meaningful relationships can be celebrated in music therapy as patients and families request songs, sing, dance (patients may *bed dance* through shuffling bottoms, moving legs, and waving hands in the air), and share stories, laughter, touch, and tears. Through songwriting, patients can also communicate meaningful thoughts and messages to others, which can connect dying patients with their families in life and potentially help families in their bereavement (O'Callaghan et al., 2013). Songs can be written for family members, friends, caring staff, spiritual faith congregations, or by a family member/friend for the patient. Positive memories about the patient's end-of-life care, which would include music therapy sessions, can help in bereavement following the deaths of both children (Lindenfelser, Grocke, & McFerran, 2008) and adults. Music therapists can also enable patients to leave tangible legacies (e.g., song compositions) and intangible legacy memories of shared sessions, which can bring comfort after the patient dies (Magill, 2009).

Music therapists can also sometimes help people with brain impairment (e.g., due to advanced brain cancer or dementia) to have more meaningful connections with others compared to when only non-music-based modalities are used. Language and music neural pathways are closely related and yet still separate (Levitin, 2006); therefore, a person trying to communicate with someone through both music and language has a greater chance of triggering preserved neural function compared to using language alone. Long-term memories also remain relatively intact when brain function is impaired, providing further opportunities for music-based connectedness.

• *Aesthetic and life-enriching experiences, creative expression, transcendence, and living until dying.* Patients at the end of life may still want to play instruments, compose songs, and engage in music appreciation (e.g., learning more about music and musicians, attending concerts, and performing for others). All of these have occurred in our day hospice music therapy group work. Music is an interest in which patients may engage and enjoy even when low in concentration and energy. Patients often request music that they have not heard for decades, and stories and humor are often shared. They may also sometimes discuss illness-related themes and provide mutual support.

• *Catharsis, dealing with loss, and transition from mortal life.* Music listening and playing can be a helpful means of releasing emotion, grieving for what is lost, and preparing for what is to come. For example, in day hospice programs, group members frequently select music that allows them to share the cumulative losses they are experiencing over time. One lady selected the Beatles' "Yesterday" and reflected on a time when "all her troubles seemed so far away," before she became unwell, and her sadness at the loss of her former life. Another group member selected John Denver's "Leaving on a Jet Plane" when she received the news of a recent and rapid decline and was mentally and psychically preparing for her own death.

Cultural Issues

My (Lucy Forrest) descriptions of work with patients from multicultural backgrounds highlight the importance of cultural sensitivity in engaging with patients and families, and the influence of significant events—such as migration, war, and traumatic loss—in palliative care (Forrest, 2000, 2011, 2014). Therefore it is important that therapists (1) acquire a broad repertoire of world music to engage clients who are potentially isolated through cultural and/or language barriers, and (2) consider when clinical work that is theoretically questionable in their own culture may be valued in another culture. These aspects are highlighted in the following story about a Chinese hospice inpatient in her mid-30s with end-stage cancer.

Sasha spoke Mandarin and little English. She lay in a darkened quiet room most of the day, did not have the energy to interact much with her family, and the English-speaking hospice staff could not offer verbal support therapies. Fortunately, I (Yun Wen) could speak Mandarin, and I had commenced a student music therapy placement in the hospice. Sasha accepted Yun Wen's offer of music therapy, requested many songs from her childhood and youth in China, and described a story about feeling abandoned when young. She was self-berating, demoralized, and felt that life was not worth living because she could not fulfill her duties as a mother. Through Yun's attentive presence and support, Sasha was able to express grief and also recall and tell humorous stories about her childhood, her grandmother, and songs on Chinese television. Yun brought this music to Sasha, and they sang together. Sasha sometimes smiled and appeared more energized, sitting up in bed. Yun Wen then invited Sasha to compose a song. Sasha decided to compose a song called "Love" for her children. Selected translated lyrics from the resultant song follow:

> Daughter, You are beautiful. . . . Your drawings are very good. Keep it up. Mummy is proud of you. Son, You are handsome. . . . You have lots of tears. Please don't cry (so much), for you are a boy. Thank you for your cranes, very pretty, I like them a lot. I really love you guys. . . .

Sasha was very proud of her song and could not wait to play the recording that she made with Yun Wen to her husband and their children through the phone. She also gave Yun Wen a picture of her happily cuddling her two beaming children to use as a CD cover. Soon after composing and recording the song, Sasha said that she had heard enough popular Chinese songs from her youth and now she wanted to hear new current popular Chinese songs. While Yun prepared new songs for the following session, Sasha died.

Yun Wen's work with Sasha highlights how music therapy can enable people to connect with the healthy and joyful part of their identity, express important messages that may assist the bereaved through legacy creation, and find a purpose in living amid the inevitability of life coming to an end. Interestingly, some of the Australian team members questioned whether Sasha's lyrical request, that her son not cry so much, would hinder his grief. Yun explained that, in Chinese culture, excessive crying is regarded as a weakness and needs to be curbed if a boy can grow into a man. It was therefore considered that Sasha's messages of love and pride to her son, alongside the encouragement to cry less, could also reflect Sasha's belief that her son had the resources to cope, and that she had hope that he would have a positive future. The team believed that these messages would likely support Sasha's son in the future.

Goals for Children and Adolescents and Their Families

Goals that music therapists can have when working with young patients and their families in palliative care may include the following:

• *Creativity, play, and fun for the child and/ or siblings and parents.* In the midst of illness, music therapy can provide normalizing opportunities for the child and family to engage in creative, fun, and playful interventions. Such interactions can be particularly important when the child is experiencing progressive disablement and is unable to engage in everyday school, family, and play activities. Familiar songs and musical games can provide experiences of success, and interventions such as instrument playing or songwriting can offer the child new and novel opportunities for creative and imaginative play, thereby shifting the focus from being/caring for a sick child to playing and having fun together. In music, family members can forget, for a brief time, that the child is sick and concentrate their energies on spending time together in a pleasurable and supportive way.

• *Enhancing attachment between the parent and child as they prepare for the final separation.* As a child becomes progressively unwell, factors such as pain and tactile sensitivity may preclude the sharing of supportive and soothing attachment behaviors such as cuddles between the parent and child. The attachment between the parent and child may also be impacted by the parents' knowledge of their child's impending death and associated anticipatory grief (O'Callaghan & Jordan, 2011).

Music can provide a means by which the child and family can be *auditorially touched.* The sound of the voice can soothe and comfort the child and nurture the parent–child attachment. An example might be the singing of gentle lullabies to *hold* the child and parent in difficult times. The music therapist can also encourage parents to incorporate simple songs and lullabies into daily life. Songs, song stories, fairytales, and imaginative play can also provide a musical means through which children and their parents can engage interactively and creatively together, strengthening the bonds of attachment.

• *Providing relief and distraction from symptoms and progressive disability.* Familiar songs, musical games, and instrumental playing can help to distract the young child from symptoms such as pain and refocus attention from what the child is no longer able to do to what he or she *can* do. With adolescents, I (Lucy Forrest) have used music, imagery, and guided relaxation to provide relief from pain and other symptoms, and I've used songwriting to explore the changes that the adolescent has experienced. Both

interventions have been observed to empower adolescents by providing a means by which they can independently address the issues they are experiencing and gain a sense of control and autonomy in a process over which they may have very little control.

• *Memory creation and expression of important messages.* Older children and adolescents may wish to share important messages with friends, family, and loved ones through songs, songwriting, audio compilation, and performance. Through their song lyrics and song choices, adolescents can choose to share their story, communicate their place in the world, and say good-bye. I (Lucy Forrest) have also audiorecorded family music therapy sessions with younger children to allow the child and/or family to listen to their sessions, either during palliative care or later in bereavement.

• *Expression of fears, anxieties, and sharing of stories.* Children may not have the words or cognitive development to understand what they are experiencing or to be able to articulate those feelings. However, through interventions such as the playing of instruments, singing of familiar songs, and the creation of song stories (Forrest, 2010), children can express those feelings and experiences. Familiar songs can create a sense of safety and security in the midst of what is often a frightening and unpredictable experience. Children can also use transient objects such as a favorite toy to tell their story, putting their fears and concerns into song and action (Dun, 1998).

• *Creating a space for the child and family to be together in music or in quiet contemplation and reflection.* Favorite songs or shared moments in improvisation can bring the child and family together in time, space, and experience. In the family home, there can be multiple distractions during music therapy, with family members doing different activities, children running in and out, visitors, the phone ringing, the sound of the radio or television, and unexpected interruptions. Music can help to bring the family together amid all these distractions and provide a shared space and focus for the child and family. And when the child is feeling tired or unwell or the family is exhausted, music therapy can be the medium that brings quiet and calm into the family home, allowing reflection and time out from the stressful grind of everyday life.

• *Continuing the story of the child with the family, in bereavement.* Music, the relationship with the music therapist, and the memories shared in music therapy can help to keep alive the memory of the child for the parents and family. Parents and siblings, classmates, and friends may also wish to continue the story of the child or adolescent in their own musical tributes and expressions. In my (Lucy Forrest) work with a young adolescent whose condition was deteriorating, an interactive song moved back and forth between the adolescent and her school friends, facilitated by the music therapist and the school music teacher, with the adolescent and her friends each adding a verse in turn. In bereavement, the music therapist and music teacher facilitated the writing and performing of a memorial song with the adolescent's school peers for their much-loved and much-missed friend. The song was recorded and presented to the adolescent's family at a special assembly.

Research

Adult Palliative Care

A Cochrane review[1] that included a meta-analysis of five end-of-life care studies (175 participants) found that there was "insufficient evidence of high quality" to support

[1] A Cochrane review is a systematic assessment of an intervention in health care. It encompasses a review of research on the intervention and, when appropriate, a meta-analysis of eligible trials. Many believe that Cochrane reviews identify gold standard health care research findings.

music therapy's effect in palliative care (Bradt & Dileo, 2010, p. 2). In addition, there were insufficient data to draw conclusions about the effects of music therapy on pain, anxiety, and other physical and psychosocial outcomes. Nonetheless, the review's meta-analysis found statistically significant findings in three studies in which music therapy improved quality of life in three domains: psychophysiological, social/spiritual well-being, and functional. For example, one randomized controlled trial (RCT) examined music therapy's effect on 25 hospice inpatients. The intervention group's anxiety, drowsiness, pain, and tiredness were significantly reduced compared to the control group that received a volunteer visit (Horne-Thompson & Grocke, 2008). In another RCT, 80 adult patients were randomly assigned to routine hospice home care (control group) or routine hospice care plus at least two music therapy sessions. The music therapy group scored significantly higher on quality-of-life scores than did the control group, and the more music therapy that was received, the higher the quality-of-life score (Hilliard, 2003).

It is important to emphasize that Cochrane reviews use four criteria to determine the risk of bias of included trials: adequate randomization; allocation concealment; the blinding of participants, assessors, and service providers; and intention-to-treat analysis (Higgins & Green, 2008). Because "it is not possible in music therapy studies to blind participants and those providing the interventions" (Bradt & Dileo, p. 5), music therapy trials cannot achieve high- quality ratings for the measurement of subjective (i.e., self-report) outcomes. Although this may seem like an unfair appraisal of music therapy research, it accurately represents the risk of bias inherent in the assessment of subjective outcomes, as research participants may be inclined to report a positive impact of the intervention to please the music therapist. This challenge is certainly not unique to music therapy research.

Arguably, findings from both music therapy RCTs and constructivist (qualitative) research are important to reveal the holistic ways in which music therapy can improve patients' lives. Constructivist research examines patients, families, and staff caregivers' subjective interpretations about what they finding meaningful in music therapy phenomena. Such research can also examine what patients are creating in palliative care music therapy. A review of 13 objectivist (quantitative), 11 constructivist (qualitative), and one mixed methods research publication from 1986 to 2009 reports substantive evidence indicating music therapy's improvement of palliative care patients' quality of life and its role in helping family caregivers (O'Callaghan, 2009). Constructivist findings, informed by session transcripts and interviews, revealed that music therapy provides palliative care patients with companionship; is a positive emotional, social, and spiritual experience; and helps family caregivers to experience meaning and empowerment (see O'Callaghan, 2009, for summaries of these studies and references).

Pediatric Palliative Care

In a study examining the use of and satisfaction with music therapy services in a home-based pediatric palliative care program, the primary caregivers were more likely to report satisfaction with the hospice care when patients received complementary therapies such as music therapy (Knapp et al., 2009). Lindenfelser, McFerran, and Hense (2012) also found that music therapy improved the physical state of children in the terminal phase of illness, fostered positive experiences for the children and families, and facilitated family communication. In bereavement research, Lindenfelser, Grocke, and McFerran (2008) found that music therapy helped to improve communication between parents and children before the children's deaths, and helped parents in their remembrance.

Research with Music Therapists and Other Staff Working in Palliative Care

The helpful effect of music therapy on staff has also been examined in palliative care settings as well as in oncology, where many patients have advanced and end-stage cancer. Using pre–post measures, Hilliard (2006) found that hospice team members improved in team building when either experiencing free-form music therapy, which included improvisation methods, or structured sessions that included guided meditation with music, lyric analysis, and movement. Grounded theory methods were used in a multisite study of 100 oncology staff members who witnessed music therapy on the hospital wards; staff were often indirectly supported by the sessions and consequently perceived that their care of patients had improved (O'Callaghan & Magill, 2009).

Applications to Other Disciplines

Combining music therapy with allied disciplines may broaden the treatments' therapeutic benefits. I (Clare O'Callaghan) have played live music to support gentle physiotherapy for well-being exercise classes in palliative care, to energize, motivate, and mitigate boredom. I have also provided live and recorded music to help patients relax and alleviate swallowing difficulties (dysphagia) due to advanced multiple sclerosis or to cope with palliative radiotherapy. Slivka and Bailey (1986) reported that conjoint family sessions with a social worker and music therapist helped support communication between young children and their parents when one of the parents was dying. The children substituted lyrics and composed new songs to express significant messages to the dying parent before death. At Caritas Christi Hospice, Melbourne, Australia, I (Clare O'Callaghan) work closely with a pastoral care art therapist to support discovery and expressions of personal meaning in patients' final days of life. In this kind of a setting the music therapist can play live music as patients create artworks, and the art therapist can help patients create CD covers of their drawings or photo collages for song compositions created in the music therapy. When significant intrapsychic distress emerges in music therapy, referrals to psychiatrists or psychologists may also be needed.

Conclusions

Music therapists work with palliative care patients and caregivers of all ages to: enable creative connections with music from their lives and experiences with unfamiliar music to alleviate distress; support and sustain; validate the well part of the person and his or her unique contribution; aid meaningful connection with significant people and existential realms; enable new awareness; and inspire aesthetic or transcendent experiences. In music therapy, joyous, connected, peaceful, and contemplative moments can be precious for dying patients and can encourage bereaved families who may share the sessions. These momentous effects are worthwhile, in and of themselves, but existing outcome tools may not be sensitive enough to detect some of the enduring benefits. Music often elicits interchanging or juxtaposed happy and sad feelings as participants relive and reintegrate memories while also being aware of, or sensing, their loss. Participants usually want the music to continue. Music can stimulate a feeling of being understood and nurtured as well as facilitate the release of pent-up emotion and grief. Music therapists can enrich the lives of people living or witnessing transitions from corporeal existence and are important members of multidisciplinary teams in end-of-life care.

REFERENCES

Aldridge, D. (Ed.). (1999). *Music therapy in palliative care: New voices*. London: Jessica Kingsley.

Bradt, J., & Dileo, C. (2010). Music therapy for end-of-life care. *Cochrane Database of Systematic Reviews, 2010*(1), CD007169.

Dileo, C., & Loewy, J. (Eds.). (2005). *Music therapy at the end of life*. Cherry Hill, NJ: Jeffrey Books.

Dun, B. (1999). Creativity and communication aspects of music therapy in a children's hospital. In D. Aldridge (Ed.), *Music therapy in palliative care: New voices* (pp. 59–67). London: Jessica Kingsley.

Forrest, L. C. (2000). Addressing issues of ethnicity and identity in palliative care through music therapy practice. *Australian Journal of Music Therapy, 11*, 23–37.

Forrest, L. C. (2010). *The interplay of attachment and withdrawal in the parent–child relationship in paediatric cancer care at the end of life: A role for music therapy*. International Symposium on Music Therapy in Supportive Cancer Care, Windsor, Canada.

Forrest, L. C. (2011). Supportive cancer care at the end of life: Mapping the cultural landscape in palliative care and music therapy. *Music and Medicine, 3*, 9–14.

Forrest, L. (2014). Your song, my song, our song: developing music therapy programs for a culturally diverse community in home-based paediatric palliative care. *Australian Journal of Music Therapy, 25*, 15–27.

Heath, B., & Lings, J. (2012). Creative songwriting in therapy at the end of life and in bereavement. *Mortality, 17*, 106–118.

Higgins, J. P. T., & Green, S. (Eds.). (2008). *Cochrane handbook for systematic reviews of interventions* (pp. 187–241). Chichester, UK: Wiley.

Hilliard, R. (2003). The effects of music therapy on the quality and length of life of people diagnosed with terminal cancer. *Journal of Music Therapy, 40*(2), 113–137.

Hilliard, R. (2005). *Hospice and palliative care music therapy: A guide to program development and clinical care*. Cherry Hill, NJ: Jeffrey Books.

Hilliard, R. (2006). The effect of music therapy sessions on compassion fatigue and team building of professional hospice caregivers. *Arts in Psychotherapy, 33*, 395–401.

Horne-Thompson, A., & Grocke, D. (2008). The effect of music therapy on anxiety in patients who are terminally ill. *Journal of Palliative Medicine, 11*, 582–590.

Knapp, C., Madden, V., Wang, H., Curtis, C.,

Sloyer, P., & Shenkman, E. (2009). Music therapy in an integrated pediatric palliative care program. *American Journal of Hospice and Palliative Medicine, 26,* 449–455.

Lee, C. (1995). *Lonely waters: Proceedings of the international conference, music therapy in palliative care.* Oxford, UK: Sobell.

Levitin, D. J. (2006). *This is your brain on music.* London: Atlantic.

Lindenfelser, K., Grocke, D., & McFerran, K. (2008). Bereaved parents' experiences of music therapy with their terminally ill child. *Journal of Music Therapy, 35,* 330–348.

Lindenfelser, K., Hense, C., & McFerran, K. (2012). Music therapy in pediatric palliative care: Family-centered care to enhance quality of life. *American Journal of Hospice and Palliative Medicine, 29,* 219–226.

Magill, L. (2009). Caregiver empowerment and music therapy: Through the eyes of bereaved caregivers of advanced cancer patients. *Journal of Palliative Care, 25,* 68–75.

Martin, J. (Ed.). (1989). *The next step forward: Music therapy with the terminally ill.* New York: Calvary Hospital.

Munro, S. (1984). *Music therapy in palliative/hospice care.* St Louis, MO: MMB Music.

O'Callaghan, C. (2009). Objectivist and constructivist music therapy research in oncology and palliative care. *Music and Medicine, 1*(1), 41–60.

O'Callaghan, C. (2010). The contribution of music therapy to palliative medicine. In G. Hanks et al. (Eds.), *The Oxford textbook of palliative medicine* (4th ed., pp. 214–221). Oxford, UK: Oxford University Press.

O'Callaghan, C., & Aasgaard, T. (2012). Arts therapies. In A. Längler, P. Mansky, & G. Seifert (Eds.), *Integrative pediatric oncology* (pp. 45–58). Berlin: Springer Verlag.

O'Callaghan, C., & Jordan, B. (2011). Music therapy supports parent–infant attachments affected by life threatening cancer. In J. Edwards (Ed.), *Music therapy in parent–infant bonding* (pp. 191–207). New York: Oxford University Press.

O'Callaghan, C., & Magill, L. (2009). Effect of music therapy on oncologic staff bystanders: A substantive grounded theory. *Journal of Palliative and Supportive Care, 7,* 219–228.

O'Callaghan, C., McDermott, F., Hudson, P., & Zalcberg, J. (2013). Sound continuing bonds with the deceased: The relevance of music, including preloss music therapy, for eight bereaved caregivers. *Death Studies, 37,* 101–125.

Pavlicevic, M. (Ed.). (2005). *Music therapy in children's hospices: Jessie's Fund in action.* London: Jessica Kingsley.

Slivka, H. H., & Magill, L. (1986). The conjoint use of social work and music therapy with children of cancer patients. *Music Therapy, 6A*(1), 30–40.

World Health Organization. (2013). *WHO definition of palliative care.* Retrieved from *www.who.int/cancer/palliative/definition/en.*

Author Index

Subject Index

Note. Italics in page numbers indicate figures or tables.